Applied Clinical Pharmacokinetics and Pharmacodynamics of Psychopharmacological Agents

Michael W. Jann • Scott R. Penzak
Lawrence J. Cohen
Editors

Applied Clinical Pharmacokinetics and Pharmacodynamics of Psychopharmacological Agents

Adis

Editors
Michael W. Jann
Department of Pharmacotherapy
University of North Texas System College of Pharmacy
Fort Worth, TX
USA

Lawrence J. Cohen
Department of Pharmacotherapy
University of North Texas System College of Pharmacy
Fort Worth, TX
USA

Scott R. Penzak
Department of Pharmacotherapy
University of North Texas System College of Pharmacy
Fort Worth, TX
USA

ISBN 978-3-319-27881-0 ISBN 978-3-319-27883-4 (eBook)
DOI 10.1007/978-3-319-27883-4

Library of Congress Control Number: 2016932526

Springer Cham Heidelberg New York Dordrecht London

Printed on acid-free paper

Adis is a brand of Springer
Springer International Publishing AG Switzerland is part of Springer Science+Business Media (www.springer.com)

Preface and Acknowledgments

The primary purpose of the *Applied Clinical Pharmacokinetics and Pharmacodynamics of Psychopharmacological Agents* text is to offer students, clinicians, scientists, and members of the pharmaceutical industry a comprehensive yet practical information resource for medications that affect the central nervous system (CNS). Part 1 presents the background for the pharmacokinetic and pharmacodynamic principles for agents that must reach the CNS to produce their clinical actions. Drug development and clinical application for the psychopharmacological agents have progressed to incorporate biomarkers, such as positron emission tomography (PET) scans, pharmacogenomics, and sophisticated mathematical modeling with population pharmacometrics. These chapters provide the readers with a foundational background of these exciting areas. Each chapter in Part 2 offers an important focus on psychopharmacological agents that reinforces the basic principles in Part 1.

The Part 2 chapters portray a broad scope of psychopharmacological agents that are available in different formulations, such as long-acting injectable antipsychotics and oral extended-release products; these formulations promote ease of dosing administration and enhance patient adherence. Some of the earliest works of pharmacokinetic-pharmacodynamic modeling occurred with the anesthetic agents, which formed the basis of analysis for the remaining psychopharmacologic medications. Pharmacodynamic parameters assessing CNS drug effects are challenging and frequently involve a variety of measurements. These measurements include patient clinical rating scales for efficacy and adverse effects, serum drug concentrations, physiologic assessments, pharmacogenomic markers, and imaging technologies.

The chapters in Part 3 concentrate on drug-drug interactions with psychopharmacological agents. Drug-drug interactions with CNS agents can occur via pharmacokinetic and/or pharmacodynamic mechanisms. Part 3 serves as a valuable resource to aid clinicians discerning clinically significant drug-drug interactions commonly encountered in patient care.

The editors wish to acknowledge our sincere appreciation to the chapter authors who contributed their time, effort, and enthusiasm, all of which made this book possible. Finally, the editors would like to thank their spouses and family members for their support during the long hours spent completing this endeavor.

Fort Worth, TX, USA

Michael W. Jann
Scott R. Penzak
Lawrence J. Cohen

Contents

About the Editors

Michael W. Jann, Pharm.D., F.C.P., F.C.C.P. is professor and chair for the Department of Pharmacotherapy at the University of North Texas System College of Pharmacy (UNTSCP) located at the UNT Health Sciences Center (UNTHSC). Professor Jann received his doctor of pharmacy degree from the University of Southern California and postdoctoral training in mental health pharmacy practice at the University of Tennessee Memphis College of Pharmacy. He has published over 230 peer-reviewed articles, abstracts, and book chapters and served as a primary investigator for numerous clinical trials in psychopharmacology. Professor Jann serves on the editorial boards of six peer-reviewed scientific journals including *CNS Drugs*, *Molecular Diagnosis & Therapy*, *The Scientific World Journal* – Pharmacology Section, *The Consultant Pharmacist*, *Journal of Clinical Pharmacology*, and *Journal of Pharmacy Practice*.

Scott R. Penzak, Pharm.D., F.C.P., is professor and vice chair for the Department of Pharmacotherapy at the University of North Texas System College of Pharmacy (UNTSCP) located at the UNT Health Sciences Center (UNTHSC). Professor Penzak received his doctor of pharmacy degree from Wayne State University and completed his postdoctoral training in infectious diseases at the University of Arkansas for Medical Science (UAMS). Prior to UNTSCP, he was the director of the Clinical Pharmacokinetics Laboratory at the NIH. He has published over 150 peer-reviewed articles, abstracts, and book chapters and served as a principal investigator on numerous pharmacokinetic and pharmacogenetic studies. Professor Penzak serves on the editorial boards of three peer-reviewed scientific journals including the *Journal of Clinical Pharmacology*, *Pharmacotherapy*, and the *International Journal of Pharmacokinetics*.

Lawrence J. Cohen, Pharm.D., B.C.P.P., F.A.S.H.P., F.C.C.P., F.C.P., F.N.A.P., is currently professor of pharmacotherapy at the University of North Texas System College of Pharmacy. Examples of Professor Cohen's previous service include global director of CNS Research for Kendle International, director of the Office of Clinical Trials for the University of Cincinnati, and director of Pharmaceutical Services for the Oklahoma Department of Mental Health and Substance Abuse Services. Professor Cohen received his doctor of pharmacy degree and postdoctoral training in psychiatric pharmacy from the University of Southern California School of Pharmacy. Professor Cohen has been a board-certified psychiatry pharmacist since the specialty was recognized. Has served on the editorial boards of *Current Psychiatry*, *Innovations in Clinical Neuroscience*, *Journal of Clinical Psychiatry* (Primary Care Companion), *Drug Benefit Trends*, *Journal of the American Medical Directors Association*, *CNS News*, and *Pharmacy Practice News*.

Editors and Contributors

Editors

Michael W. Jann, PharmD Department of Pharmacotherapy, University of North Texas System College of Pharmacy, Fort Worth, TX, USA

Scott R. Penzak, PharmD, FCP Department of Pharmacotherapy, University of North Texas System College of Pharmacy, Fort Worth, TX, USA

Lawrence J. Cohen, PharmD Department of Pharmacotherapy, University of North Texas System College of Pharmacy, Fort Worth, TX, USA

Contributors

Daniel T. Barratt, PhD Discipline of Pharmacology, School of Medicine, The University of Adelaide, Adelaide, Australia

Angela A. Boggs, PharmD, BCPP Department of Pharmacy, VA Connecticut Healthcare System, Newington, CT, USA

Douglas L. Boggs, PharmD, BCPP Department of Psychiatry, School of Medicine, Yale University, New Haven, CT, USA

Ayyappa Chaturvedula, PhD Department of Pharmacotherapy, UNT System College of Pharmacy and UNTHSC, Fort Worth, TX, USA

Janet Coller, BSc (Hon), PhD, GCert. Ed Discipline of Pharmacology, School of Medicine, The University of Adelaide, Adelaide, Australia

M. Lynn Crismon, PharmD Division of Health Outcomes and Pharmacy Practice, College of Pharmacy, The University of Texas at Austin, Austin, TX, USA

C. Lindsay DeVane, PharmD Department of Psychiatry, Medical University of South Carolina, Charleston, SC, USA

Vicki L. Ellingrod, PharmD Department of Clinical Pharmacy, College of Pharmacy, Ann Arbor, MI, USA

Department of Psychiatry, School of Medicine, University of Michigan, Ann Arbor, MI, USA

Mary H.H. Ensom, PharmD Faculty of Pharmaceutical Sciences and Distinguished University Scholar, The University of British Columbia, Vancouver, BC, Canada

Patrick J. Finley, PharmD Department of Clinical Pharmacy, School of Pharmacy, University of California, San Francisco, CA, USA

Stephanie A. Flowers, PharmD, PhD Department of Clinical Pharmacy, College of Pharmacy, University of Michigan, Ann Arbor, MI, USA

Sally R. Guthrie, PharmD Pharmacy Department, Clinical, Social, and Administrative Sciences, College of Pharmacy, University of Michigan, Ann Arbor, MI, USA

Leonard L. Howell, PhD Division of Neuropharmacology and Neurologic Diseases, Emory University School of Medicine, Imaging Center, Yerkes National Primate Research Center, Atlanta, GA, USA

Domenico Italiano, MD, PhD Department of Clinical and Experimental Medicine, University of Messina, Policlinico Universitario, Messina, Italy

Rania S. Kattura, PharmD Division of Health Outcomes and Pharmacy Practice, College of Pharmacy, The University of Texas at Austin, Austin, TX, USA

W. Klugh Kennedy, PharmD Department of Pharmacy Practice, College of Pharmacy, Mercer University, Atlanta, GA, USA

Tony K.L. Kiang, BSc (Pharm), ACPR, PhD Faculty of Pharmaceutical Sciences, The University of British Columbia, Vancouver, BC, Canada

Y.W. Francis Lam, PharmD Department of Pharmacology, University of Texas Health Science Center at San Antonio, San Antonio, TX, USA

College of Pharmacy, The University of Texas at Austin, Austin, TX, USA

Hsien-Yuan Lane, MD, PhD Department of Psychiatry, China Medical University and Hospital, Taichung, Taiwan

Jennifer Le, PharmD, MAS Department of Clinical Pharmacy, Skaggs School of Pharmacy and Pharmaceutical Sciences, University of California San Diego, San Diego, CA, USA

Kelly C. Lee, PharmD Department of Clinical Pharmacy, Skaggs School of Pharmacy and Pharmaceutical Sciences, University of California San Diego, San Diego, CA, USA

Mong-Liang Lu, MD, MS Department of Psychiatry, Wan Fang Hospital and School of Medicine, College of Medicine, Taipei Medical University, Taipei, Taiwan

Mark S. Luer, PharmD, FCPP Department of Pharmacy Practice, School of Pharmacy, Southern Illinois University, Edwardsville, IL, USA

John S. Markowitz, PharmD Department of Pharmacotherapy and Translational Research, College of Pharmacogenomics, University of Florida, Gainesville, FL, USA

Jonathan A. Nye, PhD Department of Radiology and Imaging Services, Emory University School of Medicine, Atlanta, GA, USA

Jose A. Rey, PharmD, BCPP Department of Pharmacy Practice, College of Pharmacy, NOVA Southeastern University, Fort Lauderdale, FL, USA

Carlos H. Rojas-Fernandez, BSc (Pharm) PharmD Geriatrics Pharmacotherapy, University of Waterloo, School of Pharmacy, Kitchener, ON, Canada

Andrew A. Somogyi, PhD Discipline of Pharmacology, School of Medicine, The University of Adelaide, Adelaide, Australia

Edoardo Spina, MD, PhD Department of Clinical and Experimental Medicine, University of Messina, Policlinico Universitario, Messina, Italy

David Taylor, PhD, FFRPS, FRPharmS Pharmaceutical Sciences Clinical Academic Group, Pharmacy Department, Maudsley Hospital, London, UK

Christian Teter, PharmD Department of Pharmacy Practice, University of New England, Portland, ME, USA

J. Valdes, PharmD, BCPP Department of Pharmacy Practice, Neurology and Neuropsychiatry, College of Pharmacy, NOVA Southeastern University, Palm Beach Gardens, FL, USA

Kalliopi Vallianatou, MPharm, MRPharmS Pharmacy Department, South London and Maudsley NHS Foundation Trust, Maudsley Hospital, London, UK

Chad M. VanDenBerg, PharmD Department of Pharmacy Practice, College of Pharmacy, Midwestern University, Scottsdale, AR, USA

Kristen M. Wiese, PharmD Department of Clinical Pharmacy, College of Pharmacy, University of Michigan, Ann Arbor, MI, USA

Guo Yu, PhD Pharmacotherapy and Applied Pharmacokinetics, Medical Research Center, Subei People's Hospital, Yangzhou University, Yangzhou, Jiangsu Providence, China

Part I
General Pharmacokinetic and Pharmacodynamic Principles of Psychopharmacological Agents

Scott R. Penzak
Department of Pharmacotherapy
University of North Texas
System College of Pharmacy
Fort Worth, TX
USA
e-mail: scott.penzak@unthsc.edu

Chapter 1
Pharmacokinetic Properties

Mark S. Luer and Scott R. Penzak

Abstract Pharmacokinetics is the mathematical characterization of the time course of drug absorption, distribution, metabolism, and excretion. Over the past 50 years, dramatic scientific advances have revolutionized drug development and design and clinical decision making. These include improvements in quantitating drug and metabolite concentrations in biologic matrices (plasma and tissue), measuring drug effects, and understanding how genetics, metabolic pathways, and drug transporters influences drug disposition. A major challenge for health-care professionals in clinical psychopharmacology is in understanding and adjusting for individual differences in a drug's response. Knowledge of a drug's pharmacokinetic characteristics can be leveraged to help resolve these issues and formulate rational drug therapy decisions. As an example, understanding the absorption and distribution characteristics of a drug allows one to predict the amount of an administered dose that is expected to enter the bloodstream and reach its site of action. Further, an understanding of drug metabolism and elimination allows for the prediction of drug concentrations when it is administered on a repeated basis (i.e., under steady-state conditions); this allows for the rational selection of dosing regimens. Dose and regimen selection must also take drug interactions, genetic polymorphisms, comorbid conditions, and aging into account since all of these can impact drug exposure, efficacy, and toxicity.

M.S. Luer, PharmD, FCCP (✉)
Department of Pharmacy Practice, Southern Illinois University Edwardsville School of Pharmacy, Campus Box 2000, Edwardsville, IL 62026-2000, USA
e-mail: mluer@siue.edu

S.R. Penzak, PharmD, FCP
Department of Pharmacotherapy, University of North Texas, Health Sciences Center, System College of Pharmacy, 3500 Camp Bowie Blvd, Fort Worth, TX 76107, USA
e-mail: scott.penzak@unthsc.edu

M. Jann et al. (eds.), *Applied Clinical Pharmacokinetics and Pharmacodynamics of Psychopharmacological Agents*,
DOI 10.1007/978-3-319-27883-4_1

Keywords Absorption • Distribution • Metabolism • Excretion • Cytochrome P450 • Poor metabolizer • Extensive metabolizer • Ultrarapid metabolizer • Inhibition • Induction • Drug interaction

1.1 Introduction

Pharmacokinetics is the mathematical characterization of the time course of drug absorption (A), distribution (D), metabolism (M), and excretion (E) [1]. Taken together, ADME processes relate to the intensity and time course (onset, duration, etc.) of drug action, as such their understanding is important to guiding rational drug therapy. Over the past 50 years, scientific advances have revolutionized drug development and design and clinical decision making. These include improvements in quantitating drug and metabolite concentrations in biologic matrices (plasma and tissue), measuring drug effects, and understanding how genetics, metabolic pathways, and drug transporters influences drug disposition. This chapter will provide an overview of how ADME and its applications may be used clinically to enhance the efficacy and minimize the toxicity of centrally acting pharmacologic agents.

1.2 Pharmacokinetics of CNS Active Agents

A major challenge for health-care professionals in clinical psychopharmacology is in understanding and adjusting for individual differences in a drug's response. Knowledge of a drug's pharmacokinetic characteristics can be leveraged to help resolve these issues and formulate rational drug therapy decisions. As an example, understanding the absorption and distribution characteristics of a drug allows one to predict the amount of an administered dose that is expected to enter the bloodstream and reach its site of action. Further, an understanding of drug metabolism and elimination allows for the prediction of drug concentrations when it is administered on a repeated basis (i.e., under steady-state conditions); this allows for the rational selection of dosing regimens. Dose and regimen selection must also take drug interactions, genetic polymorphisms, comorbid conditions, and aging into account since all of these can impact drug exposure, efficacy, and toxicity [2].

1.3 Principles of Pharmacokinetic Models and Relationship to Psychopharmacology

From a pharmacokinetic perspective, the body is often characterized as a series of compartments that are reversibly interconnected through a central compartment. Compartments are purely mathematical locales and do not necessarily represent a specific physiologic or anatomic area, but are fashioned when organs and tissues which display similar pharmacokinetic characteristics for a given drug are grouped together. Because of these similarities, it is assumed that a drug within each compartment is distributed homogenously, and drug movement in and out of each compartment displays consistent kinetics. By establishing these compartments, mathematical models can be created to characterize the separate aspects of ADME to describe variations in each and help predict drug actions.

Drugs that behave mathematically in the body as though they reside within a single homogenous space are described using a one-compartment model. These drugs are treated as though there is one central compartment into which they are absorbed, rapidly distributed, and eliminated. In reality, the body is not a single homogenous compartment and actual tissue concentrations will vary considerably throughout. However, in using this model, it is assumed that there is kinetic homogeneity throughout the body, and thus the rate of change of drug concentrations in one tissue will reflect a corresponding change in drug concentrations in all other tissues [3]. Typically plasma or serum drug concentration data are used as the primary reference for this compartment. Consequently, a 10 % increase in plasma drug concentrations would be reflected by a 10 % increase in tissue drug concentrations over the same time frame. For one-compartment psychopharmacologically active agents, this relative increase in tissue concentrations would include the central nervous system (CNS), which represents the site(s) of drug action.

Unfortunately, not all drugs fit well into a one-compartment model and this includes many psychopharmacologic agents. For such drugs, their tissue distribution is not necessarily rapid or uniform throughout the body; consequently, rates of change in tissue drug concentrations do not consistently match those of the central compartment. These drugs are typically described mathematically as having multiple (two or more) compartments. Such a situation can easily be observed when sufficient plasma concentrations are plotted over time following an intravenous bolus injection of a drug. Upon injection, plasma concentrations will initially be high because all of the drug is located in the blood. This is quickly followed by a period of rapid decline in plasma concentrations, due primarily to drug distribution out of the central compartment and into the tissues. This period is called the *distributive phase,* although some drug elimination (e.g., metabolism by the liver and/or excretion by the kidney) also occurs simultaneously. For drugs with three or more compartments, multiple distributive phases, each with distinct rates of decline may exist. As each distributive phase may last from minutes to hours, they can only be properly delineated with multiple plasma concentrations obtained during each phase; a process that is not typically feasible in the clinical setting. Finally as drug distribution reaches its peak, a pseudo-equilibrium is established between the individual tissues and the central compartment. The continued decline in plasma concentrations will now slow, and the subsequent changes in plasma concentrations will now largely represent drug metabolism and/or excretion. This phase is called the *elimination phase*; it is during this time that a drug's elimination half-life ($T_{1/2}$) can be calculated, and it is anticipated that subsequent changes in plasma concentrations accurately reflect changes in tissue concentrations throughout the body, similar to that of a one-compartment model.

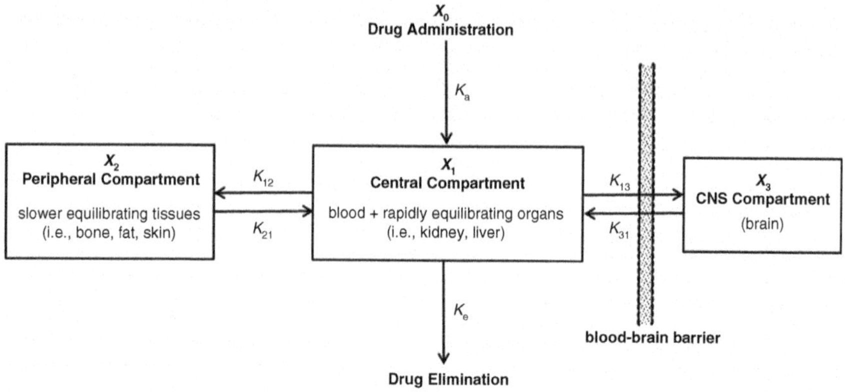

Fig. 1.1 Schematic representation of a three-compartment open model describing the kinetics of a drug that is differentially distributed between compartments. This model assumes that all drug absorption and elimination occurs via the central compartment. Arrows indicate directional movement of the drug. X_0 dose of drug, X_1 amount of drug in central compartment, X_2 amount of drug in peripheral compartment, X_3 amount of drug in CNS compartment, K_a first-order absorption rate constant, K_e elimination rate constant, and K_{12}, K_{21}, K_{13}, and K_{31} distribution rate constants of drug between compartments

For drugs acting on the CNS, pharmacokinetic modeling can be even more complicated. Let us look at an example in which a rapid intravenous bolus injection of a drug is administered into the central compartment, and the rate of drug distribution into the tissues relates principally to blood flow. In this scenario, drug concentrations in highly perfused organs and tissues such as the liver and kidney will begin to equilibrate more quickly with changes in plasma concentrations than would drug concentrations in poorly perfused tissues such as muscle and fat. These rapidly equilibrating tissues are frequently grouped together with blood since they have similar kinetic characteristics and are treated as a common central compartment where drug absorption, distribution, and elimination occur. Similarly, less well-perfused tissues are often combined into separate peripheral compartments based on their like kinetic characteristics.

Characterizing drug disposition can be difficult when considering certain organs such as the brain, which is highly perfused but is separated by a series of physiologic barriers including the blood-brain barrier (BBB) and blood-cerebral spinal fluid barriers (BCSFB). Because these barriers are lipophilic in nature, a drug's physiochemical properties can determine whether it distributes rapidly, distributes slowly, or not at all into the CNS. Consequently, the CNS may actually reside in the central compartment if a drug's distribution is rapid or a peripheral compartment if it is slower; it all depends on the drug's individual and often unique distribution characteristics.

For purposes of this discussion, psychopharmacological agents will be treated as though they reside in a dynamic system consisting of three distinct compartments (Fig. 1.1). Again, from a kinetics standpoint, these compartments are mathematical in nature and generally do not represent a distinct anatomic location. However, in this case the CNS will be treated as a compartment separate from the others. While this three-compartment model is not universally accepted for all psychopharmacologically active agents (i.e., two compartment models may best describe the disposition of certain centrally acting agents), thinking of the body as three distinct but connected compartments makes it easier to account for differences in CNS drug disposition that may result from delayed or selective tissue uptake and/or clearance that is unique to this system. While these CNS parameters are generally not determined in the clinical setting, they can be used to rationalize drug effects in the CNS that would not otherwise be predicted based solely on a measured drug concentration in the central compartment (i.e., plasma). In addition, as the different aspects of ADME are discussed in this chapter, it will be easier to refer to the effects of each parameter on the different compartments with the understanding that changes in plasma concentrations and/or tissue distributions as reflected in the traditionally calculated pharmacokinetic parameters do not necessarily indicate corresponding changes in CNS tissue concentrations.

1.4 Pharmacokinetic Processes

Drug disposition within the CNS is dependent on both the drug's physicochemical properties and its ability to permeate physiologic barriers such as the blood-brain barrier [4]. However, ADME properties each have an impact on drug concentrations in the central compartment which are ultimately what are presented to these barriers; therefore these characteristics of ADME, either individually or collectively, affect drug concentrations in the CNS.

1.4.1 Absorption

Absorption is the entry of a drug into the body, and for psychopharmacological agents, it usually refers to drug entry into the central compartment. In most cases, these agents are administered orally or intramuscularly, but some are administered transdermally, intranasally, rectally, and occasionally intravenously. Because intravenously (IV) administered drugs are delivered directly into the central compartment, absorption is considered to be 100 %, and thus it is deemed the standard by which all other routes of drug delivery are compared. This comparison is typically done by dividing the amount of drug that is quantified in the central compartment (typically measured as area under the concentration-versus-time curve [AUC]) following non-IV administration by the amount of drug measured in this compartment following direct IV administration. This comparison is expressed as a fraction or percent of drug absorbed and is called a drug's *bioavailability*, a parameter which may vary considerably depending on the route of administration [5, 6]. Differences in bioavailability are a substantial reason why the dose of a drug may differ so significantly from one route of administration to another.

In addition to the extent of drug absorption, the rate of drug absorption may also impact drug efficacy and clinical usefulness. The rate of absorption into the central compartment will influence the maximum plasma concentration (C_{max}) and the time at which it occurs (T_{max}). Importantly, while the rate of absorption by itself may have an effect on drug dosing because of its influence on C_{max}, it does not usually affect the steady-state concentrations or the overall maintenance dose. For this section on absorption, the focus will be on the oral and intramuscular routes of administration as they represent the primary routes by which psychopharmacological agents are dosed clinically.

1.4.1.1 Oral

For an oral drug, bioavailability is affected principally by its pharmaceutical formulation, gastrointestinal physiology, and susceptibility to presystemic metabolism in the GI tract and liver. The entire blood supply of the upper gastrointestinal tract passes through the liver before reaching the systemic circulation; therefore as drugs are absorbed into this blood supply, they may be metabolized partially or completely before ever reaching the central compartment. This process is called the "first-pass" effect and it can significantly limit the oral bioavailability of some drugs. Other considerations that can impact oral bioavailability include a compound's solubility, lipophilicity, susceptibility to degradation by pH extremes in the gastrointestinal tract, transport by uptake and efflux transporters such as organic anion transporting polypeptides (OATPs) and P-glycoprotein (P-gp), respectively, metabolism by cytochrome P450 (CYP) enzymes within the gastrointestinal wall, concomitant disease states, and drug interactions which could alter one or more of these factors. An example of the latter is the decreased oral absorption of the phenothiazine antipsychotics, fluphenazine and thioridazine, when they are coadministered with over-the-counter antacid medications. In one evaluation, solubility was reduced and the overall AUC and C_{max} of each phenothiazine were diminished 50 % or more [7].

Another consideration for oral dosing involves the rate and timing of drug absorption. In addition to formulation-specific characteristics of a drug such as extended-release preparations which intentionally slow the rate of absorption, alterations in gastric emptying can also affect an absorption profile since the majority of drugs are absorbed in the upper portion of the small intestine. Drugs such as metoclopramide, which decrease gastric emptying time (i.e., increase gastric emptying), can shorten the time to absorption (reduce T_{max}), whereas drugs that slow gastric emptying may delay the time to absorption (increase T_{max}). As an example, drugs with antimuscarinic activity such as the tricyclic antidepressants can significantly delay gastric emptying. This delay may result in a lag in the onset of action of co-prescribed oral medications. A similar effect can be seen with the intake of food. High-fat meals in particular can also have a dramatic effect on gastric emptying. For example, the absorption of valproic acid (VPA) is significantly delayed when coadministered with food. While, the overall bioavailability and ultimate pharmacologic effect is not altered, it can take hours longer to achieve peak concentrations when VPA is coadministered with a meal [8, 9]. In this case, the increased gastric emptying time does not actually slow the rate of absorption, but it does delay the time before absorption begins.

1.4.1.2 Intramuscular

When a drug is administered intramuscularly (IM), it avoids first-pass metabolism in the liver, potential degradation in the gastrointestinal tract, and depending on the drug's formulation, a quicker onset of action. For standard formulations of drugs in aqueous solutions, absorption by the IM route tends to be relatively fast, but the actual rate of absorption is dependent on blood flow. Differences in absorption rate may exist between individuals based on differences in body composition and sex. Differences in absorption rate may also exist between different muscle groups within the same individual. Obese or emaciated individuals may experience alterations in absorption, and females may experience slower absorption rates based on sex-related differences in the composition of subcutaneous fat. The IM administration of drugs in aqueous solutions is used when an immediate pharmacologic response is not necessary or feasible (e.g., no IV access), but a prompt effect is desired. One example is the use of a haloperidol lactate IM for the management of acutely agitated patients with moderate to severe symptoms.

In contrast to the rapid-onset and typically short-lived characteristics of standard aqueous solutions administered IM, long-acting IM depot formulations of drugs such as the antipsychotics have grown in popularity. These agents are most commonly long-chain esters (e.g., decanoate or palmitate) of the parent drug compounded in a vegetable oil. When injected, the compound forms a "depot" within the muscle and as the drug ester slowly diffuses into the bloodstream, the compound undergoes rapid hydrolysis to release the parent drug. Haloperidol decanoate in sesame oil is an example where such a formulation slows the rate of absorption considerably. For haloperidol decanoate, peak concentrations after IM administration may not be observed for up to 7 days, whereas after IM administration of fluphenazine decanoate, peak concentrations may be observed within 24 h of dosing; therefore, dosing of IM depot formulations of antipsychotics must be individualized [10]. Another formulation approach used to obtain this depot effect is the injectable suspension. These can be created by encapsulating a drug such as risperidone in a biodegradable copolymer that is slowly hydrolyzed in the body or by creating a microcrystalline salt such as olanzapine pamoate that is poorly water soluble on injection but freely dissociates in plasma [11]. Regardless of the technology used, these depot formulations exhibit a slow-release pattern of the drug into plasma and permit the administration of larger doses at less frequent intervals, with the intention of achieving better adherence and consistent and sustained plasma concentrations.

1.4.2 Distribution

After a drug is absorbed into the central compartment, it is distributed throughout the body and into the peripheral compartments. As mentioned previously, a drug's physiochemical properties can significantly impact its distribution characteristics. Larger molecules generally diffuse more slowly across plasma and cell membranes than smaller molecules. Drugs that are more hydrophilic tend to collect in the plasma, whereas drugs that are more lipophilic tend to accumulate in fatty tissues such as the brain. Finally, when drugs are highly bound to plasma proteins such as albumin or α_1-acid glycoprotein (AAG), the drug-protein complex formed in the plasma becomes so large that diffusion across plasma membranes is effectively prohibited leaving only the unbound or "free" drug capable of distributing out into tissues. As such, it is this unbound or free drug that is presented to the receptor site and is considered to be the pharmacologically active moiety [12].

When it comes to drug distribution into the CNS, the BBB and BCSFB are often considered the primary obstacles to entry. Because the BBB has capillary endothelial cells with tight intercellular junctions and is covered by a layer of glial cells, it is lipophilic in nature and usually restricts larger and more water-soluble molecules from crossing [13]. The BCSFB has comparably structured choroid plexus epithelial cells and likewise can restrict drug distribution. Previously, the BBB was considered to be the dominant barrier to CNS drug accumulation, but this has come into question as there is evidence that the BCSFB may have a surface area in the same order of magnitude as the BBB [13, 14]. The implications of this are not clear; nonetheless, it is less relevant whether a drug preferentially enters the CNS through one barrier versus another so long as clinically relevant drug concentrations are obtained at the site of action.

For a drug to distribute into the CNS after reaching systemic circulation, it must traverse the BBB and/or BCSFB via one of several pathways: simple diffusion, facilitated transport, or receptor-mediated transport [15, 16]. In terms of CNS drug distribution, the most prevalent process is simple diffusion. This bidirectional movement is governed by the drug's concentration gradient across the membrane and is impacted by drug-specific characteristics such as molecular size, lipophilicity, and protein binding as previously noted [13]. Increasing the amount of drug in the bloodstream or central compartment will result in an increase in the concentration of drug that is presented to the luminal side of the BBB or BCSFB and thus the amount of drug available for diffusion into the brain. As drug accumulates in the CNS, a pseudo-equilibrium will eventually be established as concentrations equilibrate on both sides of the barrier. Then as plasma concentrations decline secondary to redistribution, metabolism, and/or excretion, the drug will diffuse out of the CNS and back into the central compartment according to the concentration gradient. Typically, smaller, more lipophilic molecules tend to cross the BBB more readily in both directions. A classic example demonstrating this fact is a comparison of the CNS distribution of diazepam and lorazepam. Given intravenously, the more lipophilic diazepam distributes into CNS tissues more quickly than lorazepam and has a slightly more rapid onset of action [17]. However, diazepam, because of his high lipophilicity, will continue to distribute into other tissues as well. This continued distribution into other (non-CNS) tissues causes diazepam concentrations in the plasma to decline such that CNS concentrations are comparatively higher. In keeping with the concentration gradient, diazepam diffuses out of the CNS, and within 15–20 min its neuropharmacological effects can be lost. In comparison lorazepam, which is less lipophilic than diazepam, distributes out of the central compartment and into all tissues more slowly; consequently lorazepam does not display the same degree of redistribution as diazepam. Hence, when administered as an IV bolus, diazepam will have a rapid onset of action that is likely to be short-lived. Conversely, lorazepam administered as an IV bolus will have a slightly slower onset on action, yet its pharmacologic effect may persist for hours [17, 18]. This difference has led some clinicians to prefer lorazepam over diazepam for the treatment of status epilepticus although clinical data demonstrating that one drug is more efficacious than the other in this setting are conflicting [19, 20].

While most drugs gain entry to the CNS via simple diffusion, to a lesser extent drugs may enter the CNS through facilitated diffusion or passive carrier-mediated transport. This process is similar to simple diffusion in that it works along a concentration gradient, but it requires a helper protein to "facilitate" the transport process through the membrane. The greatest difference from simple diffusion is that with facilitated diffusion, the helper protein is finite in number, and thus the process is subject to being capacity limited. Examples of natural substances which utilize this method of uptake are amines, amino acids, and small peptides. Thus for drugs such as gabapentin which have been associated with neutral amino acid transport, saturable uptake into the CNS may occur [21].

The third pathway for centrally acting drugs to gain access to the CNS is receptor-mediated transport or more specifically receptor-mediated endocytosis and transcytosis [16, 22]. Receptor-mediated transport has generated a tremendous amount of interest in recent years and is aggressively being explored as a mechanism for delivering larger drug macromolecules and therapeutic proteins into the CNS. This approach capitalizes on existing transport systems in the BBB and could revolutionize treatment options for all types of neurologic disorders. At this time however, the utility of receptor-mediated transport to facilitate drug delivery in the CNS is largely investigational and mostly limited to preclinical studies [16, 22]. Further discussion of this process and its potential implications will be discussed later in this chapter.

A fourth transport system for crossing the BBB does exist, but its role in drug transport is thought primarily to limit CNS drug uptake, not facilitate it. The system is comprised of a group of naturally occurring, membrane-bound proteins that act as active efflux transporters to move substrates across membranes and against concentration gradients in an energy-dependent manner. Importantly, many drugs serve as substrates or modifiers for these transporters. One of the most prominent active efflux transporters in the BBB is P-glycoprotein (P-gp), which can significantly limit the CNS uptake of many lipophilic drugs that would otherwise be predicted to have significant distribution into the brain based on their physicochemical properties alone [23–25]. This mismatch in distribution patterns for some lipophilic drugs has been a challenge to CNS drug development for years; because a drug must not only be able to cross the BBB, it must reside in the CNS long enough to exert its desired pharmacological effects [26, 27]. In short, these efflux transporters may not be able to prevent a drug's diffusion into the CNS, but they do appear to limit its accumulation and thus minimize its effectiveness as a neuropharmacological agent. The reader is referred to Chap. 5 for a detailed description of drug transporters and the role they play in the BBB as well as overall drug therapy.

For most psychopharmacological agents which are lipophilic in nature, the concentration gradient at the BBB and BCSFB is principally what governs CNS drug disposition. In general, the rate of CNS drug uptake or loss will be proportional to this gradient, so increases or decreases in plasma concentrations will likely lead to respective changes in concentration-dependent CNS drug activity. This dynamic relationship highlights the importance of ADME, since changes in any one of the ADME parameters can alter plasma concentrations causing changes to CNS concentrations and ultimately a drug's neuropharmacological effects.

1.4.3 Metabolism

The majority of psychopharmacologically active agents are removed from the body through metabolic processes. Most drug metabolism occurs in the liver and is usually categorized as phase I or phase II reactions. Phase I involves the processes of oxidation, reduction, and hydrolysis, and phase II involves conjugation. In general, metabolism results in the biotransformation of a parent compound or drug into one or more metabolites, the purpose of which is to make the compound more polar in nature (i.e., water soluble) and thus easier to eliminate from the body by the liver and/or kidney [2, 27]. The resultant metabolite(s) may be inactive, less active, or even more pharmacologically active than the parent compound.

A drug that is metabolized may have as few as one or more than 50 metabolites, some of which may be pharmacologically and/or pharmacokinetically active. From a pharmacologic perspective, the metabolite(s) can contribute significantly to the overall efficacy and/or toxicity profile of the parent drug, and from a pharmacokinetic standpoint, the metabolite may alter (i.e., restrict or enhance) its clearance. A few examples where a metabolite is active and contributes to the drug's overall therapeutic effect are amitriptyline's conversion to nortriptyline, fluoxetine's conversion to nor-fluoxetine, and primidone's conversion to two active metabolites (phenobarbital and phenylethylmalonamide) [28–30]. In those situations when the metabolite itself is the pharmacologically active moiety, the parent drug is referred to as a prodrug. Tramadol, codeine, and fosphenytoin are each prodrugs where metabolic conversion is necessary for their desired pharmacological effect. Tramadol, for instance, is transformed to *O*-desmethyltramadol (*O*-DSMT) which is considerably more potent as a mu opioid agonist and has been shown to have a far greater analgesic effect than the parent drug, tramadol [31, 32].

Of all the metabolic pathways, the cytochrome P450 (CYP) superfamily of metabolizing enzymes is the most important to the metabolism and clearance of drugs and is a major source of variability in pharmacokinetics and plasma drug concentrations [33–38]. Table 1.1 provides an overview of many of the antipsychotics, antidepressants, anxiolytics, anticonvulsants, opioids, and hypnotics relative to their role as a CYP subfamily substrate, inhibitor, or inducer. The data compiled for this table are intended to serve as a reference point from which the discussion on metabolism will now shift to those specific intrinsic and extrinsic factors that affect CYP drug metabolism.

1.4.3.1 Genetic Variability

All enzymes involved in drug metabolism are regulated by genes and gene products (e.g., proteins and RNA). Consequently, an individual's genetic makeup plays an important role in determining the amount and activity of each enzyme system including CYP. This genetic factor accounts for significant interindividual variability in both drug metabolism and metabolite formation. Gene mutations result in enzyme variants with increased, decreased, or no activity. When a gene variant represents at least 1 % of the general population, it is considered a pharmacogenetic polymorphism [39]. Genetically, a wide spectrum of variants may occur in a population that could potentially create a broad range of enzyme activities, but in practice these variants are typically categorized into four general pharmacokinetic phenotypes:

- Poor metabolizers (PM) refer to individuals with variants resulting in highly dysfunctional or inactive CYP enzymes.
- Intermediate metabolizers (IM) refer to individuals with variants resulting in below normal CYP enzyme activity.
- Extensive metabolizers (EM) refer to individuals with the normal phenotype and represent the majority of the population. The EM is the reference phenotype by which others are compared as it is considered normal CYP enzyme activity.
- Ultrarapid metabolizers (UM) refer to individuals with variants that produce much higher than normal CYP enzyme activity [37].

Polymorphic CYP enzymes of clinical relevance for psychopharmacological agents include CYP2C9, CYP2C19, and CYP2D6 [37, 40]. While there are also variants in other important drug-metabolizing enzymes such as CYP1A2 and CYP3A4, extremes in metabolism such as PM and UM are rare [37]. The clinical impact of any pharmacogenetic polymorphism must be considered within the context of the drug(s) being used. Equivalent dosing in PM will result in higher plasma concentrations and possible toxicity relative to EM, while the opposite will occur in UM (i.e., lower plasma concentrations and a possible lack of efficacy). Differential effects also occur if the drug must be metabolically activated (i.e., prodrug); in this case PM will not convert the parent compound to its active metabolite, thus rendering the drug potentially ineffective [37, 40]. Conversely, when a prodrug is

Table 1.1 Reported psychopharmacological agents that act as substrates, inhibitors, or inducers of cytochrome P450 metabolism

CYP1A2	*CYP2B6*	*CYP2C8*	*CYP2C9*	*CYP2C19*	*CYP2D6*	*CYP3A4*
Substrates						
Amitriptyline	Bupropion	Benzphetamine	Amitriptyline	Amitriptyline	Amitriptyline	Alprazolam
Asenapine	Ketamine	Carbamazepine	Clomipramine	Citalopram	Amphetamine	Amitriptyline
Caffeine	Methadone	Phenytoin	Dronabinol	Clomipramine	Aripiprazole	Aripiprazole
Chlordiazepoxide	Sertraline	Zopiclone	Fluoxetine	Desipramine	Asenapine	Buprenorphine
Chlorpromazine			Hexobarbital	Diazepam	Atomoxetine	Buspirone
Clozapine			Imipramine	Escitalopram	Chlorpromazine	Cafergot
Imipramine			Ketamine	Hexobarbital	Clomipramine	Caffeine
Nortriptyline			Mephenytoin	Imipramine	Clozapine	Cannabinoids
Olanzapine			Phenobarbital	Lacosamide	Codeine	Carbamazepine
Perphenazine			Phenytoin	S-Mephenytoin	Desipramine	Chlordiazepoxide
Riluzole			Quetiapine	R-Mephenytoin	Dexfenfluramine	Citalopram
Tacrine			Sertraline	R-Mephobarital	Dextromethorphan	Clomipramine
Zolpidem			THC	Moclobemide	Donepezil	Clonazepam
			Valproic Acid	Nortriptyline	Duloxetine	Clorazepate
				Phenobarbital	Fluphenazine	Clozapine
				Phenytoin	Fentanyl	Cocaine
				Sertraline	Fluoxetine	Codeine
				Thioridazine	Fluvoxamine	Dextromethorphan
					Galantamine	Diazepam
					Haloperidol	Donepezil
					Hydrocodone	Dronabinol
					Iloperidone	Eszopiclone
					Imipramine	Ethosuximide
					Maprotiline	Fentanyl
					Meperidine	Flurazepam
					Methadone	Galantamine

					Methamphetamine	Haloperidol
					Methoxyamphetamine	Hydrocodone
					Minaprine	Iloperidone
					Mirtazapine	Imipramine
					Morphine	Ketamine
					Nortriptyline	Methadone
					Olanzapine	Midazolam
					Oxycodone	Mirtazapine
					Paroxetine	Modafinil
					Perphenazine	Oxycodone
					Propoxyphene	Quetiapine
					Quetiapine	Ramelteon
					Risperidone	Sertraline
					Sertraline	Sibutramine
					Thioridazine	Sufentanil
					Tramadol	Temazepam
					Trazodone	THC
					Venlafaxine	Tiagabine
						Tramadol
						Trazodone
						Triazolam
						Valproic Acid
						Zaleplon
						Ziprasidone
						Zolpidem
						Zonisamide

(continued)

Table 1.1 (continued)

CYP1A2	*CYP2B6*	*CYP2C8*	*CYP2C9*	*CYP2C19*	*CYP2D6*	*CYP3A4*
Inhibitors						
Citalopram			Fluoxetine	Citalopram	Asenapine	Fluoxetine
Fluvoxamine			Fluvoxamine	Felbamate	Bupropion	Fluvoxamine
			Modafinil	Fluoxetine	Chlorpromazine	Nefazadone
			Paroxetine	Fluvoxamine	Citalopram	Norfluoxetine
			Sertraline	Modafinil	Clomipramine	Sertraline
			Tacrine	Oxcarbazepine	Cocaine	
				Topiramate	Desipramine	
					Dozepine	
					Duloxetine	
					Escitalopram	
					Fluoxetine	
					Fluphenazine	
					Haloperidol	
					Levomepromazine	
					Methadone	
					Moclobemide	
					Nefazodone	
					Norfluoxetine	
					Paroxetine	
					Perphenazine	
					Propoxyphene	
					Sertraline	
					Thioridazine	

Inducers						
Carbamazepine	Barbiturates	Carbamazepine	Barbiturates	Barbiturates	Carbamazepine	Barbiturates
Phenobarbital	Mephenytoin	Phenytoin	Carbamazepine	Phenytoin	Ethanol	Carbamazepine
Phenytoin	Phenytoin		Primidone	St. John's wort	Phenobarbital	Ethosuximide
Primidone	Primidone		St. John's wort		Phenytoin	Modafinil
Smoking			Vigabatrin		Primidone	Oxcarbazepine
						Phenytoin
						Primidone
						St. John's wort
						Topiramate

Adapted from Refs. [33–38]

administered to an ultrarapid metabolizer, excess formation of the active metabolite may occur, resulting in possible toxicity. For example, in one evaluation of a single 30 mg dose of codeine, UM had ~50 % higher plasma concentrations of morphine and its phase II metabolites than EM [41]. The reader is referred to Chap. 6 for a detailed description of the influence of pharmacogenetics on the pharmacokinetics of psychopharmacology agents.

1.4.3.2 Substrates

Substrates are compounds or drugs that are metabolized, wholly or in part, by a particular enzymatic pathway. CYP2D6 and CYP3A4 are the most common isoforms involved in the metabolism of psychopharmacological agents, although in many cases additional isoforms are also involved. For example, the N-demethylation of sertraline principally occurs via CYP2B6 although CYP2C9, CYP2C19, CYP2D6, and CYP3A4 contribute as well [41]. This is important because if a drug is exclusively hepatically metabolized and is a substrate for only one pathway, any modulation of that pathway (i.e., inhibition or induction) would be expected to alter the pharmacokinetics of that drug. However, if a drug is only partly hepatically metabolized and/or if it is metabolized by numerous CYP isoforms, then modulation of a single metabolic pathway would be less likely to have a major impact on the drug's overall disposition. Consequently, when making therapeutic decisions, it is equally important to know which CYP isoforms are involved in a drug's metabolism as well as whether a drug is metabolized at all.

1.4.3.3 Inhibition and Induction

Another important consideration in drug metabolism is that CYP isoforms can be independently affected by other drugs or biologic compounds that result in changes in their metabolic activity. CYP inhibitors interfere with an enzyme's ability to metabolize substrates, and inducers accelerate the enzyme's metabolic activity usually through the synthesis of additional enzyme. The clinical effect of an inhibitor or an inducer is not always straightforward and depends on the extent to which an enzyme is affected and whether the substrate has alternative routes of metabolism available, which can potentially "pick up the slack" when another enzymatic pathway is inhibited.

As mentioned previously, metabolism represents a major route of elimination for many drugs. Consequently, the inhibition of metabolizing enzymes is one of the primary causes of drug interactions [42, 43]. There are several mechanisms of enzyme inhibition including competition for the catalytic binding site, allosteric (noncompetitive) interaction with the enzyme, suicide destruction of the enzyme, and competition for enzyme cofactors. The most common mechanism of inhibiting CYP metabolism is through competitive inhibition where two or more molecules compete for the same binding site. Because the interaction is competitive, the substrate K_m (defined as the substrate concentration at half the maximal velocity of an enzymatic reaction) and inhibitor K_i (inhibition constant, defined as the dissociation constant of enzyme-inhibitor complex) in conjunction with their absolute concentrations at the site of enzyme activity will determine the extent and duration of the enzyme inhibition [42]. Clinically, CYP inhibition typically results in increased plasma concentrations of a substrate medication, and if this medication has a narrow therapeutic index and/or if it is subject to capacity-limited metabolism (e.g., phenytoin), toxicity may rapidly occur. As an example, paroxetine and fluoxetine are both effective inhibitors of CYP2D6 and will inhibit the metabolism of thioridazine, a CYP2D6 substrate, thereby increasing its plasma concentrations and the risk of QTc prolongation and cardiac arrhythmias [44–47].

Enzymatic inhibition can also decrease the efficacy of a drug if the parent compound is a prodrug which requires metabolic conversion to its active component. Again, codeine is a good example because it is metabolized in part to morphine via CYP2D6 [48]. Because only a small degree of codeine is metabolized to morphine and the majority is otherwise metabolized by glucuronidation, inhibition of CYP2D6 will not significantly alter the overall pharmacokinetics of codeine, but it will reduce its metabolic conversion to morphine and thus reduce its overall analgesic activity [44]. Another consideration for inhibitory reactions involving competitive inhibition is the fact that the onset and offset of the inhibition are concentration dependent and will commence as soon as a minimum effective inhibitory concentration of the inhibitor is achieved. Depending on the dosing of the substrate and inhibitor, this interaction may occur as soon as the first dose. Conversely the inhibitory effect will dissipate once that minimum effective inhibitory concentration is no longer maintained; this is dependent upon an inhibitor's elimination half-life.

Like inhibitors, inducers also play a major role in altering substrate metabolism. However, unlike CYP inhibition, which has a relatively quick onset (i.e., hours to days), induction is a time-dependent process whose onset and offset each take place over a period of days to weeks [44, 49–51]. Clinically, induction increases substrate metabolism, which can produce different pharmacological and toxicological outcomes depending on the inherent qualities of the substrate affected. For pharmacologically active substrates (i.e., drugs for which the parent compound is pharmacologically active), induction will reduce plasma concentrations and diminish the pharmacologic effect. For prodrugs, induction will increase the substrate's conversion to its active metabolite, thereby enhancing its pharmacologic effect. Finally, induction can increase a drug's toxicity profile through enhanced activation, decreased detoxification, decreased inactivation, and/or by simply altering the balance between activation and inactivation [44, 49–52]. For example, drugs such as carbamazepine, phenobarbital, and St. John's wort significantly induce the metabolism of drugs metabolized by CYP3A4. As a result, these three CYP3A4 inducers have been implicated in the loss of therapeutic effect of concomitantly administered CYP3A4 substrates such as haloperidol [53–56]. Similarly, cigarette smoking can induce CYP1A2 and significantly reduce plasma concentrations of clozapine. In one evaluation, clozapine dose-corrected serum concentrations in smokers were 2.5 times lower compared to nonsmokers [57]. A final consideration regarding induction is that some inducers are actually capable of inducing their own metabolism. This process is called auto-induction and carbamazepine is perhaps the quintessential agent in which this phenomenon occurs. Carbamazepine auto-induction typically peaks within the first week of therapy, and the effect is elevated further following each increase in dose. Once carbamazepine is discontinued, enzymatic induction wanes over a time period that is comparable to its onset of induction. Of note, auto-induction with carbamazepine appears to be independent of prior exposure [58, 59].

1.4.4 *Excretion*

Although metabolism is the major route of elimination for most psychopharmacologically active agents, some drugs and/or their metabolites are excreted wholly or in part through renal or biliary mechanisms. Both routes of excretion correlate directly to organ function, so interference in either system by disease or drug interaction can significantly alter a drug's excretion from the body.

1.4.4.1 Renal Excretion

In general, most drug excretion occurs via the kidney and can be influenced by glomerular filtration, tubular secretion, and/or reabsorption. When a filtered compound has negligible active secretion or reabsorption, its renal clearance is essentially equivalent to the glomerular filtration rate (GFR). In the clinical arena, creatinine clearance (CrCl) or the ability of the kidney to filter creatinine is the most commonly used measure of GFR, and therefore changes in CrCl are expected to represent corresponding changes in renal function. Consequently, CrCl values are commonly used for adjusting drug dosing schedules when a drug and/or its active metabolites are excreted by the kidney. For example, the clearance of oxcarbazepine and its monohydroxy derivatives (MHD) as well as venlafaxine and *O*-desmethylvenlafaxine is reduced with renal impairment, and thus a dose reduction is recommended for each drug in patients with a CrCl <30 mL/min [60, 61].

In addition to considering GFR for drugs that undergo filtration, the step of reabsorption is one of the most important factors in determining whether the drug will be excreted renally. Lipophilic drugs tend to be reabsorbed in the proximal renal tubule, whereas hydrophilic (i.e., polar) drugs typically are not and end up being expelled in the urine. Lithium is the most prominent psychoactive drug that fits this category, as it is excreted almost 95 % unchanged by renal mechanisms. Lithium is filtered in the glomerulus and about 80 % is reabsorbed by the proximal renal tubule. Notably, lithium reabsorption is heavily governed by sodium status. Significant changes in sodium reabsorption, such as that produced by certain diuretics, can dramatically increase or decrease lithium concentrations and result in either toxicity or loss of efficacy due to its narrow therapeutic index [2, 40, 62].

1.4.4.2 Biliary Excretion

Drug excretion into the bile typically involves larger molecular weight compounds that have a strong polar group. Many are excreted as metabolites and often they are glucuronide conjugates. Typically, these compounds are secreted into bile and upon contraction of the gallbladder are expelled into the duodenum via the common bile duct where they are excreted in the feces. A drug or metabolite excreted in bile may also undergo a process termed enterohepatic circulation. This process occurs when the secreted compound is reabsorbed from the gastrointestinal tract back into the systemic circulation or when a glucuronide conjugate metabolite is converted by the β-glucuronidase enzyme present in gut bacteria back to the parent compound and then reabsorbed back into the bloodstream. The clinical importance of enterohepatic circulation is that it may extend the pharmacological effect of certain drugs and metabolites [63]. Examples of psychopharmacological agents as well as their metabolites which have been associated with enterohepatic circulation are morphine and imipramine [64, 65].

1.5 Other Factors Influencing ADME

There are numerous host and environmental factors that can impact a drug's pharmacokinetic profile. Some are constant, such as sex and genotype, whereas others are more variable or dynamic over a lifetime and include factors such age, pregnancy, drug interactions, and concomitant disease states. Genetic polymorphisms and their influences were discussed previously so the remainder of this section will briefly review other factors that can alter ADME parameters.

Sex has an effect on a number of pharmacokinetically relevant factors including body size and composition, tissue blood flow, as well as the expression of metabolizing enzymes and transporters [37, 66–69]. For some drugs, studies in women have demonstrated:

- Differences in oral drug absorption and bioavailability with increases in C_{max} and AUC [70]. Alcohol, for example, has a higher bioavailability in women versus men; this is attributed to differences in volume of distribution and gastric alcohol dehydrogenase activity between the sexes; [71].
- A tendency to metabolize some CYP3A4 substrates more rapidly than men [72].
- A higher body fat content relative to total body weight in women versus men. This is believed to explain the 40 % larger volume of distribution for diazepam – a highly lipophilic drug – in women compared to men [73].

Advanced age can also influence ADME, which has the potential to impact the pharmacokinetics of certain centrally acting agents [74]. A number of biological processes have been implicated in age-related changes in pharmacokinetics. For example, increases in gastric pH, delays in gastric emptying, decreases in gastric motility, and reductions in splanchnic blood flow have all been suggested to cause alterations in oral drug absorption. Changes in body composition (increases in total body fat, decreases in lean muscle mass, and decreases in total body water) can increase the volumes of distribution and elimination half-lives of lipophilic drugs and/or increase the plasma concentrations of hydrophilic drugs. Changes in plasma protein binding (decreases in serum albumin and increases in AAG) can change the plasma free fraction of highly protein-bound drugs. Reductions in hepatic mass and hepatic blood flow have been implicated in reductions in phase I metabolic processes as well as a decline in first-pass metabolism. Finally, a reduction in renal blood flow and GFR reduces renal drug excretion [74].

Drug interactions and disease states can each also play a major role in influencing a drug's pharmacokinetics. The entire third section of this textbook is devoted to clinically significant drug interactions with psychopharmacological agents, and the previous sections on ADME introduced the concept of how physiological conditions can impact each parameter. Taking this one step further, any pathophysiologic effects that alter gastrointestinal function, plasma protein binding, hepatic metabolism, or renal excretion can impact a drug's disposition in the body. Exactly how each disease state impacts a particular drug will depend on the individual characteristics of the drug as well as the extent of the pathology. For example, chronic liver disease and acute hepatitis each have the ability to diminish the metabolic capacity of the liver, but the degree to which drug metabolism is altered is highly variable [75]. In treating an individual with benzodiazepines for alcohol withdrawal, chlordiazepoxide, lorazepam, oxazepam, or diazepam can each be used. However, with advanced alcoholic liver disease, hepatic oxidation can be diminished, which can reduce chlordiazepoxide and diazepam metabolism resulting in prolonged sedation and respiratory depression. Conversely, lorazepam and oxazepam are glucuronidated and less affected by advanced liver disease [76, 77]. To this end, it is not sufficient to simply be aware that a drug-drug or drug-disease interaction exists; instead a comprehensive understanding of the nature and scope of all contributing factors to an interaction is necessary to determine the optimal therapeutic course of action.

1.6 Pharmacokinetic-Pharmacodynamic Relationships

The intensity of a drug's effect is largely a function of its concentration at its site of action [78]. The effect that a drug produces on the body is defined as its pharmacodynamic effect. Evaluation of pharmacokinetic-pharmacodynamic relationships informs the selection of appropriate drug therapy at optimal doses. Pharmacodynamic properties of psychopharmacological agents are considered in detail in Chap. 2.

1.7 Future Directions

One of the greatest challenges in developing new psychopharmacological agents relates to CNS drug delivery [79]. Currently, the vast majority of agents are administered systemically, and thus their delivery into the CNS is subject to the limitations of the BBB and BCSFB as described previously. Promising new drug therapies such as protein therapeutics are severely hampered because these large molecules cannot gain access to the CNS. As a result, new approaches of traversing the BBB are being explored and some of the more exciting concepts are physiological approaches to drug delivery. These approaches capitalize on endogenous nutrient transport systems in the BBB as well as methods of attaching drugs to ligands that recognize receptors expressed at the BBB [16, 22, 80, 81]. For BBB nutrient transport systems, drugs can be formulated to use carrier-mediated transporters (CMT) for glucose (GLUT1), phenylalanine (LAT1), arginine (CAT1), etc. to gain access into the CNS; however, in doing so the drugs must closely mimic the natural substrates for these transporters. Currently drugs such as L-Dopa, gabapentin, and melphalan each cross the BBB and achieve clinically relevant pharmacologic concentrations in the CNS via LAT1 by having structures similar to large neutral amino acids [80, 81]. Because the original structural characteristics of the substrate class for the targeted CMT must be retained without significantly altering its pharmacological activity, computational medicinal chemistry will be an important aspect of continued drug development in this area.

Another physiological approach for CNS drug delivery is to use receptor-mediated transcytosis (RMT) that capitalizes on the fact that naturally occurring large molecules are delivered to the CNS by specific receptors. Known receptors to date exist for insulin, transferrin, and low-density lipoprotein (LDL) and its related proteins. RMT is a three-step process for ligand transport. First, the molecules will undergo receptor-mediated endocytosis by binding to specific receptors present on the luminal side of the BBB. It then moves through the cell to the abluminal side of the BBB where it undergoes exocytosis and finally entry into the CNS. For RMT-mediated CNS drug delivery, the concept is to target specific ligands or monoclonal antibodies (mAb) for these receptors [80]. Specifically, the desired therapeutic molecules are then attached to these ligands or mAb using molecular Trojan horse (MTH) technology [82]. The ligand or mAb is then transported into the CNS and the attached therapeutic molecule essentially goes with it. Several neurotrophin and peptide combinations with mAb have already been produced using this technology [80–82]. Possibly the most promising work to date in this arena involves the LDL receptor-related proteins 1 and 2 (LRP-1 and LRP-2). Specifically a new family of peptides derived from proteins that cross the BBB using LRP-1 receptors has been designed as a new technology for delivering therapeutic agents into the CNS [80]. The technology is called Angiopep, and one agent ANG1005, a novel paclitaxel-peptide drug conjugate for the treatment of glioblastoma multiforme (GBM), was granted both orphan drug and fast track designation by the Food and Drug Association (FDA) in 2014. While this technology has not been used directly to target psychopharmacological agent delivery, the concept has the ability to deliver a broad array of neurotherapeutic agents and could be disease altering for a number of conditions.

References

1. Gibaldi M, Levy G (1976) Pharmacokinetics in clinical practice I. Concepts. JAMA 235(17):1864–1867
2. Davies SJC, Nutt D (2007) Pharmacokinetics for psychiatrics. Psychiatry 6(7):268–272

3. Gibaldi M, Perrier D (1982) One-compartment model. In: Pharmacokinetics. Marcel Dekker Inc., New York, pp 1–43
4. Badhan RK, Chenel M, Penny JI (2014) Development of a physiologically-based pharmacokinetic model of the rat central nervous system. Pharmaceutics 6(1):97–136. doi:10.3390/pharmaceutics6010097
5. Nelson E (1961) Kinetics of drug absorption, distribution, metabolism and excretion. J Pharm Sci 50:181–192
6. Rowland M, Tozer T (eds) (2011) Fundamental concepts and terminology. In: Clinical pharmacokinetics and pharmacodynamics: concepts and applications. Williams & Wilkins, Baltimore, pp 17–45
7. Moustafa MA, Babhair SA, Kouta HI (1987) Decreased bioavailability of some antipsychotic phenothiazines due to interactions with adsorbent antacid and antidiarrhoeal mixtures. Int J Pharm 36(2–3):185–189
8. Hamilton RA, Garnett WR, Kline BJ, Pellock JM (1981) Effects of food on valproic acid absorption. Am J Hosp Pharm 38(10):1490–1493
9. Chun AH, Hoffman DJ, Friedmann N, Carrigan PJ (1980) Bioavailability of valproic acid under fasting/nonfasting regimens. J Clin Pharmacol 20:30–36
10. Jann MW, Ereshefsky L, Saklad SR (1985) Clinical pharmacokinetics of the depot antipsychotics. Clin Pharmacokinet 10(4):315–333
11. Park EJ, Amatya S, Kim MS, Park JH, Seol E, Lee H, Shin YH, Na DH (2013) Long-acting injectable formulations of antipsychotic drugs for the treatment of schizophrenia. Arch Pharm Res 36(6):651–659. doi:10.1007/s12272-013-0105-7
12. Tanaka H, Mizojiri K (1999) Drug-protein binding and blood-brain barrier permeability. J Pharmacol Exp Ther 288:912–918
13. Levin VA (1980) Relationship of octanol/water partition coefficient and molecular weight to rat brain capillary permeability. J Med Chem 23:682–684
14. Johanson CE, Stopa EG, McMillan PN (2011) The blood-cerebrospinal fluid barrier: structure and functional significance. Methods Mol Biol 686:101–131
15. de Lange EC (2013) The mastermind approach to CNS drug therapy: translational prediction of human brain distribution, target site kinetics, and therapeutics effects. Fluids Barriers CNS 10:12. doi:10.1186/2045-8118-10-12
16. Xiao G, Gan L-S (2013) Receptor-mediated endocytosis and brain delivery of therapeutic biologics. Int J Cell Biol 2013:14 pages. Article ID 703545. http://dx.doi.org/10.1155/2013/703545
17. Greenblatt DJ, Ehrenberg BL, Gunderman J, Scavone JM, Tai NT, Harmatz JS, Shader RI (1989) Kinetic and dynamic study of intravenous lorazepam: comparison with intravenous diazepam. J Pharmacol Exp Ther 250(1):134–140
18. Ramsay RE, Hammond EJ, Perchalski RJ, Wilder BJ (1979) Brain uptake of phenytoin, phenobarbital, and diazepam. Arch Neurol 36:535–539
19. Alldredge BK, Gelb AM, Isaacs SM, Corry MD, Allen F, Ulrich S et al (2001) A comparison of lorazepam, diazepam, and placebo for the treatment of out-of-hospital status epilepticus. N Engl J Med 345:631–637
20. Treiman DM (1990) The role of benzodiazepines in the management of status epilepticus. Neurology 40(5 Suppl 2):32–42
21. Luer MS, Hamani C, Dujovny M, Gidal B, Cwik M, Deyo K, Fischer JH (1999) Saturable transport of gabapentin at the blood-brain barrier. Neurol Res 21(6):559–562
22. Qian ZM, Li H, Sun H, Ho K (2002) Targeted drug delivery via the transferrin receptor-mediated endocytosis pathway. Pharmacol Rev 54(4):561–587
23. Schinkel AH, Smit JJ, van Tellingen O et al (1994) Disruption of the mouse mdr1a P-glycoprotein gene leads to a deficiency in the blood-brain barrier and to increased sensitivity to drugs. Cell 77:491–502
24. Sakata A, Tamai I, Kawazu K et al (1994) In vivo evidence for ATP-dependent and P-glycoprotein-mediated transport of cyclosporin A at the blood brain barrier. Biochem Pharmacol 48(10):1989–1992

25. Schinkel AH, Wagenaar E, van Deemter L, Mol CA, Borst P (1995) Absence of the mdr1a P-glycoprotein in mice affects tissue distribution and pharmacokinetics of dexamethasone, digoxin, and cyclosporin A. J Clin Invest 96:1698–1705
26. Girardin F (2006) Membrane transporter proteins: a challenge for CNS drug development. Dialogues Clin Neurosci 8:311–321
27. Alavijeh MS, Chrishty M, Qaiser MZ, Palmer AM (2005) Drug metabolism and pharmacokinetics, the blood-brain barrier, and central nervous system drug discovery. NeuroRx® 2:554–571
28. Breyer-Pfaff U (2004) The metabolic fate of amitriptyline, nortriptyline and amitriptylinoxide in man. Drug Metab Rev 36(3–4):723–746
29. Mandrioli R, Forti GC, Raggi MA (2006) Fluoxetine metabolism and pharmacological interactions: the role of cytochrome p450. Curr Drug Metab 7(2):127–133
30. Gallagher BB, Baumel IP, Mattson RH (1972) Metabolic disposition of primidone and its metabolites in epileptic subjects after single and repeated administration. Neurology 22: 1186–1192
31. Dayer P, Desmeules J, Collart L (1997) Pharmacology of tramadol. Drugs 53(Suppl 2):18–24. doi:10.2165/00003495-199700532-00006
32. Gong L, Stamer UM, Tzvetkove MV, Altmana RB, Klein TE (2014) PharmGKB summary: tramadol pathway. Pharmacogenet Genomics 24(7):374–380. doi:10.1097/FPC.0000000 000000057
33. Davies SJ, Eayrs S, Pratt P, Lennard MS (2004) Potential for drug interactions involving cytochromes P450 2D6 and 3A4 on general adult and functional elderly psychiatric wards. Br J Clin Pharmacol 57:464–472
34. Sandson NB, Armstrong SC, Cozza KL (2005) An overview of psychotropic drug-drug interactions. Psychosomatics 46:464–494
35. Greenblatt DJ, von Moltke LL, Harmatz JS, Shader RI (1998) Drug interactions with new antidepressants: role of human cytochromes P450. J Clin Psychiatry 59(Suppl 15):19–27
36. Flockhart DA (2007) Drug interactions: cytochrome P450 drug interaction table. Indiana University School of Medicine. "/clinpharm/ddis/clinical-table/" Accessed 10 June 2015
37. Zanger UM, Schwab M (2013) Cytochrome P450 enzymes in drug metabolism: regulation of gene expression, enzyme activities, and impact of genetic variation. Pharmacol Ther 138(1):103–41. doi: 10.1016/j.pharmthera.2012.12.007. Epub 2013 Jan 16
38. Preissner S, Kroll K, Dunkel M, Goldsobel G, Kuzmann D, Senger S, Günther S, Winnenburg R, Schroeder M, Preissner R (2010) SuperCYP: a comprehensive database on Cytochrome P450 enzymes including a tool for analysis of CYP-drug interactions. Nucleic Acids Res 38(Database issue):D237–D243
39. Meyer UA (1991) Genotype or phenotype: the definition of a pharmacogenetics polymorphism. Pharmacogenetics 1:66–67
40. Chadwick B, Waller DF, Edwards JG (2005) Potentially hazardous drug interactions with psychotropics. Adv Psychiatr Treat 11:440–449
41. Kirchheiner J, Schmidt H, Tzvetkov M, Keulen JT, Lötsch J, Roots I, Brockmöller J (2007) Pharmacokinetics of codeine and its metabolite morphine in ultra-rapid metabolizers due to CYP2D6 duplication. Pharmacogenomics J 7(4):257–265, Epub 2006 Jul 4
42. Obach RS, Cox LM, Tremaine LM (2005) Sertraline is metabolized by multiple cytochrome P450 enzymes, monoamine oxidases, and glucuronyl transferases in human: an in vitro study. Drug Metab Dispos 33(2):262–270, Epub 2004 Nov 16
43. Lin JH, Lu AY (1997) Role of pharmacokinetics and metabolism in drug discovery and metabolism. Pharmacol Rev 49(4):403–449
44. Lin JH, Lu AY (1998) Inhibition and induction of cytochrome P450 and the clinical implications. Clin Pharmacokinet 35(5):361–390
45. Crewe HK, Lennard MS, Tucker GT, Woods FR, Haddock RC (1992) The effect of selective serotonin re-uptake inhibitors on cytochrome P4502D6 (CYP2D6) activity in human liver microsomes. Br J Clin Pharmacol 34:262–265
46. Reilly JG, Ayis SA, Ferrier IN, Jones SH, Thomas SH (2000) QTc-interval abnormalities and psychotropic drug therapy in psychiatric patients. Lancet 355(9202):1048–1052

47. Prozac(R) [package insert] (2011) Eli Lilly and Company, Indianapolis
48. Chen ZR, Somogyi AA, Bochner F (1988) Polymorphic O-demethylation of codeine. Lancet 32(8616):914–915
49. Moore LB, Goodwin B, Jones SA et al (2000) St. John's wort induces hepatic drug metabolism through activation of the pregnane X receptor. Proc Natl Acad Sci U S A 97(13):7500–7502
50. Markowitz JS, Donovan JL, DeVane C et al (2003) Effect of St John's wort on drug metabolism by induction of cytochrome P450 3A4 enzyme. JAMA 290(11):1500–1504. doi:10.1001/jama.290.11.1500
51. Hewitt NJ, Lecluyse EL, Ferguson SS (2007) Induction of hepatic cytochrome P450 enzymes: methods, mechanisms, recommendations, and in vitro–in vivo correlations. Xenobiotica 37(10–11):1196–1224. doi:10.1080/00498250701534893
52. Park BK, Kitteringham NR, Pirmohamed M, Tucker GT (1996) Relevance of induction of human drug-metabolizing enzymes: pharmacological and toxicological implications. Br J Clin Pharmacol 41:477–491
53. Barone GW, Gurley BJ, Ketel BL, Lightfoot ML, Abul-Ezz SR (2000) Drug interaction between St. John's wort and cyclosporine. Ann Pharmacother 34(9):1013–1016
54. Kahn EM, Schulz SC, Perel JM, Alexander JE (1990) Change in haloperidol level due to carbamazepine--a complicating factor in combined medication for schizophrenia. J Clin Psychopharmacol 10(1):54–57
55. Jann MW, Ereshefsky L, Saklad SR et al (1985) Effects of carbamazepine on plasma haloperidol levels. J Clin Psychopharmacol 5(2):106–109
56. Johannessen SI, Landmark CJ (2010) Antiepileptic drug interactions – principles and clinical implications. Curr Neuropharmacol 8(3):254–267. doi:10.2174/157015910792246254
57. van der Weide J, Steijns LS, van Weelden MJ (2003) The effect of smoking and cytochrome P450 CYP1A2 genetic polymorphism on clozapine clearance and dose requirement. Pharmacogenetics 13(3):169–172
58. Kudriakova TB, Sirota LA, Rozova GI, Gorkov VA (1992) Autoinduction and steady-state pharmacokinetics of carbamazepine and its major metabolites. Br J Clin Pharmacol 33(6):611–615
59. Browne TR, Mikati MA, Collins VA (1987) Time course of carbamazepine autoinduction (abstract). Neurology 37:100
60. Flesch G (2004) Overview of the clinical pharmacokinetics of oxcarbazepine. Clin Drug Investig 24:185–203
61. Troy SM, Schultz RW, Parker VD, Chiang ST, Blum RA (1994) The effect of renal disease on the disposition of venlafaxine. Clin Pharmacol Ther 56(1):14–21
62. Finley PR, Warner MD, Peabody CA (1995) Clinical relevance of drug interactions with lithium. Clin Pharmacokinet 29(3):172–191
63. Rollins DE, Klaassen CD (1979) Biliary excretion of drugs in man. Clin Pharmacokinet 4(5):368–379
64. Dencker H, Dencker SJ, Green A, Nagy A (1976) Intestinal absorption, demethylation, and enterohepatic circulation of imipramine. Clin Pharmacol Ther 19(5 Pt 1):584–586
65. Ouellet DM, Pollack GM (1995) Biliary excretion and enterohepatic recirculation of morphine-3-glucuronide in rats. Drug Metab Dispos 23(4):478–484
66. Beierle I, Meibohm B, Derendorf H (1999) Gender differences in pharmacokinetics and pharmacodynamics. Int J Clin Pharmacol Ther 37(11):529–547
67. Gandhi M, Aweeka F, Greenblatt RM, Blaschke TF (2004) Sex differences in pharmacokinetics and pharmacodynamics. Annu Rev Pharmacol Toxicol 44:499–523
68. Schwartz JB (2003) The influence of sex on pharmacokinetics. Clin Pharmacokinet 42(2):107–121
69. Soldin OP, Chung SH, Mattison DR (2011) Sex differences in drug disposition. J Biomed Biotechnol 2011:187103. doi:10.1155/2011/187103
70. Chen ML, Lee SC, Ng MJ, Schuirmann DJ, Lesko LJ, Williams RL (2000) Pharmacokinetic analysis of bioequivalence trials: implications for sex-related issues in clinical pharmacology and biopharmaceutics. Clin Pharmacol Ther 68(5):510–521

71. Parlesak A, Billinger MH, Bode C, Bode JC (2002) Gastric alcohol dehydrogenase activity in man: influence of gender, age, alcohol consumption and smoking in a Caucasian population. Alcohol Alcohol 37(4):388–393
72. Greenblatt DJ, von Moltke LL (2008) Gender has a small but statistically significant effect on clearance of CYP3A substrate drugs. J Clin Pharmacol 48(11):1350–1355
73. Ochs HR, Greenblatt DJ, Divoll M (1981) Diazepam kinetics in relation to age and sex. Pharmacology 23(1):24–30
74. Klotz U (2009) Pharmacokinetics and drug metabolism in the elderly. Drug Metab Rev 41(2):67–76
75. Rodighiero V (1999) Effects of liver disease on pharmacokinetics. An update. Clin Pharmacokinet 37(5):399–431
76. Greenblatt DJ (1981) Clinical pharmacokinetics of oxazepam and lorazepam. Clin Pharmacokinet 6(2):89–105
77. Peppers MP (1996) Benzodiazepines for alcohol withdrawal in the elderly and in patient is with liver disease. Pharmacotherapy 16(1):49–57
78. Derendorf H, Meibohm B (1999) Modeling of pharmacokinetic/pharmacodynamic (PK/PD) relationships: concepts and perspectives. Pharm Res 16(2):176–185
79. Pardridge WM (2005) The blood-brain barrier: bottleneck in brain drug development. NeuroRx 2(1):3–14
80. Gabathuler R (2010) Approaches to transport therapeutic drugs across the blood-brain barrier to treat brain diseases. Neurobiol Dis 37(1):48–57. doi:10.1016/j.nbd.2009.07.028, Epub 2009 Aug 5
81. Pardridge WM (2012) Drug transport across the blood–brain barrier. J Cereb Blood Flow Metab 32(11):1959–1972. doi:10.1038/jcbfm.2012.126
82. Pardridge WM, Boado RJ (2012) Reengineering biopharmaceuticals for targeted delivery across the blood–brain barrier. Methods Enzymol 503:269–292. doi:10.1016/B978-0-12-396962-0.00011-2

Chapter 2
Pharmacodynamics

Carlos H. Rojas-Fernandez

Abstract Over the past 10–15 years, there have been significant advances in our understanding of the pharmacodynamics of neuropsychopharmacological agents. Novel research techniques have allowed for the discovery of multiple receptor subtypes and have also revealed complex and ofttimes seemingly contradictory physiological effects secondary to manipulation of neural receptors. This chapter summarizes key concepts in central nervous system pharmacodynamics including brief descriptions of localization of receptor subtypes, neural pathways, as well as putative pharmacodynamic properties of drugs that affect these neural systems. The aim is to provide clinicians with an understanding of general concepts that may be applied to the relevant chapters in this book and to the literature. This chapter is arranged according to individual neural systems, yet it should be stressed that this "splitting" approach is an artificial attempt to describe, in simple terms, systems that have varying degrees of complex and hitherto not fully understood interrelationships. Indeed, any of the neural systems discussed herein merit their own chapter, if not their own book. It is for this reason that the reader should consult other chapters in this textbook, as well as relevant references for additional details in this complex and quickly evolving field.

Keywords Neuropsychopharmacology • Neurology • Psychiatry • Central nervous system

---

C.H. Rojas-Fernandez, BSc(Pharm), PharmD
Schlegel Research Chair, Geriatric Pharmacotherapy Schlegel-UW Research Institute for Ageing, Waterloo, ON, Canada

President of CRF Consulting Services, Geriatric Clinical Pharmacology, Neuropsychopharmacology, Clinical & Epidemiologic Research, Waterloo, ON, Canada
e-mail: carlos.rojas-fernandez@uwaterloo.ca

M. Jann et al. (eds.), *Applied Clinical Pharmacokinetics and Pharmacodynamics of Psychopharmacological Agents*,
DOI 10.1007/978-3-319-27883-4_2

2.1 Introduction

2.1.1 Pharmacodynamic Principles

Pharmacodynamics is the study of the effects that drugs have on the body and how these effects take place, i.e., their putative mechanism of action. Observed drug effects may be attributable to biochemical and/or physiological manipulations, and most drugs must interact with one or more macromolecular components of the organism (i.e., person) in order to exert their effects. The interactions of a drug with these components, i.e., drug receptors, result in changes in the function of that component, ultimately leading to biochemical and/or physiological responses. Proteins are ostensibly the most important class of drug receptors/ targets by virtue of their large numbers. Common examples of particular relevance to the central nervous system (CNS) include acetylcholinesterases, secretases, and proteins involved in transport processes (Na^+, K^+-ATPase). Physiological receptors, which are receptors for endogenous regulatory ligands, are also a major group of drug receptors. Drugs that bind to these receptors and mimic the effects of endogenous ligands are referred to as agonists, while drugs that bind to receptors but do not possess intrinsic activity are termed antagonists. Partial agonists are drugs possessing only partial efficacy as agonists at all concentrations; a well-known example of a partial agonist in psychopharmacology is aripiprazole [1, 2].

Lastly, there are drugs such as histamine-1 antagonists, which stabilize receptors with intrinsic constitutive activity in the absence of endogenous ligand, and are termed inverse agonists [3, 4]. The dissociation constant of a drug is a measure of the strength of the reversible interaction between a drug and its receptor and represents the affinity of one for the other, while a drug's chemical structure affects its affinity for a receptor, its intrinsic activity, and its specificity. The latter is of particular relevance, as drugs that are highly specific for receptors with limited distribution in the body have little potential for systemic adverse effects (e.g., histamine-2 receptor antagonists such as ranitidine), whereas drugs such as acetylcholinesterase inhibitors (ACHEIs) or selective serotonin reuptake inhibitors (SSRIs) carry a greater potential for systemic adverse effects given the distribution of acetylcholinesterases and serotonin (5-HT) receptors, respectively. Pharmacodynamic variability is a highly complex phenomenon, which may vary according to genetic influences, effects of diseases on the body, pharmacokinetic factors, drug-induced changes in receptors, and interactions among all of the aforementioned [5, 6].

2.1.2 The Central Nervous System as a Site for Drug Action

The CNS presents multiple challenges as well as opportunities as a site for drug action. A well-recognized challenge is the blood-brain barrier, which acts to control the microenvironment of the brain and protect it against potentially toxic substances through a complex set of transport systems and anatomical structures [7, 8]. Conversely, while there are many established sites for drug action such as the nigrostriatal dopaminergic pathway for Parkinson's disease, the mesolimbic dopaminergic pathway for schizophrenia, and others, much remains to be learned about the role of other putative pathways, intertwining pathways, and/or receptors for these and other CNS disorders. In addition, effective therapies are lacking for the treatment of cognitive impairment, which afflicts those with schizophrenia as well as those with mood and anxiety disorders.

2.1.3 Central and Peripheral Effects of Psychopharmacological Agents

As previously noted, the CNS not only encompasses a multitude of therapeutic targets for CNS diseases but is also an important source for unintended consequences, namely, adverse drug events (see respective sections below and chapters for more details). Examples include but are not limited to iatrogenic parkinsonism, sedation, cognitive impairment, insomnia, and psychosis. In addition, CNS-mediated drug effects may also lead to peripheral adverse or therapeutic effects such as tremors from dopamine blockade, gastrointestinal effects from SSRIs or ACHEIs, and decreased aggression from decreased sympathetic nervous system drive (clonidine). Direct effects of drugs in the periphery may also be observed even if the drug does not penetrate the BBB (e.g., vasodilation from psychopharmacological agents with clinically relevant alpha-1 antagonist properties such as clozapine).

2.2 CNS Pharmacodynamics: Receptor Systems

2.2.1 Serotonin

Serotonin has been localized to the gastrointestinal tract, platelets, and the brain, where it is involved in many diverse functions such as cognition, mood control, sleep-wake cycles, respiration, feeding behavior, thermoregulation, and motor control [9]. Serotonergic (5-hydroxytryptamine [5-HT]) neurons originate in the midbrain (raphe nuclei) and project widely to nearly every area of the CNS, yet the overall number of 5-HT neurons is low relative to the total number of neurons in the brain [9–13]. Specifically, the median raphe projects heavily to the dorsal hippocampus, septum, and hypothalamus; and the dorsal raphe sends projections to the ventral hippocampus, amygdala, and striatum; and both send overlapping projections to the neocortex. Additionally, both the substantia nigra (SN) and ventral tegmental areas (VTA) receive input from midbrain 5-HT neurons [14, 15]. Serotonin has been proposed to exert an overall neuromodulatory effect on the brain in addition to its contribution to synaptic transmission; it is thought that this is accomplished by 5-HT modulating the overall tone of the CNS via a regular, yet slow pattern of activity, akin to a pacemaker [9].

2.2.2 Serotonin and Drugs

The serotonin transporter (SERT) along with various serotonin receptors represent useful drug targets for diseases such as depression, anxiety, obsessive-compulsive disorder, and others. As serotonin activity in the synapse is primarily terminated by its reuptake into serotonergic terminals via the SERT, which is a high-affinity, low capacity, and saturable transporter, the SERT represents a key target for SSRIs, which lead to SERT downregulation with chronic SSRI administration [16–19]. The primary catabolic pathway for 5-HT, namely, monoamine oxidase (MAO), also presents a useful target, and in fact, some of the earliest antidepressant drugs were nonselective MAO A and B inhibitors such as tranylcypromine, which inhibits the catabolism of 5-HT and catecholamines (NE and DA), respectively [20]. In addition, multiple 5-HT receptors have been identified, all of which can be affected by various drugs [16, 18, 21, 22]. What follows is a discussion regarding 5-HT receptors that are best understood in the context of drugs which are in contemporary use.

2.2.3 5-HT_{1a} Receptor

The 5-HT_{1a} receptor is present in high density in the hippocampus, lateral septum, amygdala, cortical limbic areas, as well as in the dorsal raphe nucleus (DRN) and median raphe nucleus (MRN). It is thought that the 5-HT_{1a} receptor plays a role in emotional states as well as in cognitive function [19]. 5-HT_{1a} receptors are located postsynaptically in terminal field areas of serotonergic innervation and are also present in high density on cell soma, particularly in the DRN and MRN. In the latter areas, 5-HT_{1a} receptors function as somatodendritic autoreceptors, playing an integral role in the negative feedback modulation of neuronal serotonergic activity. In the terminal field areas such as the hippocampus, 5-HT_{1a} receptors lead to opening of potassium channels, leading to hyperpolarization, thus exerting an inhibitory effect when stimulated by 5-HT.

2.2.3.1 Presynaptic Somatodendritic 5-HT_{1a} Autoreceptors

These receptors play an important role in homeostatic control of 5-HT levels, inasmuch as activation of 5-HT_{1a} autoreceptors by endogenous 5-HT or by drugs (e.g., SSRIs) leads to neuronal hyperpolarization and a reduction in neuronal firing [23–26]. Somatodendritic 5-HT_{1a} autoreceptors also play an important and detrimental role in depressive illness, as patients with an increased activity or density of presynaptic 5-HT_{1a} receptors are more likely to develop mood disorders and to exhibit a poor response to antidepressants [27–29].

Paradoxically (at least acutely), activation of somatodendritic 5-HT_{1a} autoreceptors by 5-HT_{1a} agonists or SSRIs slows the rate of firing of serotonergic soma and reduces 5-HT neuronal activity and terminal 5-HT release, which limits the activation of postsynaptic 5-HT receptors. It has been proposed that this effect may play a role in the somewhat delayed (and possibly limited) efficacy of antidepressants. With chronic administration of SSRIs, however, $5HT_{1a}$ autoreceptors become desensitized, ultimately leading to a recovery of 5-HT cell firing at the dorsal raphe, allowing for normalized 5-HT release and increased postsynaptic 5-HT neurotransmission [30–33]. These effects translate into antidepressant and antianxiety effects vis-a-vis increased serotonergic neuronal firing rates [16, 18]. Similarly, buspirone is an example of a drug that can reduce anxiety by its partial agonist effects at the 5-HT_{1a} autoreceptor, while newer antidepressant drugs such as vortioxetine and vilazodone possess partial 5-HT_{1a} agonist properties [34, 35].

2.2.3.2 Postsynaptic 5-HT_{1a} Receptors (5-HT_{1a}-Rs)

These receptors are expressed in brain regions such as the limbic cortex, cortical forebrain, and the spinal cord and are thought to play a prominent role in cortical function. In addition, as 5-HT_{1a}-Rs are present in up to 80 % of upper cortical layers of human prefrontal cortex (PFC), activation of 5-HT_{1a}-Rs in the PFC may modulate neuronal function more distally, similar to brainstem monoaminergic nuclei [36]. Indeed, it has been suggested that 5-HT_{1a}-R agonists may enhance forebrain catecholamine release, an effect which could be involved in antidepressant actions [37, 38]. Furthermore, chronic antidepressant treatment tonically activates hippocampal 5-HT_{1a}-Rs, and selective 5-HT_{1a}-Rs agonists have demonstrated antidepressant properties in preclinical studies [21, 39, 40]. While these effects appear to contradict the aforementioned inhibitory action of 5-HT on 5-HT_{1a}-Rs, it should be noted that the functional effects of 5-HT_{1a}-Rs result in a paradoxical increase in firing activity [18, 41].

2.2.4 5-HT_{2a} Receptors

5-HT_{2a} receptors are found postsynaptically in high concentrations in the frontal cortex, parts of the limbic system (hippocampus, amygdala), the basal ganglia, and the claustrum (connected to the visual cortex). The latter is of particular interest in Parkinson's disease, as increased 5-HT_{2a} receptors in visual processing and limbic areas of the brain have recently been implicated in the genesis of visual hallucinations [42–44]. While pure 5-HT_{2a} antagonists have not been shown to be effective for these symptoms, a 5-HT_{2a} inverse agonist, pimavanserin, has recently demonstrated favorable results in the treatment of Parkinson's disease psychosis

(PDP) and, if successful in gaining regulatory approval, would represent a novel approach to the treatment of PDP [45, 46].

The 5-HT_{2a} receptor also continues to be of interest in the pharmacology of antipsychotic drugs, where $5HT_{2a}$ antagonism has been proposed to contribute to a more favorable extrapyramidal side effect profile of some drugs such as risperidone, though this property can be lost when risperidone is administered in higher doses [47]. The putative mechanism for this effect relates to the distribution of 5-HT_{2a} receptors in the basal ganglia, where antagonism of 5-HT_{2a} receptors disinhibits dopamine (DA) neurons, thus allowing for a more normalized DA release in the basal ganglia. This receptor is also important in thermoregulation, as activation of central 5-HT_{2a} receptors leads to an increase in body temperature (one of the signs of serotonin toxicity), which may be treated by administering 5-HT_{2a} antagonists such as cyproheptadine [48, 49].

2.2.5 $5HT_{2c}$ Receptors

The 5-HT_{2c} receptor is present in high density in some areas of the limbic system such as the hypothalamus, hippocampus, septum, and neocortex, as well as in the substantia nigra and the globus pallidus. 5-HT is known to be an important neurotransmitter for the central regulation of metabolism and appetite, where it has an inhibitory effect on feeding behavior, and the 5-HT_{2c} receptor is responsible for mediating the anorectic actions of 5-HT [50]. Accordingly, drugs that activate postsynaptic 5-HT receptors decrease food consumption, while those that inhibit 5-HT transmission increase food intake. Relevant examples of drugs that can decrease appetite are lorcaserin, a 5-HT_{2c} receptor agonist recently marketed as an antiobesity drug, and fenfluramine, 5-HT releaser whose effects include decreasing meal size, rate of eating (via its active metabolite, norfenfluramine), and eating between meals. Conversely, drugs with 5-HT_{2c} antagonist properties such as olanzapine are associated with weight gain [51–53]. Interestingly, there is evidence that the functional status of mesocorticolimbic DA system is under tonic and phasic inhibitory control by 5-HT. 5-HT acts via stimulation of $5HT_{2c}$ receptors, as shown by the effect of $5HT_{2c}$ antagonists, which enhance mesocorticolimbic DA function [14, 15, 54].

2.2.6 The 5-HT_3 Receptor

In the gastrointestinal tract, 5-HT regulates intestinal secretion and motility by activating 5-HT_3 receptors [55, 56]. In the CNS, 5-HT_3 receptors are located postsynaptically to 5-HT neurons (hippocampus and entorhinal cortex) and also in the PNS (spinal cord and medulla). The highest density of 5-HT_3 receptors is found in the area postrema, where the chemoreceptor trigger zone (CTZ) exists. Despite the fact that the most well-recognized role for 5-HT_3 antagonists (e.g., ondansetron) are their antinauseant and antiemetic effects, the therapeutic effect of 5-HT_3 antagonists has largely been attributed to their peripheral effects in the gastrointestinal tract, as peripherally released 5-HT by enterochromaffin cells of the gastrointestinal tract is largely responsible for increased afferent signals to the CTZ, ultimately leading to nausea and vomiting.

2.2.7 5-HT_{1d} Receptors

5-HT_{1d} receptors are found in high density in the substantia nigra, globus pallidus, and cranial blood vessels; they are involved in migraine pathobiology and may be involved in diseases of the basal ganglia [10, 57]. 5-HT_{1d} receptors are located presynaptically on 5-HT neurons where they modulate the release of 5-HT; they are also located postsynaptically, where they may affect the release of ACh and DA in the hippocampus and prefrontal cortex, respectively. The triptan family of drugs (e.g., sumatriptan, rizatriptan) has a well-established place for the treatment of migraine headaches and is believed to exert their therapeutic effects via cranial blood vessel constriction and/or inhibition of neurogenic inflammation in the dura mater [58, 59].

2.2.8 Catecholamines

Catecholamines belong to a larger group of transmitters known as monoamines. In the brain, dopamine, norepinephrine, and epinephrine are the predominant catecholamines.

Dopaminergic nuclei are found primarily in the midbrain, and groups A8 to A10 are of most relevance to contemporary neuropsychopharmacology [60]. Specifically, the A9 nucleus projects to the dorsal caudate putamen, comprising the nigrostriatal system; the A8 and A10 nuclei project to limbic and frontal cortical areas and comprise the mesolimbic and the mesocortical pathways; in addition, an intermediate projection system of interest is the tuberoinfundibular pathway which projects from hypothalamic nuclei to the median eminence of the hypothalamus; DA is released from axons of this pathway into the hypothalamic-hypophyseal portal system and is subsequently transported to the anterior pituitary gland. The nuclei groups A8 to A10 make up long projection systems and link the substantia nigra (A9) and the ventral tegmental areas (A8, A10) with the neostriatum (caudate putamen), limbic cortex (medial prefrontal, cingulated, and entorhinal areas), and additional limbic structures (nucleus accumbens, amygdaloid complex, olfactory tubercle, and piriform cortex).

With regard to noradrenergic (NA) nuclei, the locus coeruleus (LC, A6, and A4) is the most important, projecting from the midbrain widely across the brain to the cortex, limbic regions, and hindbrain. The LC-NA system plays a key role regulating energy levels, reactivity, attention, executive function, arousal, and vigilance; NA stimulation serves to enhance the signal-to-noise ratio in its target areas [61, 62].

2.2.8.1 Dopamine

In the 1950s, dopamine was identified as a potential neurotransmitter by Arvid Carlsson, which led to the dopamine hypothesis of schizophrenia [63]. Soon thereafter, the role of DA as a key neurotransmitter involved in movement, learning, pleasure, and mood became evident. There are five different dopamine receptors, D1-like (D1, D5) and D2-like (D2, D3, D4), and drugs acting at the D2 receptor have been available to treat psychotic symptoms since the 1950s. D2-R antagonists and one partial agonist (aripiprazole) are effective against psychotic and manic symptoms by virtue of their ability to antagonize the D2 receptor thereby functionally lowering the relatively high levels of DA associated with psychotic and/or manic states. D2-R antagonism in the nigrostriatal, tuberoinfundibular, and frontal cortical areas also explain the well-known side effects of DA antagonists, namely, extrapyramidal side effects, hyperprolactinemia, and cognitive impairment [47]. In addition, various sources of evidence support a role for decreased dopaminergic neurotransmission in the neuropathophysiology of depression, including the efficacy of drugs that directly act on the dopaminergic neurons or receptors [64].

Psychomotor stimulants such as amphetamines produce increased activity, euphoria, talkativeness, and a general sense of well-being. The dopamine transporter (DAT), SERT, and norepinephrine transporters (NET) represent important targets for these drugs. For example, amphetamines increase synaptic DA by blocking its uptake (as it is a substrate for the DAT) and reverse the DAT to release DA into the synapse via exchange effusion, while additional mechanisms may also contribute to its effects [65]. These drugs have an established place in the treatment of narcolepsy and attention deficit hyperactivity disorder.

2.2.8.2 NE Receptors and Drugs

Various adrenergic receptors in the CNS may be manipulated pharmacologically. Perhaps one of the earliest examples of relevance is the tricyclic antidepressants (TCAs), which, after repeated treatment, lead to a downregulation of postsynaptic beta-adrenergic receptors and presynaptic alpha-2 receptors. These effects are thought to mediate the antidepressant effect of TCAs by ultimately increasing NE neurotransmission. Specifically, antagonism of alpha-2 adrenergic autoreceptors increases NE release, and preliminary preclinical and clinical data support such an effect [17, 62, 66]. As a clinically relevant example, in a 6-week study comparing the combination of mirtazapine and paroxetine versus either agent alone, Blier et al.

noted that the combination resulted in greater improvement in depressive symptoms as measured by the MADRS ($p < 0.05$) and a faster response with combined treatment at day 7 of therapy [67, 68]. Other contemporary antidepressants such as the serotonin-norepinephrine reuptake inhibitors (SNRIs) are likewise presumed to exert their therapeutic effects in part by inhibiting reuptake of 5-HT and NE, ultimately leading to therapeutic effects similar to the combined use of SSRIs and TCAs [62, 66]. Additionally, various psychiatric states characterized by SNS hyperactivity and symptoms such as aggression may be treated with clonidine, a centrally acting alpha-2 agonist which decreases LC firing and NE release and overall CNS sympathetic output by acting at the presynaptic autoreceptor. Alpha-1-adrenergic receptor pharmacological manipulation also yields clinically important effects. For example, antagonism of central alpha-1 receptors by drugs such as prazosin or by antipsychotic drugs with alpha-1 antagonist properties will lead to sedation due to the role of NE in sleep neurobiology and the presence of these receptors in the medial preoptic area [69, 70]. Alpha-1 adrenergic receptors are also central to the signs and symptoms of posttraumatic stress disorder, and it is for these reasons that alpha-1 antagonists such as prazosin are used in the treatment of this disorder [71].

2.2.9 GABA Receptors

Gamma aminobutyric acid (GABA) is the major rapid acting inhibitory neurotransmitter in the brain. Accordingly, GABA receptors have been identified in all regions of the brain, and many neuropsychiatric disorders are associated with altered GABA function including anxiety, sleep disorders, seizure disorders, drug dependence, and schizophrenia [72–74]. Two receptor subtypes have been identified, $GABA_a$ and $GABA_b$. The $GABA_a$ receptors (chloride, ligand-gated ion channels) currently serve as the target for many CNS active drugs such as benzodiazepine receptor agonists (BZRAs), anesthetics, and others, and facilitate Cl ion influx, leading to neuronal inhibition secondary to neuronal hyperpolarization. $GABA_a$ receptors are located on neuronal terminals, where their activation inhibits neurotransmitter release, be it excitatory or inhibitory.

Considering the inhibitory nature of GABA, it is not surprising that drugs with pro-GABA properties have been widely exploited in clinical practice. The most common drugs include BZRAs, used for insomnia, anxiety, and seizures, general anesthetics, and muscle relaxants. By enhancing inhibitory neurotransmission, BZRAs cause an overall CNS depressing effect, leading to anxiolysis, and sedative/hypnotic effects. Specifically, BZRAs bind to allosteric sites distinct from the GABA-binding site on the $GABA_a$ receptor complex, as do barbiturates, alcohol, and anesthetics such as propofol; the therapeutic actions of BZRAs are attributable to an increase in the frequency of channel opening in response to endogenous GABA, whereas barbiturates may increase the duration of channel opening; these observations demonstrate that the overall end result of enhancing chloride ion flux may be achieved by overlapping, yet slightly different means [75–77]. It should be noted that unlike benzodiazepines, compounds such as zolpidem and zopiclone, which also exert their effects at the alpha-1 subunit of $GABA_a$ receptors are not effective as anticonvulsants or muscle relaxants [78]. These differences are not surprising, as preclinical models demonstrate that the alpha-1 subunit of the $GABA_a$ receptor plays a major role in the sedative, amnestic effects, part of the anticonvulsant effects, and little of the anxiolytic effects, while the alpha-2 subtype mediates anxiolytic effects and muscle relaxant effects [72].

As previously noted, $GABA_a$ receptor activation at neuronal terminals may inhibit neurotransmitter release, be it excitatory or inhibitory. These observations are congruent with recent findings suggesting a role for $GABA_a$ receptors in wakefulness [79, 80]. Indeed, mounting preclinical data have demonstrated that increasing GABA levels in the pontine reticular nucleus (PnO), oral part, increase wakefulness, though the mechanisms by which this occurs remain unclear [74]. These novel findings suggest that GABA mimetic drugs have site-specific and opposite actions on sleep and wakefulness depending on their site of action in the brain, representing a novel approach to the treatment of disorders characterized by excessive somnolence.

2.2.10 Glutamate

In contrast to GABA, glutamate is the major excitatory neurotransmitter in the CNS, being the principal fast CNS excitatory transmitter, and it is involved in normal synaptic transmission [81, 82]. There are ionotropic (AMPA, Kainate, and NMDA) and metabotropic glutamate receptors (Groups 1–3) that mediate the effects of glutamate [83, 84]. NMDA receptors (NMDARs) are essential for regulating use-dependent synaptic remodeling, long-term changes in synaptic strength, and synaptogenesis. These receptors play an important role in learning and memory, via long-term potentiation (in hippocampus) and long-term depression [85]. In addition, NMDARs are expressed in certain inhibitory GABA interneurons, whose activation aids in improving the signal-to-noise ratio in cortical circuits such as the prefrontal cortex [86].

Excessive excitotoxicity has been attributed to excessive extrasynaptic NDMAR activation leading to neuronal death in diseases such as Alzheimer's disease (AD), multiple sclerosis, and schizophrenia. Currently available NMDA antagonist drugs include memantine and amantadine and riluzole, the latter being both an NMDA antagonist and a kainate type receptor antagonist [87, 88]. Memantine is an open-channel (noncompetitive), moderate-affinity NMDAR antagonist which binds at, or near, the magnesium-binding site with strong voltage dependency and rapid blocking-unblocking kinetics [89]. This drug demonstrates a preferential blockade of excessive NMDAR activity while sparing normal synaptic function and is used in moderate to severe AD [82]. Memantine's putative mechanism of action in AD includes a possible reduction in glutamate-related excitotoxicity which is more apparent, yet still not fully delineated in more advanced stages of AD [89–91]. The drug may also have direct, yet still poorly defined effects on cognition and neuropsychiatric behaviors associated with dementia, though further investigation is necessary [92, 93].

2.2.11 Histamine

Histamine is a signaling molecule perhaps best known for its role in gastric acid secretion and in immune-based responses such as inflammation and allergies [3, 4]. In the CNS, histaminergic neurons are exclusively found in the tuberomammillary (TM) nucleus of the posterior hypothalamus and innervate widely across the brain to hypothalamic nuclei, the medial septum, the ventral tegmental area, and nucleus of the diagonal band and also in moderate density in the substantia nigra, amygdala, striatum, and cerebral cortex [94–96]. Histaminergic neurons display state-dependent spontaneous activity (i.e., pacemaker-like), have their highest firing rates during periods of wakefulness or attention, and are absent during sleep. It is currently known that three histamine receptors are expressed in the brain, namely, H_1 and H_2 (excitatory) and H_3, which is an inhibitory autoreceptor [97]. The latter is of particular importance to ongoing investigations of various CNS diseases (discussed later in this chapter under Sect. 2.2.11).

In the CNS, histamine largely acts in a manner that is consistent with its ability to increase neuronal activity [98]. As such, it is not surprising that histamine plays a key role in sleep disorders such as insomnia. Indeed, TM cells only fire during waking and are inhibited by GABA-ergic neurons in the preoptic area; the evolving role of selective, brain-penetrating H_1 antagonists such as ultra low-dose (3–6 mg) doxepin and orexin agonists and antagonists is a relevant example of drugs that specifically target the effects of histamine for treatment of sleep/wake disorders [99, 100]. In addition to its role in sleep, histamine also affects appetite by suppressing food intake (likely mediated by the ventromedial hypothalamus and also by the effects of leptin and orexin on histamine), while antagonism of the H_1 receptor leads to increases in appetite and weight gain [101, 102] (Table 2.1).

2.2.12 Acetylcholine and the Cholinergic System

Acetylcholine is a neurotransmitter with various effects in the CNS and PNS and acts as part of the autonomic nervous system [103, 104]. Within the CNS, cholinergic neurons are widely distributed from the nucleus basalis of Meynert to all parts of the neocortex and from the pedunculopontine tegmental nucleus and the dorsolateral tegmental nucleus to many areas in the CNS, the most salient of which is the thalamus; these pathways are central to sleep and cortical arousal [69, 70, 105, 106]. There is also a group of cholinergic neurons in the striatum, namely, interneurons which are of relevance in the overall functioning of the extrapyramidal system. Two

Table 2.1 Selected receptors and representative agonists and antagonists

Receptor type	Agonists	Antagonists
Serotonergic		
5-HT_{1a}	Buspirone[a], vortioxetine[b]	Pindolol[c]
5-HT_{1d}	Sumatriptan	
5-HT_{2a}	Lorcaserin	Cyproheptadine, risperidone[d], pimavanserin[e]
5-HT_{2c}	Ergotamine (also 5-HT_{2a} agonist)	Olanzapine[d], fluoxetine[d]
5-HT_{3}		Ondansetron
Catecholaminergic		
DA_2	Bromocriptine	Haloperidol[d], risperidone[d]
Alpha-2	Clonidine, tizanidine, guanfacine	Yohimbine, mirtazapine[d]
Alpha-1	Phenylephrine, midodrine	Prazosin, alfuzosin, tamsulosin
GABA		
$GABA_a$	Benzodiazepine receptor agonists (various)	Flumazenil, penicillin
Glutamate		
NMDA		Memantine, ketamine
Histamine		
Hm_1		Loratadine, doxepin (H_1 selective at doses <6 mg)
Hm_2		Ranitidine
Cholinergic		
mAChRs		
Peripheral neuronal nAChRs	Ach, nicotine	Mecamylamine
Peripheral skeletal muscle nAChRs	Ach, nicotine, succinylcholine	D-tubocurarine, vecuronium
Opioid		
Mu	Morphine	Naltrexone
Kappa	Butorphanol	Naltrexone

[a]Partial agonist
[b]Partial agonist and has various other activities including serotonin reuptake inhibition
[c]Partial agonist and beta-adrenergic antagonist
[d]Antagonist and also has other activities
[e]Inverse agonist

types of cholinergic receptors exist, namely, muscarinic (mAChR) and nicotinic (nAChR) cholinergic receptors [107].

Neuronal nAChRs represent a family of receptors with 11 neuronal subunits in mammals. In the brain, nAChR subunit expression differs according to regions. The cortex, thalamus, and dopamine neurons are endowed with abundant alpha-4 and beta-2 subunits, whereas in the hippocampus the alpha-7 subunit is highly expressed. It is likely that neuronal nAChRs exert a modulatory influence on synaptic transmission that is subtle compared to the fast synaptic transmission modulated by neuromuscular junctions and autonomic ganglia receptors in the periphery. Alpha-7 nAChRs contribute to synaptic plasticity, including long-term potentiation (i.e., learning and memory) and are associated with glutamate terminals and GABA neurons.

Nicotine promotes dopamine release by activating somatodendritic and presynaptic alpha-4-beta-2* nAChRs, and these effects are key to its reinforcement properties, which ultimately lead to dependence. This occurs within the ventral tegmental area (VTA), where nicotine also exerts its effects via GABA neurons and glutamate nerve terminals to collectively increase DA release. The VTA DA neurons project to the cortical and limbic target regions, and the nucleus accumbens is of particular relevance because it is central to reinforcement properties of drugs of abuse. Additionally, endogenous opioid and endocannabinoid transmission in reward circuitry play important roles in the behavioral effects of nicotine. Relatedly, varenicline is a partial agonist at alpha4beta2* nAChRs and is proposed to mimic the effects of nicotine while preventing nicotine from other exogenous sources (i.e., cigarettes, smokeless tobacco, etc.) to bind to the receptor [108].

Nicotinic cholinergic receptors are also of great importance to anesthesia. Indeed, neuromuscular blockade leading to muscle relaxation has been possible for about 100 years via reversible antagonism of nACHRs and has been a key adjunct to surgical anesthesia. Tubocurarine, which is part of the arrow poison used by South American Indians, represents a naturally occurring nACHR antagonist. Contemporary neuromuscular antagonists (e.g., vecuronium, pancuronium, atracurium) were developed to allow for rapid reversal of neuromuscular blockade and to produce a non-depolarizing blockade of muscle nACHRs.

Muscarinic cholinergic receptors are widely distributed in the CNS, PNS and parasympathetically innervated cardiac and gastrointestinal smooth muscle. In the CNS, the M_1 mACHR is the predominant form of mACHRs and is found postsynaptically in the cortex, hippocampus, striatum, and thalamus. Acetylcholinesterase inhibitors have been in use for over 20 years for the symptomatic treatment of Alzheimer's disease and lead to mACHR activation by increasing the availability of ACh via inhibiting its breakdown. Conversely, in Parkinson's disease, antimuscarinic drugs (e.g., benztropine) are used to restore the dopaminergic-cholinergic imbalance that results from a relative striatal excess of ACh secondary to dopaminergic neuronal loss.

2.2.13 Opioids

Opioid receptors generally mediate neuronal inhibition and include mu-opioid receptors, kappa-opioid receptors and delta-opioid receptors. These receptors are widely and differentially distributed within the CNS and PNS. The opioid system plays a pivotal role in analgesia at the supraspinal, spinal, and peripheral levels [109]. Opioid binding leads to hyperpolarization of the cell membrane secondary to activation of inwardly rectifying potassium channels, resulting in neuronal hyperpolarization.

Morphine is the prototypical relatively selective mu-opioid agonist, while endogenous ligands for this receptor include endorphins, enkephalins, and dynorphins. Analgesia from opioids is mediated largely by their central effects, where activation of the mu receptor by an agonist such as morphine results in presynaptic inhibition of glutamate release. In the periphery and dorsal horn, selective reduction of transmitter release (i.e., glutamate, substance P, CRGP) from nociceptors results from the actions of opioids at mu and delta receptors in the central terminal of A delta and C fibers. Neurons in the periaqueductal gray area and RVM, thalamus, amygdala, and somatosensory cortex are also involved in opioid analgesia. Adverse effects of opioids include respiratory depression, constipation, urinary retention, miosis, nausea, vomiting and urinary retention, drowsiness, euphoria, changes in mood, and cognitive dulling [110].

2.3 Conclusions and Future Directions

This chapter has attempted to summarize key concepts across selected aspects of CNS pharmacodynamics, yet much more could be written about a plethora of new and emerging developments in the field. The aim was to introduce the reader to some of the more well-known (or at least largely agreed upon putative mechanisms) areas of CNS pharmacodynamics, while acknowledging that much remains to be learned and that, in some cases, the literature reveals conflicting findings. With that in mind, it should be noted that common emerging themes exist, including – but not limited to – ongoing clarification of the role of receptor subtypes that may represent viable therapeutic targets for CNS diseases with the potential for decreased toxicity.

Advances have led to development of drugs such as lorcaserin, a 5-HT_{2c} receptor agonist marketed as an antiobesity agent with no appreciable effect on 5-$HT2_b$ receptors which are of central importance to valvular and pulmonary toxicity with fenfluramine [46, 50, 111]. Similarly, pimavanserin, a 5-HT_{2a} inverse agonist was developed for the treatment of Parkinson's disease psychosis, demonstrating that ongoing refinement of therapeutic targets can lead to new approaches for treating this condition that are void of well-known adverse effects associated with antipsychotic drugs. Likewise, the successful development of peripherally selective $alpha_{1a}$ antagonists such as tamsulosin and silodosin for prostatic hypertrophy, and selective antimuscarinic agents such as darifenacin, fesoterodine, and trospium for overactive bladder, also represents improvements in therapy as these drugs provide effective treatment with significantly reduced central and peripheral nervous system adverse events [112, 113]. Nonetheless, despite increasing clarity regarding the role of certain receptors such as the NDMA receptor in normal neural function and in the pathobiology of neurologic or psychiatric diseases, such advances represent only one of the multiple putative mechanisms for these diseases. It is thus becoming increasingly evident that future drug development will need to address this issue vis-a-vis development of drugs designed to be added on to existing pharmacotherapies. A salient example includes ongoing efforts to develop compounds such as alpha-7 and alpha4beta42 nicotinic cholinergic receptors to improve cognition in dementia and schizophrenia when administered as adjunct pharmacotherapy. Further, continuing developments on the mechanisms of cholinergic modulation of cognition suggest that this system is far more complex than previously thought [114, 115].

In addition to the aforementioned, notable developments in drug development include proof-of-concept studies of ketamine as a fast-acting antidepressant, new truly mixed action antidepressant drugs such as vortioxetine, and ongoing testing of triple reuptake inhibitors for depression [116–118]. There is also exciting work in serotonergic receptor pharmacology that suggests that 5-HT receptors such as 5-HT_6 and 5-HT_7 may have potential roles in the treatment of depression and cognition [22]. In addition, the histaminergic system is being investigated to determine additional roles for histamine receptors; these include the H_3 receptor and its potential role in neurodegenerative diseases, cognition, and other conditions as well as the orexins for sleep-wake disorders [97, 100]. Additional areas of promise in neuropsychopharmacology include enhancement of neuroplasticity for mood and anxiety disorders, GABA, and glutamate manipulation in schizophrenia. In conclusion, the pharmacodynamics of centrally acting agents represents a ripe and exciting area for continued research and drug development.

References

1. Tamminga CA (2002) Partial dopamine agonists in the treatment of psychosis. J Neural Transm 109(3):411–420
2. Grunder G, Kungel M, Ebrecht M, Gorocs T, Modell S (2006) Aripiprazole: pharmacodynamics of a dopamine partial agonist for the treatment of schizophrenia. Pharmacopsychiatry 39(Suppl 1):S21–S25
3. Jones BL, Kearns GL (2011) Histamine: new thoughts about a familiar mediator. Clin Pharmacol Ther 89(2):189–197
4. Simons FE (2004) Advances in H1-antihistamines. N Engl J Med 351(21):2203–2217
5. Schmith VD, Foss JF (2008) Effects of inflammation on pharmacokinetics/pharmacodynamics: increasing recognition of its contribution to variability in response. Clin Pharmacol Ther 83(6):809–811
6. Wilkinson GR (2005) Drug metabolism and variability among patients in drug response. N Engl J Med 352(21):2211–2221
7. Benarroch EE (2012) Blood-brain barrier: recent developments and clinical correlations. Neurology 78(16):1268–1276
8. Zeevi N, Pachter J, McCullough LD, Wolfson L, Kuchel GA (2010) The blood-brain barrier: geriatric relevance of a critical brain-body interface. J Am Geriatr Soc 58(9):1749–1757
9. Jacobs BL, Azmitia EC (1992) Structure and function of the brain serotonin system. Physiol Rev 72(1):165–229
10. Adell A, Celada P, Abellan MT, Artigas F (2002) Origin and functional role of the extracellular serotonin in the midbrain raphe nuclei. Brain Res Brain Res Rev 39(2–3):154–180
11. Barnes NM, Sharp T (1999) A review of central 5-HT receptors and their function. Neuropharmacology 38(8):1083–1152

12. Oleskevich S, Descarries L (1990) Quantified distribution of the serotonin innervation in adult rat hippocampus. Neuroscience 34(1):19–33
13. Smythies J (2005) Section V, serotonin system. Int Rev Neurobiol 64:217–268
14. Di Matteo V, Cacchio M, Di Giulio C, Esposito E (2002) Role of serotonin (2C) receptors in the control of brain dopaminergic function. Pharmacol Biochem Behav 71(4):727–734
15. Navailles S, De Deurwaerdere P (2011) Presynaptic control of serotonin on striatal dopamine function. Psychopharmacology (Berl) 213(2–3):213–242
16. Artigas F (2013) Serotonin receptors involved in antidepressant effects. Pharmacol Ther 137(1):119–131
17. Millan MJ (2006) Multi-target strategies for the improved treatment of depressive states: conceptual foundations and neuronal substrates, drug discovery and therapeutic application. Pharmacol Ther 110(2):135–370
18. Celada P, Puig M, Amargos-Bosch M, Adell A, Artigas F (2004) The therapeutic role of 5-HT1A and 5-HT2A receptors in depression. J Psychiatry Neurosci 29(4):252–265
19. Morrissette DA, Stahl SM (2014) Modulating the serotonin system in the treatment of major depressive disorder. CNS Spectr 19(Suppl 1):57–67; Quiz 54–57, 68
20. Yamada M, Yasuhara H (2004) Clinical pharmacology of MAO inhibitors: safety and future. Neurotoxicology 25(1–2):215–221
21. Carr GV, Lucki I (2011) The role of serotonin receptor subtypes in treating depression: a review of animal studies. Psychopharmacology (Berl) 213(2–3):265–287
22. Ramirez MJ, Lai MK, Tordera RM, Francis PT (2014) Serotonergic therapies for cognitive symptoms in Alzheimer's disease: rationale and current status. Drugs 74(7):729–736
23. Beaudet A, Descarries L (1978) The monoamine innervation of rat cerebral cortex: synaptic and nonsynaptic axon terminals. Neuroscience 3(10):851–860
24. Blier P, de Montigny C (1987) Modification of 5-HT neuron properties by sustained administration of the 5-HT1A agonist gepirone: electrophysiological studies in the rat brain. Synapse 1(5):470–480
25. Innis RB, Aghajanian GK (1987) Pertussis toxin blocks autoreceptor-mediated inhibition of dopaminergic neurons in rat substantia nigra. Brain Res 411(1):139–143
26. Sprouse JS, Aghajanian GK (1987) Electrophysiological responses of serotoninergic dorsal raphe neurons to 5-HT1A and 5-HT1B agonists. Synapse 1(1):3–9
27. Neff CD, Abkevich V, Packer JC et al (2009) Evidence for HTR1A and LHPP as interacting genetic risk factors in major depression. Mol Psychiatry 14(6):621–630
28. Stockmeier CA, Shapiro LA, Dilley GE, Kolli TN, Friedman L, Rajkowska G (1998) Increase in serotonin-1A autoreceptors in the midbrain of suicide victims with major depression-postmortem evidence for decreased serotonin activity. J Neurosci 18(18):7394–7401
29. Lemonde S, Turecki G, Bakish D et al (2003) Impaired repression at a 5-hydroxytryptamine 1A receptor gene polymorphism associated with major depression and suicide. J Neurosci 23(25):8788–8799
30. Blier P, de Montigny C (1998) Possible serotonergic mechanisms underlying the antidepressant and anti-obsessive-compulsive disorder responses. Biol Psychiatry 44(5):313–323
31. Blier P, Pineyro G, el Mansari M, Bergeron R, de Montigny C (1998) Role of somatodendritic 5-HT autoreceptors in modulating 5-HT neurotransmission. Ann N Y Acad Sci 861:204–216
32. Haddjeri N, Blier P, de Montigny C (1998) Long-term antidepressant treatments result in a tonic activation of forebrain 5-HT1A receptors. J Neurosci 18(23):10150–10156
33. Pineyro G, Blier P, Dennis T, de Montigny C (1994) Desensitization of the neuronal 5-HT carrier following its long-term blockade. J Neurosci 14(5 Pt 2):3036–3047
34. Deardorff WJ, Grossberg GT (2014) A review of the clinical efficacy, safety and tolerability of the antidepressants vilazodone, levomilnacipran and vortioxetine. Expert Opin Pharmacother 15(17):2525–2542
35. Garnock-Jones KP (2014) Vortioxetine: a review of its use in major depressive disorder. CNS Drugs 28(9):855–874

36. de Almeida J, Mengod G (2008) Serotonin 1A receptors in human and monkey prefrontal cortex are mainly expressed in pyramidal neurons and in a GABAergic interneuron subpopulation: implications for schizophrenia and its treatment. J Neurochem 107(2):488–496
37. Diaz-Mataix L, Scorza MC, Bortolozzi A, Toth M, Celada P, Artigas F (2005) Involvement of 5-HT1A receptors in prefrontal cortex in the modulation of dopaminergic activity: role in atypical antipsychotic action. J Neurosci 25(47):10831–10843
38. Hajos-Korcsok E, Sharp T (1996) 8-OH-DPAT-induced release of hippocampal noradrenaline in vivo: evidence for a role of both 5-HT1A and dopamine D1 receptors. Eur J Pharmacol 314(3):285–291
39. Cryan JF, Valentino RJ, Lucki I (2005) Assessing substrates underlying the behavioral effects of antidepressants using the modified rat forced swimming test. Neurosci Biobehav Rev 29(4–5):547–569
40. Martin P, Beninger RJ, Hamon M, Puech AJ (1990) Antidepressant-like action of 8-OH-DPAT, a 5-HT1A agonist, in the learned helplessness paradigm: evidence for a postsynaptic mechanism. Behav Brain Res 38(2):135–144
41. Celada P, Bortolozzi A, Artigas F (2013) Serotonin 5-HT1A receptors as targets for agents to treat psychiatric disorders: rationale and current status of research. CNS Drugs 27(9):703–716
42. Ballanger B, Strafella AP, van Eimeren T et al (2010) Serotonin 2A receptors and visual hallucinations in Parkinson disease. Arch Neurol 67(4):416–421
43. Huot P, Johnston TH, Darr T et al (2010) Increased 5-HT2A receptors in the temporal cortex of Parkinsonian patients with visual hallucinations. Mov Disord 25(10):1399–1408
44. Ibarretxe-Bilbao N, Junque C, Marti MJ, Tolosa E (2011) Cerebral basis of visual hallucinations in Parkinson's disease: structural and functional MRI studies. J Neurol Sci 310(1–2):79–81
45. Cummings J, Isaacson S, Mills R et al (2014) Pimavanserin for patients with Parkinson's disease psychosis: a randomised, placebo-controlled phase 3 trial. Lancet 383(9916):533–540
46. Meltzer HY, Mills R, Revell S et al (2010) Pimavanserin, a serotonin(2A) receptor inverse agonist, for the treatment of Parkinson's disease psychosis. Neuropsychopharmacology 35(4):881–892
47. Pierre JM (2005) Extrapyramidal symptoms with atypical antipsychotics: incidence, prevention and management. Drug Saf 28(3):191–208
48. Gillman PK (2011) CNS toxicity involving methylene blue: the exemplar for understanding and predicting drug interactions that precipitate serotonin toxicity. J Psychopharmacol 25(3):429–436
49. Isbister GK, Buckley NA (2005) The pathophysiology of serotonin toxicity in animals and humans: implications for diagnosis and treatment. Clin Neuropharmacol 28(5):205–214
50. Meltzer HY, Roth BL (2013) Lorcaserin and pimavanserin: emerging selectivity of serotonin receptor subtype-targeted drugs. J Clin Invest 123(12):4986–4991
51. Zhang JY, Kowal DM, Nawoschik SP, Lou Z, Dunlop J (2006) Distinct functional profiles of aripiprazole and olanzapine at RNA edited human 5-HT2C receptor isoforms. Biochem Pharmacol 71(4):521–529
52. Gunes A, Melkersson KI, Scordo MG, Dahl ML (2009) Association between HTR2C and HTR2A polymorphisms and metabolic abnormalities in patients treated with olanzapine or clozapine. J Clin Psychopharmacol 29(1):65–68
53. Roerig JL, Steffen KJ, Mitchell JE (2011) Atypical antipsychotic-induced weight gain: insights into mechanisms of action. CNS Drugs 25(12):1035–1059
54. Alex KD, Pehek EA (2007) Pharmacologic mechanisms of serotonergic regulation of dopamine neurotransmission. Pharmacol Ther 113(2):296–320
55. Aapro M (2005) 5-HT(3)-receptor antagonists in the management of nausea and vomiting in cancer and cancer treatment. Oncology 69(2):97–109

56. Machu TK (2011) Therapeutics of 5-HT3 receptor antagonists: current uses and future directions. Pharmacol Ther 130(3):338–347
57. Roth BL, Willins DL, Kristiansen K, Kroeze WK (1998) 5-Hydroxytryptamine2-family receptors (5-hydroxytryptamine2A, 5-hydroxytryptamine2B, 5-hydroxytryptamine2C): where structure meets function. Pharmacol Ther 79(3):231–257
58. Tfelt-Hansen P, De Vries P, Saxena PR (2000) Triptans in migraine: a comparative review of pharmacology, pharmacokinetics and efficacy. Drugs 60(6):1259–1287
59. Loder E (2010) Triptan therapy in migraine. N Engl J Med 363(1):63–70
60. Williams SM, Goldman-Rakic PS (1998) Widespread origin of the primate mesofrontal dopamine system. Cereb Cortex 8(4):321–345
61. El Mansari M, Guiard BP, Chernoloz O, Ghanbari R, Katz N, Blier P (2010) Relevance of norepinephrine-dopamine interactions in the treatment of major depressive disorder. CNS Neurosci Ther 16(3):e1–e17
62. Hamon M, Blier P (2013) Monoamine neurocircuitry in depression and strategies for new treatments. Prog Neuropsychopharmacol Biol Psychiatry 45:54–63
63. Iversen SD, Iversen LL (2007) Dopamine: 50 years in perspective. Trends Neurosci 30(5):188–193
64. Dunlop BW, Nemeroff CB (2007) The role of dopamine in the pathophysiology of depression. Arch Gen Psychiatry 64(3):327–337
65. Sulzer D, Sonders MS, Poulsen NW, Galli A (2005) Mechanisms of neurotransmitter release by amphetamines: a review. Prog Neurobiol 75(6):406–433
66. Gillman PK (2007) Tricyclic antidepressant pharmacology and therapeutic drug interactions updated. Br J Pharmacol 151(6):737–748
67. Blier P, Gobbi G, Turcotte JE et al (2009) Mirtazapine and paroxetine in major depression: a comparison of monotherapy versus their combination from treatment initiation. Eur Neuropsychopharmacol 19(7):457–465
68. Blier P, Ward HE, Tremblay P, Laberge L, Hebert C, Bergeron R (2010) Combination of antidepressant medications from treatment initiation for major depressive disorder: a double-blind randomized study. Am J Psychiatry 167(3):281–288
69. Watson CJ, Baghdoyan HA, Lydic R (2010) Neuropharmacology of sleep and wakefulness. Sleep Med Clin 5(4):513–528
70. Watson CJ, Baghdoyan HA, Lydic R (2012) Neuropharmacology of sleep and wakefulness: 2012 update. Sleep Med Clin 7(3):469–486
71. Miller LJ (2008) Prazosin for the treatment of posttraumatic stress disorder sleep disturbances. Pharmacotherapy 28(5):656–666
72. Rudolph U, Knoflach F (2011) Beyond classical benzodiazepines: novel therapeutic potential of GABAA receptor subtypes. Nat Rev Drug Discov 10(9):685–697
73. Tyson JA, Anderson SA (2014) GABAergic interneuron transplants to study development and treat disease. Trends Neurosci 37(3):169–177
74. Olsen RW, Sieghart W (2009) GABA A receptors: subtypes provide diversity of function and pharmacology. Neuropharmacology 56(1):141–148
75. Whiting PJ (2003) The GABAA receptor gene family: new opportunities for drug development. Curr Opin Drug Discov Devel 6(5):648–657
76. Blednov YA, Jung S, Alva H et al (2003) Deletion of the alpha1 or beta2 subunit of GABAA receptors reduces actions of alcohol and other drugs. J Pharmacol Exp Ther 304(1):30–36
77. Reynolds DS, Rosahl TW, Cirone J et al (2003) Sedation and anesthesia mediated by distinct GABA(A) receptor isoforms. J Neurosci 23(24):8608–8617
78. Morin AK, Jarvis CI, Lynch AM (2007) Therapeutic options for sleep-maintenance and sleep-onset insomnia. Pharmacotherapy 27(1):89–110
79. Brevig HN, Watson CJ, Lydic R, Baghdoyan HA (2010) Hypocretin and GABA interact in the pontine reticular formation to increase wakefulness. Sleep 33(10):1285–1293
80. Watson CJ, Soto-Calderon H, Lydic R, Baghdoyan HA (2008) Pontine reticular formation (PnO) administration of hypocretin-1 increases PnO GABA levels and wakefulness. Sleep 31(4):453–464

81. Bleich S, Romer K, Wiltfang J, Kornhuber J (2003) Glutamate and the glutamate receptor system: a target for drug action. Int J Geriatr Psychiatry 18(Suppl 1):S33–S40
82. Chen HS, Lipton SA (2006) The chemical biology of clinically tolerated NMDA receptor antagonists. J Neurochem 97(6):1611–1626
83. Benarroch EE (2011) NMDA receptors: recent insights and clinical correlations. Neurology 76(20):1750–1757
84. Zorumski CF, Izumi Y (2012) NMDA receptors and metaplasticity: mechanisms and possible roles in neuropsychiatric disorders. Neurosci Biobehav Rev 36(3):989–1000
85. Malenka RC, Bear MF (2004) LTP and LTD: an embarrassment of riches. Neuron 44(1):5–21
86. Wang H, Stradtman GG 3rd, Wang XJ, Gao WJ (2008) A specialized NMDA receptor function in layer 5 recurrent microcircuitry of the adult rat prefrontal cortex. Proc Natl Acad Sci U S A 105(43):16791–16796
87. Zarate CA, Manji HK (2008) Riluzole in psychiatry: a systematic review of the literature. Expert Opin Drug Metab Toxicol 4(9):1223–1234
88. Mathew SJ, Manji HK, Charney DS (2008) Novel drugs and therapeutic targets for severe mood disorders. Neuropsychopharmacology 33(9):2080–2092
89. McKeage K (2009) Memantine: a review of its use in moderate to severe Alzheimer's disease. CNS Drugs 23(10):881–897
90. Chohan MO, Iqbal K (2006) From tau to toxicity: emerging roles of NMDA receptor in Alzheimer's disease. J Alzheimers Dis 10(1):81–87
91. Francis PT, Parsons CG, Jones RW (2012) Rationale for combining glutamatergic and cholinergic approaches in the symptomatic treatment of Alzheimer's disease. Expert Rev Neurother 12(11):1351–1365
92. Fox C, Crugel M, Maidment I et al (2012) Efficacy of memantine for agitation in Alzheimer's dementia: a randomised double-blind placebo controlled trial. PLoS One 7(5):e35185
93. Maidment ID, Fox CG, Boustani M, Rodriguez J, Brown RC, Katona CL (2008) Efficacy of memantine on behavioral and psychological symptoms related to dementia: a systematic meta-analysis. Ann Pharmacother 42(1):32–38
94. Baronio D, Gonchoroski T, Castro K, Zanatta G, Gottfried C, Riesgo R (2014) Histaminergic system in brain disorders: lessons from the translational approach and future perspectives. Ann Gen Psychiatry 13(1):34. doi:10.1186/s12991-014-0034-y, eCollection 2014
95. Shan L, Bao AM, Swaab DF (2015) The human histaminergic system in neuropsychiatric disorders. Trends Neurosci 38(3):167–177
96. Tashiro M, Mochizuki H, Iwabuchi K et al (2002) Roles of histamine in regulation of arousal and cognition: functional neuroimaging of histamine H1 receptors in human brain. Life Sci 72(4–5):409–414
97. Ellenbroek BA, Ghiabi B (2014) The other side of the histamine H3 receptor. Trends Neurosci 37(4):191–199
98. Haas HL, Sergeeva OA, Selbach O (2008) Histamine in the nervous system. Physiol Rev 88(3):1183–1241
99. Rojas-Fernandez CH, Chen Y (2014) Use of ultra-low-dose (</=6 mg) doxepin for treatment of insomnia in older people. Can Pharm J (Ott) 147(5):281–289
100. Mieda M, Sakurai T (2013) Orexin (hypocretin) receptor agonists and antagonists for treatment of sleep disorders. Rationale for development and current status. CNS Drugs 27(2):83–90
101. He M, Deng C, Huang XF (2013) The role of hypothalamic H1 receptor antagonism in antipsychotic-induced weight gain. CNS Drugs 27(6):423–434
102. Deng C, Weston-Green K, Huang XF (2010) The role of histaminergic H1 and H3 receptors in food intake: a mechanism for atypical antipsychotic-induced weight gain? Prog Neuropsychopharmacol Biol Psychiatry 34(1):1–4
103. Cuello AC, Sofroniew MV (1984) The anatomy of the CNS cholinergic neurons. Trends Neurosci 7(3):74–78
104. Wenk GL (1997) The nucleus basalis magnocellularis cholinergic system: one hundred years of progress. Neurobiol Learn Mem 67(2):85–95

105. Benarroch EE (2012) Effects of acetylcholine in the striatum. Recent insights and therapeutic implications. Neurology 79(3):274–281
106. Benarroch EE (2013) Pedunculopontine nucleus: functional organization and clinical implications. Neurology 80(12):1148–1155
107. Hurst R, Rollema H, Bertrand D (2013) Nicotinic acetylcholine receptors: from basic science to therapeutics. Pharmacol Ther 137(1):22–54
108. Jimenez-Ruiz C, Berlin I, Hering T (2009) Varenicline: a novel pharmacotherapy for smoking cessation. Drugs 69(10):1319–1338
109. Benarroch EE (2012) Endogenous opioid systems: current concepts and clinical correlations. Neurology 79(8):807–814
110. Lutz PE, Kieffer BL (2013) Opioid receptors: distinct roles in mood disorders. Trends Neurosci 36(3):195–206
111. Hutcheson JD, Setola V, Roth BL, Merryman WD (2011) Serotonin receptors and heart valve disease – it was meant 2B. Pharmacol Ther 132(2):146–157
112. DuBeau CE (2009) Therapeutic/pharmacologic approaches to urinary incontinence in older adults. Clin Pharmacol Ther 85(1):98–102
113. Wagg AS (2012) Antimuscarinic treatment in overactive bladder: special considerations in elderly patients. Drugs Aging 29(7):539–548
114. Hasselmo ME, Sarter M (2011) Modes and models of forebrain cholinergic neuromodulation of cognition. Neuropsychopharmacology 36(1):52–73
115. Sarter M, Paolone G (2011) Deficits in attentional control: cholinergic mechanisms and circuitry-based treatment approaches. Behav Neurosci 125(6):825–835
116. Pizzagalli DA (2011) Frontocingulate dysfunction in depression: toward biomarkers of treatment response. Neuropsychopharmacology 36(1):183–206
117. Carlson PJ, Diazgranados N, Nugent AC et al (2013) Neural correlates of rapid antidepressant response to ketamine in treatment-resistant unipolar depression: a preliminary positron emission tomography study. Biol Psychiatry 73(12):1213–1221
118. Nugent AC, Diazgranados N, Carlson PJ et al (2014) Neural correlates of rapid antidepressant response to ketamine in bipolar disorder. Bipolar Disord 16(2):119–128

Chapter 3
Positron Emission Tomography (PET) Use in Pharmacology

Jonathon A. Nye and Leonard Howell

Abstract Positron emission tomography (PET) is a sensitive and specific noninvasive imaging technology used to measure the 3-dimensional distribution of molecules and their functional outcome over time. This is achieved by detecting the annihilation photons resulting from the decay of radioisotopes (i.e., oxygen-15, nitrogen-13, carbon-11, fluorine-18) chemically labeled to biologically active molecules. The functional fate of these radiolabeled molecules may be determined by examining the images formed from the 3-dimensional reconstruction of the decay events. The approximate sensitivity of PET is picomolar, which permits the injection of molecular masses far below that known to disturb most physiological processes. This methodology is known as the "tracer technique" and is the basic analysis principle used to extract quantitative information from PET images. PET has the ability to provide valuable information related to functional processes of the body including blood flow, transport rates, receptor density, and drug occupancy. This chapter focuses on the physics of PET and its use in answering questions related to pharmacology. The basic principles of PET imaging will be reviewed followed by methods to derive quantitative information related to physiology from the image data. The application of compartmental modeling will be discussed in detail as will potential pitfalls that can occur during data collection.

Keywords Positron emission tomography (PET) • Tracer technique • Compartmental modeling • Dosimetry • Radioisotopes

J.A. Nye, PhD (✉)
Department of Radiology and Imaging Services, Emory University School of Medicine, 1841 Clifton Road NE, Room 205, Atlanta, GA 30329, USA
e-mail: jnye@emory.edu

L. Howell, PhD
Division of Neuropharmacology and Neurologic Diseases, Yerkes National Primate Research Center, Emory University, Atlanta, GA USA
e-mail: lhowell@emory.edu

M. Jann et al. (eds.), *Applied Clinical Pharmacokinetics and Pharmacodynamics of Psychopharmacological Agents*,
DOI 10.1007/978-3-319-27883-4_3

Positron emission tomography (PET) is a sensitive and specific noninvasive imaging technology used to measure the 3-dimensional distribution of molecules and their functional outcome over time. This is achieved by detecting the annihilation photons resulting from the decay of radioisotopes (i.e., oxygen-15, nitrogen-13, carbon-11, fluorine-18) labeled to biologically active molecules. The functional fate of these radiolabeled molecules may be determined by examining the images formed from the 3-dimensional reconstruction of the decay events. The approximate sensitivity of PET is picomolar, which permits the injection of molecular masses far below that known to disturb most physiological processes. This methodology is known as the "tracer technique" and is the basic analysis principle used to extract quantitative information from PET images.

The design of the biochemically active molecule depends on the system to be studied and may be endogenous or an analogue to the functional system. As an example, the most widely used radiotracer in PET is fluorine-18 labeled glucose ([F-18]FDG). In the synthesis of this compound, a hydroxyl group is replaced with an F-18 atom resulting in a nonnatural analogue of glucose. The analogue nature of [F-18]FDG is advantageous as the radiotracer completes only a few metabolic steps compared to glucose and eventually becomes trapped within a cell following phosphorylation. The in vivo fate of [F-18]FDG can be modeled by assigning compartments to processes that lead to the trapping of [F-18]FDG [1]. The rate constants describing the movement of [F-18]FDG between these compartments are solved for using principles of pharmacology, which allow for the estimation of regional glucose metabolism. PET has the ability to provide valuable information related to functional processes of the body including blood flow, transport rates, receptor density, and drug occupancy.

This chapter focuses on the physics of PET and its use in answering questions related to pharmacology. The basic physical principles of PET imaging will be reviewed followed by methods to derive quantitative information related to physiology from the image data. The application of compartmental modeling will be discussed in detail as will potential pitfalls that can occur during data collection.

3.1 Physical Principles of PET Imaging

PET takes advantage of the unique characteristics of positron decay. The purpose of the decay is to shed positive charge and reach a stable energy state. This decay process results in a daughter isotope with an atomic number one less than the parent. For example, the positron decay of fluorine-18 results in stable oxygen-18. Upon decay of the positron, the particle will expend its kinetic energy through scatter and ionization events up to a distance of approximately 1–2 mm from the decay origin. Once the positron has expended its kinetic energy, it meets its antiparticle, an electron and annihilates. The annihilation results in two nearly colinear 511 keV photons. Detection of these photons is accomplished by a ring of detectors; therefore, a pair of annihilation photons is ideally detected by opposing detectors which

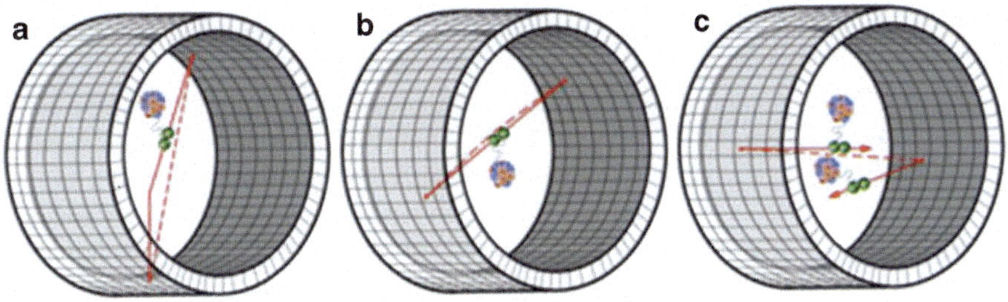

Fig. 3.1 Three types of events recorded by a 3D PET scanner are shown. The annihilation event occurs several millimeters from the decay origin. The *dotted line* represents the line of response, along which the scanner assigns the decay event. (**a**) Scatter event, one annihilation photon undergoes Compton scattering before reaching the detector. (**b**) True event, both annihilation photons reach opposing detectors uninhibited. (**c**) Random event, two unrelated annihilation photons from separate decay events reach the detectors

is called coincidence detection. The two opposing detectors form a line in space, called a line of response (LOR), along which it is highly probable the original decay event occurred. If a sufficient number of these events are recorded, the information can be used to estimate the location of radioactive sources in a 3-dimensional volume. This process is called tomography, where 2D projections are collected over many angles and used to recreate the 3-dimensional distribution of the radioactive sources.

For a subject injected with a radiotracer that emits positrons, the resulting annihilation photons are detected by a cylindrical ring of scintillation crystals. Scanners are made of several rings sandwiched together, and all detectors are continuously monitoring for photons. The number of photons intercepting these detectors will depend on the mode of operation. In 2-dimensional mode, annihilation photons detected are restricted to a single detector ring by lead collimation placed between each ring. In 3-dimensional mode, the lead collimation is absent and annihilation events are free to cross between rings, substantially increasing sensitivity of detection but also presenting additional challenges (Fig. 3.1).

The process of detection is not perfect and is statistically bound by the conversion of light to electrical signal; thus, a PET scanner will accept a range of photon energies (450–600 keV). The photons detected in the scintillation crystals are converted to an electrical signal, and from that signal, the photon energy, location, and time of its arrival at the detector are recorded. Knowing the time is critical. If two opposing detectors recorded an event within a very short coincidence timing window (i.e., a few nanoseconds), then there is a high probability that the photons originated from a single annihilation event. These events are assigned to an LOR and called prompt coincidence events.

In recording the energy of the detection event, it is important to know whether the annihilation photon interacted with tissue in the body prior to its detection. If the recorded energy is 511 keV, then it is overwhelmingly likely the photon did not interact with tissue in its flight to the detector. Events with less energy suggest the photon lost energy by scattering in the body and that its current line of trajectory does not include the origin of the annihilation event.

There are four categories of prompt coincidence events: true, random, scatter, and multiple. True events (Fig. 3.1b) occur when both photons originate from a single annihilation source and intercept the detectors at their original energy, 511 keV. These events occur within the coincidence timing window and are the most desirable. The reconstruction of these events will estimate the distribution of the radioactive sources in the imaged volume. Random events (Fig. 3.1c) may also occur in the coincidence timing window; however, their occurrence results from two 511 keV photons that originated from separate annihilation events. The resulting LOR does not accurately represent the location of an annihilation event. These events are random in time and space and add a uniform background to the image. Fortunately, the randomness in time can be exploited by choosing a coincidence window of which true events cannot occur; thus, the random rate can be measured directly during the data acquisition process.

A scatter event (Fig. 3.1a) is when one of the annihilation photons interacts with tissue resulting in a transfer of energy to the tissue and a change in trajectory from its original path. The greater the angle of scatter from its original trajectory, the greater the amount of energy transferred to the tissue. If enough energy is lost in the scatter event, that photon's energy will fall below the accepted photon energy range of the scintillation detectors and the event will not be recorded. If a scattered photon is recorded, then it will be assigned an LOR. Again, this LOR will not include the origin of the original annihilation event. The recording of scatter events increases the background causing a loss of image contrast. These events cannot be measured during the data collection and therefore are modeled using specialized software. The last event type is a multiple event, which is a combination of a true and random event resulting in three detected events within the coincidence window. These combinations of events result in three possible LORs, but it is unknown which is the true LOR. Typically one can be eliminated because one of the LORs is outside the field of view. What is left over is a random and true LOR. Correction of the randoms should reveal the true LOR. Overall, these events are rare.

There is one event that is not recorded in the prompt dataset: an attenuation event. Attenuation is the loss of annihilation events because they are either absorbed in the tissue or scattered outside the detector plane. Attenuation depends on the total path length traveled by the annihilation photons. Therefore, photons originating from the center of an object have a greater probability of being attenuated compared to those originating from the periphery of the object. The result of attenuation is a depressed signal in center of the image compared to the periphery. Estimating these lost events is relatively straightforward and can be accomplished by collecting transmission data of the object as explained in the next section.

The spatial resolution of PET is limited by a few primary physical factors: detector size, positron range, and non-colinearity of the annihilation photons. Discrete detectors are used to monitor photons which are constructed as long rectangular columns focused at the center of the scanner. Their size range from

4–8 mm on the face and 20–30 mm in depth. The limiting resolution of a detector is approximately half the size on the face, or about 3–4 mm. Secondly, during a decay event, the positrons carry kinetic energy and travel a finite distance expending that energy into surrounding tissue before annihilating with an electron. The higher the kinetic energy of the positron, the greater the distance traveled from its decay origin. This distance adds uncertainty to the location of the original decay site and contributes to resolution degradation in the reconstructed image. Lastly the majority of annihilation events do not result in perfectly colinear 511 keV photons because some residual momentum is left with the positron at the time of annihilation. The loss in spatial resolution of non-colinear photons is ~0.2 % of the detector ring diameter, which for an 80 cm ring can be as high as 2 mm. These three physical factors of the detection process limit the intrinsic resolution of a PET scanner to approximately 6 mm in an 80 cm detector ring. Constructing a scanner with smaller detectors and a smaller ring diameter will improve the intrinsic resolution, but as the size decreases, the positron range will eventually dominate the resolution degradation.

Objects smaller than the spatial resolution of the PET system can still be resolved in an image, but the measured radioactivity concentration and contrast are diminished compared to the truth. The spatial resolution of a system is measure by placing a point object in the scanner field of view and collecting an image. The resulting image is a sphere with an intensity profile that is Gaussian, having a full width of 3–4 mm at half maximum (FWHM). This is called the system's point spread function. A PET system is able to correctly measure the true radioactivity concentration when the measured object is greater than twice the resolving volume (2 × FWHM) of the system. When imaging volumes are smaller than the resolving volume of the PET systems, the pixel intensities in the reconstructed image no longer represent the true concentration. This physical effect is called the partial volume problem. However, this loss in signal can be modeled and corrected using methods of partial volume correction.

3.2 Corrections and Image Formation

The basic approach to image formation is the process of using 2D projections to estimate the 3D distribution of radioactivity in a structure. This can be done using stacks of 2D or fully 3D projection data. The image formation process is called reconstruction, and two general methods are available: (1) a direct inversion process called filtered back projection (FBP) and (2) an iterative process called maximum likelihood expectation maximization. The former algorithm requires fewer computational recourses compared to expectation maximization but is limited by assumptions that include geometric invariance across the field of view, noiseless data, perfect corrections for true events, and no gaps in the tomographic projections. These assumptions are not necessary for expectation maximization because the physics of the photon interactions and scanner geometry among other aspects can be included in the algorithm during reconstruction. However, before the projection data can be reconstructed into an image, corrections need to be made to address random events, scatter events, and attenuation effects in the prompt dataset.

As briefly discussed above, random events are random in time and space. These events are measured in two ways: (1) direct measurement using a delayed window or (2) estimated from the single 511 keV count rates between opposing detectors. The estimate of randoms is obtained for all LORs and subtracted from the prompt dataset resulting in the sum of the true and scatter coincidence events. Ideally, a randoms fraction <10 % of the prompt rate is considered desirable, as this rate will not overly tax the counting electronics. Scatter in a dataset leads to a reduction in contrast and resolution. The distribution of scatter in an image is dependent on the structure of the object, and the probability of scatter is higher for LORs that pass through the center of an object. Thus, a reconstructed image without scatter correction will have the appearance of higher radioactivity at the center of the object. Scatter correction is a difficult problem because the source of a scattering event depends on the radioactivity distribution and attenuating structures of the object. PET instruments are not sensitive enough to measure scatter directly; thus, scatter is estimated using knowledge of the radioactive and structural source distributions. The algorithms that are most commonly used are the single scatter simulation, convolution scatter correction methods, and a Gaussian fitting technique. Two fundamental difficulties can result in the application of these algorithms. First, these methods operate on measured data collected inside the field of view; thus, sources of radioactivity outside the field of view are unknown. Scatter from outside the field of view is typically overcome by calculating the shape of the scatter profile and then scaling to scattered radioactivity measured outside the object. The second difficulty is estimating scatter at low count rates where scaling of the profile can be erroneous due to increased uncertainty in the detected scatter events. The total scatter in the prompt dataset depends on the mode of operation. The scatter signal comprises approximately 10–15 % of the prompt dataset in 2D imaging and 40–50 % of the prompt dataset in 3D imaging. Scatter correction is performed by subtracting the estimated scatter from the prompt dataset resulting in the sum of true coincidence events.

Attenuation correction estimates the loss of signal in a dataset due to photons absorbed in the object or scattered outside the field of view. For a 20 cm diameter object, this signal loss can be as high as a factor of ×7 in the center of the object. For PET, attenuation of an object depends on the total path length traveled along an LOR. The total attenuation can be measured directly by placing a source of radioactivity at the edge of the field of view and acquiring counts with and without the object in the scanner. The logarithm of the ratio of these measurements will give the attenuation factor for a given line of response. Traditionally, the transmission scan is accomplished using an external sealed radioactive source (Ge-68, Cs-137, Co-57) that is rotated around the object for several minutes. In modern clinical PET systems, the transmission scan is acquired using a computed tomography (CT) scanner. These hybrid (PET/CT) systems provide two major advantages compared to traditional systems. First, the CT provides anatomical detail that can be fused with the

PET reconstruction for localization and correlation of radiotracer uptake with anatomy. Second, CT imaging is a high photon statistical process that provides nearly noiseless data when compared to external rotating sources, thereby minimizing the propagation of transmission data noise into the reconstructed image. Attenuation correction is performed by multiplying the true coincidence events by a set of attenuation correction factors.

When randoms, scatter, and attenuation corrections have been made to the data, the final result should be a dataset made up of true events. FBP requires that the corrections to randoms, attenuation, and scatter be performed perfectly prior to reconstruction. There are additional corrections needed to meet the requirements for filtered back projection, including scanner geometry and detector efficiency. Although great effort is spent in instrument calibration and computational resources to generate these corrections, invariably a breakdown does occur in the FBP assumptions, and the results can be observed in the image. Poisson noise in the individual lines of response results in streaks in the images radiating out from the center of the field of view. This is most apparent outside the object where both positive and negative streaks occur. Some level of image artifacts due to the FBP process should be acceptable to take advantage of the fast reconstructions offered by this algorithm.

The iterative reconstruction process is not constrained by the same assumptions as FBP but does have drawbacks. The process of iterative reconstruction can incorporate many aspects of the imaging process into the algorithm to compute the most likely source distribution that created the prompt dataset. The iterative process begins with a guess of the source distribution. The scanning process is then simulated by forward projecting the guess to create a simulated prompt dataset. The simulated dataset is then compared to the measured prompt dataset, and a correction for the guess image is created. The guess image is then updated, and the process occurs repeatedly through several iterations until the simulated data match, or closely match, the measured dataset. The advantage of the iterative reconstruction process is the inclusion of the corrections (i.e., randoms, scatter, and attenuation). Poisson count statistics and other physical scan processes are factored into the scanning simulation step of the algorithm. The result is an image that is much more accurate, as noted by a visual improvement in contrast and noise compared to FBP. The drawback of the iterative method is a substantial increase in computational time. The process of simulating the scanner physics is time consuming, and increasing the number of corrections adds to the computing time. A second drawback is deciding how many iterations are necessary for the simulated data to be considered matched to the measured dataset. Because the decay and acquisition process follow well-known Poisson distributions, the decision can be made by probabilistically comparing the datasets. In general, there are a number of iterations that when exceeded result in an incremental improvement in the guess image; thus, a fixed number of iterations is chosen for practical reasons. The choice of using FBP or iterative reconstruction is often a legacy matter, but as computation power increases, iterative reconstruction has become preferred.

3.3 Quantification

PET offers the possibility of absolute quantitative measurements of radiotracer concentration in vivo. This implies that the voxel intensities are directly proportional to the radioactivity concentration. There are several methods of image processing to extract physiologically relevant data from PET images, from the simplistic data normalizations to mathematical modeling of radiotracer time-courses. Whatever the needed information from the analysis of image data, it is desirable that the process be easily reproducible and reliable across subjects with various biological states. This would permit studying populations or the progression/inhibition of biological states in an individual before and after treatment. The purpose of this section is to describe techniques to quantify PET image data.

3.3.1 Standardized Uptake Value

The standardized updake value (SUV) is a dimensionless quantity (g/mL) that is calculated by normalizing the measured radiotracer concentration in a target tissue to the ratio of the administered radioactivity and subject mass. This normalizing step is an attempt to compensate for the inter- and intra-subject variation and offers a fast and easy method of comparing radiotracer uptake in a target. The SUV is a function of time as the compound distributes and concentrates in tissues. Generally, given enough time post injection, the radiotracer will reach peak uptake or transient equilibrium. It is at one of these time points that SUV is typically evaluated. For a radiotracer evenly distributed throughout the body, the SUV would equate to one everywhere. An SUV value greater than one suggests that a physiological mechanism is actively involved in the concentration of a radiotracer. But SUVs are subject to variability from a number of sources such as the duration of the scan, physical decay correction, biological variations or nonsteady-state processes, inaccuracies in body weight (i.e., presence of fat), image noise, and scanner cross-calibration.

3.3.2 Target to Reference Tissue Ratios

The ratio of target-to-reference tissue regions improves the robustness of the quantification because it does not require calibration of the scanner. Secondly, the PET data do not need to be corrected for physical decay of the labeled radioisotope. The target tissue contains the molecular target, whether a transporter process, receptor site, or other cellular process. The reference tissue is a region that does not include the molecular target or has a negligible concentration. For example, the target tissue may be a region in the brain that expresses a receptor that exhibits specific binding for the radiotracer, but this receptor is absent in the reference region. Some challenges are present with this method, as a tissue or region exhibiting negligible specific binding may not be available. Secondly, the target-to-reference tissue ratios are a function of time; therefore, care must be taken in selecting the most appropriate time point.

3.3.3 Kinetic Analysis

Quantitative image data from PET allows relationships to be inferred that relate the kinetics and distribution of a radiotracer to one or more physiological processes in the body. This usually requires dynamic imaging (acquiring multiple images of the radiotracer distribution over time) to observe the movement of radiotracer from region to region or its change within a region over time. Physiological information regarding processes responsible for the radiotracer's dynamic distribution can then be estimated with the help of a mathematical model. This concept has been used to determine a number of physiologically meaningful parameters such as blood flow, cellular metabolism, and receptor density. The mathematical model may be carried out using several approaches such as compartment modeling, graphical transformation, and evaluating the system at equilibrium.

The process of collecting dynamic PET data starts at the time of injection and extends for a duration long enough to capture the biochemical process of interest. The interval of successive images, or frames, should be on the order of the temporal changes of the radiotracer distribution. At the time of injection, the radiotracer enters the bloodstream through a peripheral vein and is quickly pumped though the pulmonary vasculature and the rest of the body. Early images of the radiotracer contain information primarily influenced by blood flow and interstitial tissue exchange and must be collected rapidly because the distribution changes quickly. Each successive pass of the radiotracer through the system is characterized by radiotracer leaving the blood and concentrating in the peripheral tissue for one reason or another. Over time the accumulated radioactivity is sensitive to differences in cell physiology. Therefore, a dynamic PET acquisition begins with short time frames to capture blood flow-dependent changes followed by gradually lengthening time frames to capture slower processes occurring within the tissues.

It is desirable to image for as long as the relative radiotracer distribution continues to change. However, the total imaging time is limited by physical, physiological, and practical considerations. First, the physical half-life of the labeling isotope limits the useful imaging time to approximately 3–4 half-lives. After more than about 4 half-lives, the reduced number of collected counts increases image noise, decreases image contrast, and leads to a less accurate estimate of the amount of radiotracer in tissue. Physiological factors such as organs that metabolize, concentrate, and excrete the radiotracer can confound image interpretation in areas surrounding those tissues. Lastly, practical limitations such as use of scanner time and patient or subject comfort will impose limits on the duration of an imaging study.

Considering these limitations, it is reasonable to assume that no matter the biochemical process of interest, approximately 2 h of useful imaging time (including positioning and transmission scanning) is available to collect information.

3.3.3.1 Compartment Modeling to Described PET Data

The reconstructed radioactivity concentration contained within a region or voxel in the PET image arrives from a combination of multiple signals including that from arterial blood and tissue. The influence of one signal versus the other depends on a variety of physiological mechanisms including transport from the plasma to the interstitial tissues and changes in the molecular state such as metabolism or binding to receptors. Each of these physiological spaces or states is assigned to a compartment. Each of these compartments varies over time in the region or voxel and can be described by a series of coupled first-order differential equations. The coefficients, representing the rate of radiotracer exchange between compartments, are assumed to be invariant over the duration of the study. The rate of exchange of radiotracer between compartments could be very interesting physiologically. For example, it could represent a metabolic rate, the rate that the radiotracer binds to a specific site which in turn is proportional to the number of binding sites, or the rate at which a radiotracer crosses a capillary membrane, which is in turn proportional to the amount of blood flowing into that capillary or tissue. The goal of modeling is to choose an appropriate number of compartments and their associated rate constants to permit the elucidation of pharmacokinetic parameter values that are of physiological importance.

The sophistication of the compartment model in PET imaging is limited due to spatial and temporal sampling as well as noise in the image. Image noise is the largest confounding factor and is influenced by a large number of variables in the processing of PET data, including camera sensitivity, radiotracer uptake, scan duration, reconstruction parameters and image corrections, and the size of the region of interest. One, two, or three compartments are generally sufficient to describe PET data. A series of compartments might consist of (1) free radiotracer in blood plasma, (2) free radiotracer in extracellular space, and (3) radiotracer in intracellular space. The free radiotracer in plasma is generally considered the first compartment and is measured from arterial blood (see Sect. 3.3.3.2). The compartments representing the extracellular and intracellular space are commonly referred to as "tissue" compartments; therefore, the above example is also termed a two-tissue compartment model where the plasma compartment is inferred. The exact physiological meaning of the rate constants assigned to the compartments will depend on the modeling assumptions and compartment definitions. For example, a two-tissue compartment model linked by four rate constants is typically sufficient describing a radiotracer that binds to a receptor site in the brain (Fig. 3.2a, b).

Often the number of compartments corresponds to the number of physical spaces within the tissue but may also represent a state. These physiological

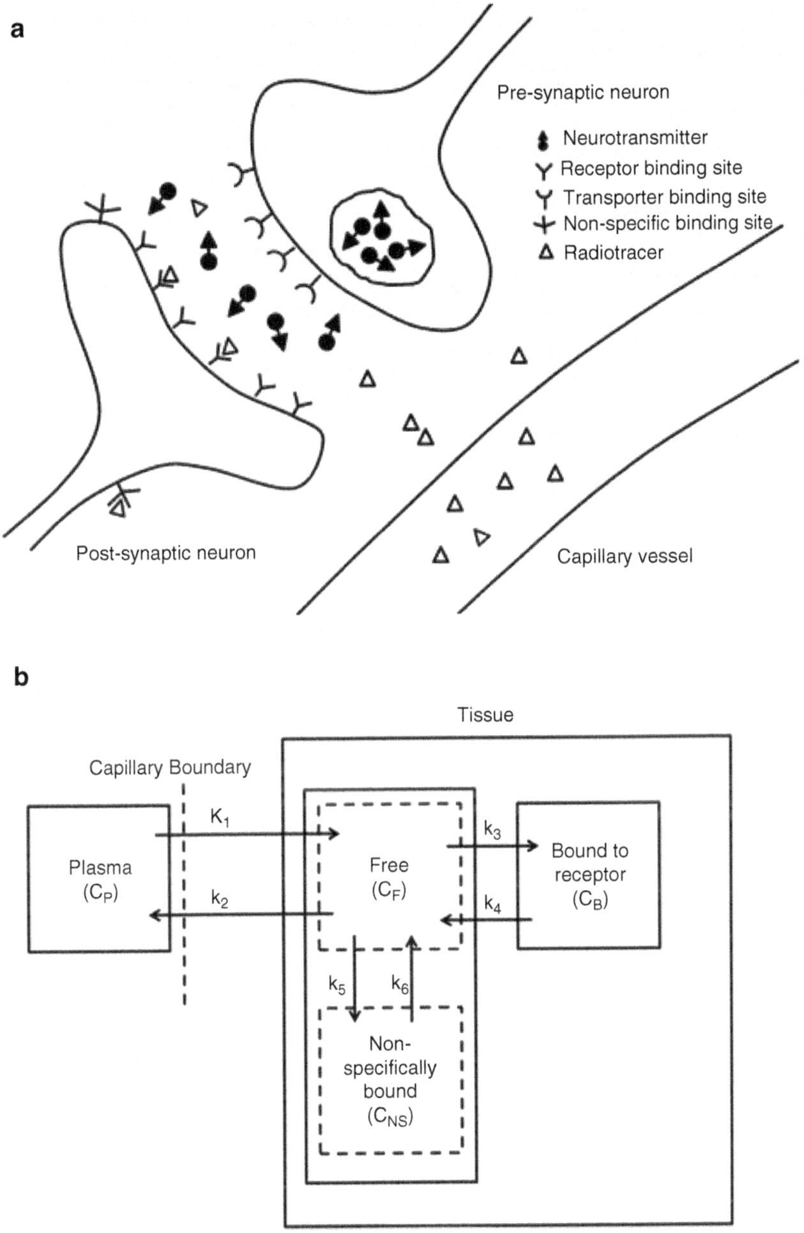

Fig. 3.2 Simplistic representation of the binding of a radiotracer selective for a receptor on the postsynaptic neuron (**b**) A two-tissue compartment model depicting the process in (**a**). The compartments consist of (1) radiotracer in the plasma supplying the tissue, C_P; (2) free radiotracer in the extracellular space, or bound to a nonspecific site, C_{F+NS}; and (3) radiotracer bound to the target receptor, C_B. The rates of exchange between compartments are denoted by the arrows and their associated constants (K_1, k_2, k_3, k_4). The compartment model is considered reversible because the radiotracer is free to leave the bound state and reenter the extracellular space

differences, and others like them, must be considered in the compartment model because they affect how the rate constants are interpreted. The physical scale of the situation depicted in Fig. 3.1 is on the order of 10 μm. A PET scanner, with resolution on the order of mm, cannot distinguish between a radiotracer in the different compartments; thus, the measured PET signal at any given time is the total of the radioactivity in all compartments. The contribution of modeling is to infer how the radiotracer is being transported between the compartments by using mathematical modeling as a basis for understanding the dynamic data measured by the scanner.

The constants describing the rates of exchange between compartments are obtained by solving a coupled series of differential equations (Eqs. 3.1 and 3.2). The measured PET signal is the weighted sum of the blood (C_P), extracellular (C_{F+NS}), and bound compartments (C_B) (Eq. 3.3). The weighting factors (V_P, V_F, V_B) are the fraction of an image pixel that each of the compartments occupies. There are more constants than available equations; therefore, the problem is mathematically underdetermined, and there is not be a single unique set of rate constants that describe the measured data. In the model's application, the rate constants are determined simultaneously using iterative methods, and the solution is restricted to physiologically relevant values. Equations for the model depicted in Fig. 3.1 are:

$$\frac{\mathrm{d}C_F}{\mathrm{d}t} = K_1 C_P - k_2 C_{F+NS} - k_3 C_{F+NS} + k_4 C_B \tag{3.1}$$

$$\frac{\mathrm{d}C_B}{\mathrm{d}t} = k_3 C_{F+NS} - k_4 C_B \tag{3.2}$$

$$PET = V_P C_P + V_F C_{F+NS} + V_B C_B \tag{3.3}$$

If the radiotracer freely exchanges between compartments for a sufficient length of time, and the radioactivity concentration in the plasma is held constant, the concentrations in the extracellular and intracellular spaces eventually reach equilibrium. At this point the individual compartment concentrations do not change, and the left side of Eqs. 3.1 and 3.2 are zero. At equilibrium, it is very difficult to accurately separate the individual influx and efflux rate constants for each compartment because of the underdetermined nature of the problem. However, the ratio of rate constants is considered unique and useful for representing the ratio of concentrations of radiotracer in two compartments. The equilibrium ratio is termed a volume of distribution and can be calculated as an appropriate combination of rate constants. By convention, the total volume of distribution, V_T, is the ratio of the radioactivity concentrations in the tissue to that in plasma. For the two-tissue compartment model in Fig. 3.2, V_T is the summation of the distribution volumes in the free compartment and cellular compartments (since V_F and V_B are equal in this case). The distribution volume in the free compartment is also referred to as the non-displaceable distribution volume,

$V_{ND} = C_F/C_P$. The relationship to the rate constants can be derived from Eqs. 3.1 and 3.2 and the equilibrium condition as:

$$V_T = \frac{C_{F+NS}}{C_P} + \frac{C_B}{C_P} = \frac{K_1}{k_2} + \frac{K_1 k_3}{k_2 k_4} = \frac{K_1}{k_2}\left(1 + \frac{k_3}{k_4}\right) \approx \frac{C_T}{C_P} \tag{3.4}$$

where the last approximate equality arises from Eq. 3.4, assuming V_P is small and $V_F = V_B$. The analysis techniques below can be used to quantitatively determine combinations of rate constants even if the system under investigation is not in equilibrium. In this case, a quantitative value can be derived from the dynamic PET data that is directly related to the physiology being studied.

In the brain, the compartment model for receptor imaging has two-tissue compartments. The first corresponds to the radiotracer residing in extracellular space and the second corresponds to the radiotracer bound to the receptor target. The latter tissue compartment is not defined in space but a change in state of the radiotracer from "free" to "bound." The rate constants describing the movement of the radiotracer in the receptor model are as follows: K_1 [mL/g/min] and k_2 [1/min] represent the unidirectional fractional rate constants, corresponding to the influx and efflux of radioligand diffusion across the blood brain barrier, respectively. k_2 is the rate that tracer leaves the extracellular compartment for the plasma, $k_3 = k_{on}B_{avail}$ since this is a tracer experiment, and $k_4 = k_{off}$, the off rate from the transporter [2]. The kinetic parameter of interest is the number of available receptors for binding (B_{avail}) in a brain region compared to that in the free space,

$$\frac{(V_T - V_{ND})}{V_{ND}} = \frac{C_B}{C_{F+NS}} = \frac{k_3}{k_4} = \frac{k_{on} B_{avail}}{k_{off}} = \frac{B_{avail}}{K_D} \tag{3.5}$$

where K_D is the disassociation constant. This term is commonly referred to as binding potential (BP).

For a radiotracer that is trapped in a cellular process, whether by incorporation into another molecule, the model has at least one compartment that is irreversible (Fig. 3.3). In this case, the concept of equilibrium distribution volume is not useful. Instead, the rate at which the radiotracer is incorporated into protein is more relevant and related to the rate that the radiotracer enters the irreversible compartment. The flux into the extracellular space is the product of the blood flow and extraction fraction (the probability that a radiotracer molecule will cross the capillary membrane during a single pass through the capillary). The flow and extraction fraction product is the unidirectional rate constant K_1 in the compartment model. Multiplying this quantity by the radiotracer arterial plasma concentration gives an estimate of the rate of transfer of radiotracer into tissue. Let K_1 represent the rate of glucose delivery to the free space. Then the net rate of glucose delivery across the cell membrane can be determined by multiplying K_1 by the fraction of

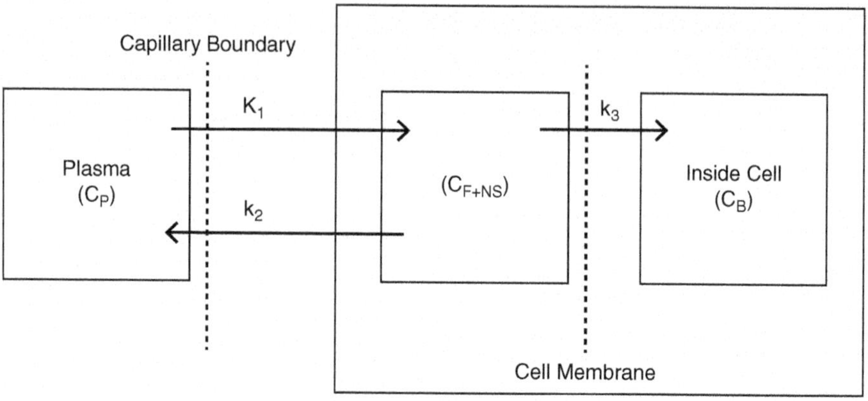

Fig. 3.3 A two-tissue compartment model representing the trapping of a radiotracer in a cell

radiotracer that leaves the free space and enters the cell. This quantity represents the net influx of a radiotracer into the cell.

$$K_{\text{influx}} = K_1 \frac{k_3}{k_2 + k_3} \tag{3.6}$$

This is represented in Fig. 3.3.

3.3.3.2 Input Function

The concentration of the radiotracers in tissue depends on the time varying concentration of the radiotracers in arterial blood. The input function can be determined by measuring arterial blood samples. Following a bolus injection, blood samples are initially drawn at a high frequency and as the dose distributes throughout the body, blood samples are collected less frequently. The blood is then centrifuged to separate blood cells and proteins from the plasma. Only radioactivity contained in the plasma fraction is measured because it represents the amount of radiotracer that is free to cross the capillary boundary and enter the tissue.

Another technique to derive a suitable input function is to measure it directly from image data. This technique entails placement of a large ROI over an arterial structure, such as the left ventricle, aorta, or another large artery. If number and proportion of labeled metabolites in blood are known or they are rapidly and efficiently excreted from the bloodstream, this approach may permit comparisons between kinetic parameter estimates and actual arterial samples [3, 4].

A third technique to estimate an input function is the reference region approach which is widely used in receptor imaging [5]. A reference region is defined as a tissue region that is identical in all aspects to the region of interest except there are negligible specific binding sites. This technique provides several advantages compared to arterial sampling including reduction in discomfort to the patient, need for fewer personnel, and reduced errors in the compartment model parameter estimates because the reference region and region of interest are derived from the same image data. The reference procedure introduces a second compartment model that describes the delivery of radioligand to the interstitial space of the reference region. This in turn permits construction of a mathematical model that describes the plasma input in terms of the reference region and the estimation of kinetic parameters.

3.3.3.3 Modeling Assumptions

There are a number of implicit assumptions made when using compartment models to describe the kinetics of a radiotracer in a complex biological system. The first and most important assumption is that the mass of injected radiotracer (labeled and unlabeled) is a trace amount. That is, its concentration is negligible to the extent that is does not alter in any way the process that it is intended to mimic. This is equivalent to saying that so little compound is administered that it does not produce even the slightest pharmacological effect. This assumption is met when the specific activity, which is radioactivity divided by the total mass (GBq/micromole), of the tracer is sufficiently high. Second, the endogenous molecule mimicked by the radiotracer must be at steady state throughout the duration of the experiment. This condition is met if there are no changes in external factors such as administration of compounds that alter the physiological state or compete with the radiotracer for binding in the tissue. Thirdly, the mixing of the radiotracer with other molecules in the compartment must occur at a substantially faster rate than its exchange between compartments. Often this assumption is referred to as instantaneous mixing. Lastly, the labeled isotope does not change the behavior of the radiotracer in relation to the stable label. For example, [C-11]raclopride is expected to behave exactly as raclopride containing stable carbon. This is termed the isotope effect.

3.3.4 Graphical Transformation

A common approach to estimating kinetic parameters that is often performed in parallel with compartmental modeling is graphical analyses because it is simple and does not require complete knowledge of the underlying physiology of the system. Current graphical methods only require knowledge that the radiotracer is either freely reversible in all compartments or irreversibly trapped by at least one compartment, regardless of the number. In both cases, transformations are performed on the time and measured radioactivity so that, when plotted, the graph approaches a straight line at later time points.

The Patlak plot is a graphical method that has been used in analyzing [F-18] FDG data because it assumes at least one compartment is irreversibly trapped [6, 7]. This compartment would represent the phosphorylation of [F-18]FDG. This graphical approach estimates fractional uptake rate of [F-18]FDG described in the two-tissue compartment model (Fig. 3.3). The approach works, because after the reversible compartments reach quasi-equilibrium, the change in radioactivity levels in tissue is due solely to trapping in the irreversible compartment. The data transformation described by Patlak is such that when equilibrium in the reversible and plasma compartments is achieved, the plot approaches a straight line and the slope of the line is the influx constant, K_{influx}. A second graphical approach is applicable when all compartments are reversible and is referred to as Logan analysis [8, 9]. Such an analysis may be appropriate for tracers that are reversible, such as receptor binding studies. Following the graphical transformation, the slope of the linear region is the distribution volume. Both the Patlak and Logan graphical transformation methods can be used with a reference tissue input if arterial blood is not measured.

3.4 Application of PET in Pharmacology

The PET tracer technique permits the characterization of in vivo drug interactions with specific protein targets while not perturbing the physiological system. Choosing an appropriate radiotracer, of high affinity for a target of interest, can provide insights into neurochemical interactions related to behavioral observations. Some of these insights include drug interactions with neurotransmitter receptors and transporters, changes in cerebral blood flow, and alterations of cerebral metabolism. A straightforward application of PET is characterization of the radiotracer uptake kinetics and biodistribution, including overall magnitude (SUV), time-to-peak uptake, and the washout phase. This simplistic analysis has lead to several notable contributions including radiolabeling of cocaine and methylphenidate with carbon-11 to examine their in vivo kinetics in humans [10, 11]. These psychostimulants have roughly equal affinity for all three monoamine transporter systems (dopamine, serotonin, and norepinephrine); however, their kinetics vary considerably. The washout phase of methylphenidate is substantially slower than cocaine, and this observation is thought to contribute to differences in abuse potential between these agents despite their similar binding profiles. Radiolabeling of drugs has led to a number of insights into how behavioral outcomes relate to drug kinetic profiles and their interactions and continues to be a powerful technique with PET [12, 13].

Compartment modeling analysis can lead to a deeper understanding of underlying physiological processes in vivo by estimating rate constants that govern radiotracer uptake. One aspect is calculation of binding potential, which is related to the total number of available binding sites and plays an essential role examining the acute and chronic integrity of protein targets [2]. Furthermore, binding potential may be calculated in the presence of competitive drug binding to determine occupancy at the target site [14]. Occupancy experiments are generally conducted in two steps, an initial study in the presence of no drugs to measure the baseline density followed by exposure to the drug then immediately repeating the study to measure the density with drug on board. The ratio of the measured binding potential between these two states can be used to calculate the occupancy of drug in the target tissue,

$$\text{Occupancy } \% = 100 \times \left(1 - \frac{BP_{\text{drug on-board}}}{BP_{\text{baseline}}}\right)$$

Calculation of occupancy has been crucial in determining the relationship between drug concentration in vivo and pharmacological onset. For many psychostimulants, it has been determined using PET that a minimum drug occupancy of at least 65 to 75 % is needed to observe behavioral changes [11, 15, 16]. These experiments can be conducted in a single session starting with an initial baseline phase followed by a drug chase that displaces the baseline signal [17, 18].

Similar to the occupancy protocol, PET has been used to measure drug-induced endogenous neurotransmitter release. In this case, the drug administered evokes release of endogenous neurotransmitters that compete with the radiotracer for binding. The classic case is displacement of [C-11]raclopride from D2/D3 receptors by release of dopamine after administration of amphetamine or similar analogues. This experiment is different than drug occupancy described above because the displacement action is due to competitive interactions with an endogenous molecule rather than an exogenously administered drug. Again, the binding potential can be calculated using compartmental modeling concepts and the difference between the baseline and drug induction are typically compared.

Lastly, assessments in changes of cerebral metabolism are useful for monitoring changes in brain activity under various drug actions. The actual calculation of regional cerebral glucose metabolism is complicated by the need for arterial blood sampling to determine the input function. Secondly, FDG imaging does not follow the complete glucose metabolic pathway, and a conversion factor is needed to relate FDG metabolism to glucose metabolism, called the lumped constant. FDG data are compared using SUV quantitation or by group analysis packages such as statistical parametric mapping [19]. Hyper- and hypometabolic changes can be determined in these studies compared to a baseline or normal control population [20]. These techniques have been used extensively in studies of acute and chronic drug interactions [16, 20–23].

PET offers a great value in translational sciences from simple experiments to measure brain penetrability of radiolabeled drugs and their biodistribution to more sophisticated studies including calculation of occupancy using radiotracer displacement protocols.

3.5 Challenges to Using PET

The uptake and distribution of radiolabled molecules will depend, in part, on the laboratory conditions during the study including the environment, normal physiology, and use of anesthetics. These factors add variability to the outcome measurement and anticipating such pitfalls can improve the quality of the data. Below is a brief discussion of some particular challenges.

PET imaging requires that the subject be still throughout the exam. Motion on the order of the resolution of the scanner (by as little as a few millimeters) degrades the achievable reconstructed resolution, reduces contrast, and may lead to the erroneous application of attenuation correction. In dynamic PET imaging, scan durations may be in excess of 1 h, and invariably a subject will shift a small amount to ease discomfort over this duration. A motion event may be voluntary or involuntary. For example, motion such as moving an arm to tend to an itch or respiratory motion during normal breathing. Additional movement may result from the subject's physiological state such as muscle tremors or forgetting instructions. It is desirable to correct for motion events as best as possible by either closely monitoring the subject or using software tools. In brain imaging there are generally two types of motion to consider: (1) motion between the emission (PET) and attenuation scans and (2) motion within an emission frame. The former is relatively easy to address using software to align the transmission data with the emission data and re-reconstruct the PET images. The latter presents more challenges and has been addressed by subdividing the emission data into shorter frame durations, throwing out the time duration that included the motion or incorporating more sophisticated motion correction algorithms in the reconstruction. Head restraints help prevent a great deal of these troubles but not all.

With the exception of a few laboratories, anesthesia is used in the preclinical imaging environment to sedate animals and maintain the quiescent state needed for PET imaging. There is ample evidence showing that anesthesia alters the physiological state of an animal including blood flow, metabolism, and neurotransmitter expression in the brain [24–26]. A large number of commonly used anesthetics including ketamine and isoflurane have been shown to alter brain homeostasis. Many of the effects listed above are dose and species dependent. Minimizing physiological alterations secondary to anesthetics generally entails careful monitoring and simplifying laboratory procedures so they can be easily replicated.

A well-controlled environment including warming devices and monitoring equipment is crucial to a successful study. Control of these conditions is most important in animal imaging, where the mouse, rat, or nonhuman primate is sedated during the study. A reduction in an animal's core body temperature results in constriction of blood vessels and redistribution of blood to conserve vital functions. These changes will alter the uptake of radiotracers, generally reducing the contrast.

3.6 Dosimetry

Radiation dosimetry refers to the amount of energy deposited in an organ and the whole body (i.e., dose) resulting from the internal administration of radionuclides. This information is important in assessing deterministic (e.g., cataract, radiotoxicity) and stochastic (cancer induction) effects from radiation exposure. Some regulatory bodies limit the amount of internally deposited radiation dose; therefore, estimating internal dose from radiopharmaceutical injections may be warranted. The purpose of this section is to provide an overview of how absorbed dose is estimated for internally deposited radiolabeled molecules.

The absorbed dose is a function of the radiotracer's kinetics, the number and energy of the emitted radiations, and the organ sizes and positions. The latter can be obtained from anatomical imaging (either CT or MR); however, capturing the radiotracer kinetics for calculation of individual absorbed doses requires long scan times and is not feasible in a clinical setting. Thus, methodology has been developed to estimate dose based on anthropomorphic phantoms that is then extrapolated to populations of subjects. The following sections briefly describe the Medical Internal Radiation Dose Committee (MIRD) method and present published absorbed dose results for some common radiotracers used in PET research.

3.6.1 Acquisition Protocols and Calculation of Time Activity Curves

Serial whole-body scans spanning from the head to mid-thigh are used to gather the radiotracer kinetics for absorbed dose calculations. Bed durations are typically short following administration of the radioactivity to measure the blood pool changes and then gradually increase to capture longer retention kinetics within organs. Fast excretion kinetics may necessitate that scans begin at the mid-thigh rather than the head in order to capture the initial elimination of the tracer and its metabolites by the kidney before it is taken up into tissue. As with compartment modeling, the total scan duration that a subject can tolerate is limited to about 2 h. Information beyond this point is estimated by extrapolation assuming only physical decay beyond the last measured data point or by using more sophisticated methods of curve fitting and compartment modeling.

3.6.2 Absorbed Dose

To standardize the dose calculation, Stabin et al., 1996, published the MIRDOSE software which calculates the internally deposited dose from the number of decays that take place in each organ [27]. The software includes the International Commission on Radiological Protection (ICRP) GI tract model and Cloutier dynamic bladder model (ICRP 30) which account for radioactivity moving through these excretory systems [28, 29]. The software provides the absorbed dose and effective dose per unit of administered radioactivity as detailed in the MIRD primer [30]. The MIRDOSE code has since been updated to comply with FDA 510k rules and renamed OLINDA/EXM [31]. OLINDA contains all the features of MIRDOSE with some additions such as an expansion of the radionuclide library, the ability to change organ masses to better match patient populations, and updates to absorbed fractions of marrow, bone, and skin.

The organ dose result from the MIRD schema is reported in units of equivalent dose as defined by the ICRP that are then normalized by the administered radioactivity [mSv/mBq]. The equivalent dose (Sv) is the absorbed dose (Gy) multiplied by a weighting factor called the relative biological effectiveness (RBE). The RBE is proportional to the amount of energy needed to produce a biological effect relative to a standard (200 keV x-rays). It is an empirical weighting factor that ranges from 1, for x-rays, to 20, for alpha particles. For establishing annual limits, the ICRP introduced the effective dose to take into account the probability of stochastic effects such as cancer caused by radiation-induced cell mutations. The effective dose is a sum of the individual organ contributions to the whole-body stochastic radiation burden, for which each organ is multiplied by a weighting factor proportional to an organ's susceptibility to cancer induction [32]. This effective dose is used in comparisons of radiation risk and for recording cumulated radiation burden. It is also of interest to know which organ receives the highest equivalent dose. This organ is referred to as the critical organ. Often the limit for an individual organ dose is reached before the limit established for the whole body. The US Food and Drug Administration in Title 21 CFR Part 361 suggests limits for whole-body radiation dose to adult research subjects to less than 30 mSv for a single injection and 50mSv annually. A single organ cannot receive more than 50 mSv in a single injection and 150 mSv annually. These constraints on dose will limit the maximum number of injections for research subjects.

The whole-body effective dose per unit administered radioactivity for a variety of Fluorine-18 labeled compounds typically ranges between 0.015 and 0.025 mSv/MBq (6–10 mSv for 370 MBq). The whole-body dose is a function of isotope half-life, but the reduction in dose from using short-lived isotopes is often offset by the need to inject more activity to provide suitable counting statistics in the image. The dose per administered activity is roughly greater by a factor of 3 for the ^{18}F-labeled compounds.

3.7 Conclusions

The application of compartmental modeling in PET provides a simplified mathematical interpretation of the time varying uptake of radiotracers that is used to extract physiological information. Prior to application of a model, it is important to understand both the biochemical behavior of the injected radiotracer and underlying physiology of the disease. This information is crucial for choosing an appropriate number of compartments and rate constants and in the interpretation of the estimated parameters. A well-constructed model will give more insight into the physiological mechanisms that characterize a disease and be more sensitive to changes in the disease state.

References

1. Reivich M, Kuhl D, Wolf A et al (1979) The [18F]fluorodeoxyglucose method for the measurement of local cerebral glucose utilization in man. Circ Res 44:127–137
2. Mintun MA, Raichle ME, Kilbourn MR et al (1984) A quantitative model for the in vivo assessment of drug binding sites with positron emission tomography. Ann Neurol 15: 217–227
3. Raylman RR, Caraher JM, Hutchins GD (1993) Sampling requirements for dynamic cardiac PET studies using image-derived input functions. J Nucl Med 34:440–447
4. Hoekstra CJ, Hoekstra OS, Lammertsma AA (1999) On the use of image-derived input functions in oncological fluorine-18 fluorodeoxyglucose positron emission tomography studies. Eur J Nucl Med 26:1489–1492
5. Lammertsma AA, Hume SP (1996) Simplified reference tissue model for PET receptor studies. Neuroimage 4:153–158
6. Patlak CS, Blasberg RG, Fenstermacher JD (1983) Graphical evaluation of blood-to-brain transfer constants from multiple-time uptake data. J Cereb Blood Flow Metab 3:1–7
7. Patlak CS, Blasberg RG (1985) Graphical evaluation of blood-to-brain transfer constants from multiple-time uptake data. Generalizations. J Cereb Blood Flow Metab 5:584–590
8. Logan J, Fowler JS, Volkow ND et al (1996) Distribution volume ratios without blood sampling from graphical analysis of PET data. J Cereb Blood Flow Metab 16:834–840
9. Logan J, Fowler JS, Volkow ND et al (1990) Graphical analysis of reversible radioligand binding from time-activity measurements applied to [N-11C-methyl]-(−)-cocaine PET studies in human subjects. J Cereb Blood Flow Metab 10:740–747
10. Volkow ND, Wang GJ, Fischman MW et al (1997) Relationship between subjective effects of cocaine and dopamine transporter occupancy. Nature 386:827–830
11. Volkow ND, Wang GJ, Fowler JS et al (1996) Relationship between psychostimulant-induced "high" and dopamine transporter occupancy. Proc Natl Acad Sci U S A 93:10388–10392
12. Kimmel HL, Negus SS, Wilcox KM et al (2008) Relationship between rate of drug uptake in brain and behavioral pharmacology of monoamine transporter inhibitors in rhesus monkeys. Pharmacol Biochem Behav 90:453–462
13. Volkow ND, Ding YS, Fowler JS et al (1996) Cocaine addiction: hypothesis derived from imaging studies with PET. J Addict Dis 15:55–71
14. Laruelle M, Slifstein M, Huang Y (2002) Positron emission tomography: imaging and quantification of neurotransporter availability. Methods 27:287–299
15. Howell LL, Murnane KS (2008) Nonhuman primate neuroimaging and the neurobiology of psychostimulant addiction. Ann N Y Acad Sci 1141:176–194
16. Howell LL, Murnane KS (2011) Nonhuman primate positron emission tomography neuroimaging in drug abuse research. J Pharmacol Exp Ther 337:324–334
17. Votaw JR, Howell LL, Martarello L et al (2002) Measurement of dopamine transporter occupancy for multiple injections of cocaine using a single injection of [F-18]FECNT. Synapse 44:203–210
18. Endres CJ, Kolachana BS, Saunders RC et al (1997) Kinetic Modeling of [11C]Raclopride: combined PET-Microdialysis studies. J Cereb Blood Flow Metab 17:932–942
19. Friston KJ, Frith CD, Liddle PF et al (1991) Comparing functional (PET) images: the assessment of significant change. J Cereb Blood Flow Metab 11:690–699
20. Henry PK, Murnane KS, Votaw JR et al (2010) Acute brain metabolic effects of cocaine in rhesus monkeys with a history of cocaine use. Brain Imaging Behav 4:212–219
21. Volkow ND, Fowler JS, Wang GJ et al (2004) Dopamine in drug abuse and addiction: results from imaging studies and treatment implications. Mol Psychiatry 9:557–569
22. Volkow ND, Fowler JS, Wolf AP et al (1991) Changes in brain glucose metabolism in cocaine dependence and withdrawal. Am J Psychiatry 148:621–626
23. Volkow ND, Wang GJ, Ma Y et al (2005) Activation of orbital and medial prefrontal cortex by methylphenidate in cocaine-addicted subjects but not in controls: relevance to addiction. J Neurosci 25:3932–3939

24. Kaisti KK, Metsähonkala L, Teräs M et al (2002) Effects of surgical levels of propofol and sevoflurane anesthesia on cerebral blood flow in healthy subjects studied with positron emission tomography. Anesthesiology 96:1358–1370
25. Matsumura A, Mizokawa S, Tanaka M et al (2003) Assessment of microPET performance in analyzing the rat brain under different types of anesthesia: comparison between quantitative data obtained with microPET and ex vivo autoradiography. Neuroimage 20:2040–2050
26. Alstrup AK, Smith DF (2013) Anaesthesia for positron emission tomography scanning of animal brains. Lab Anim 47:12–18
27. Stabin MG (1996) MIRDOSE: personal computer software for internal dose assessment in nuclear medicine. J Nucl Med 37:538–546
28. ICRP (1988) Radiation dose to patients from radiopharmaceuticals. Publication 53. 18/1–4
29. Cloutier RJ, Watson EE, Rohrer RH et al (1973) Calculating the radiation dose to an organ. J Nucl Med 14:53–55
30. Loevinger R, Berman M (1968) A formalism for calculation of absorbed dose from radionuclides. Phys Med Biol 13:205–217
31. Stabin MG, Sparks RB, Crowe E (2005) OLINDA/EXM: the second-generation personal computer software for internal dose assessment in nuclear medicine. J Nucl Med 46:1023–1027
32. Harrison JD, Streffer C (2007) The ICRP protection quantities, equivalent and effective dose: their basis and application. Radiat Prot Dosimetry 127:12–18

Chapter 4
Population Pharmacokinetics

Ayyappa Chaturvedula

Abstract Population pharmacokinetics is the study of sources and correlates of variability in drug exposure and response. The study of population pharmacokinetics represents an important aspect of drug development and plays a key role in finding the right dose to inform product labeling decisions. Application of novel mathematical and statistical tools to the study of population pharmacokinetics has revolutionized the drug development process. Pharmacostatistical models composed on pharmacokinetic, pharmacodynamic, disease progression, trial design aspects, and econometrics are widely used in decision-making at every stage of drug development. Nonlinear mixed-effects modeling methodology enables the analysis of sparsely collected pharmacokinetic and pharmacodynamic data from large-scale late-stage clinical trials to understand drug exposure–response relationships. Regulatory authorities such as the US FDA and EMEA have supported and worked with pharmaceutical industry to bring about a successful culture of change in drug development, which has evolved into a concept called model-based drug development (MBDD). MBDD uses modeling and simulation to implement a "learn and confirm" paradigm. This chapter is intended to provide the reader with a basic understanding of the various methods involved in population pharmacokinetics with an emphasis on the current gold standard of nonlinear mixed-effects modeling methodology.

Keywords Population pharmacokinetics • Nonlinear mixed-effects modeling (NONMEM) • Pharmacokinetics • Pharmacodynamics • Pharmacometrics

A. Chaturvedula, PhD
Department of Pharmacotherapy, UNT System College of Pharmacy and UNTHSC, Fort Worth, TX 76107, USA
e-mail: Ayyappa.chaturvedula@unthsc.edu

M. Jann et al. (eds.), *Applied Clinical Pharmacokinetics and Pharmacodynamics of Psychopharmacological Agents*,
DOI 10.1007/978-3-319-27883-4_4

Population pharmacokinetics is defined as the study of the variability in plasma drug concentrations between individuals when standard dosage regimens are administered [1]. Studying the sources and correlates of variability in plasma concentrations provides clinicians with important information for designing appropriate dosing regimens. Important sources of interindividual variability in drug exposure may be due to various factors such as food, drug–drug interactions, pathophysiological conditions, and patient demographics.

During the course of new drug development, it is imperative to understand the safety and efficacy of a new chemical entity by taking into account experimental results from preclinical and clinical studies. Clinical development of a drug includes phase I–IV studies in which a candidate compound progresses through studies in healthy volunteers to clinical trials in patient populations. These trials typically require collection of several plasma concentrations followed by pharmacokinetic data analysis (compartmental or non-compartmental methods) and statistical analysis to test the study hypothesis. This method is known as standard, two-stage population pharmacokinetic analysis. The methodology first requires the estimation of individual pharmacokinetic parameters and then calculation of the summaries that represent population parameters (mean and standard deviation); this is followed by hypothesis testing via statistical analysis. This classical clinical pharmacological approach is somewhat limited to the early phase clinical trials with healthy populations where extensive pharmacokinetic sampling is feasible. It is logistically impossible to collect such data in large-scale clinical trials (phase III) where only sparse samples (1–2 samples per subject) are collected at intermittent clinical visits. Data collected in this manner is not amenable to traditional pharmacokinetic analysis; nonetheless, these trials contain plasma concentration data from the relevant patient population in which the drug will ultimately be used.

Lack of pharmacokinetic methodology to analyze sparse data limits the utility of routine therapeutic drug monitoring from actual patient populations. Other approaches such as naïve pooling and naïve averaging of the data have been proposed to handle sparse sample data but were shown to result in large biases in parameter estimates or to lack the inference on variability [2].

The pioneering work by Drs. Sheiner and Beal on nonlinear mixed-effects modeling (NLME) approaches set the stage for sparse sample pharmacokinetic data analysis. The NLME approach is a parametric model-based approach to study population pharmacokinetics. The NLME approach provides unbiased mean pharmacokinetic parameters as well as the estimate of variability by partitioning total variability in parameters into between-subject variability and residual variability [3]. The software developed to implement this analytical approach was named after the analytical method (nonlinear mixed-effects modeling (NONMEM™)) by the University of Southern California and is currently licensed and managed by Icon Development Solutions (Baltimore, MD). Currently, NONMEM™ is considered the gold standard for population pharmacokinetic analysis; however, other software options that use different algorithms for parameter estimation are also available. These include Monolix (Lixoft, France), Phoenix (Certara, USA), ADAPT (BMSR, University of Southern California, USA), and Pmetrics (LAPK, University of

Southern California, USA). Of note, it is now common in the pharmacometrics community to use the term NONMEM to describe the software program as opposed to the NLME analytical approach. Also, for purposes of clarification, the terms "population pharmacokinetics" and "NLME approach" are used interchangeably.

The objective of the current chapter is to describe the basic principles of population pharmacokinetic modeling. This will include basic terminology, statistical concepts of error structures, mixed-effects modeling, and methodology used to build a population pharmacokinetic model. An in-depth mathematical discussion is beyond the scope of this text. For a more extensive discourse, the reader is referred to reviews by Ene et al., Bonate et al., and Giltinan et al., as well as the NONMEM™ user guide (Icon Development Solutions Inc., MD, USA) [2, 4, 5].

4.1 Basic Terminology and Concepts

The term "model" in this chapter refers to a mathematical model that describes the pharmacokinetics or pharmacodynamics of a drug. These mathematical models originate from various compartmental model assumptions and are generally in the form of differential equations that describe the temporal profile of plasma concentrations that result from a particular dosage regimen. For example, the pharmacokinetic profile of a drug that is administered as an IV bolus and follows first-order elimination from a one-compartment model can be described by the following mathematical equation:

$$C_j = \frac{\text{Dose}}{\text{Vd}} e^{-\frac{\text{CL}}{\text{Vd}} * t} \tag{4.1}$$

where Cj represents the concentration at the jth time point and CL and Vd represent clearance and volume of distribution, respectively; t is the time elapsed between dose ingestion and plasma sample collections. The above model consists of dose as input, time as an independent variable, concentration as a dependent variable, and CL and Vd as pharmacokinetic parameters. When a clinical pharmacokinetic experiment is conducted, post-dose plasma samples are collected from an individual at various time points. These data (longitudinal) are then fit to a model such as that described by Eq. 4.1 to estimate individual pharmacokinetic parameters CL and Vd. The process of estimating the parameters by fitting a model to the data is called "modeling." Once the appropriate pharmacokinetic model is fit to the data and pharmacokinetic parameters are estimated, Eq. 4.1 can be used to calculate the resulting plasma concentrations from various inputs (i.e., dose and dosing frequency); this process is referred to as pharmacokinetic simulation. Modeling and simulation have become a vital component of clinical pharmacology and drug development programs, as they provide the tools for building predictive pharmacostatistical models. These predictive models are based on prior preclinical and clinical information and assist investigators in planning future confirmatory (phase III) clinical trials with a greater probability of success [6]. Pharmacometrics can be defined as the branch of science that is concerned with the interplay between mathematical models of biology, pharmacology, disease, and physiology. Pharmacometric data are used to describe and quantify interactions between xenobiotics and patients, including both beneficial and adverse effects [7]. This ideology has given birth to a new approach to developing drugs called model-based drug development (MBDD) [8]. MBDD involves the application of various mathematical and statistical modeling and simulation tools to assist in key drug development decisions, such as dosage selection and clinical trial design.

Pharmacokinetic modeling and simulation are both math and statistic intensive, and a basic appreciation of both is necessary. These topics are briefly addressed here but do not represent an exhaustive review of either subject. For more information, readers are referred to detailed texts on linear algebra, calculus, mathematical statistics, and probability theory. Nevertheless, a brief refresher is provided in this section on the required terminology. Random variables are real-valued functions of a sample space with a probability distribution function. The value of the random variable is determined by the outcome of a particular experiment. Random variables can be discrete, such as categorical scoring for a pharmacodynamic effect or continuous such as plasma concentrations. Expectation of a random variable and a function of a random variable can be calculated from probability theory for both discrete and continuous random variables, representing a weighted average of the possible values that it can take [9]. Random variables can have several probability distributions such as Bernoulli, binomial, Poisson, geometric, hypergeometric, and negative hypergeometric for discrete variables and uniform, normal, exponential, gamma, chi-squared, and Cauchy for continuous variables. Central limit theorem provides the theoretical basis that many random phenomena obey – at least approximately – a normal probability distribution [9]. Normal distribution of a continuous random variable is applicable to many assumptions in population pharmacokinetic modeling. A univariate, normal-variable distribution can be characterized by the mean and variance of that distribution. Multivariate normal-variable distribution can be characterized by a mean and a variance–covariance matrix [4, 9].

4.1.1 Methods for Studying Population Pharmacokinetics

Pharmacokinetic parameters in a population differ between individuals due to intrinsic and extrinsic factors. Intrinsic factors include age, weight, gender, genetics, and metabolic status of individuals, and extrinsic factors include concomitant medications, comorbid conditions, and food. An individual pharmacokinetic model consists of individual pharmacokinetic parameters, while a population pharmacokinetic model consists of population pharmacokinetic parameters and variability parameters. Variability parameters of interest include between-subject variability, between-occasion variability, and residual variability arising from errors in analytical methods, sampling, dosing, etc. For this introductory text, we will not detail the intercession variability. Traditionally, various methods have been applied to the study of population pharmacokinetics. Although some methods are more common than others, we will discuss a variety of such methods to provide a complete picture of their use in the study of population pharmacokinetics. When drug administration and sampling schedules are identical in all subjects in a study, one can take average plasma concentrations across the same time points and fit a model to the mean data. This approach is called naïve average data approach (NAD). It is not a reliable method for estimating population pharmacokinetic parameters because the averaging may completely smooth the pharmacokinetic variability and completely change the temporal pharmacokinetic profile (bi-peak phenomenon in individual pharmacokinetic profile may not be shown in a population average profile). Moreover, this method does not provide any information on the between-subject variability. This approach is currently only being used for preclinical experiments because other sources of variability such as variability between animals or between occasions are less than those observed in a clinical setting [2].

In situations where the sampling schedules are different between individuals, a naïve pooled approach (NPA) can be used. Using this approach, plasma concentrations from all subjects are pooled and fit to a model as if they originated from a single individual [10]. This approach can provide reliable population pharmacokinetic parameter data but as with NAD, it does not provide information on parameter variability. However, this approach has been shown to provide biased estimates when there is higher between-subject variability and heterogeneity in the sampling schedules. A standard two-stage (STS) approach involves the fitting of individual pharmacokinetic data and summarizing mean and variance data to determine population parameters. This method is applicable in situations where extensive sampling is performed; however, simulation studies show that this method provides upward biases in the variability parameters [3, 11, 12].

An NLME approach has been proposed as the appropriate theoretical mathematical framework for analyzing longitudinal pharmacokinetic data from clinical pharmacology studies [5, 10]. The NLME takes a midway compared to STS, NPD, and NPA approaches to appropriately pool the samples from various individuals and fit a population model with parameters of typical pharmacokinetic parameters and variability parameters. This approach can handle sparse samples in individuals (2–3 per subject) and nonuniform study designs and thus can be applied to data from late phase clinical trials and data from routine clinical practice. Some important features of NLME that differ from traditional methods discussed above include (1) collection of relevant pharmacokinetic information from a target population, (2) identification and measurement of variability in drug exposure during development, and (3) determination of the sources and estimating the magnitude of unexplained variability in the patient population [13]. It is vital to prospectively plan a population pharmacokinetic study with regard to study design (sample size, covariate selection), methodology, and analytical plan. The US FDA recommends population pharmacokinetic study designs that include single-trough, multiple-trough, and full-population pharmacokinetic sampling designs. The single-trough design has limited utility in that it only allows for inferences on drug clearance – and only if the samples are collected around the time of the true trough concentration of the drug. This design will not be useful in estimating other pharmacokinetic parameters such as absorption rate constant. The multiple-trough design consists of two or more blood samples obtained near the time of the trough concentration under steady-state conditions. The full-population pharmacokinetic sampling design involves the collection of multiple post-dose samples (typically 1–6) at various times that may differ between individuals [13].

Pharmacokinetic variability was once considered a nuisance variable when it came to data analysis; however, it is now appreciated that the magnitude of random variability is important because drug safety and efficacy are inversely proportional to the unexplainable variability in a drug's pharmacokinetic and pharmacodynamic profile. The model shown in Eq. 4.1 must take into account errors in individual observations. A correct representation of the model is as follows:

$$C_j = \frac{\text{Dose}}{\text{Vd}} e^{-\frac{\text{CL}}{\text{Vd}} * t} + \varepsilon_j \tag{4.2}$$

where ε_j is the error associated with the plasma concentration at the jth time point; generally the errors are assumed to be independent and have a normal distribution with a mean of zero and some (unknown) variance (σ^2). The same model in a population context will have at least another level of variability in addition to the residual error as described above in Eq. 4.2. This additional level of variability is referred to as between-subject variability (BSV) which occurs at the pharmacokinetic parameter level. Interindividual differences in pharmacokinetic parameters must be accounted for in a population model. A typical population model for a group of subjects administered an IV bolus dose is written as follows:

$$C_{ij} = \frac{\text{Dose}_i}{\text{Vd}_i} e^{-\frac{\text{CL}_i}{\text{Vd}_i} * t_{ij}} + \varepsilon_{ij} \tag{4.3}$$

where C_{ij} represents plasma concentration in the ith subject at the jth time point; Dose_i and t_{ij} represent individual dose and time of sample collection, respectively; CL_i and Vd_i represent individual clearance and volume of distribution, respectively. In a population model, we will mathematically relate the individual pharmacokinetic parameters to the population parameters as shown in the equations below:

$$\text{CL}_i = \text{TVCL} * e^{\eta_{1i}} \tag{4.4}$$

$$\text{Vd}_i = \text{TVVd} * e^{\eta_{2i}} \tag{4.5}$$

where TVCL and TVVd are the typical values for population clearance and volume of distribution, respectively; η_i represents the difference between the population parameter and the individual parameter on a logarithmic scale. One can understand this by simply rearranging the variables in Eq. 4.4 or Eq. 4.5:

$$\eta_{1i} = \text{LOG}(\text{CL}_i) - \text{LOG}(\text{TVCL}) \tag{4.6}$$

The LOG in Eq. 4.6 is a natural logarithm, and η_i is the difference between an individual pharmacokinetic parameter and a typical population value. One can see from this equation that η_i can be either a positive or a negative value because a person can have a clearance value that is greater or less than the population average. The η_i is a vital concept to population modeling and mixed-effects concepts; it is discussed in greater detail below.

4.1.2 Fixed Effects, Random Effects, and Mixed Effects

Fixed effects are those variables whose levels represent an exhaustive set of all possible levels. Random effects are variables whose levels do not exhaust the set of possible levels, and each level is equally representative of the other levels [4]. Fixed effects are those that can be measured in an experiment; they include dosages and covariates such as age, gender, race, and creatinine clearance. Fixed effect parameters relate these fixed effects to the population pharmacokinetic parameters in a quantitative manner. For example, if one wants to relate creatinine clearance measured in individuals to the population clearance of a drug given as an IV bolus, then the population model is written as below:

$$C_{ij} = \frac{\text{Dose}_i}{\text{Vd}_i} e^{-\frac{\text{CL}_i}{\text{Vd}_i} * t_{ij}} + \varepsilon_{ij} \quad (\text{without covariate}) \tag{4.3}$$

$$\text{CL}_i = \left(\text{TVCL} * \left(\frac{\text{CRCL}_i}{120} \right)^{\theta} \right) * e^{\eta_{1i}} \quad (\text{with covariate}) \tag{4.7}$$

CRCL_i and θ in Eq. 4.7 represent the individual measured creatinine clearance and effect of creatinine clearance on the typical population estimate of clearance (TVCL), respectively. The individual creatinine clearance is normalized to a reference value of 120 mL/min in this case. The θ in Eq. 4.7 is a fixed effect parameter. The covariate submodel can be in the form of additive, proportional, exponential, or power models [14]. Typical values for pharmacokinetic parameters in the model are also considered a special case of fixed effects, because they do not vary between individuals. Random effect parameter quantifies the random unknown variability in the pharmacokinetic parameters and residual variability in the concentrations. Random effects in the population model include between-subject random effects, which are quantified by between-subject variability, and residual random effects, which are quantified by residual variability or intraindividual variability. Because plasma concentrations are a result of multivariate normal distributions of pharmacokinetic parameters (i.e., multiple parameters in the model have different distributions), the parameters that quantify the random effects are represented in a variance–covariance matrix or covariance matrix. The η_i is assumed to be normally distributed with a mean of zero and a variance of ω_i^2. The population model in Eq. 4.3 will include the following covariance matrix to quantify random effects:

$$\begin{pmatrix} \omega_1^2 & \omega_2\omega_1 \\ \omega_1\omega_2 & \omega_2^2 \end{pmatrix}$$

where ω_1^2 and ω_2^2 represent the variances in η_{1i} and η_{2i} in the population, which represents between-subject variability in clearance and volume of distribution, respectively. The $\omega_2\omega_1$ or $\omega_1\omega_2$ represent covariance between clearance and volume of distribution. Covariance matrices are generally represented as lower triangular matrices because the upper triangular elements are the same as the lower triangular matrix elements. The individual parameter estimates in nonlinear mixed-effects modeling are estimated using Bayesian methodology, and they are generally referred to as empirical Bayes estimates (EBEs). The use of the phrase "empirical Bayes" emphasizes that the parameters for the prior distribution are estimated from the data and are used as if they were known to obtain the posterior distribution [15]. When there is less information in an individual, the model assumes the person to be a typical individual, and the individual parameters shrink toward population parameters. The opposite occurs when there is more information in an individual subject, which means more samples were collected for that person at informative time points. If the population model is adequate, the quality of the individual parameter estimates will depend heavily on the observed data. The variance of EBE distribution will shrink toward zero as the quantity of information at the individual level is reduced; this phenomenon is defined as η-shrinkage. Similarly, in cases where data are less informative, the individual weighted residual (IWRES; discussed below) distribution shrinks toward zero, which is defined as ε-shrinkage and is sometimes called "overfitting" [15].

The residual error (i.e., the difference between model predicted and observed concentration) can have a structure. Most important error structures encountered in pharmacokinetic modeling include additive, proportional, and combination errors. Additive error has the following structure:

$$y_{ij} = ipred_{ij} + \varepsilon_{ij} \tag{4.8}$$

where y_{ij} is the observed data in the ith individual at the jth time point; $ipred_{ij}$ is the predicted concentration in the ith individual at the jth time point and ε_{ij} is the random effect with a mean of zero and a variance of σ^2. Additive error is also called homoscedastic error; this error is not dependent on the magnitude of the prediction (higher or lower concentration). Proportional error, as the name indicates, is proportional to the magnitude of the concentration in the following way:

$$y_{ij} = ipred_{ij}\left(1 + \varepsilon_{ij}\right) \tag{4.9}$$

This is also equivalent to $y_{ij} = ipred_{ij} + ipred_{ij} * \varepsilon_{ij}$.

In this type of error, the higher the concentration, the greater the error, but the coefficient of variation (ratio of the standard deviation to the mean) is constant. Thus, it is also called a constant coefficient variation model. In this model there is an interaction between residual error (ε_{ij}) and between-subject variability (η), due to the dependency of $ipred_{ij}$ on the EBEs. A proper estimation algorithm method that accounts for η-ε interaction should be used to avoid biases in parameter estimation, which will be discussed below. A combination error model combines the additive and proportional error models and is also sometimes called a "slope and intercept" model as shown below:

$$y_{ij} = ipred_{ij}\left(1+\varepsilon_{1ij}\right)+\varepsilon_{2ij} \tag{4.10}$$

where ε_{1ij} and ε_{2ij} represent proportional and additive error components, respectively.

A mathematical model containing both fixed and random effects is called a mixed-effects model. Mixed-effects models can describe a linear or nonlinear relationship between an independent variable and a dependent variable. If the function describing this relationship is a linear model, then it is a linear mixed-effects model and is commonly used to assess bioequivalence data, QTc data, and dose-response relationships [16]. The functions that relate the plasma concentrations (dependent variables) to time (independent variables) are nonlinear as in Eq. 4.3, and nonlinear mixed-effects modeling (NONMEM) methodology is applied. As mixed-effects modeling includes random effect parameters, the optimization methods play an important role in estimating the parameters of the model. Several basic estimation algorithms that are commonly used in NONMEM methodology will be discussed below.

4.2 Estimation Methods Used in NONMEM

Parameter estimation in mixed-effects models is complex; hence ordinary least square-based methods are not optimal when residual variance is dependent on the model parameters [4]. Although estimation methods discussed thus far have focused on those available in NONMEM™, other software packages with slightly different (or the same) algorithms are also available. Most of the NLME methods use maximum likelihood approach for parameter estimation. Likelihood is a conditional probability of an event occurring, given that another event has occurred. The probability of the data to which the model is being fit is written as a function (likelihood function) of model parameters; the maximum likelihood estimates (MLEs) represent where this probability is maximum. Several mathematical approximations were developed to calculate likelihood function to linearize the random effects, due to the nonlinear dependence on the observations [2].

The first-order (FO) approximation was the first to be used and takes a first-order Taylor series expansion of the population model with respect to the random effects around zero. Currently FO is not recommended due to the availability of better approximations such as first-order conditional estimation (FOCE) and first-order conditional estimation with interaction (FOCEI). FOCE takes a first-order Taylor series expansion around the conditional estimates of the interindividual random effect (η_i), instead of zero. The FOCEI method accounts for the interaction between the between-subject and within-subject variability components and should be used when heteroscedastic error models (e.g., proportional error) are used.

A number of newer NLME methods have been introduced based on expectation–maximization principles such as stochastic approximation expectation maximization (SAEM), Monte Carlo importance sampling (IMP, IMPMAP), and Markov chain Monte Carlo (MCMC) Bayesian methods in the newer versions of NONMEM™. The EM-based methods are advantageous because they do not use linearized approximations (e.g., FO, FOCE) and therefore can theoretically induce less bias. MCMC Bayesian methods do not provide point estimates but provide a series of fixed effect parameters that are distributed according to their ability to fit the data. A comparison among FOCEI, ITS, IMP, IMPMAP, and Bayesian methods in a simulated, complex, target-mediated drug disposition model showed that newer methods performed similarly to FOCEI in parameter bias and standard error of the estimate (SE) [17]. It is important to realize that the calculated objective function value that represents the global fit statistic to the data cannot be compared between estimation algorithms, as the method of calculation varies significantly. For instance, the NONMEM™ software calculates the objective function in first-order approximation estimation methods as equivalent to −2* log likelihood, which is approximately distributed to the chi-square ($\chi 2$) statistic with q degrees of freedom, where q is the number of parameters in the model. NONMEM™ objective function can be used for hypothesis testing for hierarchical models, such as covariate analysis; this process is called log likelihood ratio testing. The objective function, calculated using the SAEM method in NONMEM™, cannot be used for hypothesis testing; however, the parameters do represent maximum likelihood estimates. In the newer version of NONMEM™ software, multiple estimation methods can be used where SAEM is used for parameter estimation and important sampling-based methods (IMP, IMPMAP) for hypothesis testing and calculation of asymptotic standard error of parameters. Readers are referred to the NONMEM™ technical guide for mathematical derivations and further information on the differences in objective functions [18–20].

4.2.1 General Principles of Population Pharmacokinetic Model Development

Population pharmacokinetic models are hierarchical in nature in that they have a structural pharmacokinetic model, a covariate submodel, and a statistical model. The structural model consists of the compartmental model equation that describes the temporal profile of plasma concentrations. The statistical model includes submodels that may incorporate between-subject variability or interindividual variability, residual variability or intraindividual variability, and between-occasion variability. The structural model is generally based on a prior understanding of a drug's pharmacokinetics from preclinical studies or phase I studies where extensive sampling was performed.

When only sparse data are available, the ability to identify a more complex compartmental model is compromised. For example, data from a drug that is optimally described by a two-compartment model may fit a one-compartment model better if plasma concentrations are missing during the drug's distribution phase. Identifiability of a model and its parameters is an important consideration when framing a structural model. Structural identifiability is the ability to uniquely estimate a model's parameters. Parameter identifiability is the ability to estimate a structurally identifiable model [4].

Let us consider a compartmental model that consists only of plasma concentration samples, yet we desire to estimate both renal and nonrenal clearance. It is impossible to separate these two parameters unless either the urine compartment or the nonrenal compartment (metabolite) is sampled. These identifiability issues arise quickly when the model gets complicated such as parent drug–metabolite models where both a parent drug and its metabolite are modeled in an integrated model such as in Fig. 4.2. In this model, it is not possible to estimate all three parameters: (1) metabolite formation rate, (2) volume of the metabolite compartment, and (3) metabolite elimination rate [21]. Generally, some assumptions involving the metabolic fraction or volume of metabolite compartments are made so that only two of the three parameters are estimated. Statistical models consist of between-subject variability in pharmacokinetic parameters and residual variability that cannot be explained by the between-subject variability. An exponential error model is generally used for between-subject variability in pharmacokinetic parameters to represent the log-normal distribution because negative values for pharmacokinetic parameters are not meaningful. Residual error models were discussed in the previous section, namely, proportional, additive, and combination error models.

First, a base model that includes a structural model with random effect parameters will be finalized. Generally, the base model will not contain any covariates. However, it is now common to include weight as a covariate for volume and clearance parameters based on established allometric scaling methods [22, 23]. The base model provides individual pharmacokinetic parameters (EBEs), which are used to evaluate potential covariate relationships using plots of EBEs versus covariates such as age, weight, and gender. When a large number of covariates are present, several screening methods are proposed, which use generalized additive modeling and Wald's approximation to the likelihood ratio test [24, 25]. It is important to have an extensive discussion between the clinical and pharmacometrics teams to determine which covariates should be included in the model; this should be determined by clinical relevance and final utility of the model. Covariate modeling represents the model-based hypothesis testing framework and actually represents the act of finding sources and correlates of variability as per the definition of population pharmacokinetics. Two important methods currently used in covariate modeling are stepwise addition and full model estimation [26–28].

Stepwise covariate modeling includes a forward addition step where covariates are progressively added based on their statistical significance and a backward elimination step where each of the covariate parameters entered in the forward addition step are removed, and the statistical result is evaluated. As mentioned, the objective function that is used as global goodness of fit is a χ^2 statistic. For hierarchical models, the drop in objective function value by 3.84 points with an addition of one new parameter addition compared to the base model (no covariates) is statistically significant (α=0.05). When a significant covariate is removed from the model, the objective function must increase by a similar magnitude. In stepwise addition, generally, a lower significance step is selected (α=0.05 or lower) compared to backward elimination (α=0.01 or higher); this is done to control for false positives. There is an automated computer program that performs stepwise covariate modeling (SCM); it is available in PsN tools [29]. For nonhierarchical models, Akaike criterion can be used for model selection [30].

For full model evaluation, it is recommended to add clinically relevant covariates and to construct a full model without statistical significance and then reduce the model by backward elimination. In this approach clinical relevance and utility of the covariate in clinical practice are more important than statistical significance [27, 31]. In cases where there is no covariate available but the base model shows clear multimodal distribution of EBEs, one can apply mixture models to assign an individual to two or more models. Mixture modeling helps to explain such multimodal distributions, and also the probability of each mixture population is estimated as a parameter [32]. The objective function value (OFV) that is minimized in mixture model is the sum of the OFVs for each patient (OFV_i), which in turn is the sum across the k subpopulations ($OFV_{i,k}$). The individual probability of belonging to a subpopulation can be calculated using the OFV in that individual together with the total probability in the population [33]. An example of mixture model for risperidone is discussed in the subsequent sections.

4.2.2 Evaluation of a Population Model

Population pharmacokinetic model development involves fitting several (100 or more) models with varying structural, statistical, and covariate models to come up with a parsimonious model that has no redundant parameters and is also an irreducible model. Several model diagnostics are commonly used to make decisions at every stage of modeling. Commonly used diagnostics include likelihood-based objective function value modulation, basic goodness of fit plots, residual plots, standard error of estimates, and normalized predicted distribution errors (NPDE). The likelihood objective function value is a global objective measure of model fit and can be used to retain a parameter in the model using the LRT method for hierarchical models. It is important to recognize that the LRT method theoretically does not apply to parameters with boundary conditions such as between-subject variability parameters and absorption lag time. However, the LRT method is applicable for inclusion decisions for covariance parameters (covariance can be a positive or negative value).

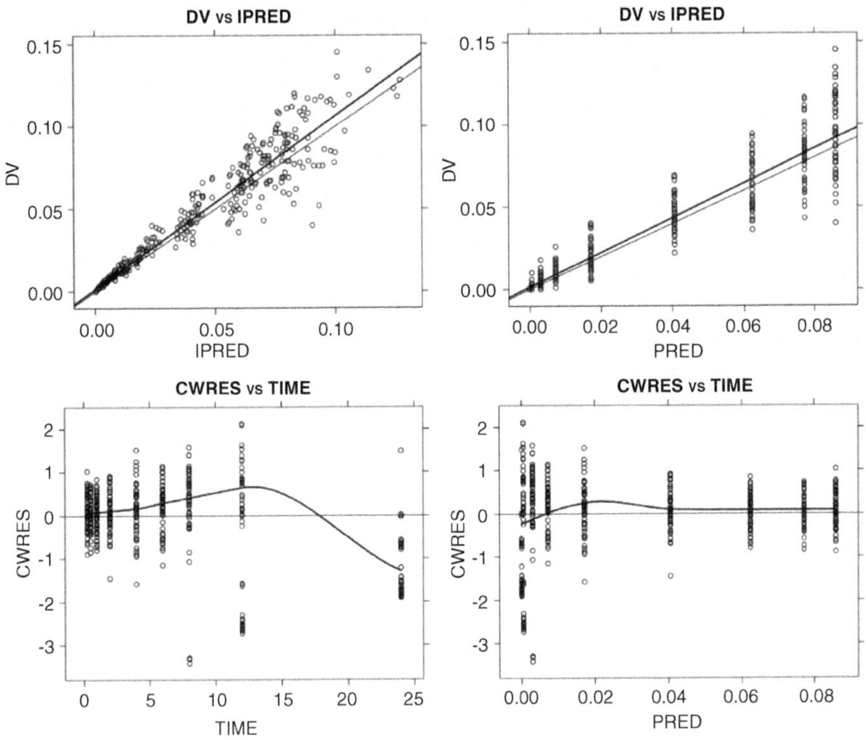

Fig. 4.1 Basic goodness of fit plots in population pharmacokinetic model evaluation. Plots in *top panel* have a line of identity (*lighter solid line*) and a regression line (*darker solid line*) as trend line. Plots in *bottom panel* have a (*lighter solid*) *horizontal line* at zero and a (*darker solid*) smooth line as trend line. The data was simulated from a one-compartment IV bolus model in NONMEM and refitted to the model to generate these plots

Diagnostic plots are generally created using XPOSE library in R software, which is created specifically for evaluating population pharmacokinetic models [34, 35]. These plots will enable the modeler to visually inspect whether the model-predicted concentrations match the observed data and to also check model assumptions such as normality of random effects, statistical outliers, and covariate relationships.

Population modeling results in individual predictions (IPRED), population predictions (PRED), residuals (RES, IWRES, CWRES, WRES, etc.), and EBEs. These variables are used along with covariates and time after dose to prepare diagnostic plots or goodness of fit (GOF) plots. The most commonly reported plots for population pharmacokinetic models and those recommended by regulatory guidance agencies are discussed here. PREDs account for explainable between-subject variability by covariates, and IPREDs have additional between-subject variability [14]. A plot of observed data (DV) versus IPRED and PRED shows any structural model misspecifications or need of covariates to explain variability. A line of identity (solid line in Fig. 4.1 with a slope of one) and trend line (dark solid line in Fig. 4.1, preferably a regression line) are recommended for DV versus IPRED or PRED plots. Any deviations between the line of identity and trend line represent potential model misspecification. The DV versus PRED plots are more sensitive to covariate effects and the modeler looks for perceivable differences and lack of correlations before and after inclusion of a particular covariate. The DV versus IPRED plots can look artificially better in case of shrinkage (>30 %). Commonly calculated residuals in population modeling include individual weighted residuals (IWRES), weighted residuals (WRES), and conditional weighted residuals (CWRES).

Residual is defined as the difference between observed concentration and predicted concentration in an individual. WRES is calculated as the ratio of residual-to-weight (generally variance) and is calculated based on FO approximation. WRES is not appropriate to use with FOCE or FOCEI approximations to the true model. CWRES is calculated based on FOCE approximation and have better qualities in identifying model misspecification [36]. The time after dose versus CWRES or IWERS plot with a horizontal line at 0 and a trend line is recommended for checking the independence of the residuals with the independent variable, which is a fundamental assumption in regression analysis. The trend line (preferably a smooth line) should be horizontal and must not show any trends (Fig. 4.1, bottom panel). The same should be the case with PRED versus residual plots. It is also suggested that any individual observations with an absolute CWRES > 6 be identified as statistical outliers, as the CWRES has a mean of zero and unit variance [31]. The SE is generated from the variance–covariance matrix during the minimization process; 95 % confidence intervals of the parameters can be calculated as the parameter estimate ± 2*SE. Generally, SE greater than or equal to 50 % represents a parameter with high imprecision [30]. The histograms and Q–Q (quantile–quantile) plots of EBEs are used to check the assumption of normality. If all points fall on the line of unity, then the normality assumption is satisfied (Fig. 4.2). NPDE is a simulation-based diagnostic that is used for model discrimination. By derivation, NPDE follows a standard normal distribution (normal distribution with mean of 0 and standard deviation of 1); any deviations from the model-predicted NPDE indicate a misspecification of the model [37]. Some other plots that are commonly used in population pharmacokinetic model development include IPRED versus time after dose, parameter versus parameter correlations, and EBE versus EBE plots [38].

Once a final model is selected, several computing-intensive statistical methods are used for qualification and validation. These include visual predictive check (VPC), numerical predictive check (NPC), bootstrapping, cross-validation, and jack-knifing methods. VPC is a simulation-based diagnostic that takes into account all the model components (structural, fixed, and random effects) and is used to make model comparisons, suggest model improvements, and support appropriateness of a model. VPC is conducted by first simulating several datasets with the same design aspects as the clinical trial that generated the observed data used for model development. Then percentiles (5th, 50th, and 95th) of the all simulated concentrations (not to be confused with IPRED or PRED) and overlaying in a plot with observed data percentiles for the same. The entire distribution

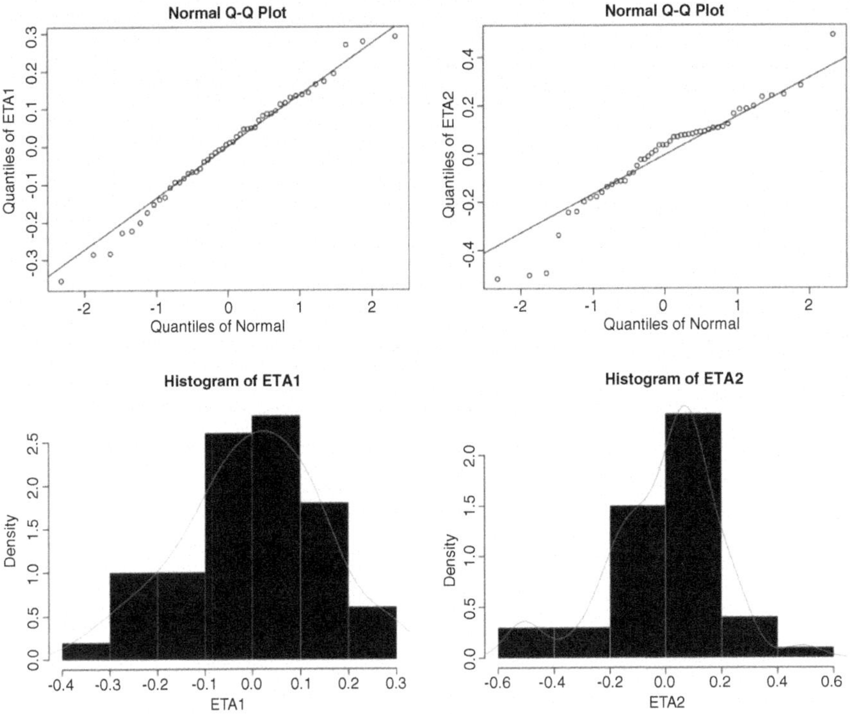

Fig. 4.2 Histograms and Q–Q plots of the between-subject random effects from the same model in Fig. 4.1 to check the assumption of normality. A probability density curve was added to the histogram. Any deviation from the line of unity in Q–Q plot represents the deviation from the normality assumption. ETA1 and ETA2 represent the random effect parameters on clearance and volume of distribution, respectively

of the observed data should match the predicted data from the model [39]. When there are major differences in study design, such as different doses and sample collection times, it is recommended to use standardized VPC and prediction-corrected VPC, which are preferred over traditional VPCs [40, 41]. Numerical predictive check is very similar to VPC except instead of a visual display of concentrations, a metric (i.e., AUC) is calculated from simulated datasets and compared to the observed data. Bootstrapping is a resampling-based technique where original data are resampled to create several bootstrap samples; the final model is then fit to all the samples to calculate the nonparametric CIs of the parameters and distributions. These CIs are generally considered more reliable than the parametric SE-based CIs calculated from the variance–covariance matrix. Please refer to extensive descriptions on the cross-validation and jack-knifing techniques that can identify influential subjects and provide a more robust evaluation of the predictive capabilities of a model [42, 44].

4.2.3 Population Pharmacokinetic Modeling of Antipsychotics

In this section, several examples of population pharmacokinetic modeling applied to antipsychotic drugs are reviewed. Feng et al. reported an integrated population pharmacokinetic model for risperidone after oral administration from highly sparse sampling measurements from the CATIE study [43]. Risperidone is an atypical antipsychotic with selected antagonistic properties at serotonin 5-HT2 and dopamine D2 receptors [44]. The structural model was a one-compartment model with first-order absorption for risperidone that was linked to the active metabolite (9-hydroxy risperidone) compartment by formation clearance. The fraction of parent drug converted to metabolite was estimated as a function of parent clearance. Due to identifiability issues, it was assumed that the volume of the metabolite compartment was the same as that of the parent compartment. In this study, a total of 1236 plasma risperidone and 9-hydroxy risperidone concentrations were collected in 490 subjects. A clear multimodal distribution in individual risperidone clearance parameters was observed in the base model; this was likely due to the fact that risperidone is metabolized by the polymorphic cytochrome P 450 (CYP) 2D6 enzyme [45]. Therefore, a mixture modeling approach in the clearance parameter was utilized to capture the CYP2D6 polymorphism and explain the multimodal distribution in risperidone clearance. The mixture model was able to capture the CYP2D6 poor metabolizers (PM), intermediate metabolizers (IM), and extensive metabolizers (EM) successfully. The probability of being a PM, IM, or EM was estimated at 41 %, 52 %, and 7 %, respectively. The final model identified age as a significant covariate affecting 9-hydroxyrisperidone clearance.

Data from the above investigation suggest that older individuals may experience higher exposure to the active 9-hydroxy metabolite, thereby placing them at risk for toxicity. Combination error models with additive and proportional components were separately estimated for risperidone and its 9-hydroxy metabolite. Sherwin et al. applied the above model to data from 28 children and adolescents and successfully described the data, thereby suggesting that this model may be potentially useful for individualizing risperidone therapy in this population [46].

Thyssen et al. studied the population pharmacokinetics of oral risperidone in children, adolescents, and adults [47]. The modeling was conducted using a pooled dataset of 304 pediatric and 476 adult subject plasma concentration samples. Different models were developed for risperidone and active antipsychotic fraction (calculated as risperidone plus 9-hydroxyrisperidone concentrations at each sample collection time point). The structural model consisted of two compartments with first-order absorption, with body weight added as a covariate on clearance, and volume parameters based on allometric principles. Testing for statistical significance by LRT was not performed. In contrast to the study conducted by Feng et al. [43] mixture modeling was employed to describe the oral bioavailability of risperidone. Data from two subpopulations, representing PMs and EMs were modeled. Age and creatinine clearance were identified as significant covariates affecting the risperidone clearance. The probability of being an EM or a PM was estimated at 19 % and 81 %, respectively. Simulations from the model showed that risperidone and the active antipsychotic fraction were similar in children, adolescents, and adults.

Like risperidone, clozapine is another atypical antipsychotic; it is used in the treatment of refractory schizophrenia. After oral administration, clozapine is extensively metabolized by CYP1A2 to form the pharmacologically active metabolite, norclozapine. Ismail et al. characterized the population pharmacokinetics of clozapine and norclozapine in an integrated model [48]. Data from this investigation were collected retrospectively and fit to a final model that included one compartment for the parent compound and one compartment for the metabolite. The volume for the metabolite compartment was fixed to twice the amount of the parent compartment to avoid the identifiability issue. The fraction of conversion of clozapine to norclozapine was estimated separately for tablet and suspension formulations and found to be 0.015 and 0.4, respectively. Age and gender were significant covariates affecting the clearance of norclozapine. Different absorption rate constants were estimated for different formulations, with tablet and suspension formulations displaying a more rapid absorption compared to tablet formulations [48].

4.3 Summary and Conclusion

Population pharmacokinetic modeling provides valuable tools for studying the pharmacokinetics of drugs in a real world patient population. Model development is typically performed in a stepwise manner in which a hierarchical model is built that contains both structural and statistical components. Population pharmacokinetic modeling involves an understanding and mastery of several key disciplines, including math, statistics, pharmacology, and pharmacokinetics. Expertise in all of these disciplines must be carefully applied to concentration versus time data to synthesize appropriate population pharmacokinetic models that can be used to optimize drug therapy.

Acknowledgment The author would like to express his sincere gratitude and thanks to Mr. Raj Thatavarthi and Mr. Karthik Lingineni at GVK Biosciences Pvt., Ltd., for helping in procuring literature and plots.

References

1. Aarons L (1991) Population pharmacokinetics: theory and practice. Br J Clin Pharmacol 32:669–670
2. Ette EI, Williams PJ, Ahmad A (2007) In: Williams PJ, Ette EI (eds) Pharmacometrics: the science of quantitative pharmacology, John Wiley & Sons Inc, Hoboken, pp 265–285

3. Sheiner LB, Beal SL (1980) Evaluation of methods for estimating population pharmacokinetics parameters. I. Michaelis-Menten model: routine clinical pharmacokinetic data. J Pharmacokinet Biopharm 8:553–571
4. Bonate PL (2011) Pharmacokinetic and pharmacodynamic modeling and simulation, 2nd edn. Springer Science+Business Media, LLC, New York, NY, USA
5. Giltinan MD, David M (1885) Nonlinear models for repeated measurement data (Chapman & Hall/CRC monographs on statistics & applied probability). Springer, New York, NY, USA
6. Sheiner LB (1997) Learning versus confirming in clinical drug development. Clin Pharmacol Ther 61:275–291
7. Barrett JS, Fossler MJ, Cadieu KD et al (2008) Pharmacometrics: a multidisciplinary field to facilitate critical thinking in drug development and translational research settings. J Clin Pharmacol 48:632–649
8. Lalonde RL, Kowalski KG, Hutmacher MM et al (2007) Model-based drug development. Clin Pharmacol Ther 82:21–32
9. Ross S (2014) A first course in probability, 9th edn. Pearson Education Limited, Harlow, England
10. Sheiner LB (1984) The population approach to pharmacokinetic data analysis: rationale and standard data analysis methods. Drug Metab Rev 15:153–171
11. Sheiner LB, Beal SL (1981) Evaluation of methods for estimating population pharmacokinetic parameters. II. Biexponential model and experimental pharmacokinetic data. J Pharmacokinet Biopharm 9:635–651
12. Sheiner LB, Beal SL (1983) Evaluation of methods for estimating population pharmacokinetic parameters. III. Monoexponential model: routine clinical pharmacokinetic data. J Pharmacokinet Biopharm 11:303–319
13. The US FDA (1999) www.fda.gov. [Online]. http://www.fda.gov/Drugs/GuidanceComplianceRegulatoryInformation/Guidances/ucm064982.htm
14. Mould D, Upton R (2012) Basic concepts in population modeling, simulation, and model-based drug development. CPT Pharmacometrics Syst Pharmacol 1:e6
15. Savic RM, Karlsson MO (2009) Importance of shrinkage in empirical bayes estimates for diagnostics: problems and solutions. AAPS J 11:558–569
16. Florian JA, Tornøe CW, Brundage R et al (2011) Population pharmacokinetic and concentration—QTc models for moxifloxacin: pooled analysis of 20 thorough QT studies. J Clin Pharmacol 51:1152–1162
17. Gibiansky L, Gibiansky E, Bauer R (2012) Comparison of Nonmem 7.2 estimation methods and parallel processing efficiency on a target-mediated drug disposition model. J Pharmacokinet Pharmacodyn 39:17–35
18. Beal SL, Sheiner LB (1992) NONMEM users guide- part VII. Conditional estimation methods. University of California, San Francisco
19. Bauer RJ (2013) NONMEM 7 technical guide. ICON Development Solutions Ellicott City, Maryland
20. Wang Y (2007) Derivation of various NONMEM estimation methods. J Pharmacokinet Pharmacodyn 34:575–593
21. Bertrand J, Céline M, Laffont CM et al (2011) Development of a complex parent-metabolite joint population pharmacokinetic model. AAPS J 13:390–404
22. Anderson BJ, McKee D, Holford NH (1997) Size, myths and the clinical pharmacokinetics of analgesia in paediatric patients. Clin Pharmacokinet 33:313–327
23. Holford NH (1996) A size standard for pharmacokinetics. Clin Pharmacokinet 30:329–332
24. Mandema JW, Verotta D, Sheiner LB (1992) Building population pharmacokinetic– pharmacodynamic models. I. Models for covariate effects. J Pharmacokinet Biopharm 20:511–528

25. Kowalski KG, Hutmacher MM (2001) Efficient screening of covariates in population models using Wald's approximation to the likelihood ratio test. J Pharmacokinet Pharmacodyn 28:253–275
26. Wählby U, Jonsson EN, Karlsson MO (2002) Comparison of stepwise covariate model building strategies in population pharmacokinetic-pharmacodynamic analysis. AAPS PharmSci 4:E27
27. Gastonguay M (2004) A full model estimation approach for covariate effects: inference. AAPS meeting abstract W4354
28. Gastonguay M (2011) Full covariate models as an alternative to methods relying on statistical significance for inferences about covariate effects: a review of methodology and 42 case studies. PAGE Abstract
29. Lindbom L, Ribbing J, Jonsson EN (2004) Perl-speaks-NONMEM (PsN) – a Perl module for NONMEM related programming. Comput Methods Programs Biomed 75:85–94
30. Boeckmann AJ, Sheiner LB, Beal SL (2003) NONMEM user guide- part V, NONMEM Project Group, University of California, San Francisco.
31. Byon W, Smith MK, Chan P et al (2013) Establishing best practices and guidance in population modeling: an experience with an internal population pharmacokinetic analysis guidance. CPT Pharmacometrics Syst Pharmacol 2:e51
32. Frame B (2007) Mixture modeling with NONMEM V. Pharmacometrics: the science of quantitative pharmacology. Science+Business Media, LLC, New York, NY, USA. pp 723–757
33. Carlsson KC, Savic RM, Hooker AB et al (2009) Modeling subpopulations with the $MIXTURE subroutine in NONMEM: finding the individual probability of belonging to a subpopulation for the use in model analysis and improved decision making. AAPS J 11:148–154
34. Jonsson EN, Karlsson MO (1999) Xpose – an S-PLUS based population pharmacokinetic/pharmacodynamic model building aid for NONMEM. Comput Methods Programs Biomed 58:51–64
35. R: a language and environment for statistical. R (2014) http://www.R-project.org/
36. Hooker AC, Staatz CE, Karlsson MO (2007) Conditional weighted residuals (CWRES): a model diagnostic for the FOCE method. Pharm Res 24:2187–2197
37. Comets E, Brendel K, Mentré F (2008) Computing normalised prediction distribution errors to evaluate nonlinear mixed-effect models: the npde add-on package for R. Comput Methods Programs Biomed 90:154–166
38. Jonsson NE, Hooker A. xpose.sourceforge.net/bestiarium_v1.0.pdf. xpose.sourceforge.net. [Online] xpose.sourceforge.net
39. Karlsson MO, Holford NH. (2008) A tutorial on visual predictive checks. PAGE 17 abstract: 1434.
40. Wang DD, Zhang S (2012) Standardized visual predictive check versus visual predictive check for model evaluation. J Clin Pharmacol 52:39–54
41. Bergstrand M, Hooker AC, Wallin JE, Karlsson MO (2011) Prediction-corrected visual predictive checks for diagnosing nonlinear mixed-effects models. AAPS J 13:143–151
42. Colby E, Bair E (2013) Cross-validation for nonlinear mixed effects models. J Pharmacokinet Pharmacodyn 40:243–252
43. Feng Y, Pollock BG, Coley K et al (2008) Population pharmacokinetic analysis for risperidone using highly sparse sampling measurements from the CATIE study. Br J Clin Pharmacol 66:629–639

44. Leysen JE, Gommeren W, Eens A et al (1988) Biochemical profile of risperidone, a new antipsychotic. J Pharmacol Exp Ther 247:661–670
45. Fang J, Bourin M, Baker GB (1999) Metabolism of risperidone to 9-hydroxyrisperidone by human cytochromes P450 2D6 and 3A4. Naunyn Schmiedebergs Arch Pharmacol 359:147–151
46. Sherwin CM, Saldaña SN, Bies RR et al (2012) Population pharmacokinetic modeling of risperidone and 9-hydroxyrisperidone to estimate CYP2D6 subpopulations in children and adolescents. Ther Drug Monit 34:535–544
47. Thyssen A, Vermeulen A, Fuseau E et al (2010) Population pharmacokinetics of oral risperidone in children, adolescents and adults with psychiatric disorders. Clin Pharmacokinet 49:465–478
48. Ismail Z, Wessels AM, Uchida H et al (2012) Age and sex impact clozapine plasma concentrations in inpatients and outpatients with schizophrenia. Am J Geriatr Psychiatry 20:53–60

Chapter 5
Drug Transporters

Scott R. Penzak

Abstract Membrane transporters are present in a variety of anatomical locations and organ systems throughout the body. Transporters control the absorption, distribution, intracellular penetration, and excretion of numerous drugs. ATP-binding cassette (ABC) and solute carrier (SLC) superfamilies comprise the majority of clinically relevant transport proteins. In intestinal and liver epithelia, transport proteins control the access of certain medications to systemic circulation. In the kidney, transporters may facilitate or impair drug excretion depending on their specific location and function. However, it is at the blood-brain barrier (BBB) where membrane transporters regulate access of endogenous and exogenous compounds to the central nervous system (CNS). This chapter will review the common drug transport proteins in the intestine and liver as they impact the systemic exposure of drugs that exert their primary pharmacologic effects in the CNS; drug transporters in the kidney that may influence the excretion of such agents will also be addressed. The primary focus of this chapter will be drug transport of centrally acting agents at the BBB, primarily via the efflux transporter and *ABCB1* gene product, P-glycoprotein (P-gp). Additional transport proteins will be considered for their documented or putative involvement in drug interactions involving centrally acting medications. Lastly, approaches to circumvent the influence of drug efflux at the BBB will be considered, including modulation of centrally located membrane transporters. Approaches to developing drugs that bypass the effects of efflux transporters at the BBB will also be discussed.

Keywords Drug transport • Blood-brain barrier (BBB) • P-glycoprotein (P-gp) • Organic anion transporting polypeptide (OATP) • *ABCB1* • Central nervous system (CNS) • Depression • Schizophrenia • Analgesia • Epilepsy

S.R. Penzak, PharmD, FCP
Department of Pharmacotherapy, University of North Texas, Health Sciences Center, System College of Pharmacy, 3500 Camp Bowie Blvd – RES 411A, Fort Worth, TX 76107, USA
e-mail: scott.penzak@unthsc.edu

M. Jann et al. (eds.), *Applied Clinical Pharmacokinetics and Pharmacodynamics of Psychopharmacological Agents*,
DOI 10.1007/978-3-319-27883-4_5

Membrane transporters are present in a variety of anatomical locations and organ systems throughout the body. In their various roles, these transporters control the absorption, distribution, intracellular penetration, access to organs, and excretion of many drugs. Currently, more than 400 transport proteins have been identified, which primarily include transporters from the ATP-binding cassette (ABC) and solute carrier (SLC) superfamilies [1]. In intestinal and liver epithelia, transport proteins can control the access of medications to systemic circulation [2]. In the kidney, transporters may facilitate or impair drug excretion depending on their specific location and function [3]. However, it is at the blood-brain barrier (BBB) where membrane transporters regulate access of numerous endogenous and exogenous compounds to the central nervous system (CNS) [4]. The blood-cerebrospinal fluid (CSF) barrier also contains transport systems that can control permeability of the choroid plexus (CP) membrane to xenobiotics [5]. Accordingly, the ability of drug transporters to regulate access of medications to the CNS is particularly important for drugs that exert pharmacologic effects (efficacy and/or toxicity) on receptor systems located in the brain. Indeed, a number of agents used for the treatment of schizophrenia, seizure disorders, depression, pain, and anxiety are substrates for transport proteins present at the BBB, particularly P-glycoprotein. P-glycoprotein (P-gp) is an efflux transporter and *ABCB1* gene product that has been studied more than any other transporter [4, 6]. Pharmacologic modulation (inhibition or induction) of P-gp at the BBB has the potential to alter the distribution characteristics of substrate medications and either enhance or reduce their penetration into the CNS; this may result in clinically relevant drug-drug interactions. In addition, *ABCB1* genetic polymorphisms impact P-gp expression, which has the potential to influence drug entry into the CNS [7].

This chapter will review the common drug transport proteins in the intestine and liver as they impact the systemic exposure of drugs that exert their primary pharmacologic effects in the CNS; drug transporters in the kidney that may influence the excretion of such agents will also be addressed. However, the primary focus of this chapter will be drug transport of centrally acting agents at the BBB, primarily via P-gp. Data from humans, animals, and in vitro cellular systems will be assessed with regard to specific transport mechanisms that influence drug access to the brain. Individual transport proteins will be considered for their documented or putative involvement in drug interactions involving centrally acting medications. Lastly, approaches to circumvent the influence of drug efflux at the BBB will be considered, including modulation of centrally located membrane transporters. Approaches to developing drugs that bypass the effects of efflux transporters at the BBB will also be discussed.

5.1 Presystemic Drug Transport in the Gastrointestinal Tract

Orally administered medications that exert their pharmacologic effects in the central nervous system (CNS) must first achieve adequate systemic concentrations prior to distribution across the BBB. This process involves absorption via the gastrointestinal (GI) tract and passage through the liver. A number of variables can influence drug absorption, including GI pH, presystemic intestinal metabolism, gastric emptying time, drug solubility and permeability, presence or absence of food, and drug transport processes [2, 8].

A number of uptake and efflux transporters have been identified in human enterocytes [2]. Uptake transport proteins are located on the apical (luminal) or basolateral (abluminal; blood) cell membranes and facilitate xenobiotic uptake into enterocytes – a gradient-mediated process that largely tends to potentiate drug absorption [2]. The major uptake transporters include the two solute carrier superfamilies, SLC and SLCO (2). The SLCO family consists of the organic anion transporting polypeptides (OATP) such as OATP1A2, OATP2B1, OATP3A1, and OATP4A1. The SLC superfamily contains a large number of transporters including organic anion transporters (OAT), organic cation transporters (OCT), the electroneutral organic cation transporters (OCTN), the equilibrative nucleoside transporters (ENT), and others [2]. There is currently a paucity of information with regard to which psychoactive agents, if any, are transported by these intestinal uptake proteins in the GI tract [2].

Similar to uptake transporters, efflux transport proteins are also located on the apical and basolateral membranes of enterocytes; however, unlike uptake transporters, efflux transport proteins, at the apical membrane, extrude drugs from enterocytes and pump them back into the intestinal lumen, thereby reducing their absorption [2]. Efflux transporters expressed in intestinal tissue include members of the ATP-binding cassette superfamily, which includes P-glycoprotein (P-gp), multidrug resistance proteins 1–6 (MRP1-MRP6), and breast cancer-related protein (BCRP) [9, 10].

Numerous preclinical studies using in vitro cellular systems and *mdr1* (ABCB1) knockout mice (mice lacking *mdr1*, which subsequently do not express P-gp) have documented the involvement of P-gp on drug absorption [11]. A general finding in these studies is that the absence or pharmacologic inhibition of intestinal P-gp results in reduced efflux and increased absorption of P-gp substrates; this may result in increased toxicity or enhanced efficacy of the substrate medication. A potentially clinically relevant example of such an interaction in humans is the 1.5-fold increase in the AUC of the antidepressant and P-gp substrate paroxetine ($P<0.5$) that occurred when it was coadministered with the P-gp inhibitor itraconazole [12]. However, despite its role as an efflux transporter in intestinal tissue, P-gp does not always significantly limit the absorption of orally administered substrate medications [13, 14]. To clarify, just because a drug is a P-gp substrate does not automatically imply that it will be poorly absorbed through the GI tract secondary to P-gp-mediated efflux. Many drugs that are well-described P-gp substrates display reasonably good bioavailability; this is likely due to saturation of intestinal P-gp at clinically relevant doses of these agents (where GI drug concentrations are in the mg/mL range) [15]. Examples of centrally acting P-gp substrates that achieve adequate oral availability include aripiprazole, risperidone, lamotrigine, and citalopram [16–19]. Typically, drugs that are most likely to experience reduced absorption secondary to P-gp-mediated efflux include those that are poorly water soluble, dissolve slowly, and are large in size [20]. Examples of centrally acting agents that meet these criteria are rare, with paliperidone being an exception [21]. Conversely, induction of intestinal P-gp would be expected to reduce the bioavailability of substrate medications, potentially compromising their pharmacologic activity in the CNS. It also bears mentioning that anatomical sites beyond the GI tract (brain, liver, and kidney) are likely to encounter lower plasma concentrations of orally administered P-gp substrates (i.e., ng/mL) that do not saturate this transporter and are amenable to P-gp-mediated efflux and subsequent drug interactions [22].

Intestinal P-gp can influence the absorption of substrate medications by effluxing substrate medications into the intestinal lumen and reducing absorption; the co-role of intestinal CYP3A4-mediated metabolism must also be considered for drugs that are substrates for both of these intestinal proteins. In such cases, a drug is absorbed into the enterocyte and is then extruded back into the intestinal lumen prior to presystemic metabolism by CYP3A4. After extrusion into the lumen, the drug is once again passively absorbed where it reencounters CYP3A4 [23]. Thus, intestinal CYP3A4 "sees" the drug multiple times; this increases intracellular contact time between the drug and CYP3A4 and augments the degree of intestinal metabolism that the drug undergoes [23]. Thus, P-gp (and presumably other intestinal efflux proteins) works in concert with CYP3A4 to protect the body from potentially dangerous foreign substances, which include medications. A number of centrally acting medications including diazepam, aprepitant, aripiprazole, buspirone, haloperidol, methadone, ondansetron, pimozide, risperidone, ziprasidone, and zolpidem are substrates for P-gp and CYP3A4 (to varying degrees) [21, 24–32]. Since the majority of these agents are readily orally bioavailable (>60 % in most cases), it is unlikely that P-gp, under normal conditions, potentiates the presystemic metabolism of these agents by CYP3A4. Nonetheless, it is possible that induction of P-gp by agents such as St. John's wort, rifampin, or other P-gp inducers may enhance the CYP3A4-mediated metabolism of these agents and lower their bioavailability upon oral administration.

Intestinal absorption may also be influenced by single nucleotide polymorphisms (SNPs) in the genes that encode for various transport proteins in the GI tract [33]. This is most notably appreciated among the *ABCB1* gene, which encodes for P-glycoprotein. The presence of T alleles at positions 3435, 2677, and 1236 has generally been associated with decreased expression and increased plasma concentrations of a number of substrate medications, although it bears mentioning that opposite results have also been reported in which C,G, and C alleles at these respective positions correlated with increased absorption of the P-gp substrate digoxin [34–36]. Lazarowski et al. reported persistently subtherapeutic plasma concentrations of the P-gp substrate anticonvulsant medications, phenytoin and phenobarbital, in a patient with refractory epilepsy who overexpressed *ABCB1* [37]. These data suggest that drug absorption was limited in this patient secondary to increased intestinal P-gp-mediated efflux, which resulted in inadequate drug exposure and uncontrolled epilepsy. In a separate report exemplifying the impact of intestinal P-gp expression on the absorption of psychoactive medications, a higher fluvoxamine concentration/dose ratio was found among men with depression who possessed the

3435 TT versus the CC genotype ($P=0.026$) [38]. A detailed discussion on the pharmacogenomics of *ABCB1* and other transporter genes potentially involved in drug absorption is beyond the scope of this chapter but can be found in several recent reviews [2, 7, 39, 40].

In general, drug interactions arising from intestinal P-gp inhibition tend to be overstated. Drug interactions due to P-gp inhibition at the intestinal level are more likely to be clinically relevant for those centrally acting medications that are given as small oral doses or have slow dissolution and/or diffusion rates [41]. Conversely, drug interactions due to induction of intestinal P-gp are far more plausible, even if there aren't readily available examples that involve psychoactive medications [42–44].

5.2 Presystemic Drug Transport in the Liver

Similar to transport proteins in the intestine, transporters in the liver can affect the amount of an oral dose that ultimately reaches systemic circulation [2]. Uptake transport proteins in the liver are located on the basolateral (sinusoidal) membrane of hepatocytes and control substrate access to the liver [45]. These proteins include OCT1, OAT2, OATP1B1, OATP1B3, OATP2B1, OATP1A2, and sodium-taurocholate cotransporting polypeptide (NTCP) [2]. Pharmacologic inhibition of these transporters can lead to elevated plasma concentrations and possible toxicity of substrate medications. A notable example of this is the 2.1-fold elevation in rosuvastatin AUC that occurred with concurrent administration of lopinavir-ritonavir [46]. The mechanism of this interaction was presumed to involve inhibition of hepatic uptake of rosuvastatin via OATP1B1 by lopinavir-ritonavir. Although an important uptake transporter in the liver, OATP1B1 has not been shown to transport centrally acting medications such as antidepressants, antipsychotics, anxiolytics, anticonvulsants, or centrally acting pain medications [45, 47].

In contrast to uptake transporters in the liver, efflux transporters extrude drugs from the hepatocyte either into the bile or back into the blood [1, 2, 45]. P-glycoprotein, MRP2, BCRP, bile salt export pump (BSEP), and multidrug and toxin extrusion protein 1 (MATE1) are located at the apical (canalicular) membrane of hepatocytes facing the bile duct lumen where they extrude drugs into the bile, thereby facilitating their removal from plasma [1, 2, 45]. Multidrug resistance protein 3, MRP4, and MRP6 are also efflux transporters; however, they are located at the basolateral membrane of the hepatocyte where they pump drug back into the blood [1, 2, 45].

Unlike the respective processes of efflux and metabolism that occur in the intestine, in the liver, drugs enter into the hepatocyte (via passive diffusion or active transport) and undergo intracellular trafficking where they are exposed to phase I and phase II metabolic enzymes prior to encountering P-gp and other canalicular transport proteins [20, 41]. Therefore, only drugs that are not significantly metabolized in the liver yet undergo considerable biliary excretion via P-gp will be susceptible to drug interactions resulting from P-gp modulation; examples of such medications are relatively rare and include digoxin and fexofenadine [22]. Examples of psychoactive medications reported to potentiate digoxin toxicity, potentially due to P-gp inhibition, include fluoxetine and tramadol [48, 49]. However, since these putative interactions are based on case reports and not formal pharmacokinetic investigations, it remains speculative whether observed changes in digoxin plasma concentrations were due to P-gp modulation, and if so, at what anatomical location the interaction occurred (i.e., intestine vs. liver vs. kidney). Although current information suggests that drug transport processes in the liver do not significantly contribute to efficacy, toxicity, or drug interactions with psychoactive medications, this may change as new information becomes available and new drugs are developed.

5.3 Drug Transport in the Kidney

Secretory transport proteins located on basolateral and apical (luminal) membranes of the proximal tubule play a significant role in the disposition of numerous medications [3]. Cationic drug secretion is largely mediated by organic cation transporter 2 (OCT2), which is located on the basolateral membrane, and the multidrug and toxin extrusion proteins MATE1 and MATE2/2K, which are located on the apical membrane. Conversely, weakly acidic drugs tend to be transported by OAT1 and OAT3 on the basolateral membrane and MRP2 and MRP4 on the apical membrane. P-glycoprotein and BCRP, which transport a large number of structurally and chemically unrelated compounds, are also located on the luminal membrane where they secrete drugs from the proximal tubular cell into the urine [50, 51]. Variability in the expression and activity of membrane transporters in the kidney can contribute to interpatient heterogeneity in drug exposure and response. Modulation of transport proteins in the kidney, where one medication alters the secretion or reabsorption of another, is a well-recognized mechanism by which drug-drug interactions can occur.

Despite the high level of drug transport that takes place in the kidney, psychoactive agents do not appear to be appreciably affected by alterations in drug transport processes. This is likely because psychoactive medications have not been identified as substrates for common renal tubular transporters such as OCT2, OAT1, MRP4, OAT3, BCRP, MATE1, and MATE2K [3, 52]. Nonetheless, a number of centrally acting agents have been shown to inhibit transporters involved in renal elimination. These include amantadine, amitriptyline, chlorpromazine, clonidine, cocaine, desipramine, diphenhydramine, and doxepin [3]. Similarly, flurazepam, imipramine, ketamine, and phencyclidine have been found to inhibit OCT2 [3]. Multidrug and toxin extrusion proteins MATE1 and MATE2K are also inhibited by several psychoactive agents including amantadine, chlorpheniramine, desipramine, and imipramine [3]. Clinically relevant transport-mediated drug interactions at the site of the kidney have not been routinely observed with these agents.

Although a number of psychoactive agents have been identified as substrates for P-gp, renal P-gp does not appear to be a significant source of pharmacokinetic variability or an important site for drug interactions involving these medications. This may be due to the fact that, as in the liver, renal P-gp does not "see" drugs, drug metabolites, or drug conjugates until intracellular trafficking has occurred, at which point compounds are excreted into the urine by P-gp [20, 41]. Thus, medications that are secreted into the urine unchanged are most likely to be affected by P-gp modulation in the kidney. Since the majority of centrally acting agents are extensively metabolized by phase I and II enzymatic systems, they do not fall into this category. This likely explains why P-gp modulation in the kidney does not appear to be a common mechanism by which drug interactions occur with psychoactive medications.

5.4 Drug Transport in the Brain

Drug transport into and out of the brain is largely regulated by the BBB and blood-CSF barrier. The BBB serves as both a physical and metabolic interface between the microenvironment of the brain and systemic circulation [6, 53]. It consists of a single layer of adjacent brain capillary endothelial cells that contain very tight junctures (zonulae occludens) between them. This monolayer of endothelial cells contains a dearth of fenestrae and pinocytotic vesicles, which restricts brain uptake of endogenous and exogenous substances [6]. It was largely held that drug transport across the BBB was solely dependent on the physiochemical properties of the xenobiotic such as molecular weight, lipophilicity, and state of ionization [6]. It is now clear that ABC transport proteins, particular P-gp and to a lesser extent MRPs and BCRP, limit the brain uptake of a number of lipophilic drugs that would otherwise be expected to diffuse across the capillary endothelium and into the brain [6, 54].

A number of membrane transporters have been identified at both the apical (luminal) and basolateral (abluminal) cell membranes of the brain capillary endothelium (Figs. 5.1, 5.2, and 5.3) [4]. Only drug efflux proteins that are located at the luminal (apical) cell membrane of the brain capillary endothelium are in the appropriate position to extrude drugs back into the blood and restrict drug uptake into the brain [4]. Apically located transporters include P-gp, MRP1, MRP2, MRP4, MRP5, and BCRP [6]. Additional transporters, including several MRPs, appear to be located at the basolateral membrane. The exact cellular location of MRPs in brain capillary endothelial cells is unclear, as is the specific role of basolaterally located transporters, although it has been suggested that transporters located at the basolateral membrane may function in concert with those located at the apical membrane [4].

The epithelial blood-CSF barrier, located at the choroid plexuses and outer arachnoid membrane, also functions, along with the BBB to control brain entry of certain nutrients and xenobiotics [5]. The choroid plexus differs in that it contains fenestrated, readily permeable capillaries facing the blood side of cells (basal location); these cells are enveloped by a monolayer of tightly conjoined epithelial cells, which face the CSF (apical location) [5].

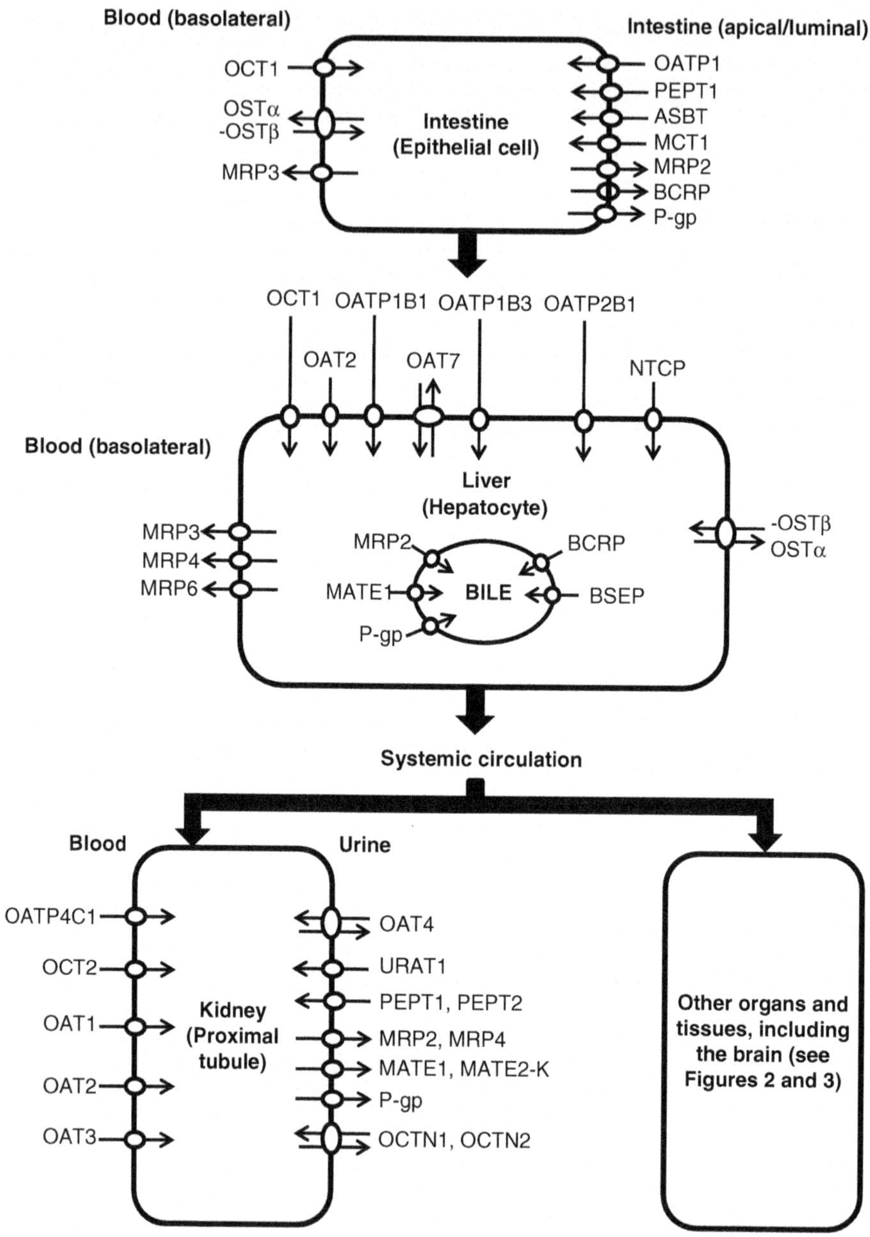

Fig. 5.1 Transport proteins in intestinal epithelia, hepatocytes, and kidney proximal tubules. Transport proteins of potential clinical relevance to centrally acting medications are included in the organs presented. Only root names of the transport proteins are defined below; individual families, subfamilies, and isoforms are not addressed here but are listed in the figure. The reader is referred to Refs [1–3, 23, 45, 47] for detailed reviews of drug transport protein function, activity, and clinical relevance in intestinal, hepatic, and kidney tissue. *OCT* organic cation transporter, *OSTα-OSTβ* heteromeric organic solute, *MRP* multidrug resistance protein transporter, *OATP* organic anion

Drug transporters that control the influx and efflux of drugs at the blood-CSF barrier have been identified, yet exploration of the identity, location, and function of these transporters at the blood-CSF barrier has only recently begun, and much information remains to be learned. To this end, drug entry into the brain primarily depends on the physical barriers of the BBB and blood-CSF barrier and the affinity of drugs for the membrane transporters located at each of these sites [55–60]. It is the interplay between these factors that govern drug exposure response in the brain.

5.4.1 *Drug Transporter-Mediated Efflux in the Brain: Examples of Clinical Relevance*

P-glycoprotein (P-gp) is the most extensively studied of the ATP-binding cassette (ABC) proteins, which also include the multidrug resistance proteins (MRPs) and breast cancer resistance protein (BCRP) [41, 51]. P-gp is principally expressed at

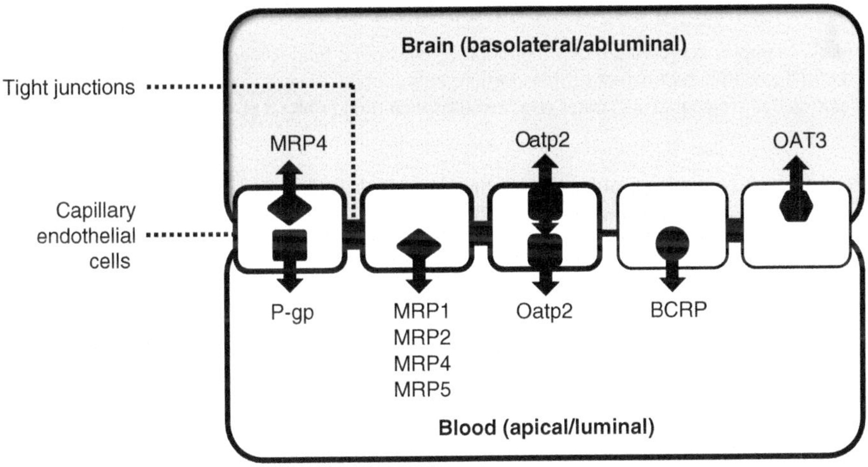

Fig. 5.2 Localization of drug transporters on brain capillary endothelial cells of the blood-brain barrier (BBB). Please see Fig. 5.1 legend for root names of transport proteins contained within this figure. *Arrows* indicate directional movement of substrates (i.e., brain to blood or vice versa)

transporting polypeptide, *PEPT* peptide transporter, *ASBT* ileal apical sodium/bile acid cotransporter, *MCT* monocarboxylic acid transporter, *BCRP* breast cancer-related protein, *P-gp* P-glycoprotein, *OAT* organic anion transporter, *NTCP* sodium/taurocholate cotransporting peptide, *BSEP* bile salt export pump, *MATE* multidrug and toxin extrusion pump, *OAT* organic anion transporter, *URAT* urate transporter, *OCTN* organic cation/ergothioneine transporter. *Arrows* pointing inward to the organ are uptake transporters (i.e., OATP, PEPT1, ASBT, and MCT1 in the intestines); *arrows* pointing away from an organ are efflux transporters (i.e., BCRP and P-gp in the liver). In the liver, 5 transport proteins extrude drug into the bile (MRP2, MATE1, BCRP, BSEP, and P-gp)

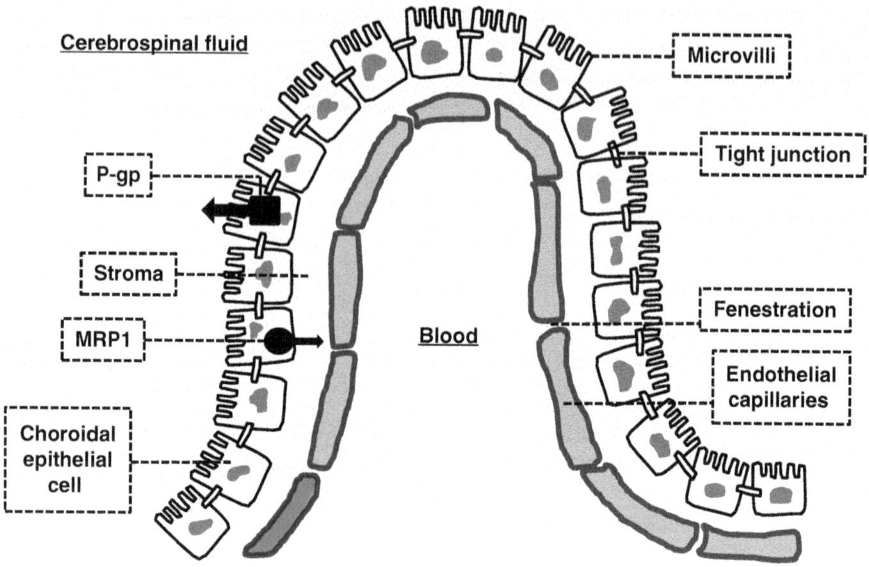

Fig. 5.3 Graphic representation of the blood-cerebrospinal fluid (blood-CSF) barrier. Please see Fig. 5.1 legend for root names of transport proteins contained within this figure. *Arrows* indicate directional movement of substrates (i.e., cerebrospinal fluid to blood or vice versa)

the luminal (apical) membrane of capillary endothelial cells of the human brain (under normal physiologic conditions) where it functions to pump substrate medications back into systemic circulation [51, 61–63]. Of note, in certain pathologic states (i.e., epilepsy), P-gp expression and its localization in the BBB may be altered, as will be discussed in greater detail below. Genetic polymorphisms can also alter the degree of P-gp expression at the BBB, which can impact drug access to the brain.

One of the most important models for studying the impact of drug transport at the BBB involves the use of genetically deficient animals (i.e., aforementioned "knockout mice") [4]. In a classic example, the impact of P-gp in preventing CNS-mediated toxicity was serendipitously realized in a scenario in which *mdr1a* knockout mice (mice devoid of P-gp expression at the BBB) were administered the antiparasitic and well-recognized neurotoxic drug, ivermectin, to treat a mite infection [64]. When *mdr1a* knockout mice received ivermectin, they developed severe neurologic toxicity and nearly all the animals died. When ivermectin was quantitated in brain tissue of the *mdr1a* knockout mice, it was present in 10–100-fold higher concentrations compared to wild-type mice that expressed functional P-gp [64]. As a result of this study, and further data in Collies and other dog breeds that exhibit severe ivermectin neurotoxicity, P-gp became widely accepted as a "gatekeeper" at the BBB that impeded brain penetration of potentially toxic compounds [65, 66].

Analgesia In addition to its protective role in preventing CNS toxicity, P-gp-mediated efflux has also been observed to impact drug efficacy in both animals and humans; this has been effectively illustrated with opiate analgesics [53]. A number

Table 5.1 Examples of clinically relevant psychoactive medications that are substrates and/or inhibitors of P-glycoprotein [1, 4–6, 21, 51, 53, 63]

Substrates	Inhibitors
Antipsychotics	
Amisulpride, aripiprazole, chlorpromazine, clozapine, fluphenazine, haloperidol, loxapine, lurasidone, mesoridazine, olanzapine, paliperidone, perphenazine, pimozide, quetiapine, risperidone, thioridazine, thiothixine, ziprasidone	Aripiprazole, chlorpromazine, clozapine, fluphenazine, haloperidol, loxapine, lurasidone, mesoridazine, olanzapine, paliperidone, perphenazine, pimozide, quetiapine, risperidone, thioridazine, thiothixine, ziprasidone
Antidepressants	
Amitriptyline, paroxetine, clomipramine, doxepin, imipramine, trimipramine, citalopram, escitalopram, fluoxetine, fluvoxamine, venlafaxine, duloxetine, nefazodone, trazodone	Amitriptyline, paroxetine, clomipramine, doxepin, imipramine, trimipramine, fluoxetine, venlafaxine, nefazodone, trazodone
Analgesics (and antidiarrheals with opioid receptor activity)	
Morphine, methadone, fentanyl, loperamide, diphenoxylate, tramadol, hydromorphone, oxycodone, hydrocodone, meperidine, codeine, butorphanol, pentazocine	Tramadol, loperamide, diphenoxylate, meperidine, butorphanol, pentazocine
Anticonvulsants	
Phenytoin, phenobarbital, carbamazepine, lamotrigine, valproate, gabapentin, topiramate, felbamate	
Antianxiety agents	
Chlordiazepoxide, clonazepam, diazepam, lorazepam, buspirone	
Sedative/hypnotics	
Zolpidem, melatonin, flurazepam, eszopiclone	Flurazepam
Drugs for the treatment of attention deficit hyperactivity disorder	
Methylphenidate, atomoxetine, clonidine	
Agents for the treatment of Alzheimer's disease	
Donepezil, galantamine	Donepezil
Antiaddiction agents	
Buprenorphine, naloxone	

of opioid analgesics (and antidiarrheals that act upon peripheral opioid receptors) have been identified as P-gp substrates [53, 67]. Such agents include morphine, fentanyl, methadone, loperamide, diphenoxylate, and others (Table 5.1). Several studies in mice showed improved brain access and greater analgesic effect with morphine in mdr1a or mdr1a/b knockout mice [68–70]. Similar results in mice lacking functional P-gp were also observed for fentanyl and methadone [70]. Consistent with these reports, investigators have shown that selectively blocking P-gp in wild-type rats with an inhibitor such as GF120918 increases extracellular fluid concentration and analgesic efficacy of morphine and methadone [71, 72]. Preclinical data such as these have led to "proof of concept" studies in humans with the antidiarrheal agent, loperamide [73]. Loperamide acts upon peripheral opioid receptors to reduce

GI motility and exert its antidiarrheal effect [74, 75]. At clinically relevant doses, loperamide does not cross the BBB due to its strong affinity for P-gp; therefore, it is void of CNS effects typically associated with centrally acting opiates (analgesia, euphoria, respiratory depression, drowsiness, etc.) [76]. Sadeque et al. administered a 16 mg dose of loperamide with and without the P-gp inhibitor quinidine 600 mg to 8 healthy male volunteers [73]. In the presence of quinidine, loperamide produced a statistically significant reduction in ventilator response to carbon dioxide (i.e., respiratory depression) ($P<0.001$) that was not explained by increased loperamide plasma concentrations. Results from this study demonstrate the ability of P-gp to prevent CNS side effects – and possibly thwart the abuse potential – of loperamide, which can be reversed by the P-gp inhibitor quinidine [73].

In a separate investigation in healthy volunteers, the effect of quinidine on the CNS-mediated pharmacodynamic effects of loperamide was found to be influenced by *ABCB1* genotype [77]. Individuals with the G2677T(A)/C3435T haplotype experienced a more pronounced increase in mitotic effects when quinidine 800 mg was coadministered with loperamide 24 mg. These results are consistent with previous data that show that this haplotype is associated with reduced P-gp activity [35]. As such, the clinical relevance of P-gp inhibition at the BBB is likely to vary between individuals based upon their genetic predisposition, thereby making it difficult to predict the clinical significance of P-gp-mediated drug interactions on a case-by-case basis.

Not all opiates that are P-gp substrates are susceptible to interactions with P-gp inhibitors at the human BBB [78]. Fentanyl and methadone were both subject to P-gp-mediated brain extrusion in mice; however, neither drug, when administered intravenously to healthy human subjects, produced changes in respiration or miosis when coadministered with quinidine [70, 79]. One reason for these disparate results may lie in the fact that fentanyl is a relatively lipophilic drug that would be predicted to permeate the endothelial lining of the BBB to a greater extent than other, comparatively less lipophilic opiate analgesics such as morphine [80]. As a result, for more lipophilic drugs, such as fentanyl, P-gp-mediated efflux may be less pronounced [6]. Another potential reason why various P-gp substrates and inhibitors may interact differently with regard to their BBB-penetrating characteristics involves the presence of multiple P-gp binding sites [81]. A number of substrate binding sites throughout the transmembrane domains of P-gp have been recognized, and these sites differentially interact with P-gp substrates and inhibitors; therefore, the ability of a drug (i.e., quinidine) to inhibit P-gp may depend upon the specific P-gp substrate (i.e., loperamide vs. fentanyl) with which it is coadministered [81, 82]. To illustrate, both colchicine and quercetin were found to enhance the transport of the P-gp substrate rhodamime-123; in contrast, these medications were found to inhibit the transport of the P-gp substrate Hoechst 33342 [81]. The affinity of a particular drug for P-gp (i.e., strong vs. weak substrate) also undoubtedly contributes to a drug's susceptibility to P-gp-mediated drug interactions at the BBB as does the potential contribution of transport proteins in addition to P-gp (such as MRPs and BCRP). A "one size fits all" approach then cannot be used to predict transport-mediated interactions with opiate analgesics at the BBB. The ability to predict these types of interactions should become easier as more data become available regarding the transport characteristics of specific opiate analgesic/P-gp inhibitor combinations.

Seizure Disorders Approximately 20–40 % of patients receiving therapy for seizure disorders are resistant to anticonvulsant therapy [83, 84]. Despite the fact that anticonvulsants act by different pharmacological mechanisms, most patients who are resistant to anticonvulsant therapy are resistant to multiple, if not all available anticonvulsant medications [85]. The potentially severe clinical consequences of uncontrolled epilepsy include a shortened lifespan and neurological and psychiatric disorders [85, 86]. Uncovering the mechanism(s) responsible for anticonvulsant drug resistance is of great interest. One potential mechanism is localized overexpression of drug transporters such as P-gp, which can limit the access of anticonvulsants to epileptogenic brain regions [87]. The following anticonvulsant medications have been identified as substrates for P-gp and/or MRPs: phenytoin, phenobarbital, carbamazepine, topiramate, valproate, and lamotrigine [88]. As stated earlier, under normal physiologic conditions, P-gp is primarily expressed by capillary endothelial cells; however, animal data have shown that repeated seizures induce overexpression of P-gp in different cell types of the brain, including perivascular astrocytes, parenchymal astrocytes, and neurons [89–91]. These data are consistent with those of Tishler et al. who found that brain expression of *ABCB1* (formerly *MDR1*) is significantly increased in patients with intractable partial (predominantly) temporal lobe epilepsy [92]. In addition to P-gp, a number of MRPs were also found to be overexpressed in brain capillary endothelial cells and/or astrocytes in patients resistant to anticonvulsant therapy [93–98]. BCRP does not appear to be overexpressed in brain tissue in anticonvulsant drug-resistant patients. These data, along with those of others, have led researchers to hypothesize that overexpressed multidrug resistance transporters reduce the extracellular concentration of anticonvulsant medications in the localized area of the brain expressing epileptogenic pathology [4]. This idea is supported by data from Rizzi et al. who observed a 30 % decrease in the brain/plasma ratio of phenytoin in rodents with increased hippocampal *ABCB1* mRNA after kainite-induced seizures [99].

For direct proof of principle regarding the role of enhanced P-gp activity at the BBB and antiepileptic drug resistance (AED) resistance, several studies in rat models showed that administration of the P-gp inhibitor tariquidar improved seizure control in phenytoin and phenobarbital-treated chronic epileptic rats [100, 101]. This led to the conduct of several pilot studies using the P-gp inhibitor verapamil in human subjects with AED-resistant seizure disorders [102, 103, 105, 106]. Due to the small size of these studies and the lack of double-blinded placebo-controlled investigations, it is not possible to determine whether verapamil or other P-gp inhibitors may have a future role as adjunct agents for the treatment of AED-resistant epilepsy. Further evidence supporting the role of P-gp overexpression and AED resistance is the fact that levetiracetam, a non-substrate for P-gp, was highly effective in treating patients with epilepsy who were unresponsive to previous antiseizure medications – all of which were presumably P-gp substrates [104].

Overexpression of P-gp as well as other drug transporters at the BBB and in parenchymal glial cells in the brain likely contributes to AED resistance. One potential strategy to combat this phenomenon involves the use of antiseizure medications that are not substrates for P-gp, such as levetiracetam. Another involves the administration of add-on therapy with P-gp inhibitors such as verapamil, in hopes that they can enhance the CNS penetration of AEDs and improve seizure control; however, this approach is premature at this time and requires data from large well-controlled trials before it can be supported. Lastly, new drug formulations that circumvent the influence of drug transporters at the BBB may prove useful for the treatment of patients with AED-resistant seizure disorders.

In addition to seizure activity increasing drug transporter expression in brain tissue, overexpression of drug transporters at the BBB has also been postulated to arise secondary to anticonvulsant administration; however, data from several preclinical studies suggest that this is not the case. Long-term administration of phenytoin and phenobarbital, respectively, did not induce the expression of P-gp in the brain in rats [105]. Similarly, 7-day administration of therapeutic doses of phenytoin and carbamazepine did not alter *ABCB1* mRNA in the hippocampus of mice [99]. These data suggest that seizure activity in the brain, as discussed above, and not anticonvulsant drug therapy is responsible for overexpression of drug transporters in the brain [4, 6].

Functional genetic polymorphisms in genes that encode for drug transporters at the BBB (i.e., *ABCB1and ABCC2*) represent another mechanism by which enhanced transporter expression and reduced access of anticonvulsants to epileptogenic brain regions may occur [106, 107]. Numerous studies have investigated the relationship between AED and the *ABCB1* polymorphism (C to T) at position 3435 [108]. The first of these studies, performed by Siddiqui et al., found that patients with drug-resistant epilepsy, defined as ≥4 seizures during the previous year despite trials with >3 anticonvulsant medications at maximally tolerated doses, were more likely to possess the *ABCB1* 3435 CC genotype versus the TT genotype (odds ratio, 2.66; 95 % confidence interval, 1.32–5.38; $P=0.006$) [107]. This study involved 200 AED-resistant patients, 115 AED-responsive patients, and 200 control subjects without epilepsy. These data are consistent with previous data that show that the 3435 CC genotype is associated with increased P-gp expression and activity in a number of in vitro and in vivo investigations (although conflicting evidence has also been reported) [34–36]. This increase in P-gp expression at the BBB is postulated to reduce AED access to the brain, resulting in AED resistance [107].

Since the initial study by Siddiqui et al., numerous investigations have been conducted assessing the influence of *ABCB1* polymorphisms on AED resistance [107, 109–120]. Most of these studies assessed the role of C3435T on AED resistance and they reported conflicting results, with some studies identifying a relationship between 3435 CC and AED resistance, some identifying a relationship between 3435 TT and AED resistance, and some not finding any relationship at all. To address discordant results among the studies, at least 6 meta-analyses have been performed to date, with only the most recent showing a significant relationship between 3435C and AED-resistant epilepsy [108, 121–125]. A meta-analysis reported on results from 38 studies involving 8716 patients. An association between the 3435C allele and AED resistance in patients experiencing >10 seizures per year was observed [108]. The association was most notable in Caucasians, adults, and in patients treated with multiple medications.

In addition to C3435T, G2677T and C1236T (which are in linkage disequilibrium with C3435T) have also been associated with P-gp expression and activity and have been assessed in AED resistance [126]. Although the 3435, 2677, 1236 CGC haplotype has traditionally been associated with increased P-gp activity (and the TTT haplotype with comparatively less P-gp activity), a study conducted in Japanese patients with AED drug resistance found that the TTT haplotype was associated with carbamazepine-resistant epilepsy [127]. These results would appear counterintuitive, considering that the TTT haplotype would be expected to be associated with reduced P-gp expression and increased penetration of carbamazepine into epileptogenic brain tissue. Similar results were observed by Subenthiran et al. who reported a significant association between 2677TT and 3435TT and resistance to carbamazepine monotherapy in 314 Malaysian patients [128]. Given the overall lack of consistency in data describing the association between *ABCB1* and AED resistance, other transporters, such as *ABCC2*, may represent additional avenues of drug resistance in patients with seizure disorders.

ABCC2, which encodes for the MRP2 transporter, has been assessed in a small number of studies of AED resistance [126, 129, 130]. *ABCC2* C24T and C3972T were associated with AED resistance in 537 Chinese patients [129]. Similarly, another study in 221 German patients with epilepsy (103 responders and 118 non-responders to first-line AED therapy) found that nonresponders were more likely to carry the "T" allele of the C24T variant of the *ABCC2* gene [130]. These data are surprising in that the *ABCC2* 24T allele has been associated with reduced activity in vitro, and reduced MRP2 activity would be expected to correlate with adequate AED penetration into the brain and a reduced incidence of AED resistance [131]. A number of postulated mechanisms for these results have been put forth, most notably the likelihood that other drug transporter genes (i.e., *ABCB1*) are upregulated in the presence of the low-function *ABCC2* 24T allele.

In conclusion, the pharmacogenomics of drug transporters at the BBB represents a complex area where study results are often counterintuitive or in disagreement. Numerous reasons exist for disparity between studies attempting to characterize the roles of *ABCB1* and *ABCC2* on P-gp expression at the BBB and anticonvulsant drug activity. These include a variety of covariates such as compensatory upregulation of other transport proteins; differences in transporter expression between tissues (i.e., the BBB vs. the liver or intestine); types of drugs being studied (i.e., stronger vs. weaker P-gp substrates); the presence of drug-drug interactions; ethnicity of the study populations, which may display differential haplotype frequencies; and polymorphisms in drug metabolizing enzymes (i.e., cytochrome P450) that may impact systemic drug exposure.

5.4.2 Depression

Approximately 30–50 % of patients with depression exhibit an incomplete response to antidepressant medications of adequate dose and duration [132]. Common antidepressant drug classes include selective serotonin reuptake inhibitors (SSRIs), tricyclic antidepressants (TCAs), serotonin-norepinephrine reuptake inhibitors (SNRIs), and tetracyclic antidepressants, all of which must cross the BBB to exert their pharmacologic effects. Evolving evidence suggests that P-gp may impede the uptake of antidepressant medications into the CNS, thereby contributing to the high degree of treatment failure associated with current antidepressant regimens [133]. It has also been postulated that P-gp inhibition by antidepressant medications contributes to their antidepressant activity by altering glucocorticoid penetration across the BBB, resulting in reduced hypothalamic-pituitary-adrenal (HPA) axis activity [134].

It remains controversial which antidepressants are substrates and/or inhibitors of P-gp and whether or not P-gp contributes to treatment-resistant depression (TRD) [133]. The interaction between antidepressants and P-gp can be attributed to the use of different in vitro assays; lack of a validated, highly reliable predictive screening model to identify P-gp substrates and inhibitors; interlaboratory differences that yield disparate results despite use of a common assay; differences in data interpretation between investigators; use of different cell lines for P-gp experiments; differences in knockout mouse models (single- vs. double knockout mice); and animal dosing strategies (single-dose vs. chronic drug administration) [133]. These inconsistencies represent challenges to understanding the complex relationship between P-gp expression at the BBB and patients with TRD.

Despite uncertainty as to which antidepressants are P-gp substrates, emerging clinical data suggest that P-gp plays a role in antidepressant drug response. A PET study using [^{11}C]-verapamil observed increased P-gp function in patients being treated for major depression [38]. Reasons for the increase in P-gp activity may include *ABCB1* induction due to chronic antidepressant therapy, increased P-gp expression secondary to cytokines resulting from immune activation, or functional SNPS in the *ABCB1* gene [135–140]. A number of studies have been conducted to assess the influence of *ABCB1* polymorphisms on TRD, with the prevailing hypothesis being that low-function SNPs will be associated with greater CNS penetration of antidepressant medications and improved clinical response.

The most compelling data supporting a relationship between predicted P-gp activity and antidepressant efficacy was reported by Uhr and colleagues [141]. The authors investigated the relationship between remission rates in 443 depressed Caucasian patients treated with antidepressants and 95 SNPs in *ABCB1*. Eleven rare intronic SNPs, presumably associated with reduced P-gp activity and greater CNS antidepressant penetration, were associated with a 7.7-fold greater chance of remission ($P<0.001$) after 5 weeks of therapy with P-gp substrate antidepressants that included citalopram, paroxetine, amitriptyline, and venlafaxine [141]. This association was not due to differences in plasma concentrations or antidepressant drug doses, and no association was found between *ABCB1* SNPs and remission in subjects receiving the non-P-gp substrate, mirtazapine. Of particular interest, these findings were reproduced by Sarginson et al. for the P-gp substrate paroxetine and the non-P-gp substrate mirtazapine [142]. However, a large retrospective analysis failed to replicate the findings of Uhr and colleagues with regard to a potential relationship between *ABCB1* SNPS and citalopram [143].

A number of additional studies have investigated the association between *ABCB1* SNPs and antidepressant clinical response and toxicities; however, despite the positive pharmacogenetic results discussed above, there is a prevailing disagreement in the literature regarding the involvement of different *ABCB1* SNPs and antidepressant drug response. Reasons for disparity in study results are similar to those discussed for the relationship between AED resistance and P-gp; they include differences in ethnicities of studied populations, the unlikelihood that an individual SNP or gene is responsible for antidepressant drug response, the role of other transporters at the BBB besides P-gp, uncertainty regarding the degree to which a drug is a substrate for P-gp (strong vs. week), and the possible contribution of P-gp inhibition by antidepressant medications to their mechanism of action in the CNS [133].

Hypothalamic-pituitary-adrenal (HPA) axis hyperactivity is a consistent finding in patients suffering from depression [144]. Patients typically have elevated plasma cortisol and ACTH, which is indicative of HPA axis dysregulation [145]. This compromised negative feedback inhibition process is hypothesized to result from P-gp-mediated efflux of endogenous glucocorticoids at the BBB (or in neuronal tissue), thereby preventing the glucocorticoids from binding to their receptors within the CNS. Pariante and coworkers hypothesize that P-gp inhibition at the BBB by antidepressant medications allows endogenous glucocorticoids (i.e., cortisol) greater access to the CNS, subsequently restoring normal HPA axis function and reducing depressive symptoms [134]. This hypothesis is supported by data in mice in which desipramine reduced basal and activated HPA axis activity [146]. This theory has been challenged based on (1) uncertainty regarding whether antidepressant medications could achieve concentrations at the BBB high enough to inhibit P-gp to a clinically relevant degree, (2) failure to demonstrate that acute or chronic desipramine administration leads to increased glucocorticoid penetration into the brain secondary to P-gp inhibition in an in situ mouse model, and (3) a dearth of in vivo data supporting this hypothesis in humans [133, 147]. The primary impact of P-gp on antidepressant activity would appear to be related to its ability to limit access of antidepressant medications to the CNS.

Despite the absence of prospective, controlled, adequately powered trials to characterize the role of *ABCB1* gene variants on antidepressant activity, it is conceivable that pharmacologic inhibition of P-gp at the BBB may augment antidepressant efficacy in patients with TRD [133]. Anecdotal evidence suggests that adjunctive treatment with the P-gp inhibitor verapamil produced a beneficial effect in severely depressed patients refractory to SSRI treatment [148]. This approach also appears to be supported by data which show that the addition of an antipsychotic medication such as aripiprazole, olanzapine, quetiapine, or risperidone can be used to enhance antidepressant treatment response in patients with TRD [149]. Since some of these antipsychotics have been shown to inhibit P-gp in vitro, it has been speculated that this is the mechanism by which these antipsychotic medications augment antidepressant treatment response (i.e., by enhancing CNS penetration of antidepressant medications secondary to P-gp inhibition). Further supporting this premise are data which show that risperidone coadministration with sertraline resulted in a trend toward increased brain concentrations of sertraline in of CF1 mice [150]. The ability of antipsychotics to achieve P-gp inhibitory concentrations at the BBB, which is usually in the micromolar range, has been called into question [53]. Nonetheless, these observations are largely preclinical and anecdotal. Controlled studies are necessary to determine the role, if any, of P-gp inhibition in improving antidepressant treatment efficacy in TRD.

5.4.3 Schizophrenia

Schizophrenia that is resistant to antipsychotic therapy (pharmacoresistant schizophrenia) is prevalent in approximately 13–50 % of all schizophrenic patients and by definition continues despite combination drug therapy [151–154]. Because most typical and atypical antipsychotics are, to varying degrees, substrates for P-gp (Table 5.1), and these medications require brain access to exert their pharmacologic activity, it has been postulated that P-gp may contribute to pharmacoresistant schizophrenia by limiting penetration of these drugs into the CNS. It has also been hypothesized that low P-gp activity at the BBB is associated with increased penetration of psychotropic medications into the brain and subsequent toxicities such as cognitive impairment, weight gain, and polydipsia [155–157].

In a similar investigative process as that observed with anticonvulsant medications, a number of studies have assessed the influence of *ABCB1* polymorphisms (primarily C3435T, G2677T, and C1236T) on antipsychotic efficacy and toxicity [155–166]. Lin et al. observed a relationship between the 3435T allele, olanzapine plasma concentrations, and a reduction in positive symptoms of schizophrenia which include hallucinations, delusions, thought disorders, and movement disorders [158]. The investigators also reported a similar relationship between the linked SNPs, C1236T and G2677T and olanzapine dose-response. The authors speculate that enhanced brain access with the *ABCB1* T alleles may have led to the improved drug response with olanzapine. However, the authors also caution that because of the small sample size ($n=41$), their results should be considered preliminary. Similar results were reported by Bozina et al. who observed a significantly better initial treatment response to olanzapine in 117 female schizophrenic patients who possessed a 2677 T allele [160]. Results from this investigation are noteworthy in that subjects had not received chronic antipsychotic therapy and were not receiving concurrent antipsychotic medications, each of which have the potential to modulate P-gp activity and confound study results. The all-female population eliminated any sex-related differences in olanzapine treatment response that may exist.

In addition to olanzapine, several studies also observed positive relationships between *ABCB1* genotypes and risperidone treatment response [157, 162, 167]. Xing and coworkers found that the percentage improvement in the brief psychiatric rating scale (BPRS) in 130 Chinese patients (85 female) treated with risperidone was better in patients with the 1236 TT genotype [162]. These results are not unexpected, considering that numerous preclinical studies have shown that risperidone has a greater affinity for P-gp than most other typical or atypical antipsychotic medications. Consistent with these findings, the 1236 TT genotype was associated with increased improvement during risperidone therapy in 45 Portuguese patients with autism spectrum disorder [167]. Nonetheless, as has been noted in studies with antiseizure and antidepressant medications, results from other studies with antipsychotics have failed to identify a relationship between P-gp activity (as represented by *ABCB1* genotype) and drug response [159, 168, 169].

In contrast to the above results, Nikisch et al. observed significantly lower plasma and CSF concentrations of the P-gp substrate quetiapine in 22 German schizophrenic patients possessing the TT genotype at positions 3435, 2677, and 1236 [164]. The *ABCB1* 2677TT carriers exhibited a 2.6-fold lower quetiapine plasma concentration compared to noncarriers and a 5.4-fold lower quetiapine CSF concentration compared to noncarriers after 4 weeks of quetiapine therapy. The comparatively lower concentration in the CSF versus the plasma suggests that the low CSF concentration could not be explained solely on the basis of reduced drug diffusion into the CSF from the plasma – but likely occurred due to active drug efflux at the BBB. These results, which show reduced CNS penetration and poorer treatment response with TT genotypes at positions 3435, 2677, and 1236, are in opposition to those previously reported with olanzapine and risperidone, which showed greater treatment response (and better presumed CNS penetration) in TT individuals at at least one of these positions [158, 160, 162]. Reasons for these disparate results may be due to ethnic differences in the treatment populations, differences in transport characteristics of the studied medications, and the possibility that other transport proteins (i.e., MRPs) are upregulated in the presence of low-activity *ABCB1* genotypes.

In addition to drug response, several studies have noted relationships between *ABCB1* SNPS and toxicity with antipsychotic medications. A hallmark of each of these studies is that the reported toxicity occurred more frequently in subjects possessing the low-activity (T) allele [155–157]. Yasui-Furukori et al. noted a relationship between the 3435 TT genotype and poor improvement in cognitive function in a study of 31 acutely exacerbated schizophrenic patients receiving bromperidol, a structurally related analogue to haloperidol [155]. The authors speculate that higher brain concentrations of bromperidol in patients with the 3435 TT genotype would be expected to be associated with worsening cognitive function [155]. In a separate study, a significant relationship was identified between *ABCB1* TT variants at positions 3435 and 2677 and weight gain with risperidone after 4 months of treatment in 108 female schizophrenic patients of Croatian descent [157]. Presence of 3435 and 2677 T variants was not associated with weight gain secondary to olanzapine treatment in this study. This may be due to the fact that olanzapine is an intermediate substrate for P-gp compared to risperidone, which is a strong substrate [170, 171]. Shinkai and colleagues reported that polydipsia occurred more frequently in 84 schizophrenic polydipsic patients with the 3435 T allele compared with 247 non-polydipsic controls (odds ratio = 1.46; 95 % CI = 1.03–2.07; P = 0.0.35) [156]. The authors speculate that the C3435T polymorphism may play a role in the pathophysiology of polydipsia in schizophrenia, presumably by allowing greater brain penetration of antipsychotic medications which is believed to contribute to this disorder.

In addition to genetically controlled differences in P-gp expression at the BBB and in neuronal tissue, concomitant administration of P-gp-modulating medications is another mechanism by which the pharmacologic response of antipsychotic medications may be impacted, especially in patients with pharmacoresistant schizophrenia [172]. Patients with pharmacoresistant schizophrenia typically receive multiple psychotropic medications including antipsychotics, antidepressants, and mood-stabilizing anticonvulsants such as carbamazepine [172]. Chronic therapy with certain medications may modulate P-gp activity and alter the CNS penetration (and the subsequent efficacy and/or toxicity profile) of antipsychotic medications. To illustrate, chlorpromazine can act as both an inhibitor and inducer of P-gp-mediated efflux, depending on the medication with which it is coadministered [173]. Assuming that other medications can also differentially affect P-gp-mediated transport, chronic polypharmacy in patients with pharmacoresistant schizophrenia may be associated with transport-mediated drug interactions that either positively or negatively influence antipsychotic drug response. A number of factors likely influence such putative interactions, including *ABCB1* genotype, ethnicity, diet, age, gender, and specific medications that are being coadministered. Large, prospective, randomized, carefully controlled trials are necessary to ferret out the influences of these factors on antipsychotic drug response in patients with pharmacoresistant schizophrenia.

5.5 Conclusions and Future Directions

In recent years, a remarkable amount of progress has been made in understanding the role of transport proteins, especially P-gp, on drug absorption and disposition. One of the most interesting and difficult areas to study involves the role of efflux transporters as "gatekeepers" that control drug distribution across the BBB and into the CNS. While the ability of efflux transporters, P-gp in particular, to protect the brain from xenobiotic-induced toxicity is well-recognized, P-gp is also capable of hindering the pharmacologic activity of drugs that must gain CNS access to exert their pharmacologic activity. A number of approaches have been suggested to deal with this phenomenon. First and foremost, however, is the need to gain a better understanding of drug transport at the BBB.

Despite the increase in transporter information that has become available in the biomedical literature over the last decade, the optimal approach to in vitro and animal testing to determine whether a drug is a P-gp substrate or modulator remains unclear, as does a standardized manner in which to interpret such data [4]. While information on MRPs, BCRP, OATPs, and OATs has increased recently, it still lags significantly behind P-gp. More information is needed with regard to the regulation, genetics, substrates, and modulators of these membrane transporters. Detailed information is necessary regarding the potential overexpression of these transporters when P-gp expression/activity is reduced or absent. While clearly a daunting task, large, well-controlled studies are necessary to elucidate the role of multiple transporters (and their various polymorphisms) on drug disposition and drug interactions. Such studies will need to take numerous additional factors into account such as ethnicity, sex, diet, smoking, concurrent medications, disease states, and age to determine the impact of various transport proteins on psychoactive drug responses. A multiple logistic regression approach with large sample sizes will likely be necessary to identify the combination of factors that can potentially influence drug distribution into the CNS.

In the meantime, several approaches have been suggested to circumvent the influence of P-gp on drug transport at the BBB. One such tactic includes direct pharmacologic inhibition, as was mentioned earlier with regard to the P-gp inhibitor verapamil in combination with AEDs and antidepressants. This approach though can only be used to enhance, as opposed to reduce, brain drug delivery and it allows for little control over the extent and duration of barrier opening [174]. Moreover, most inhibitors aren't selective for a specific protein, which may result in unwanted side effects. Conversely, targeting transporter regulation by modulating the effects of inflammatory mediators (i.e., cytokines such as tumor necrosis factor-α [TNF-α], interleukin-1 β [IL-1 β], and interleukin-6 [IL-6]), mediators of oxidative stress such as reactive oxygen species, and nuclear receptors including the pregnane X receptor (PXR) can be turned off for brief, controlled time periods [174].

Attention has focused on developing new molecular entities that do not interact with P-gp or other efflux transporters [175]. Drugs that are not substrates for membrane transporters at the BBB would be expected to reach therapeutic concentrations at their site of activity in the brain. While this has the potential to be therapeutically advantageous, such medications will need to be carefully developed and studied to avoid untoward toxicities when such medications have unfettered brain access. A current example of a medication that is not a P-gp substrate and is active against AED-resistant epilepsy is levetiracetam [104]. Drug-containing nanoparticles with the capability of passing through the luminal membrane of the BBB represent another means by which drug formulations may be developed that circumvent the actions of centrally located efflux transporters.

In conclusion, centrally located membrane transporters restrict drug delivery to the brain and can compromise the efficacy of psychoactive medications. When pharmacologically inhibited or minimally expressed due to genetic polymorphisms, these same transporters may allow unopposed brain access to certain drugs resulting in toxicity. An evolving understanding of these phenomena, as well as novel therapeutic strategies is necessary to improve CNS drug delivery and optimize the safety and efficacy of psychoactive pharmacotherapy.

References

1. Giacomini KM, Huang SM, Tweedie DJ et al (2010) Membrane transporters in drug development. Nat Rev Drug Discov 9:215–236
2. Shugarts S, Benet LZ (2009) The role of transporters in the pharmacokinetics of orally administered drugs. Pharm Res 26:2039–2054
3. Morrissey KM, Stocker SL, Wittwer MB et al (2013) Renal transporters in drug development. Annu Rev Pharmacol Toxicol 53:503–529

4. Löscher W, Potschka H (2005) Role of drug efflux transporters in the brain for drug disposition and treatment of brain diseases. Prog Neurobiol 76:22–76
5. Lee G, Dallas S, Hong M et al (2001) Drug transporters in the central nervous system: brain barriers and brain parenchyma considerations. Pharmacol Rev 53:569–596
6. Löscher W, Potschka H (2005) Blood–brain barrier active efflux transporters: ATP-binding cassette gene family. NeuroRx 2:86–98
7. Yoo H-D, Lee Y-B (2011) Interplay of pharmacogenetic variations in ABCB1 transporters and cytochrome P450 enzymes. Arch Pharm Res 34:1817–1828
8. Tozer TN, Rowland M (2006) Extravascular dose and systemic absorption. In: Introduction to pharmacokinetics and pharmacodynamics. Lippincott Williams & Wilkins, Baltimore, pp 105–136
9. Choudhuri S, Klaassen CD (2006) Structure, function, expression, genomic organization, and single nucleotide polymorphisms of human ABCB1 (MDR1), ABCC (MRP), and ABCG2 (BCRP) efflux transporters. Int J Toxicol 25:231–259
10. Kosters A, Karpen SJ (2008) Bile acid transporters in health and disease. Xenobiotica 38:1043–1071
11. Van Waterschoot RA, Schinkel AH (2011) A critical analysis of the interplay between cytochrome P450 3A and P-glycoprotein: recent insights from knockout and transgenic mice. Pharmacol Rev 63:390–410
12. Yasui-Furukori N, Saito M, Niioka T et al (2007) Effect of itraconazole on pharmacokinetics of paroxetine: the role of gut transporters. Ther Drug Monit 29:45–48
13. Kim RB, Fromm MF, Wandel C et al (1998) The drug transporter P-glycoprotein limits oral absorption and brain entry of HIV-1 protease inhibitors. J Clin Invest 101:289–294
14. Lee CGL, Gottesman MM (1998) HIV protease inhibitors and the MDR1 multidrug transporter. J Clin Invest 101:287–288
15. Lin JH (1999) Role of pharmacokinetics in the discovery and development of indinavir. Adv Drug Deliv Rev 39:33–49
16. Winans E (2003) Aripiprazole. Am J Health Syst Pharm 60:2437–2445
17. He H, Richardson JS (1995) A pharmacological, pharmacokinetic and clinical overview of risperidone, a new antipsychotic that blocks serotonin 5-HT2 and dopamine D2 receptors. Int Clin Psychopharmacol 10:19–30
18. Rambeck B, Wolf P (1993) Lamotrigine clinical pharmacokinetics. Clin Pharmacokinet 25:433–443
19. Van Harten J (1993) Clinical pharmacokinetics of selective serotonin reuptake inhibitors. Clin Pharmacokinet 24:203–220
20. Lin JH, Yamazaki M (2003) Role of P-glycoprotein in pharmacokinetics: clinical implications. Clin Pharmacokinet 42:59–98
21. Name of website: DrugBank. Available from: http://www.drugbank.ca/drugs/DB01267. Accessed 18 July 2014
22. Penzak SR (2005) Mechanisms of drug interactions II: transport proteins. In: Piscitelli SC, Rodvold KA (eds) Drug interactions in infectious diseases, 2nd edn. Human Press, Totowa, pp 41–82
23. Benet LZ (2009) The drug transporter- metabolism alliance: uncovering and defining the interplay. Mol Pharm 6:1631–1643
24. Name of website: Indiana University, Division of Clinical Pharmacology, P450 Drug Interaction Table. http://medicine.iupui.edu/clinpharm/ddis/main-table/. Accessed 18 July 2014
25. Crismon ML, Argo TR, Buckley PF (2014) Schizophrenia. In: DiPiro JT, Talbert RL, Yee GC et al (eds) Pharmacotherapy: a pathophysiologic approach, 9th edn. McGraw-Hill, New York, pp 1019–1045
26. Name of website: Micromedex 2.0. DRUGDEX Evaluations. http://www.micromedexsolutions.com.proxy.hsc.unt.edu/micromedex2/librarian/ND_T/evidencexpert/ND_PR/evidencexpert/CS/F912E4/ND_AppProduct/evidencexpert/DUPLICATIONSHIELDSYNC/63B994/ND_PG/evidencexpert/ND_B/evidencexpert/ND_P/evidencexpert/PFActionId/

evidencexpert.DisplayDrugdexDocument?docId=0229&contentSetId=31&title=Diazepam&servicesTitle=Diazepam&topicId=pharmacokineticsSection. Accessed 19 July 2014
27. Name of website: Micromedex 2.0. DRUGDEX evaluations. http://www.micromedexsolutions.com.proxy.hsc.unt.edu/micromedex2/librarian/ND_T/evidencexpert/ND_PR/evidencexpert/CS/11248C/ND_AppProduct/evidencexpert/DUPLICATIONSHIELDSYNC/6005E9/ND_PG/evidencexpert/ND_B/evidencexpert/ND_P/evidencexpert/PFActionId/evidencexpert. DisplayDrugdexDocument?docId=2303&contentSetId=31&title=Aprepitant&servicesTitle=Aprepitant&topicId=pharmacokineticsSection. Accessed 19 July 2014
28. Name of website: Micromedex 2.0. DRUGDEX evaluations. http://www.micromedexsolutions.com.proxy.hsc.unt.edu/micromedex2/librarian/ND_T/evidencexpert/ND_PR/evidencexpert/CS/54400D/ND_AppProduct/evidencexpert/DUPLICATIONSHIELDSYNC/EF9157/ND_PG/evidencexpert/ND_B/evidencexpert/ND_P/evidencexpert/PFActionId/evidencexpert. DisplayDrugdexDocument?docId=2467&contentSetId=31&title=Buspirone+Hydrochloride&servicesTitle=Buspirone+Hydrochloride&topicId=pharmacokineticsSection. Accessed 19 July 2014
29. Name of website: Micromedex 2.0. DRUGDEX evaluations. http://www.micromedexsolutions.com.proxy.hsc.unt.edu/micromedex2/librarian/ND_T/evidencexpert/ND_PR/evidencexpert/CS/EC38F4/ND_AppProduct/evidencexpert/DUPLICATIONSHIELDSYNC/89C445/ND_PG/evidencexpert/ND_B/evidencexpert/ND_P/evidencexpert/PFActionId/evidencexpert. DisplayDrugdexDocument?docId=0482&contentSetId=31&title=Methadone+Hydrochloride&servicesTitle=Methadone+Hydrochloride&topicId=pharmacokineticsSection. Accessed 19 July 2014
30. Langtry HD, Benfield P (1990) Zolpidem. A review of its pharmacodynamic and pharmacokinetic properties and therapeutic potential. Drugs 40:291–313
31. Christofaki M, Papaioannou A (2014) Ondansetron: a review of pharmacokinetics and clinical experience in postoperative nausea and vomiting. Expert Opin Drug Metab Toxicol 10:437–444
32. Balant-Gorgia AE, Balant L (1987) Clinical pharmacokinetics of potential candidates for plasma concentration monitoring. Antipsychotic drugs. Clin Pharmacokinet 13:65–90
33. Misaka S, Müller F, Fromm MF (2013) Clinical relevance of drug efflux pumps in the gut. Curr Opin Pharmacol 13:847–852
34. Nakamura T, Sakaeda T, Horinouchi M et al (2002) Effect of the mutation (C3435T) at exon 26 of the MDR1 gene on expression level of MDR1 messenger ribonucleic acid in duodenal enterocytes of healthy Japanese subjects. Clin Pharmacol Ther 71:297–303
35. Kurata Y, Ieiri I, Kimura M et al (2002) Role of human MDR1 gene polymorphism in bioavailability and interaction of digoxin, a substrate of P-glycoprotein. Clin Pharmacol Ther 72:209–219
36. Chinn LW, Kroetz DL (2007) *ABCB1* pharmacogenetics: progress, pitfalls, and promise. Clin Pharmacol Ther 81:265–269
37. Lazarowski A, Sevlever G, Taratuto A et al (1999) Tuberous sclerosis associated with MDR1 gene expression and drug-resistant epilepsy. Pediatr Neurol 21:731–734
38. Fukui N, Suzuki Y, Sawamura K et al (2007) Dose-dependent effects of the 3435 C>T genotype of ABCB1 gene on the steady-state plasma concentration of fluvoxamine in psychiatric patients. Ther Drug Monit 29:185–189
39. Franke RM, Gardner ER, Sparreboom A (2010) Pharmacogenetics of drug transporters. Curr Pharm Des 16:220–230
40. Cascorbi I (2006) Role of pharmacogenetics of ATP-binding cassette transporters in the pharmacokinetics of drugs. Pharmacol Ther 112:457–473
41. Lin JH (2003) Drug-drug interaction mediated by inhibition and induction of P-glycoprotein. Adv Drug Deliv Rev 55:53–81
42. Greiner B, Eichelbaum M, Fritz P et al (1999) The role of intestinal P-glycoprotein in the interaction of digoxin and rifampin. J Clin Invest 104:147–153
43. Westphal K, Weinbrenner A, Zschiesche M et al (2000) Induction of P-glycoprotein by rifampin increases intestinal secretion of talinolol in human beings: a new type of drug/drug interaction. Clin Pharmacol Ther 68:345–355

44. Hebert MF, Roberts JP, Prueksaritanont T et al (1992) Bioavailability of cyclosporine with concomitant rifampin administration is markedly less than predicted by hepatic enzyme induction. Clin Pharmacol Ther 52:453–457
45. Niemi M, Pasanen MK, Neuvonen PJ (2011) Organic anion transporting polypeptide 1B1: a genetically polymorphic transporter of major importance for hepatic drug uptake. Pharmacol Rev 63:157–181
46. Kiser JJ, Gerber JG, Predhomme JA et al (2008) Drug/drug interaction between lopinavir/ritonavir and rosuvastatin in healthy volunteers. J Acquir Immune Defic Syndr 47:570–578
47. Kalliokoski A, Niemi M (2009) Impact of OATP transporters on pharmacokinetics. Br J Pharmacol 158:693–705
48. Leibovitz A, Bilchinsky T, Gil I et al (1998) Elevated serum digoxin level associated with coadministered fluoxetine. Arch Intern Med 158:1152–1153
49. Product Information: ULTRAM(R)ER extended-release oral tablets, tramadol hcl extended-release oral tablets. PriCara, Raritan, 12/00/2005
50. Ni Z, Bikadi Z, Rosenberg MF et al (2010) Structure and function of the human breast cancer resistance protein (BCRP/ABCG2). Curr Drug Metab 11:603–617
51. Schinkel AH, Jonker JW (2003) Mammalian drug efflux transporters of the ATP binding cassette (ABC) family: an overview. Adv Drug Deliv Rev 55:3–29
52. Launay-Vacher V, Izzedine H, Karie S et al (2006) Renal tubular drug transporters. Nephron Physiol 103:97–106
53. Linnet K, Broeng Ejsing T (2008) A review on the impact of P-glycoprotein on the penetration of drugs into the brain. Focus on psychotropic drug. Eur Neuropsychopharmacol 18: 157–169
54. Golden PL, Pollack GM (2003) Blood–brain barrier efflux transport. J Pharm Sci 92:1739–1753
55. Cornford EM, Hyman S (1999) Blood–brain barrier permeability to small and large molecules. Adv Drug Deliv Rev 36:145–163
56. Pardridge WM (1999) Blood–brain barrier biology and methodology. J Neurovirol 5:556–569
57. Tsuji A, Tamai I (1999) Carrier-mediated or specialized transport of drugs across the blood–brain barrier. Adv Drug Deliv Rev 36:277–290
58. Segal MB (2000) The choroid plexuses and the barriers between the blood and the cerebrospinal fluid. Cell Mol Neurobiol 20:183–196
59. Spector R (2000) Drug transport in the mammalian central nervous system: multiple complex systems. A critical analysis and commentary. Pharmacology 60:58–73
60. Graff CL, Pollack GM (2004) Drug transport at the blood–brain barrier and choroid plexus. Curr Drug Metab 5:95–108
61. Cordon-Cardo C, O'Brien JP, Casals D et al (1989) Multidrug-resistance gene (P-glycoprotein) is expressed by endothelial cells at the blood–brain barrier sites. Proc Natl Acad Sci U S A 86:695–698
62. Demeule M, Regina A, Jodoin J et al (2002) Drug transport to the brain: key roles for the efflux pump P-glycoprotein in the blood–brain barrier. Vascul Pharmacol 38:339–348
63. Sun H, Dai H, Shaik N et al (2003) Drug efflux transporters in the CNS. Adv Drug Deliv Rev 55:83–105
64. Schinkel AH, Smit JJ, van Tellingen O et al (1994) Disruption of the mouse mdr1a P-glycoprotein gene leads to a deficiency in the blood–brain barrier and to increased sensitivity to drugs. Cell 77:491–502
65. Paul AJ, Tranquilli WJ, Seward RL et al (1987) Clinical observations in collies given ivermectin orally. Am J Vet Res 48:684–685
66. Neff MW, Robertson KR, Wong AK et al (2004) Breed distribution and history of canine mdr1-1Delta, a pharmacogenetic mutation that marks the emergence of breeds from the collie lineage. Proc Natl Acad Sci U S A 101:11725–11730
67. De Boer AG, van der Sandt ICJ, Gaillard PJ (2003) The role of drug transporters at the blood–brain barrier. Annu Rev Pharmacol Toxicol 43:629–656

68. Xie R, Hammarlund-Udenaes M, de Boer AG et al (1999) The role of P-glycoprotein in blood–brain barrier transport of morphine: transcortical microdialysis studies in mdr1a (–/–) and mdr1a (+/+) mice. Br J Pharmacol 128:563–568
69. Zong J, Pollack GM (2000) Morphine antinociception in enhanced in mdr1a gene-deficient mice. Pharm Res 17:749–753
70. Thompson SJ, Koszdin K, Bernards CM (2000) Opiate-induced analgesia is increased and prolonged in mice lacking P-glycoprotein. Anesthesiology 92:1392–1399
71. Letrent SP, Pollack GM, Brouwer KR et al (1999) Effects of a potent and specific P-glycoprotein inhibitor on the blood–brain barrier distribution and antinociceptive effect of morphine in the rat. Drug Metab Dispos 28:827–834
72. Rodriguez M, Ortega I, Soengas I et al (2004) Effect of P-glycoprotein inhibition on methadone analgesia and brain distribution in the rat. J Pharm Pharmacol 56:367–374
73. Sadeque AJM, Wandel C, He H et al (2000) Increased drug delivery to the brain by P-glycoprotein inhibition. Clin Pharmacol Ther 68:231–237
74. Heykants J, Michiels M, Knaeps A et al (1974) Loperamide (R 18553), a novel type of antidiarrheal agent. Arzneimittelforschung 24:1649–1653
75. Doser K, Meyer B, Nitsche V et al (1995) Bioequivalence evaluation of two different oral formulations of loperamide (Diarex lactab vs Immodium capsules). Int J Clin Pharmacol Ther 33:431–436
76. Schinkel AH, Wagenaar E, Mol CAAM et al (1996) P-glycoprotein in the blood–brain barrier of mice influences the brain penetration and pharmacological activity of many drugs. J Clin Invest 97:2517–2524
77. Skarke C, Jarrar M, Schmidt H et al (2003) Effects of ABCB1 (multidrug resistance transporter) gene mutations on disposition and central nervous effects of loperamide in healthy volunteers. Pharmacogenetics 13:651–660
78. Skarke C, Jarrar M, Erb K et al (2003) Respiratory and miotic effects of morphine in healthy volunteers when P-glycoprotein is blocked by quinidine. Clin Pharmacol Ther 74:303–311
79. Dagenais C, Graff CL, Pollack GM (2004) Variable modulation of opioid brain uptake by P-glycoprotein in mice. Biochem Pharmacol 67:269–276
80. Upton RN (2002) Theoretical aspects of P-glycoprotein mediated drug efflux on the distribution volume of anaesthetic-related drugs in the brain. Anaesth Intensive Care 30:183–191
81. Shapiro AB, Ling V (1997) Positively cooperative sites for drug transport by P-glycoprotein with distinct drug specificities. Eur J Biochem 250:130–137
82. Yasuda K, Lan LB, Sanglard D, Furuya K, Schuetz JD, Schuetz EG (2002) Interaction of cytochrome P450 3A inhibitors with P-glycoprotein. J Pharmacol Exp Ther 303:323–332
83. Kwan P, Brodie MJ (2000) Early identification of refractory epilepsy. N Engl J Med 342:314–319
84. Chang BS, Lowenstein DH (2003) Epilepsy. N Engl J Med 349:1257–1266
85. Luna-Tortós C, Fedrowitz M, Löscher W (2008) Several major antiepileptic drugs are substrates for human P-glycoprotein. Neuropharmacology 55:1364–1375
86. Sperling MR (2004) The consequences of uncontrolled epilepsy. CNS Spectr 9:98–99
87. Löscher W, Potschka H (2005) Drug resistance in brain diseases and the role of drug efflux transporters. Nat Rev Neurosci 6:591–602
88. Löscher W, Potschka H (2002) Role of multidrug transporters in pharmacoresistance to antiepileptic drugs. J Pharmacol Exp Ther 301:7–14
89. Volk HA, Burkhardt K, Potschka H, Chen J et al (2004) Neuronal expression of the drug efflux transporter P-glycoprotein in the rat hippocampus after limbic seizures. Neuroscience 123:751–759
90. Volk HA, Löscher W (2005) Multidrug resistance in epilepsy: rats with drug-resistant seizures exhibit enhances brain expression of P-glycoprotein compared with rats with drug-responsive seizures. Brain 2005(128):1358–1368
91. Volk HA, Potschka H, Löscher W (2005) Immunohistochemical localization of P-glycoprotein in rat brain and detection of its increased expression by seizures are sensitive to fixation and staining variables. J Histochem Cytochem 53:517–531

92. Tishler DM, Weinberg KT, Hinton DR et al (1995) MDR1 gene expression in brain of patients with medically intractable epilepsy. Epilepsia 36:1–6
93. Sisodiya SM, Lin WR, Squier MV et al (2001) Multidrug resistance protein 1 in focal cortical dysplasia. Lancet 357:42–43
94. Sisodiya SM, Lin WR, Harding BN et al (2002) Drug resistance in epilepsy: expression of drug resistance proteins in common causes of refractory epilepsy. Brain 125:22–31
95. Dombrowski SM, Desai SY, Marroni M et al (2001) Overexpression of multiple drug resistance genes in endothelial cells from patients with refractory epilepsy. Epilepsia 42:1501–1506
96. Aronica E, Gorter JA, Jansen GH et al (2003) Expression and cellular distribution of multidrug transporter proteins in two major causes of medically intractable epilepsy: focal cortical dysplasia and glioneuronal tumors. Neuroscience 118:417–429
97. Aronica E, Gorter JA, Ramkema M et al (2004) Expression and cellular distribution of multidrug resistance-related proteins in the hippocampus of patients of with mesial temporal lobe epilepsy. Epilepsia 45:441–451
98. Sisodiya SM, Martinian L, Scheffer GL et al (2003) Major vault protein, a marker of drug resistance, is upregulated in refractory epilepsy. Epilepsia 2003:1388–1396
99. Rizzi M, Caccia S, Guiso G et al (2002) P-glycoprotein in rodent brain: functional implications for pharmacoresistance. J Neurosci 22:5833–5839
100. Brandt C, Bethmann K, Gastens AM et al (2006) The multidrug transporter hypothesis of drug resistance in epilepsy: proof-of-principle in a rat model of temporal lobe epilepsy. Neurobiol Dis 24:202–211
101. Van Vliet EA, van Schaik R, Edelbroek PM et al (2007) Region-specific overexpression of P-glycoprotein at the blood–brain barrier affects brain uptake of phenytoin in epileptic rats. J Pharmacol Exp Ther 332:141–147
102. Nicita F, Spalice A, Papetti L et al (2014) Efficacy of verapamil as an adjunctive treatment in children with drug-resistant epilepsy: a pilot study. Seizure 23:36–40
103. Asadi-Pooya AA, Razavizadegan SMA, Abdi-Ardekani A et al (2013) Adjunctive use of verapamil in patients with refractory temporal lobe epilepsy: a pilot study. Epilepsy Behav 29:150–154
104. Betts T, Yarrow H, Greenhill L et al (2003) Clinical experience of marketed levetiracetam in an epilepsy clinic – a one year follow up study. Seizure 12:136–140
105. Seegers U, Potschka H, Löscher W (2002) Lack of effects of prolonged treatment with phenobarbital or phenytoin on the expression of P-glycoprotein in various rat brain regions. Eur J Pharmacol 451:149–155
106. Kerb R, Hoffmeyer S, Brinkmann U (2001) ABC drug transporters: hereditary polymorphisms and pharmacological impact in MDR1, MRP1, and MRP2. Pharmacogenomics 2:51–64
107. Siddiqui A, Kerb R, Weale ME et al (2003) Association of multidrug resistance in epilepsy with a polymorphism in the drug-transporter gene ABCB1. N Engl J Med 348:1442–1448
108. Li M, Tan J, Yang X et al (2014) The ABCB1-C3435T polymorphism likely acts as a risk factor for resistance to antiepileptic drugs. Epilepsy Res 108:1052–1067
109. Alpman A, Ozkinay F, Tekgul H et al (2010) Multidrug resistance 1 (MDR1) gene polymorphisms in childhood drug-resistant epilepsy. J Child Neurol 25:1485–1490
110. Di Q, Wang L, Xu L et al (2011) Association between the C3435T polymorphism of human multidrug resistance 1 gene and refractory epilepsy. Chin J Neuromed 10:127–131
111. Ebid AH, Ahmed MM, Mohammed SA (2007) Therapeutic drug monitoring and clinical outcomes in epileptic Egyptian patients: a gene polymorphism perspective study. Ther Drug Monit 29:305–312
112. Haerian BS, Lim KS, Mohamed EH et al (2004) Lack of association of ABCB1 and PXR polymorphisms with response to treatment in epilepsy. Seizure 20:387–394
113. Haerian BS, Lim KS, Tan HJ et al (2011) Association between ABCB1 polymorphism and response to sodium valproate treatment in Malaysian epilepsy patients. Epileptic Discord 13:65–75

114. Hajnsek S, Basic S, Poljakovic Z et al (2004) The effect of MDR1 gene C3435T polymorphism in pharmacotherapeutic efficacy in epilepsy. Neurol Croat 53:69–78
115. Hung CC, Jen Tai J, Kao PJ et al (2007) Association of polymorphisms in NRNR1I2 and ABCB1 genes with epilepsy treatment responses. Pharmacogenomics 8:1151–1158
116. Hung CC, Tai JJ, Lin CJ et al (2005) Complex haplotypic effects of the ABCB1 gene on epilepsy treatment response. Pharmacogenomics 6:411–417
117. Kwan P, Baum L, Wong V et al (2007) Association between ABCB1 C3435T polymorphism and drug-resistant epilepsy in Han Chinese. Epilepsy Behav 11:112–117
118. Kwan P, Wong V, Ng PW et al (2009) Gene-wide tagging study of association between ABCB1 polymorphisms and multidrug resistance in epilepsy in Han Chinese. Pharmacogenomics 10:723–732
119. Sanchez MB, Herranz JL, Leno C et al (2010) Genetic factors associated with drug-resistance of epilepsy: relevance of stratification by patient age and aetiology of epilepsy. Seizure 19:93–101
120. Soranzo N, Cavalleri GL, Weale ME et al (2004) Identifying candidate causal variants responsible for altered activity of the ABCB1 multidrug resistance gene. Genome Res 14:1333–1344
121. Bournissen FG, Moretti ME, Juurlink DN et al (2009) Polymorphism of the MDR1/ABCB1 C3435T drug-transporter and resistance to anticonvulsant drugs: a meta-analysis. Epilepsia 50:898–903
122. Haerian BS, Lim KS, Tan CT et al (2011) Association of ABCB1 gene polymorphisms and their haplotypes with response to antiepileptic drugs. A systematic review and meta-analysis. Pharmacogenomics 12:713–725
123. Haerian BS, Roslan H, Raymond AA et al (2010) ABCB1 C3435T polymorphism and the risk of resistance to antiepileptic drugs in epilepsy: a systematic review and meta-analysis. Seizure 19:339–346
124. Leschziner GD, Andrew T, Leach JP et al (2007) Common ABCB1 polymorphisms are not associated with multidrug resistance in epilepsy using a gene-wide tagging approach. Pharmacogenet Genomics 17:217–220
125. Nurmohamed L, Garcia-Bournissen F, Buono RJ et al (2010) Predisposition to epilepsy – does the ABCB1 gene play a role? Epilepsia 51:1882–1885
126. Subenthiran S, Abdullah NR, Josepj JP et al (2013) Linkage disequilibrium between polymorphisms of ABCB1 and ABCB2 to predict the treatment outcome of Malaysians with complex partial seizures on treatment with carbamazepine mono-therapy at the Kuala Lumpur hospital. PLoS One 8:e64827
127. Seo T, Ishitsu T, Ueda N et al (2006) ABCB1 polymorphisms influence the response to antiepileptic drugs in Japanese epilepsy patients. Pharmacogenomics 7:555–561
128. Subenthiran S, Abdullah NR, Muniandy PK et al (2013) G2677T polymorphism can predict treatment outcome of Malaysians with complex partial seizures being treated with carbamazepine. Genet Mol Res 12:5937–5944
129. Qu J, Zhou BT, Yin JY et al (2012) ABCB2 polymorphisms and haplotype are associated with drug resistance in Chinese epileptic patients. CNS Neurosci Ther 18:647–651
130. Ufer M, Mosyagin I, Muhle H et al (2009) Non-response to antiepileptic pharmacotherapy is associated with the ABCB2 -24C>T polymorphism in young and adult patients with epilepsy. Pharmacogenet Genomics 19:353–362
131. Haenisch S, Zimmerman U, Dazert E et al (2007) Influence of polymorphisms of ABCB1 and ABCB2 on mRNA and protein expression in normal and cancerous kidney cortex. Pharmacogenomics 7:56–65
132. Fava M, Davidson KG (1996) Definition and epidemiology of treatment-resistant depression. Psychiatr Clin North Am 17:179–200
133. O'brien FE, Dinan T, Griffen BT et al (2012) Interactions between antidepressants and P-glycoprotein at the blood–brain barrier: clinical significance of in vitro and in vivo findings. Br J Pharmacol 165:289–312
134. Pariante CM, Thomas SA, Lovestone S et al (2004) Do antidepressants regulate how cortisol affects the brain? Psychoneuroendocrinology 29:423–447

135. Bauer B, Hartz AMS, Fricker G et al (2004) Pregnane X receptor up-regulation of P-glycoprotein expression and transport function at the blood–brain barrier. Mol Pharmacol 66:413–419
136. Narang VS, Fraga C, Kumar N et al (2008) Dexamethasone increases expression and activity of multidrug resistance transporters at the rat blood–brain barrier. Am J Physiol Cell Physiol 295:C440–C450
137. Bauer B, Hartz AMS, Miller DS (2007) Tumor necrosis factor alpha and endothelin-1 increase P-glycoprotein expression and transport activity at the blood–brain barrier. Mol Pharmacol 71:667–675
138. Yu CH, Kastin AJ, Tu H et al (2007) TNF activates P-glycoprotein in cerebral microvascular endothelial cells. Cell Physiol Biochem 20:853–858
139. Liptrott NJ, Penny M, Bray PG et al (2009) The impact of cytokines on the expression of drug transporters, cytochrome P450 enzymes and chemokine receptors in human PBMC. Br J Pharmacol 156:497–508
140. Lin KM, Chiu YF, Tsai IK et al (2011) ABCB1 gene polymorphisms are associated with the severity of major depressive disorder and its response to escitalopram treatment. Pharmacogenet Genomics 21:163–170
141. Uhr M, Tontsch A, Namendorf C et al (2008) Polymorphisms in the drug transporter gene ABAB1 predict antidepressant treatment response in depression. Neuron 57:203–209
142. Sarginson JE, Lazzeroni LC, Ryan HS et al (2010) ABCB1 (MDR1) polymorphisms and antidepressant response in geriatric depression. Pharmacogenet Genomics 20:467–475
143. Peters EJ, Slager SL, Kraft JB et al (2008) Pharmacokinetic genes do not influence response or tolerance to citalopram in the STAR*D sample. PLoS One 3:e1872
144. Pariante CM, Lightman SL (2008) The HPA axis in major depression: classical theories and new developments. Trends Neurosci 31:464–468
145. Carroll BJ, Cassidy F, Naftolowitz D et al (2007) Pathophysiology of hypercortisolism in depression. Acta Psychiatr Scand Suppl 443:90–103
146. Yau JLW, Noble J, Thomas S et al (2007) The antidepressant desipramine requires the ABCB1 (Mdr1)-Type p-glycoprotein to upregulate the glucocorticoid receptor in mice. Neuropsychopharmacology 32:2520–2529
147. Mason BL, Thomas SA, Lightman SL et al (2011) Desipramine treatment has minimal effects on the brain accumulation of glucocorticoids in P-gp-deficient and wild-type mice. Psychoneuroendocrinology 36:1351–1360
148. Clarke G, O'Mahony SM, Cryan JF et al (2009) Verapamil in treatment resistant depression: a role from the P-glycoprotein transporter? Hum Psychopharmacol 24:217–223
149. Phillip NS, Carpenter LL, Tyrka AR et al (2010) Pharmacologic approaches to treatment resistant depression: a re-examination for the modern era. Expert Opin Pharmacother 11:709–722
150. Wang JS, DeVane CL, Gibson BB et al (2006) Population pharmacokinetic analysis of drug-drug interactions among risperidone, bupropion, and sertraline in CF1 mice. Psychopharmacology (Berl) 183:490–499
151. Conley RR, Buchanan RW (1997) Evaluation of treatment-resistant schizophrenia. Schizophr Bull 23:663–674
152. Meltzer HY (1992) Treatment of the neuroleptic-nonresponsive schizophrenic patient. Schizophr Bull 18:515–542
153. Juarez-Reyes MG, Shumway M, Battle C et al (1995) Effects of stringent criteria on eligibility for clozapine among public mental health clients. Psychiatr Serv 46:801–806
154. Essock SM, Hargreaves WA, Covell NH et al (1996) Clozapine's effectiveness for patients in state hospitals: results from a randomized trial. Psychopharmacol Bull 32:683–697
155. Yasui-Furukori N, Saito M, Nakagami T et al (2006) Association between multidrug resistance 1 (MDR1) gene polymorphisms and therapeutic response to bromperidol in schizophrenic patients: a preliminary study. Pro Neuropsychopharmacol Biol Psychiatry 30:286–291
156. Shinkai T, De Luca V, Utsunomiya K et al (2008) Functional polymorphism of the human multidrug resistance gene (MDR1) and polydipsia-hyponatremia in schizophrenia. Neuromolecular Med 10:362–367

157. Kuzman MR, Medved V, Bozina N et al (2008) The influence of 5-HT_{2C} and MDR1 genetic polymorphisms on antipsychotic-induced weight gain in female schizophrenic patients. Psychiatry Res 160:308–315
158. Lin YC, Ellingrod VL, Bishop JR et al (2006) The relationship between P-glycoprotein (PGP) polymorphisms and response to olanzapine treatment in schizophrenia. Ther Drug Monit 28:668–672
159. Kastelic M, Koprivšek J, Plesničar BK et al (2010) MDR1 gene polymorphisms and response to acute risperidone treatment. Prog Neuropsychopharmacol Biol Psychiatry 34:387–392
160. Bozina N, Kuzman MR, Medved V et al (2008) Associations between MDR1 gene polymorphisms and schizophrenia and therapeutic response to olanzapine in female schizophrenic patients. J Psychiatr Res 42:89–97
161. Alenius M, Wadelius M, Dahl ML et al (2008) Gene polymorphism influencing treatment response in psychotic patients in a naturalistic setting. J Psychiatr Res 42:884–893
162. Xing Q, Gau R, Li H et al (2006) Polymorphisms of the ABCB1 gene are associated with the therapeutic response to risperidone in Chinese schizophrenic patients. Pharmacogenomics 7:987–993
163. Suzuki Y, Tsuneyama N, Fukui N et al (2013) Impact of the ABCB1 gene polymorphism on plasma 9-hydroxyrisperidone and active moiety levels in Japanese patients with schizophrenia. J Clin Psychopharmacol 33:411–414
164. Nikisch G, Baumann P, Oneda B et al (2011) Cytochrome P450 and ABCB1 genetics: association with quetiapine and norquetiapine plasma and cerebrospinal fluid concentrations and with clinical response in patients suffering from schizophrenia. A pilot study. J Psychopharmacol 25:896–907
165. Vijayan NN, Mathew A, Balan S et al (2012) Antipsychotic drug dosage and therapeutic drug response in schizophrenia is influences by ABCB1 genotypes: a study from a south Indian perspective. Pharmacogenomics 13:1119–1127
166. Moons T, de Roo M, Claes S et al (2011) Relationship between P-glycoprotein and second generation antipsychotics. Pharmacogenomics 12:1193–1211
167. Correia CT, Almeida JP, Santos PE et al (2010) Pharmacogenetics of risperidone therapy in autism: association analysis of eight candidate genes with drug efficacy and adverse drug reactions. Pharmacogenomics J 10:418–430
168. Jovanovic N, Bozina N, Lovric M et al (2010) Effect of CYP2D6, CYP3A5, and MDR1 genetic polymorphisms on the pharmacokinetics of risperidone and its active moiety. J Clin Pharmacol 50:659–666
169. Takao T, Tachikawa H, Kawanishi Y et al (2006) Association of treatment-resistant schizophrenia with the G2677A/T and C3435T polymorphisms in the ATP-binding cassette subfamily B member 1 gene. Psychiatr Genet 16:47–48
170. Mahar Doan KM, Humphreys JE, Webster LO et al (2002) Passive permeability and P-glycoprotein-mediated efflux differentiate central nervous system (CNS) and non-CNS marketed drugs. J Pharmacol Exp Ther 303:1029–1037
171. Boulton DW, DeVane CL, Liston HL et al (2002) Human recombinant P-glycoprotein specificity for atypical antipsychotics. Life Sci 71:163–169
172. Bebawy M, Chetty M (2008) Differential pharmacological regulation of drug efflux and pharmacoresistant schizophrenia. Bioessays 30:183–188
173. Bebawy M, Morris MB, Roufogalis BD (2001) Selective modulation of P-glycoprotein-mediated drug resistance. Br J Cancer 85:1998–2003
174. Hartz AMS, Bauer B (2010) Regulation of ABC transporters at the blood-brain barrier: new targets for CNS therapy. Mol Interv 10:293–304
175. Schinkel AH (1999) P-glycoprotein, a gatekeeper in the blood-brain barrier. Adv Drug Deliv Rev 36:179–194

Chapter 6
Pharmacogenomics

Kristen M. Wiese, Stephanie A. Flowers, and Vicki L. Ellingrod

Abstract Pharmacogenomics is a rapidly growing field dedicated to identifying genetic markers that will allow practitioners to identify safe and effective therapy that is tailored to the individual patient. As a result, pharmacogenomic testing has the potential to optimize drug therapy for a variety of disease states. The landmark Sequenced Treatment Alternatives to Relieve Depression trial, commonly known as the STAR*D trial, showed that only a disappointing 30 % of patients experience remission from depression symptoms with their initial trial of antidepressant therapy. Furthermore, other studies have shown that 70 % of patients not remitting after their first medication trial may endure symptoms for months before experiencing relief secondary to drug therapy. In the future it is hoped that advancing pharmacogenomics research will help identify the safest and most effective medication for each patient—not only for the treatment of depression but for other disease states as well. Currently pharmacogenomic testing is not widely implemented; however, this is likely to change as clinicians become increasingly familiar with this field. This chapter will familiarize clinicians with the field of pharmacogenomics by (1) building a simple understanding of how genetic variability can alter drug response, (2) discussing current approaches in pharmacogenomics research, (3) describing helpful resources for practitioners, (4) providing an overview of the clinical application of pharmacogenomics and the associated issue of reimbursement, and (5) reviewing opinions on the future of pharmacogenomics in the clinical setting.

Kristen M. Wiese and Stephanie A. Flowers contributed equally to this work.

K.M. Wiese, PharmD • S.A. Flowers, PharmD, PhD
Department of Clinical Pharmacy, College of Pharmacy,
University of Michigan, 428 Church Street, Ann Arbor, MI 48109, USA
e-mail: kmwiese@umich.edu; fstephan@umich.edu

V.L. Ellingrod, PharmD, FCCP (✉)
Department of Clinical Pharmacy, College of Pharmacy,
Ann Arbor, MI, USA

Department of Psychiatry, School of Medicine, University of Michigan,
428 Church Street, Ann Arbor, MI 48109, USA
e-mail: vellingr@med.umich.edu

M. Jann et al. (eds.), *Applied Clinical Pharmacokinetics and Pharmacodynamics of Psychopharmacological Agents*,
DOI 10.1007/978-3-319-27883-4_6

Keywords Pharmacogenomics • Personalized medicine • Pharmacogenetics • Individualized therapy • Single-nucleotide polymorphism (SNP) • Genome-wide association studies (GWAS) • Genotype • Whole-exome sequencing (WES)

Pharmacogenomics is a rapidly growing field dedicated to identifying genetic markers that will allow practitioners to identify safe and effective drug therapy tailored to the individual patient. As such, pharmacogenomics is a key component of personalized medicine, which is a broad term encompassing preventative, diagnostic, and treatment strategies based on the molecular profile of the individual.

The potential for pharmacogenomics to make a significant impact on the practice of pharmacy is impressive. As an example, for those with depression, the landmark Sequenced Treatment Alternatives to Relieve Depression trial, commonly known as the STAR*D trial, showed that only a disappointing 30 % of patients experience remission from depression symptoms with their initial trial of antidepressant therapy [1, 2]. Furthermore, other studies have shown that 70 % of patients not remitting after their first medication trial may endure symptoms for months before experiencing relief secondary to drug therapy [3]. In the future it is hoped that advancing pharmacogenomics research will help identify the safest and most effective medication for each patient starting a new course of drug therapy. Patients, practitioners, and third-party payers would all be expected to benefit from the impressive amount of time, money, and frustration saved by eliminating this trial and error period.

Currently pharmacogenomics is not widely applied by clinicians; however, with the constant expansion of personalized medicine tailoring therapies and diagnostics to the individual, knowing when pharmacogenomics tests are appropriate, where to order them, and how to interpret and apply the results will be important tools for healthcare practitioners in the near future. The following chapter objectives are structured to familiarize clinicians with pharmacogenomics by (1) building a simple understanding of how genetic variability can alter drug response, (2) discussing current approaches in pharmacogenomics research, (3) describing helpful resources for practitioners, (4) providing an overview of the clinical application of pharmacogenomics and the associated issue of reimbursement, and (5) reviewing opinions on the future of pharmacogenomics in the clinical setting.

6.1 Objective 1: Genetic Variability and Drug Response

Interindividual variation in the DNA sequence occurs approximately once every 300 base pairs, or in roughly ten million locations [4]. By far the most common source of genetic variation, and the source of the above estimate, refers to single-nucleotide polymorphisms (SNPs), commonly referred to as "snips."

SNPs occur when one of the four DNA base pairs (adenine [A], cytosine [C], thymine [T], or guanine [G]) is substituted for another. In pharmacogenomics literature, SNPs are often designated by their position on the gene of interest and include some indication of the more common base pair, for example, 109T>C or T109C. In this instance the SNP occurs at position 109 on the gene, and the most common nucleotide found is thymine, followed by cytosine. Therefore, 109T and 109C are different variants of this fictional gene and may occur on one or both alleles (or stands of DNA). In some situations, sets of SNPs that are inherited together due to close proximity on the DNA strand are studied as a group, or haplotype.

Another mechanism of genetic variation that has demonstrated importance in drug response is called a copy number variant (CNV). This type of mutation is observed when large sections of DNA are repeated (or deleted altogether) in an individual's genome. Whereas SNPs are estimated to occur at roughly ten million locations on the human genome, far fewer regions of variable copy number have been identified [4, 5]. In a 2006 analysis of 270 individuals, only 1447 regions of variable copy number greater than 1 thousand base pairs were identified [5]. The estimated occurrence of CNVs per individual has been quoted at anywhere from 11 to 140 [6].

The presence of an SNP or CNV alone is not enough to confer impact on clinical outcome with respect to drug response. In fact, the vast majority of SNPs and CNVs likely have no impact on pharmacogenomics. As illustrated in the upcoming examples of pharmacogenomics research, genetic variants that are most likely to impact drug response often have one of the following characteristics: they change the activity of enzymes important for medication metabolism, they occur in a site important to the mechanism of action (such as in the binding pocket of a drug target or a change in the promoter region of the gene that regulates expression), or they impact a medication's side effect profile. The outcomes that are measured and assumed to be due to genetic variability are called phenotypes. Phenotypes are a reflection of the impact of a person's genotype. Common phenotypes in pharmacogenomic studies include treatment response, tolerability, side effects, and drug pharmacokinetics.

An additional consideration unique to pharmacogenomics research is variant frequency. Genetic variants often differ in occurrence by ethnicity, and for a study to be feasible with respect to participant size, a variant typically needs to be present in at least 5 % of the general population. Otherwise, the number of study participants necessary to show a statistically significant impact becomes unattainable for many investigators (in the thousands depending on expected clinical impact). Examples of methods used in pharmacogenomics research to detect and analyze SNPs, haplotypes, and CNVs will be discussed in more detail in the following section.

6.2 Objective 2: Current Approaches in Pharmacogenomic Research

6.2.1 Targeted Genotyping

The targeted genotyping method is employed when a predetermined SNP is linked to a disease or drug response phenotype. Identification of candidate genes is particularly useful when disease pathophysiology or drug mechanism of action is known. Often for these studies, one or more genes are sequenced, and a few SNPs are examined in relation to the identified phenotype.

An example of utilizing a candidate gene approach in pharmacogenomics of mental health is defining the mechanism of antidepressant-associated sexual dysfunction (SD). Sexual dysfunction is a frequently described side effect of antidepressants, specifically those associated with the serotonergic pathway [7]. Selective serotonin reuptake inhibitors (SSRIs) are first-line agents for the treatment of depression but have a reported SD rate that approaches 40 % [8]. Males typically describe a decrease in desire and ability to achieve orgasm, while females report a decrease in arousal that is attributed to SSRI use. As a result of SD, clinicians report decreased compliance with antidepressant treatment [9]. Most research on SSRI-associated SD has focused on the *5-HTTLPR* variant, which is a 44 base pair insertion/deletion in the promoter of the gene *SLC6A4* [10, 11]. This gene encodes a serotonin transporter 5-HTT and, due to its involvement in the serotonergic pathway, is a logical gene to interrogate by the candidate gene approach in this population. Upon sequencing the *SLC6A4* loci, analysis showed that the longer *5-HTTLPR* variant (44 bp insertion present) is associated with greater SSRI efficacy; however, the long allele is also associated with greater SD in carriers [12–15]. Clinically, we may find that although homozygous carriers of the long *5-HTTLPR* variant respond well to antidepressant therapy, compliance may become an issue as the patient is likely to experience SD [11, 16].

6.2.2 Genome-Wide Association Studies (GWAS)

The majority of pharmacogenomics research has generally focused on genes related to drug metabolism. However, as sequencing technology improves along with our understanding of disease pathophysiology, we find a greater need to understand additional pathways that may determine treatment response. GWAS uses array chip technology to associate specific phenotypes with genetic variants, or SNPs, across the entire genome [17]. Unlike candidate gene studies, the GWAS method does not require prior knowledge of the pathophysiology of the disease state and has the potential to identify novel candidate variants.

GWAS design requires several elements. DNA is required from a large phenotypically relevant population in addition to the ability to detect polymorphic alleles that can be genotyped and have adequate coverage of the genome [18]. Importantly, GWAS also requires rigorous statistical methodology to determine genetic associations [19]. For many recent GWA studies, the few common associated SNPs show a small effect size and explain small portions of genetic risk [20]. Aside from monogenic diseases, or an inherited disease controlled by a single pair of genes, the genetic cause of more complex disease may need to consider a graded quantitative genetic risk that includes the involvement of high-risk and low-risk genes. In many cases, researchers feel that current GWAS methods are only the first step in the identification of target genes [21]. Additionally GWAS investigations can examine the accumulation of gene variants in a specific network that may result in complex disease.

Genome-wide association studies have been widely utilized to identify target genes responsible for varying treatment response phenotypes in psychiatric medicine. The STAR*D trial, previously mentioned, provided the largest cohort of DNA from patients with major depressive disorder (MDD) [2]. One of STAR*D's goals was to determine the effectiveness of alternate therapies for patients who were nonresponders to initial antidepressant treatment, and a genetic portion of the trial examined how differences in patient response may be explained in part by pharmacogenetics [22].

To do this, researchers examined DNA sequences from 68 suspect genes collected from 1297 STAR*D participants, comparing those who responded to treatment with citalopram as opposed to nonresponders [23]. This initial analysis established a response relationship with a variant of the *HT2RA* gene (rs7997012), which is a serotonin receptor. A later analysis of the STAR*D trial expanded the population to include 1816 patients and duplicated the analysis between the citalopram responders and nonresponders [24]. This study reproduced the previous association with the *HT2RA* variant and treatment response but additionally found an association of the *GRIK4* gene variant (rs1954787) with the higher likelihood of treatment response. This was the first report that highlighted the role of *GRIK4*, a glutamate receptor, in the pathogenesis and treatment outcome of MDD.

6.2.3 Whole-Exome Sequencing (WES)

Out of the approximate three billion base pairs that configure the human genome, only 1 % of this sequence actually translates into protein [25]. An exon is the protein-coding portion of the gene and the exome consists of all the genome's exons. Therefore, whole-exome sequencing is a technique in which genomic DNA binds to a predefined target of sequences that correspond to the protein-coding portion of the genome. As next-generation sequencing platforms become cheaper and more available, it is now possible to cost-effectively target variation in the coding portion of the genome [26]. The obvious drawbacks to WES are that structural changes and intergenic and promoter sequences that may influence gene transcription or splice variants will be excluded from analysis. Additionally, our current understanding of the genome limits our analysis as parts of the genome not currently recognized as translatable will not be interrogated by this method [27]. Despite these limitations, WES has been shown to be highly effective at identifying high-penetrance exonic mutations causing disease.

Much like the GWAS STAR*D trial, which examined the genetics of nonresponders to SSRIs, WES has also been employed to investigate pharmacogenomics of antidepressant treatment. Wong and colleagues compared the effectiveness of fluoxetine and desipramine therapy in a prospective pharmacogenetic study in first-generation Mexican Americans to identify specific SNPs that correlated with treatment response [28]. Although the study showed that fluoxetine was generally more effective after 8 weeks of treatment, whole-exome sequencing was performed for 36 treatment responders and 29 subjects who did not respond to treatment.

Pharmacogenetic analysis showed that exm-rs1321744 achieved significance for the treatment remission group. Interestingly, the location of the variant suggests an epigenetic function, as it's situated in a brain-methylated DNA immunoprecipitation sequencing site, which further implicates its functional role in antidepressant treatment response.

6.2.4 *Whole-Genome Sequencing*

Most loci identified by genome-wide association analysis do not result in amino acid substitutions in proteins or may not even locate to an exome sequence [29]. Instead, these mutations can potentially alter gene expression and translational activity or affect gene splicing. Current array-based methodologies such as WES identify common allele variants in a population, but these may only have minor effects on phenotype or have variable penetrance due to epigenetic confounders. Whole-genome sequencing offers the most comprehensive picture of an individual's genome by providing both uncommon variant sequence data as well as structural data. As the cost of genome sequencing continues to decrease, experts predict a shift from array-based technologies to whole-genome sequencing approaches [30]. Whole-genome sequencing analysis requires redundant sequencing of millions of short DNA fragments [31]. Construction of the genome can be performed de novo but is more commonly done with the aid of the reference genome. The most important element of whole-genome sequencing is the quality of the genome assembly defined by the assembly and alignment algorithms.

Whole-genome sequencing is now employed to identify variants in pharmacogenomic biomarkers for commonly prescribed drugs [32]. Mizzi and colleagues analyzed whole-genome sequences from 482 unrelated individuals of mixed ethnic backgrounds. Analysis revealed over 400,000 variants in 231 pharmacogenes associated with the absorption, distribution, metabolism, excretion, and toxicity (ADMET) of several drugs. Of these variants, 26,807 were in exon sequences and regulatory regions, whereas 16,487 were previously undetected. Interestingly, when authors focused their analysis on defined pharmacogenes, *CYP2D6*, *CYPC9*, *VKORC1*, *UGT1A1*, and *TPMT*, 11 novel exonic variants were revealed that reached a frequency of over 1 %. These data emphasize the potential of whole-genome sequencing to capture several novel and potentially important ADMET-associated variants in patients.

6.2.5 *Copy Number Variant*

In addition to identifying sequence changes in the genetic code, current genomic research also focuses on structural changes in genetic representation of genes (duplications, deletions) such as copy number variations (CNVs) [5, 6]. When CNVs are at least 1 kb in length, vary from the reference genome, and are identified in a population at a frequency of at least 1 %, they are called copy number polymorphisms (CNPs) [5, 33]. CNVs are common in the human population, affect about 15 % of the genome, and are likely to result in the change of expression levels of genes in or close to the effected regions [34]. With specific regard to psychiatric illness, CNVs have been shown to contribute to conditions such as Alzheimer's disease, schizophrenia, and autism [35–37].

CYP2D6 is a highly polymorphic gene that encodes an enzyme responsible for metabolizing 25 % of currently used drugs [38]. Included in this list of substrates are SSRIs, tricyclic antidepressants, and some antipsychotics. To date there are 75 individual variant *CYP2D6* alleles documented in the Human Cytochrome P450 Allele Nomenclature Database (http://www.cypalleles.ki.se), which include those with normal, reduced, and nonfunctional enzymatic activity levels resulting from different combinations of SNPs. In addition to SNPs, CNVs of *CYP2D6* wild-type and variant alleles have been observed resulting in increased expression levels of this enzyme in vivo [39]. Carriers of multiple functional alleles of *CYP2D6* can result in rapid metabolization of substrates, and standard dosing recommendations for *CYP2D6*-metabolized medications may not suffice.

6.3 Objective 3: Pharmacogenomics Resources

There are a multitude of online resources available regarding the research and clinical implementation of pharmacogenetics.

6.3.1 HapMap Project

The HapMap Project (www.hapmap.org) is an international collaboration of scientists and different funding agencies that have developed a haplotype map of the human genome. This resource is designed to describe common patterns of DNA sequence variations, where they occur on the chromosome, and how they are distributed in different populations. These data are devised to be a resource for researchers to identify genes affecting disease, drug response, and environmental health.

6.3.2 The 1000 Genomes Project

The goal of The 1000 Genomes Project (www.1000genomes.org/) is to discover and locate genetic variants that have frequencies of at least 1 % in various populations. Although the title stipulates 1000 genomes, the project intends to combine the light sequencing (4× coverage) data from a total of 2500 genomes to provide an accurate picture of estimated variants and genotypes that were not sequenced directly. This project was designed with the intent that individual researchers will utilize the 1000 Genomes dataset to expand their personal data to include millions of additional variants beyond those genotyped directly by the investigator. This process is entirely computational and requires no genotyping cost. The additional genotype data allows investigators to localize phenotype-associated loci and target associated genes more precisely.

6.3.3 The Psychiatric GWAS Consortium (PGC)

The PGC (http://www.med.unc.edu/pgc) is the largest psychiatric consortium that serves as a repository for the genome-wide genetic data for over 170,000 subjects submitted by over 500 investigators from at least 80 institutions. As discussed earlier, GWAS data analysis requires large sample sizes to identify robust genetic associations, and obtaining this data for investigators can be a challenge. The PCG repository of genetic data can be used by individual investigators to conduct mega-analysis of gene associations of psychiatric disorders. Initially, analysis was focused on autism, attention-deficit hyperactivity disorder, bipolar disorder, major depressive disorder, and schizophrenia but has expanded to encompass other disorders in addition to CNV analysis.

PGC is also involved in the Psych Chip project where they are conducting new genotyping of large numbers of new cases and controls. To accomplish this, the Infinium® PsychArray BeadChip from Illumina (http://products.illumina.com/) was developed in collaboration with the PCG in order to evaluate genetic variants associated with common psychiatric disorders. The PsychArray BeadChip, or the Psych Chip, is a SNP array that contains 250,000 exome variants selected by the PGC, high-density sequencing coverage of loci associated with psychiatric illness, and genome-wide common variants that allow comparison to other GWAS studies.

6.3.4 PharmGKB

PharmGKB (www.pharmgkb.org) is a knowledge base and resource center that contains and disseminates clinical information about pharmacogenomics and drug response. In 2009, a collaboration between PharmGKB and Pharmacogenomics Research Network (PRN) created the Clinical Pharmacogenetics Implementation Consortium (CPIC). The purpose of CPIC is to develop clinical guidelines from the interpretation of rigorous laboratory genetic testing into applicable instructions for clinicians to implement pharmacogenetic information into practice. Guidelines can either focus on specific genes or drugs and encompass directions on how to assign phenotypes to genotypes in addition to drug-specific prescribing recommendations. CPIC guidelines are published in peer-reviewed journals and are periodically updated with supplemental data; these guidelines and additional resources are located on the CPIC webpage (http://www.pharmgkb.org/page/cpic).

6.4 Objective 4: Current Clinical Applications of Pharmacogenomics and Reimbursement

As discussed in objective 3, there are multiple resources that provide dosing recommendations for psychiatric medications based on genetic profile, but there is very little guidance on when to order a genetic test. The following examples will address this knowledge gap by illustrating how providers are currently employing pharmacogenomics in a clinical setting. Additional considerations, such as the quality control regulation of laboratories that offer genetic testing, and the issue of insurance reimbursement will also be discussed.

At this time, the mood stabilizer carbamazepine is the only medication used in psychiatric medicine that includes a labeling recommendation to obtain genetic testing prior to use in individuals of Asian ancestry [40]. This recommendation was added to the product packaging label based on research showing that patients of East Asian descent were at an increased risk of developing a serious, potentially life-threatening rash when taking carbamazepine [41]. At least 5 % of this risk was attributed to carrying a particular variant of the human leukocyte antigen allele: HLA-B*1502 [42]. This allele is present at a much greater frequency in East Asians (10–15 %), as compared to those of Japanese or Korean (<1 %) descent [43]. This situation provides a fairly straightforward example of when SNPs distant from the site of a medication's mechanism of action significantly impact a drug's side effect profile.

Outside of this recommendation for carbamazepine, how do healthcare providers know when to order genetic testing to guide drug therapy? Many would consider the following two situations: (1) for patients being treated with medication for a new indication in order to avoid multiple medication trials and (2) for patients who are refractory to treatment with a particular medication for the dual purpose of determining the cause of suboptimal treatment response and assisting with the selection of a different medication. A common focus of genetic tests offered by commercial laboratories to improve medication use is the analysis of drug metabolizing enzyme activity, most often enzymes within the cytochrome P450 family.

As part of the genetic testing process, samples (usually blood or saliva) are sent to laboratories where the DNA is sequenced and analyzed for the presence of multiple SNPs and CNVs that have been associated with variable drug response in pharmacogenomics studies. The results of these assays are then interpreted to classify the genotyped individual as a poor, intermediate, extensive, or ultrarapid metabolizer of medications metabolized by the tested enzyme. In this classification system, extensive metabolizers are considered to have an average level of metabolizing capacity, while poor and intermediate metabolizers have a lower metabolic capacity. Poor or intermediate metabolizers typically have higher plasma concentrations of substrate medications, experience more side effects, and require lower-than-normal doses. Alternatively, ultrarapid metabolizers have higher-than-normal enzyme activity resulting in reduced efficacy; these patients may require higher-than-average doses of drugs metabolized by the tested enzyme.

After classifying the metabolizing status of each tested enzyme, a report will typically be sent to the ordering healthcare professional that describes the dosing recommendations made by organizations such as CPIC or the Dutch Pharmacogenetics Working Group [44, 45]. Consider the following example situation: you just diagnosed a 45-year-old woman with depression. This is her first diagnosed episode, and her comorbid conditions include migraines and chronic back pain. She tells you that her sister has had depression for the past several years and that she is still struggling to find a medication that works well for her. She is worried this will happen to her so you broach the topic of pharmacogenomics and she agrees to genetic testing.

The test results return and you note that her CYP2D6 status is classified as extensive (or normal), but that her CYP2C19 status is classified as poor. Your first impression was to select nortriptyline to simultaneously target her migraine, mood, and pain symptoms, but you know that this medication is metabolized in part by CYP2C19. You refer to the report and read that CPIC recommends considering a 50 % reduction in the recommended starting nortriptyline dose in patients with this genetic profile and to utilize therapeutic drug monitoring to guide dose adjustments [46]. In this situation, pharmacogenomic testing alerted a practitioner to initiate and titrate treatment more cautiously than standard recommendations dictate. Additionally, the provider is now aware that medications the patient may take in the future which are metabolized by CYP2C19, such as diazepam, may be present in higher-than-average plasma concentrations, and lower starting doses may be prudent.

Like TDM for lithium, genetic testing can be a helpful tool to improve medication use when it is implemented correctly. Unlike lithium TDM, genetic tests do not need to be repeated unless new variants are found to impact the response of medications your patient is currently receiving or plans to receive in the future. Another dissimilarity between pharmacogenomics tests and the majority of labs used in healthcare decisions (such as lipid and blood glucose screening) is that the provider has to select the lab that will perform the pharmacogenomic testing. In most cases, clinicians cannot simply write an order for pharmacogenomics testing and instruct the patient to visit the genetic test retailer nearest them.

This leads to the question: how do you select a pharmacogenomics laboratory to sequence your patient's DNA, and who is regulating these tests? The Food and Drug Administration (FDA) has the authority to regulate the clinical validity of pharmacogenomics tests. However, so far the FDA has only exercised this authority over genetic tests sold as kits [47]. Therefore, clinicians may wish to refer to resources such as PharmGKB for current literature and guideline summaries prior to determining how applicable specific test results may be to their patient. The Centers for Medicare and Medicaid Services (CMS) also regulates laboratory testing through the Clinical Laboratory Improvement Amendments (CLIA) [48]. CLIA certification is focused on analytical validity and the overall quality of laboratory practices [49]. Practitioners planning to order genetic tests may wish to consider selecting facilities that have CLIA certification because it ensures that an independent body has approved their employees' training and analytical laboratory quality.

CLIA certification is also necessary for reimbursement from Medicare and Medicaid [48]. Currently there are very few pharmacogenomics tests that are covered by insurance. As noted in a detailed review of pharmacogenomic reimbursement, Milligan stated that private third-party payers tend to take cues from Medicare with respect to what tests should be covered [50]. Pharmacogenomics tests for many medications are not covered because they are considered experimental and lack established clinical value [51]. However, as time progresses the costs of these tests will decrease, and the body of evidence supporting the relationship between genetic variation and drug response will accumulate. It is reasonable to predict that personalized drug prescribing will be a cost effective, reimbursable means of improving drug response in the future.

6.5 Objective 5: Future of Pharmacogenomics

Several issues complicate the widespread adoption of genetic testing in psychiatric pharmacy. As noted in many reviews, there is an absence of large, prospective randomized clinical trials comparing the cost and outcomes of patients treated with or without pharmacogenomics-based medication algorithms in the field of mental health. Some speculate that a large-scale study necessary to prove the cost/benefits analysis of pharmacogenomics within the mental health arena will never be attempted due to unacceptably high costs [52].

In 2009, a retrospective analysis of the STAR*D trial attempted to assess whether the benefits of pharmacogenomics testing outweighed the costs [53]. For this study, the author used genotype data from one SNP in a serotonin gene that was previously associated with citalopram response in combination with a rather complex cost analysis assessment that assumed that patients entered treatment at age 40 and were followed over the course of their lifetime [23, 53]. The authors concluded that the genetic testing for this one SNP was not cost effective [53]. However, the authors did state that incorporating multiple genetic variants into a cost-benefit analysis might improve the predictive power of a pharmacogenomics test and push the cost-benefit analysis in favor of testing [53].

This comment leads to several important considerations regarding the future of pharmacogenomics testing. First, like any new technology, the cost of running sequencing assays is steadily decreasing. Costs are already below $100 for the reagents used to analyze about 500,000 SNPs [52]. Furthermore, it is highly likely that incorporating more loci of genetic variability will improve the predictive power of pharmacogenomics.

No discussion of pharmacogenomics would be complete without addressing the ethical issues associated with collecting and storing DNA. Patient uncertainty regarding the use and confidentiality of collected DNA may become a substantial barrier to the widespread adoption of genetic testing once reimbursement is no longer an issue. In the research setting, patient rights are protected via a detailed informed consent process, which informs individuals that they are surrendering their DNA for current and future genetic testing. Alternatively, "tiered" approaches to genetic research are being used where patients can consent to have their DNA studied for the current trial in which they are participating but decline consent for future research [54].

When genetic information is used for diagnosis or treatment decisions, there is concern that test results could be used to discriminate against individuals when they seek future employment or health insurance. The United States enacted a law in 2008 to protect individuals from this type of discrimination. It is called the Genetic Information Nondiscrimination Act (GINA). GINA contains two parts that expressly prohibit health insurance providers from using genetic information to make eligibility or coverage decisions. In addition, GINA forbids employers from making employment decisions based on an individual's genetic profile [55]. There are a few uncovered groups in this act, such as those serving in the military or those working for employers with less than 15 employees. Furthermore, GINA does not apply to any other insurance type, such as life or disability insurance.

6.6 Conclusion

As the cost of genetic testing decreases and evidence supporting the utility of pharmacogenomics in drug prescribing continues to grow, it will be increasingly important for clinicians to understand the resources available to them for interpreting the quality and relevance of pharmacogenomic test results. This chapter was designed to provide an introduction to the application of pharmacogenomics in the mental health field. The interested reader is referred to the websites discussed throughout the chapter and those listed here:

1. PharmGKB: www.pharmgkb.org
2. CPIC dosing guidelines: http://www.pharmgkb.org/page/cpic
3. 1000 Genomes: www.1000genomes.org/
4. The Psychiatric GWAS Consortium: http://www.med.unc.edu/pgc
5. HapMap Project: www.hapmap.org
6. Dutch Pharmacogenetics Working Group: http://www.pharmgkb.org/page/dpwg
7. CLIA lab certification: http://www.cms.gov/Regulations-and-Guidance/Legislation/CLIA/index.html?redirect=/clia/
8. GINA: http://www.genome.gov/24519851

References

1. Rush AJ, Trivedi MH, Wisniewski SR et al (2006) Acute and longer-term outcomes in depressed outpatients requiring one or several treatment steps: a STAR*D report. Am J Psychiatry 163:1905–1917
2. Trivedi MH, Rush AJ, Wisniewski SR et al (2006) Evaluation of outcomes with citalopram for depression using measurement-based care in STAR*D: implications for clinical practice. Am J Psychiatry 163:28–40

3. Gelenberg AJ, Freeman MP, Markowitz JC et al (2010) Practice guideline for the treatment of patients with major depressive disorder. Retrieved from: http://psychiatryonline.org/pb/assets/raw/sitewide/practice_guidelines/guidelines/mdd.pdf
4. Genetics Home Reference, U.S. National Library of Medicine (2015) What is the International HapMap Project? (2014). Retrieved from: http://ghr.nlm.nih.gov/handbook/genomicresearch/hapmap
5. Redon R, Ishikawa S, Fitch KR et al (2006) Global variation in copy number in the human genome. Nature 444:444–454
6. Ouahchi K, Lindeman N, Lee C (2006) Copy number variants and pharmacogenomics. Pharmacogenomics 7:25–29
7. Clayton AH, Montejo AL (2006) Major depressive disorder, antidepressants, and sexual dysfunction. J Clin Psychiatry 67 Suppl 6:33–37
8. Higgins A, Nash M, Lynch AM (2010) Antidepressant-associated sexual dysfunction: impact, effects, and treatment. Drug Healthc Patient Saf 2:141–150
9. Kennedy SH, Rizvi S (2009) Sexual dysfunction, depression, and the impact of antidepressants. J Clin Psychopharmacol 29:157–164
10. Barr CS, Newman TK, Schwandt M et al (2004) Sexual dichotomy of an interaction between early adversity and the serotonin transporter gene promoter variant in rhesus macaques. Proc Natl Acad Sci U S A 101:12358–12363
11. Strohmaier J, Wüst S, Uher R et al (2011) Sexual dysfunction during treatment with serotonergic and noradrenergic antidepressants: clinical description and the role of the 5-HTTLPR. World J Biol Psychiatry 12:528–538
12. Lesch KP, Bengel D, Heils A et al (1996) Association of anxiety-related traits with a polymorphism in the serotonin transporter gene regulatory region. Science 274:1527–1531
13. Gillihan SJ, Rao H, Wang J et al (2010) Serotonin transporter genotype modulates amygdala activity during mood regulation. Soc Cogn Affect Neurosci 5:1–10
14. Zanardi R, Serretti A, Rossini D et al (2001) Factors affecting fluvoxamine antidepressant activity: influence of pindolol and 5-HTTLPR in delusional and nondelusional depression. Biol Psychiatry 50:323–330
15. Peters EJ, Slager SL, McGrath PJ, Knowles JA, Hamilton SP (2004) Investigation of serotonin-related genes in antidepressant response. Mol Psychiatry 9:879–889
16. Bishop JR, Ellingrod VL, Akroush M et al (2009) The association of serotonin transporter genotypes and selective serotonin reuptake inhibitor (SSRI)-associated sexual side effects: possible relationship to oral contraceptives. Hum Psychopharmacol 24:207–215
17. Daly AK (2010) Genome-wide association studies in pharmacogenomics. Nat Rev Genet 11:241–246
18. Yang TH, Kon M, DeLisi C (2013) Genome-wide association studies. Methods Mol Biol 939:233–251
19. Hayes B (2013) Overview of statistical methods for genome-wide association studies (GWAS). Methods Mol Biol 1019:149–169
20. No authors listed (2010) On beyond GWAS. Nat Genet 42:551
21. Edwards SL, Beesley J, French JD et al (2013) Beyond GWASs: illuminating the dark road from association to function. Am J Hum Genet 93:779–797
22. Laje G, Perlis RH, Rush AJ et al (2009) Pharmacogenetics studies in STAR*D: strengths, limitations, and results. Psychiatr Serv 60:1446–1457
23. McMahon FJ, Buervenich S, Charney D et al (2006) Variation in the gene encoding the serotonin 2A receptor is associated with outcome of antidepressant treatment. Am J Hum Genet 78:804–814
24. Paddock S, Laje G, Charney D et al (2007) Association of GRIK4 with outcome of antidepressant treatment in the STAR*D cohort. Am J Psychiatry 164:1181–1188
25. Lander ES (2011) Initial impact of the sequencing of the human genome. Nature 470:187–197
26. Bao R, Huang L, Andrade J et al (2014) Review of current methods, applications, and data management for the bioinformatics analysis of whole exome sequencing. Cancer Inform 13:67–82

27. Rabbani B, Teki M, Mahdieh N (2014) The promise of whole-exome sequencing in medical genetics. J Hum Genet 59:5–15
28. Wong ML, Dong C, Flores DL et al (2014) Clinical outcomes and genome-wide association for a brain methylation site in an antidepressant pharmacogenetics study in Mexican Americans. Am J Psychiatry 171:1297–1309
29. Cirulli ET, Goldstein DB (2010) Uncovering the roles of rare variants in common disease through whole-genome sequencing. Nat Rev Genet 11:415–425
30. Yu Y, Wu B, Wu J et al (2012) Exome and whole-genome sequencing as clinical tests: a transformative practice in molecular diagnostics. Clin Chem 58:1507–1509
31. Ng PC, Kirkness EF (2010) Whole genome sequencing. Methods Mol Biol 628:215–226
32. Mizzi C, Peters B, Mitropoulou C et al (2014) Personalized pharmacogenomics profiling using whole-genome sequencing. Pharmacogenomics 15:1223–1234
33. Sebat J, Lakshmi B, Troge J et al (2004) Large-scale copy number polymorphism in the human genome. Science 305:525–528
34. Estivill X, Armengol L (2007) Copy number variants and common disorders: filling the gaps and exploring complexity in genome-wide association studies. PLoS Genet 3:1787–1799
35. Hooli BV, Kovacs-Vajna ZM, Mullin K et al (2014) Rare autosomal copy number variations in early-onset familial Alzheimer's disease. Mol Psychiatry 19:676–681
36. Merikangas AK, Segurado R, Cormican P et al (2014) The phenotypic manifestations of rare CNVs in schizophrenia. Schizophr Res 158:255–260
37. Coe BP, Witherspoon K, Rosenfeld JA et al (2014) Refining analyses of copy number variation identifies specific genes associated with developmental delay. Nat Genet 46:1063–1071
38. Zhou SF, Liu JP, Lai XS (2009) Substrate specificity, inhibitors and regulation of human cytochrome P450 2D6 and implications in drug development. Curr Med Chem 16:2661–2805
39. Hosono N, Kato M, Kiyotani K et al (2009) CYP2D6 genotyping for functional-gene dosage analysis by allele copy number detection. Clin Chem 55:1546–1554
40. National Institutes of Health (2008) DailyMed – CARBAMAZEPINE- carbamazepine tablet CARBAMAZEPINE- carbamazepine tablet, chewable. Retrieved from: http://dailymed.nlm.nih.gov/dailymed/drugInfo.cfm?setid=c13bc0b8-7900-4ef4-98ed-e1315a08d95d
41. Ferrell PB, McLeod HL (2008) Carbamazepine, HLA-B*1502 and risk of Stevens-Johnson syndrome and toxic epidermal necrolysis: US FDA recommendations. Pharmacogenomics 9:1543–1546
42. Hung SI, Chung WH, Jee SH et al (2006) Genetic susceptibility to carbamazepine-induced cutaneous adverse drug reactions. Pharmacogenet Genomics 16:297–306
43. U.S. Food and Drug Administration (2013) Postmarket drug safety information for patients and providers – information for healthcare professionals: dangerous or even fatal skin reactions – carbamazepine (marketed as Carbatrol, Equetro, Tegretol, and generics). Retrieved from: http://www.fda.gov/Drugs/DrugSafety/Postmarket.DrugSafetyInformationforPatientsandProviders/ucm124718.htm
44. PharmGKB. DPWG: Dutch Pharmacogenetics Working Group. Retrieved from: https://www.pharmgkb.org/page/dpwg
45. PharmGKB. CPIC: clinical pharmacogenetics implementation consortium. Retrieved from: https://www.pharmgkb.org/page/cpic
46. Hicks JK, Swen JJ, Thorn CF et al (2013) Clinical pharmacogenetics implementation consortium guideline for CYP2D6 and CYP2C19 genotypes and dosing of tricyclic antidepressants. Clin Pharmacol Ther 93:402–408
47. National Human Genome Research Institute (2015) Regulation of genetic tests. Retrieved from: http://www.genome.gov/10002335
48. Centers for Medicare & Medicaid Services (2014) Clinical laboratory improvements amendments (CLIA). Retrieved from: http://www.cms.gov/Regulations-and-Guidance/Legislation/CLIA/index.html?redirect=/clia/
49. Genetics Home Reference, U.S. National Library of Medicine (2014) How can consumers be sure a genetic test is valid and useful? Retrieved from: http://ghr.nlm.nih.gov/handbook/testing/validtest

50. Robert J, Milligan RJ (2008) Coverage and reimbursement for pharmacogenomic testing. Jurimetrics J 48:137–165
51. Priority Health (2010) Pharmacogenomic testing. Retrieved from: https://www.priorityhealth.com/provider/manual/auths/~/media/documents/medical-policies/91570.pdf
52. Crettol S, de Leo J, Hiemke C, Eap CB (2014) Pharmacogenomics in psychiatry: from therapeutic drug monitoring to genomic medicine. Clin Pharmacol Ther 95:254–257
53. Perlis RH, Patrick A, Smoller JW et al (2009) When is pharmacogenetic testing for antidepressant response ready for the clinic? A cost-effectiveness analysis based on data from the STAR*D study. Neuropsychopharmacology 34:2227–2236
54. Santa Clara University (2008) Pharmacogenomics, ethics, and public policy. Retrieved from: http://www.scu.edu/ethics/practicing/focusareas/medical/pharmacogenomics.html
55. Genetics Home Reference, U.S. National Library of Medicine (2015) The genetic information nondiscrimination act (GINA). (2014). Retrieved from: http://ghr.nlm.nih.gov/spotlight=thegeneticinformationnondiscriminationactgina

Part II
Clinical Pharmacokinetics and Pharmacodynamics of Psychopharmacological Drug Classes

Michael W. Jann, PharmD
Department of Pharmacotherapy
University of North Texas
System College of Pharmacy
Fort Worth, TX
USA
e-mail: Michael.jann@unthsc.edu

Chapter 7
Antipsychotics

Michael W. Jann and W. Klugh Kennedy

Abstract Antipsychotic medications have been used for the treatment of patients with schizophrenia, schizoaffective, bipolar disorders, and other psychotic conditions. Antipsychotics administration can occur by various routes that includes oral, sublingual, intramuscular, and inhalation. Long-acting depot antipsychotics offer the clinician an additional option for chronic disease management. Most antipsychotics are metabolized by the hepatic CYP enzymes except ziprasidone and paliperidone. Antipsychotics are either substrates or inhibitors of P-glycoprotein. A "therapeutic" plasma concentration range has been recommended for antipsychotics except for asenapine, iloperidone, and lurasidone due to their recent entrance into clinical practice. Each antipsychotic agent possesses a different pharmacodynamic profile with receptor binding that accounts for their varying therapeutic effects regarding daily doses and their different adverse event characteristics. The antipsychotic doses are at the lower therapeutic range that achieves a dopamine receptor subtype 2 (D2) blockade of 65–85 % as measured by the PET technology. Yet, routine daily practice exceeds these low doses based upon the patient's clinical response and tolerability indicating the limitations of linking pharmacokinetic and pharmacodynamic models with complex psychiatric diseases such as schizophrenia. Other pharmacodynamic effects include QT/QTc prolongation, prolactin changes, anticholinergic, sedation, and cardiovascular actions. Population pharmacokinetic analysis has been extended to antipsychotics, yielding some interesting findings regarding pharmacokinetic and pharmacodynamic models.

M.W. Jann, PharmD (✉)
Department of Pharmacotherapy, University of North Texas System College of Pharmacy (UNTSCP) and University of North Texas Health Science Center (UNTHSC), Fort Worth, TX, USA
e-mail: Michael.jann@unthsc.edu

W.K. Kennedy, PharmD
Department of Pharmacy Practice, College of Pharmacy, Mercer University, Atlanta, GA, USA

M. Jann et al. (eds.), *Applied Clinical Pharmacokinetics and Pharmacodynamics of Psychopharmacological Agents*,
DOI 10.1007/978-3-319-27883-4_7

Keywords Long-acting depot • Flip-flop • Plasma concentrations • Receptors • Positron emission tomography (PET)

7.1 Introduction

The advent of antipsychotics ushered into the treatment of various psychiatric disorders that contain psychotic symptoms is an important intervention to improve patient care. The psychiatric conditions that commonly employ the use of antipsychotics include schizophrenia and bipolar disorders. These diseases are chronic in nature with relapses and remissions over the patient's lifetime. Antipsychotics also have been used to treat depression, various anxiety disorders, and other psychiatric illnesses. Antipsychotics have been grouped into several categories: typical, atypical, and dopamine stabilizers (e.g., aripiprazole). The typical agents are the older drugs (e.g., chlorpromazine) and have been used for greater than (e.g., chlorpromazine) 35 years to treat patients. The atypical agents have become the first-line medications for the treatment of patients with schizophrenia and bipolar disorders. Whereas a mutual definition of atypical agents remains to be elucidated, it is generally accepted by clinicians that these agents produce little or negligible extrapyramidal side effects, efficacy in treating the negative and cognitive symptoms, a relative absence of tardive dyskinesia, and moderate serum prolactin increases at therapeutic dosages.

The clinical pharmacokinetics of antipsychotics has been extensively studied due to the technological advances in assay methodology that allow for the accurate detection and measurement of plasma drug concentrations (see Chap. 1). However, the routine monitoring for clinical utility of antipsychotic drug concentrations continues to be of questionable use. The wide interpatient variability of antipsychotic agents poses challenges for clinicians to interpret these findings applied to direct patient care. Identification and validation of a "therapeutic" range for these agents enhance usage of serum concentration monitoring to maximize efficacy while minimizing adverse effects. Drug-drug interactions or suspicion of excessive drug serum concentrations despite modest drug dosages can be reasonable explanations for obtaining a sample. Linking serum concentrations to pharmacodynamic effects at the receptor level have been applied to dosages and dopamine receptor (D2) blockade determined by positron emission tomography (PET; see Sect. 7.4.1).

This chapter will present the clinical pharmacokinetics and pharmacodynamics of antipsychotics with a focus on the atypical agents and includes only a selected number of the typical agents [1]. For a more detailed review of the older typical agents, the reader is referred to the other resources [2].

7.2 Clinical Pharmacokinetics

7.2.1 *Absorption*

7.2.1.1 Oral Administration and Bioavailability

The pharmacokinetic properties of selected typical and atypical antipsychotics are presented in Table 7.1. The physiologic mechanism for antipsychotic drug absorption is passive diffusion through the gastrointestinal (GI) membranes. P-glycoprotein (Pgp; see Chap. 1) is present in the GI tract, and all antipsychotic agents were reported to be Pgp substrates in varying magnitudes [1, 3]. As a result, Pgp can also influence antipsychotic drug absorption rates contributing to the interpatient variability found with these agents. The time-to-maximal serum or plasma concentrations (T_{max}) for the majority of both typical and atypical antipsychotics normally occur between 1 and 5 h (data not shown) from capsule and immediate-release tablet formulations [4, 5]. Several agents have been formulated as oral disintegrating tablets (olanzapine, risperidone, aripiprazole). Asenapine must be given sublingually to achieve a bioavailability of at least 30 %; oral administration is associated with less than 2 % systemic availability [6, 7]. A slightly longer T_{max} was reported for olanzapine (mean 6 h) [4]. Quetiapine extended-release (ER) tablet had a mean T_{max} of 5 h (versus a mean of 2 h for the immediate release), while paliperidone extended-release capsule reported a mean T_{max} of 24 h [8, 9].

The effect of food was shown to increase ziprasidone's bioavailability up to 60 % [10]. A high fat meal had the greatest impact increasing ziprasidone area under the plasma concentration-time curve (AUC). A high fat meal also increased quetiapine AUC and peak plasma concentration (C_{max}) by 15 % and 25 %, respectively [11]. Lurasidone is recommended to be taken with at least a 350 Kcal meal independent of fat content to ensure maximum exposure [12]. Food decreased the absorption rate of risperidone but not the extent [13]. Food did not significantly affect the absorption rate of the other antipsychotics [1, 2].

7.2.2 *Inhalation*

An inhalation device was developed to administer loxapine via inhalation for patients who refuse oral or intramuscular antipsychotic administration. Single doses of 0.625–10 mg given to healthy volunteers produced a mean T_{max} of 5 min [14]. Although this route has a faster T_{max} compared to other administration routes including intramuscular loxapine [15], additional clinical studies should be explored to determine the feasibility of inhalation antipsychotic therapy for agitated patients.

Table 7.1 Summary of the mean clinical pharmacokinetic parameters of the antipsychotics

Drug	$T_{½}$ (h)	CL (L/h)	Vd	Primary metabolic pathway	Metabolite	Therapeutic concentrations (ng/mL)
First-generation typical antipsychotics				*CYP enzymes*		
Chlorpromazine	11.8	919	980–2000 L	1A2, 2D6, 3A4	7-Hydroxychlorpromazine	30–300
Fluphenazine	13.0	571–4821 L	10,500	1A2	7-Hydroxfluphenazine	0.5–2.0
Enthanate	4 days		62,000 L			
Decanoate	14 days					
Haloperidol	20.0	33–49	9.5 L/kg	1A2, 2D6, 3A4	Reduced haloperidol	5–17
Decanoate	21 days					
Mesoridazine	9–30	N.A.	N.A.	2D6	Mesoridazine sulfoxide	150–1000
Perphenazine	9.4	49–183	9.8–26.7 L/kg	1A2, 2D6	N-Desmethylperphenazine 7-Hydroxyperphenazine	0.6–2.4
Thioridazine	6.5	0.59 L/kg/h	6700 L	1A2, 2D6, 3A4	Mesoridazine	200–2000
Second-generation atypical antipsychotics						
Asenapine (sl)	24	0.867 (L/min)	1700 L	1A2, UGT	N-Desmethylasenapine	N.R.
Aripiprazole	75	3.4 L/h	4.9 L/kg	2D6, 3A4	Dehydroaripiprazole	150–300
Decanoate	29.9–46.5 days					
Clozapine	9–17	9–53	2–7 L/kg	1A2, 3A4, (2D6 minor), 2C19 (minor)	Desmethylclozapine	350–600 ng/mL

Iloperidone	14	47–102	2527 L	2D6, 3A4, 1A2 (minor)	P88-8991, P95-12113	N.R.
Decanoate	28 days					
Lurasidone	29–37	3.9 L/min	6137 L	3A4	ID-14283, ID-14326	N.R.
Olanzapine	33	26	16 L	1A2, UGT, 2D6 (minor)	10-N-glucuronide	20–80
Pamoate	30 days				4′-N-desmethylolanzapine	
Paliperidone	24	1.4–8.2	70–192 L	UGT, 2D6 (minor), 3A4 (minor)	None	20–52
Palmitate	25–49 days					
Quetiapine (IR)	6	55–87	513–700 L	3A4, 2D6 (minor)	N-Dealkyalquetiapine (norquetiapine)	70–170
Risperidone	22	5.0 mL/min/kg	1.0 L/kg	2D6 3A4 (minor)	9-Hydroxyrisperidone	20–60
Microspheres	3–6 days					
Ziprasidone	4–10	5.08 mL/min/kg	1.03 L/kg	Aldehyde oxidase, 3A4 (minor) 1A2 (minor)	Dihydroziprasidone	50–160

$T_{1/2}$ elimination half-life, *CL* clearance, *CYP* cytochrome P450, *Vd* volume of distribution, *L* liters, *h* hours, *N.R.* not reported

7.2.3 *Intramuscular (IM) Administration*

Acute Treatment The administration of IM antipsychotics is designated for agitated and psychotic patients who refuse oral administration. Generally, IM administration achieves higher plasma drug concentrations than the oral route due to the bypassing of the gastrointestinal absorption barriers.

Haloperidol remains a commonly used agent with established pharmacokinetic parameters [16]. The T_{max} of haloperidol takes place after 20 min (faster than oral administration) with a C_{max} about twice the amount of the oral route [17, 18]. Haloperidol IM doses can be repeated every 30 min for several doses to manage very agitated patients. Based upon the bioavailability data of the IM haloperidol, a conversion factor of 1.0–1.5 times higher than the IM dose is suggested for converting patients to the oral dose [19]. IM ziprasidone also has a C_{max} of about 30 min [20]. Olanzapine IM administration compared to the oral route has a T_{max} of 30 min with a 2–5-fold higher C_{max} [21]. Peak plasma aripiprazole concentrations were achieved at 0.5 h, and a 90 % higher AUC was reached in the first 2 h with the IM formulation compared to oral aripiprazole [22]. The elimination half-lives from IM antipsychotic administration do not significantly differ from oral administration [1, 5, 6].

Long-Acting Depot Treatment A number of long-acting injectable (LAI) depot antipsychotics are available worldwide. Depot agents were developed to enhance patient adherence to treatment. The older typical antipsychotic, fluphenazine enanthate, was the first depot agent introduced in 1964, and then over the next decade, a variety of agents such as fluphenazine decanoate, haloperidol decanoate, and others became available. The chemical characteristic that all of these molecules have in common is the presence of a terminal alcoholic group (–OH), which allows the combination with carboxylic acid by esterification. These esters display very low solubility in water but are highly soluble in oil. Therefore, sesame oil or viscoleo was used, and after injection into the muscle, a depot of drug is formed that slowly diffuses into the bloodstream. The LAI atypical agents lack the –OH group requiring other strategies to produce a depot preparation [23]. The methods used were drug encapsulation in a biodegradable polymer (risperidone, iloperidone, aripiprazole) or an aqueous suspension of an insoluble compound in water (olanzapine pamoate, paliperidone palmitate). The absorption rate for depot formulations is slower than their elimination rate; thus, the time needed to achieve steady-state conditions is a function of the absorption rate. A principle referred to as "flip-flop" kinetics [23, 24].

The T_{max} and $T_{1/2}$ of fluphenazine enanthate slightly differ from fluphenazine decanoate with a T_{max} of 2–3 days and shorter elimination $T_{½}$ of 3.5–4 days [23]. Fluphenazine decanoate has an earlier T_{max} than other LAIs due to its manufacturing process where "free" fluphenazine is present. The elimination half-life of LAIs shown in Table 7.1 displays a range between 21 and 46.5 days except for risperidone microspheres which has a shorter half-life of 3–6 days. Due to their formulations, risperidone and aripiprazole LAIs are unable to include initial “loading” dose approach, and oral supplementation is recommended for 2–3 weeks after starting LAI therapy [23, 24]. The T_{max} for risperidone LAI occurs at 4–5 weeks [25]. Both aripiprazole decanoate and long-acting iloperidone injection (a crystalline salt structure like paliperidone palmitate) are given on a monthly basis [26, 27]. Recently, a new paliperidone LAI formulation has been approved the US FDA for an administration once every 3 months by injection. The T_{max} occurs between 30 and 33 days with elimination half-lives from the deltoid and gluteal injection sites between 84–95 days and 118–139 days, respectively (Package Insert, Invega Trinza™, Janssen Pharmaceuticals, 2015). The extended time period for the 3-month injection is due to the nanocrystal technology, increased drug concentration, and larger injection volume up to 2.6 mL.

A loading dose approach saturates the tissue compartment due to the agent’s large volume of distribution (*Vd*; see Sect. 7.2.4). A conversion factor of 1.6 times the oral fluphenazine dose administered weekly during the first month has been recommended for fluphenazine decanoate [23]. After the initial month, the fluphenazine decanoate dosing interval can be increased to every 2 weeks for 1 month and then every 4 weeks afterward. Various loading dose methods were described for haloperidol decanoate; these include multiplying the oral dose by 10, 20, or 30 times the oral daily dose given during the first month divided into 2 injections [28]. A weekly 100 mg dosing method can be used for less stable patients for 4 weeks, then every 2 weeks for 1 month, and then every 4 weeks [29]. The time interval can be shortened to 2–3 days for the first two injections, and in specialized forensic units, a loading dose of up to 300 mg can be given weekly for 3 weeks [30]. Paliperidone palmitate is given in the deltoid muscle (28 % higher Cps versus gluteal muscle) 234 mg and then a second injection of 156 mg with a ±4-day window [31]. Olanzapine pamoate loading dose is based on the oral dose for stable patients. For patients taking olanzapine 10 mg daily, the pamoate formulation can be given 210 mg every 2 weeks or 405 mg every 4 weeks. When oral olanzapine 15–20 mg daily is used, the pamoate is dosed 300 mg every 2 weeks. After 8 weeks, dosing can be individually titrated based on the oral daily dose with the highest dose of 300 mg every 2 weeks [24].

7.2.4 Distribution

Antipsychotics are highly lipophilic agents that need to enter the central nervous system (CNS) by penetrating the blood-brain barrier (BBB). These drugs directly bind to tissue components and can readily penetrate or accumulate within the adipose tissue. This principle is one of the aspects that allows for the LAIs loading dose method in dosing initiation. From Table 7.1, antipsychotics have a wide and a large volume of distribution (Vd) with values greater than 1.0 L/kg indicating widespread diffusion throughout the body. The large Vd contributes to the wide interpatient pharmacokinetic variability of these agents [1, 2, 5, 6]. Serum concentration profiles of antipsychotics from single-dose pharmacokinetic studies display a biphasic or triphasic exponential decline as the drug enters various body compartments prior to elimination. Antipsychotics bind to the CNS and peripheral receptors that lead to their therapeutic and adverse side effect profile. Plasma or serum concentration represents the amount of drug in the peripheral compartment but not in the tissue compartments.

7.2.5 Protein Binding

All of the antipsychotics are highly protein bound (>90 %) with the exception of quetiapine (83 %) and paliperidone (74 %) [1, 2, 4, 5]. These agents are bound to various plasma proteins albumin and alpha-one acid glycoprotein (AAG) to varying degrees. For example, olanzapine was reported to be bound to AAG and albumin by 77 % and 90 %, respectively [32]. Theoretically, when two different antipsychotics are used during treatment, protein-binding displacement could occur resulting in an increase of "free" drug into the system for one or both agents. In vitro models reported that when thioridazine was added to plasma from patients taking haloperidol or fluphenazine, increased free concentrations of haloperidol and fluphenazine of 50 % and 30 %, respectively, were found [33, 34]. Displacement reactions could also possibly occur when antipsychotics are coadministered with warfarin or digoxin, and these types of studies are a regulatory agency requirement for the drug approval process. Nonetheless, the clinical significance of protein-binding displacement interactions may be minimal as antipsychotics exhibits a low extraction ratio such as clozapine (mean 0.17 ± 0.11), and most display a wide therapeutic safety index for this type of potential drug-drug interaction [35–37].

7.2.6 CNS Distribution

Based on pharmacokinetic and pharmacodynamics models, drug concentration in the cerebrospinal fluid (CSF) represents the amount of medication presented in the brain that becomes available to the CNS receptors (see Chaps. 3 and 4). As previously mentioned, antipsychotics are highly lipophilic and must pass through the BBB. Also located in the BBB is the Pgp efflux transporter that has been shown to transport all antipsychotics to varying degrees [2, 38]. Pgp-mediated efflux contributes toward the CNS accessibility of these agents and influences their therapeutic and adverse effect profile (see Chap. 6).

Due to their invasive nature, studies of antipsychotic drug distribution into the CSF are challenging to complete in patients with psychiatric disorders. Only a few studies have been conducted. Antipsychotic drug CSF concentrations are lower than the plasma concentrations. The mean CSF/serum thioridazine concentration ratio was reported to be 0.010 (range 0.005–0.26) in 48 patients [39]. Fluphenazine CSF/plasma concentration ratios were ported in six patients taking the LAI decanoate; four patients had a ratio of 0.02, one patient 0.18, and one patient 0.85 (this patient did not experience any significant adverse effects) [40]. CSF haloperidol concentrations measured in ten patients had an equal amount of drug (10 %) as the amount of free haloperidol assayed in the serum [17]. Olanzapine CSF and serum concentrations were measured in 37 outpatients taking 2.5–25 mg daily for at least 14 days [41]. Smoking and other factors were included in the data analysis. The mean serum olanzapine concentration was 34.0 ± 19.7 ng/mL, and the mean CSF olanzapine concentration was 6.9 ± 3.3 ng/mL (20 %). A strong linear correlation between serum and CSF olanzapine concentrations was found ($r = 0.93$, $p < 0.05$). This was the first study that also examined the influence of Pgp gene expression and reported that patients with the carriers of the ABCB1 1236 T/2677 T/3435 T haplotype had higher mean serum olanzapine concentrations (influencing drug absorption rates; see Sect. 7.2.1) of 37.3 ± 21.0 ng/mL versus 22.5 ± 7.9 ng/mL ($p = 0.035$) and 1.8 times higher CSF concentrations (4.7 ± 2.4 ng/mL versus. 2.6 ± 0.8 ng/mL, $p = 0.018$) [42].

7.2.6.1 P-Glycoprotein (Pgp)

The relationship between Pgp and antipsychotics has been described elsewhere, but as previously indicated, antipsychotics are Pgp substrates by varying extents [2, 38]. Pgp is located in the GI tract, liver, kidney, and BBB; therefore, the ABCB1 SNP could impact the antipsychotic drug distribution (see Chap. 6). Drugs that are substrates of Pgp also often overlap with CYP3A4 [42]. The ABCB1 gene that encodes Pgp has most of this research investigating three SNPs, C1236T, G2677T/A, and C3534T, and their relationship with antipsychotic drug concentrations [43]. As mentioned in the Sect. 7.2.6, olanzapine serum and CSF concentrations were reported to be significantly ($p = 0.01$) higher in patients with ABCB1 1236 T/2677 T/3435 T haplotype [41]. Significantly higher quetiapine AUC was found in pharmacokinetic study in healthy volunteers ($N = 24$) with the ABCB1 genotypes C3435T not the C1236T SNPs and was suggested that the polymorphic C3435T SNP may influence plasma concentrations [44]. Two studies reported that median clozapine plasma concentrations were about 1.6-fold higher in patients with the C3435T haplotypes compared to the other patients [45, 46]. Several studies have reported that ABCB1 SNPs variants were not associated with steady-state plasma concentration of risperidone and 9-hydroxyrisperidone metabolite [47, 48]. Based upon these limited studies, it appears that the Pgp T haplotypes may influence plasma concentrations in some but not all antipsychotics. The role of Pgp and its SNPs in antipsychotics continue to be explored.

7.2.7 Metabolism and Elimination

Agents with pharmacologically active metabolites are notable considerations when clinicians evaluate patients for treatment. Antipsychotic metabolites are listed in Table 7.1 as 7-hydroxy, desalkyl, N-desmethyl, and other prefixes that do not include the parent compound name [1]. The complete metabolite name can be derived by including the name of the parent drug such as 7-hydroxychlropromazine. Of note, thioridazine is converted to mesoridazine, and risperidone is metabolized to 9-hydroxyrisperidone (known as paliperidone). Haloperidol is transformed to a reduced haloperidol which is partially converted back to haloperidol [49]. A similar metabolic profile occurs with clozapine where it is converted to clozapine N-oxide and also is partially converted back to the parent drug clozapine, but its major metabolite is desmethylclozapine [50]. The perphenazine metabolite N-dealkylperphenazine is present in concentrations of 1.5–2.0 times that of the parent drug with the 7-hydroxymetabolite about 50 % of the parent drug [51]. Iloperidone and lurasidone have reported metabolite identification [52, 53]. Quetiapine is converted to norquetiapine (via N-dealkylation) which binds to the norepinephrine reuptake transporter (NET) and is suggested to possess antidepressant properties [54]. Paliperidone is primarily metabolized by phase II glucuronidation and is renally eliminated, while ziprasidone is metabolized by aldehyde oxidase [55, 56].

The elimination half-lives of the antipsychotics are presented in Table 7.1 [1, 2, 4, 5]. These values originate from the most commonly reported studies and show the wide interpatient variability in the elimination of antipsychotics as a result of the variability in Vd and CL. The depot antipsychotics also have elimination half-lives that can be measured in days. Fluphenazine enanthate has a shorter elimination half-life compared to the decanoate and can be dosed every 2 weeks [23]. The other depot agents are commonly given every 4 weeks. However, when patients have been on LAIs for extended time periods, antipsychotic drug concentrations may persist for prolonged time periods. Haloperidol and fluphenazine plasma concentrations remained detectable for up to 12 weeks post depot drug cessation when patients were treated with these agents for greater than 6 months [57, 58]. Clinicians should continue to monitor patients for potential adverse side effects for 2–3 months after depot agents are discontinued.

7.2.7.1 CYP Metabolism and Polymorphism

Phase I hepatic oxidative metabolism by cytochrome P450 (CYP) enzymes represents the major pathway of metabolism and elimination for many antipsychotics as shown in Table 7.1 [59–61]. There are some exceptions such as paliperidone and ziprasidone as previously mentioned. Phase II glucuronidation is also an important pathway that contributes to antipsychotic disposition, but very few studies have been conducted to specifically determine its impact in psychopharmacology compared to oxidative phase I metabolism [62]. Olanzapine is primarily metabolized by glucuronidation to its 10-N-glucuronide, but CYP1A2 also significantly contributes to its metabolism [63]. Genetic variations in different CYP enzymes occur and can impact drug disposition in various populations (see Chap. 6). CYP2D6 polymorphisms may impact antipsychotic disposition for those agents where this enzyme is metabolized by this pathway. Table 7.1 lists the antipsychotics that are CYP2D6 substrates: chlorpromazine, haloperidol, perphenazine, thioridazine, aripiprazole, clozapine, iloperidone, and risperidone. These agents except perphenazine are also metabolized by other CYP enzymes (e.g., CYP3A4). The contributions of CYP2D6 polymorphisms and multiple CYPs on drug metabolism are additional factors that contribute to the wide interpatient variability found with antipsychotics. It is beyond the scope of this chapter to review every study examining CYP2D6 polymorphisms and antipsychotic drug disposition. For example, clearance of chlorpromazine and clozapine was not associated with CYP2D6 EMs versus PMs [64, 65]. This chapter will present selected studies where CYP2D6 polymorphisms display a significant impact on specific antipsychotics.

Perphenazine disposition is primarily influenced by CYP2D6 and CYP1A2 [66]. This agent serves as an interesting example as one of the early antipsychotics whose pharmacokinetic profile was examined based upon CYP2D6 genetic variants. A single-dose pharmacokinetic study with perphenazine 6 mg in healthy volunteers ($N=12$, 6 EMs and 6 PMs) reported significantly higher C_{max} in the PMs (2.4 ± 0.6 nmol/L versus 0.7 ± 0.3 nmol/L, $p<0.05$) and AUC (18.5 ± 6.2 nmol/L-h versus 4.5 ± 2.5 nmol/L-h, $p<0.001$) [67]. Median perphenazine serum concentrations per dose at steady state were found to be significantly higher in psychiatric patients who were PMs compared to EMs (0.195 nmol/L-mg versus 0.098 nmol/L-mg, $p<0.01$) [68]. In another study in psychiatric patients, three groups were identified based upon genotype: EMs without two mutant alleles, EMs with one mutant allele, and PMs with two mutant alleles [69]. Mean perphenazine clearance significantly differs between the three groups (EMs without 754 ± 385 L/h, EMs with 454 ± 279 L/h, PMs 250 ± 30 L/h, $p<0.01$).

Metabolism of thioridazine to mesoridazine occurs via CYP2D6. Thioridazine is converted via N-demethylation and 5-sulfoxidation by CYP1A2 and CYP3A4 [70]. A single thioridazine 25 mg dose was given to healthy volunteers ($N=13$ EMs and $N=6$ PMs) where the mean thioridazine AUC was about 4 times greater in the PMs compared to the EMs (709 ± 425 nmol/L-h versus 3179 ± 420 nmol/L-h, $p<0.001$) [71]. Mean mesoridazine AUC did not significantly differ between the PMs and the EMs. Mesoridazine conversion to sulforidazine may be partly influenced by CYP2D6, and its pharmacokinetics has been described from oral and intramuscular administration [72–75]. Thioridazine, mesoridazine, and sulforidazine steady-state concentrations have been described in psychiatric patients ($N=76$) with a median thioridazine dose of 150 mg/day for at least 15 days (median 170 days) [75]. Patients were genotyped for CYP2D6 and CYP2C9 status. PM patients ($N=5$) with the CYP2D6 genotype *4/*4 and *6/*6 had significantly higher dose-corrected plasma thioridazine concentrations compared to other populations with greater than 1 active gene ($N=19$, *1/*4 and *1/*3) and the functional wild-type CYP2D6 *1 allele ($N=47$). The mean dose-corrected thioridazine concentration for the PM group was 15.2 nmol/L-mg compared to the 1 active gene 7.2 nmol/L-mg and the functional CYP2D6 group 4.0 nmol/L-mg ($p<0.01$).

With renewed interest in loxapine, which can be administered by inhalation, metabolism of loxapine has been revisited. Loxapine is converted to amoxapine (an antidepressant) and loxapine N-oxide via CYP3A4. Loxapine is also metabolized to

7-hydroxyloxapine by CYP2D6 and 8-hydroxyloxapine by CYP1A2 [76]. The in vitro D2 (see Sect. 7.3) potency of 7-hydroxyloxapine was reported to be similar to haloperidol or trifluoperazine, whereas amoxapine and 8-hydroxyloxapine are less potent than loxapine [77]. Loxapine disposition dependent upon CYP2D6 genetic variants remains to be determined. Loxapine is also a P-glycoprotein substrate; however, the influence of ABCB1 SNPs on its disposition has not been evaluated [78].

Haloperidol has a complex metabolic profile with the involvement of multiple CYP enzymes shown in Fig. 7.1. Haloperidol is converted to a reduced haloperidol metabolite by the reductase enzyme and is partially converted by about 25 % back to haloperidol by CYP2D6 [19, 49]. Haloperidol is metabolized by CYP2D6, CYP1A2, and CYP3A4 to two metabolites. Therefore, the CYP2D6 polymorphism can influence two potential metabolic pathways. An early study in healthy volunteers phenotyped for CYP2D6 with debrisoquine reported the mean haloperidol elimination half-life to be significantly longer in PMs than EMs (29.4 ± 4.2 h versus 16.3 ± 6.4 h, $p < 0.01$) and slower clearance (1.16 ± 0.36 L/h versus 2.49 ± 1.31 L/h, $p < 0.05$) [79]. In a separate study, the metabolic ratio of dextromorphan to dextrorphan, a marker of CYP2D6 activity, was reported to significantly correlate with steady-state haloperidol concentrations [80]. Mutated CYP2D6 alleles have been identified that result in a lack of enzyme activity. These include CYP2D6*3, CYP2D6*4, CYP2D6*5, CYP2D6*6, and CYP2D6*10 [81]. The *10 allele is present in about 50 % of Asians and the *3 and *4 alleles are rarely identified. However, the relationship between haloperidol plasma concentrations in Japanese patients and CYP2D6*10 allele has been inconsistent [81, 82]. In Caucasian patients, haloperidol was reported to have a dose-dependent inhibitory effect on CYP2D6 and influence steady-state haloperidol plasma concentrations which is suggested to enhance potential drug interactions with other drugs that undergo CYP2D6 metabolism [83].

Risperidone and 9-hydroxyrisperidone concentration/dose (C/D) ratios were compared in patients genotyped with CYP2D6*1*1 (reference) versus patients with the CYP2D6*3, CYP2D6*4, CYP2D6*5, or CYP2D6*6 alleles [84]. After oral risperidone administration, the mean C/D ratios of risperidone, 9-hydroxyrisperidone, and risperidone + 9-hydroxyrisperidone were significantly greater in patients without the functional reference alleles (e.g., mean C/D risperidone 1.15 ± 2.10 ng/mL/mg/day versus 8.18 ± 4.73 ng/mL/mg/day, $p < 0.01$). A similar finding was found with patients treated with the risperidone LAI (mean C/D 0.12 ± 0.03 ng/mL/mg/day versus 0.86 ± 0.71, $p < 0.01$). A later study investigated CYP2D6 IM patients genotyped into three subgroups treated with risperidone [85]. Patients with the nonfunctional allele (def) or reduced-function allele (red) had significantly higher median risperidone serum concentrations that were 4.5- and 3.4-fold higher, respectively, than patients with the functional allele ($p < 0.01$). CYP2D6 was found to be the only enzyme that correlated with risperidone dose or plasma concentrations, whereas CYP2C9, CYP3A4, and ABCB1 status did not correlate [48, 86].

Aripiprazole metabolism to dehydroaripiprazole (OPC-14857) occurs via CYP3A4 and CYP2D6 with the metabolite having an equal pharmacologic activity

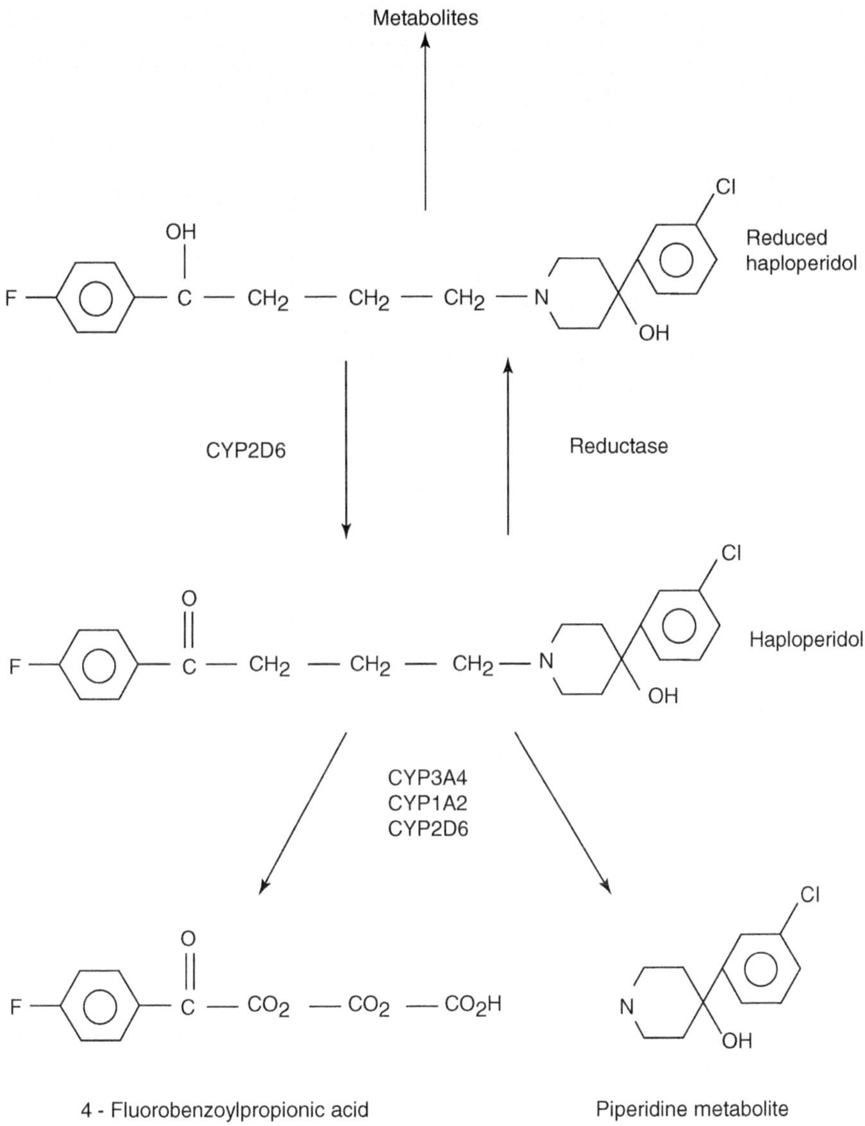

Fig. 7.1 Metabolism of haloperidol (With permission from Perel et al. [1], p. 819)

to the parent drug [87]. Healthy Japanese volunteers were genotyped by CYP2D6 status as EMs (N=9), IMs (N=9), and PMs (N=2). Then, a pharmacokinetic study conducted with a single 6 mg dose and then 3 mg/day for 14 days [88]. The mean pharmacokinetic parameters in the IMs and PMs groups did not significantly differ from the Caucasian EMs population shown in Table 7.1. Among the Japanese groups, the mean aripiprazole clearance was significantly greater in the EMs versus

IMs and PMs (4142 ± 553 mL/h versus 2451 ± 631 mL/h and 2983 mL/h, $p < 0.01$) in the single-dose study. The mean elimination half-life for the EMs was significantly shorter than the IMs and PMs (45.8 ± 8.6 h versus 75.6 ± 16.3 h, 65.8 h; $p < 0.05$). The mean aripiprazole elimination half-life reported in Japanese PMs patients resembles the general population presented in Table 7.1. The 3 mg/day dose given for 14 days was associated with a significantly higher mean AUC obtained over 24 h for total drug concentration (aripiprazole + OPC-14857) in PMs compared to EMs (731.5 ± 397.0 ng • h/mL versus 977.2 ± 396.6 ng • h/mL, $p < 0.01$). Steady-state aripiprazole and dehydroaripiprazole plasma concentrations and CYP2D6*10 allele status were compared in Japanese patients with schizophrenia [89]. Patients were genotyped into three groups: zero, one, and two *10 alleles. The C/D ratios of aripiprazole were significantly higher ($p < 0.001$) in patients with the two *10 alleles compared to patients with the one or zero *10 alleles (19.0 ± 6.8 ng/mL/mg versus 12.7 ± 4.4 ng/mL/mg and 9.0 ± 2.9 ng/mL/mg, respectively). Similar results were reported for the dehydroaripiprazole and total drug concentrations. A further analysis of CYP3A5 genotype and the ABCB1 genotype revealed an unlikely impact on of polymorphism in those genes on aripiprazole plasma concentrations in the Japanese patients [90].

Olanzapine disposition was shown to not be impacted by CYP2D6 polymorphism in a previous study; its metabolism occurs via CYP1A2, CYP1A expression regulator AHR, UGT, and FMO systems [63]. Caffeine is used as a phenotypic tool for CYP1A2 metabolism. A significant correlation was not found between olanzapine clearance and caffeine clearance ($r = 0.19$, $p = 0.56$) when compared in healthy volunteers who were CYP2D6 PMs and EMs [91]. However, a later study reported that olanzapine clearance was significantly correlated ($p < 0.05$) to caffeine and its metabolite ratios measured in plasma ($r = 0.701$), two saliva time points of 6 ($r = 0.644$) and 10 (0.701) hours, and two urinary time points of 8 ($r = 0.745$) and 24 ($r = 0.701$) hours [92]. Application of phenotype and genotype information was suggested to be used in optimizing olanzapine dosage in patients with schizophrenia [93]. CYP1A2 metabolism occurs with clozapine (see Table 7.1), and clearance was reported to be significantly correlated with caffeine N1 and N7 demethylation ($r = 0.89$ and $r = 0.85$, respectively; $p < 0.005$) indicating that the CYP1A2 enzyme has a significant role in clozapine disposition [94].

7.2.7.2 Population Pharmacokinetics

The application of population pharmacokinetic (Pop PK) analysis has been used for antipsychotic medications in patient applications and drug development. The principles of Pop PK have been described in Chap. 4. An early study using a Pop PK regression-pharmacokinetic-statistical model was conducted with haloperidol in patients with schizophrenia. It was reported that haloperidol clearance was influenced by the covariates carbamazepine and smoking with only a variability of 36 % in the population left unexplained [95]. A subsequent analysis in Japanese patients reported that antiepileptics (e.g., carbamazepine, phenobarbital, phenytoin) significantly influenced haloperidol clearance [96]. An additional finding was that age (persons > 55 years) also affected haloperidol clearance, but concurrent administration of CYP2D6 substrates (e.g., thioridazine) did not. Risperidone and 9-hydroxyrisperidone (9-OH-R) metabolite plasma concentrations were analyzed by Pop PK methodology with data collected from the CATIE clinical trial, which was conducted in patients with schizophrenia [97]. Risperidone and 9-OH-R plasma concentrations, representing risperidone dosage adjustments, could be predicted with Pop PK with observed and predicted parent and metabolite plasma concentrations being highly correlated ($r=0.96$, $p<0.0001$ and $r=0.92$, $p<0.0001$, respectively).

Covariates were found to have significant effects on olanzapine plasma concentrations using the Pop PK mixed-effects regression model which included smoking, carbamazepine, and lamotrigine [98]. Using a one-compartment model with first-order absorption, the apparent clearance of aripiprazole was found to be significantly impacted by CYP2D6 status as IM metabolizers had about 60 % lower drug clearance than EM [99]. CYP2D6 status did not affect dehydroaripiprazole clearance. However, CYP2D6 PMs were not included in this study as it may have been difficult to identify a significant number of patients expressing this phenotype. From a routine therapeutic drug monitoring (TDM) program with clozapine, a Pop PK analysis was conducted examining clozapine and desmethylclozapine plasma concentrations [100]. A one-compartment model with first-order absorption and elimination best described the data and reported that smoking and gender (males) had significantly lower clozapine and desmethylclozapine plasma concentrations. Based upon the series of studies in patients treated in the clinical setting, Pop PK has revealed a variety of covariates that can significantly influence antipsychotic clearance and highlighted possible applications to patient care such as dose adjustments based on plasma concentration predictions.

Risperidone and 9-OH-R plasma concentrations from bipolar patients during drug development were analyzed by the Pop PK approach [101]. A two-compartment disposition model was used from the single-dose trials. A depot compartment model from the risperidone dose via a zero-order process with the final amount of drug absorbed split into two models that accounts for risperidone and 9-OH-R concentrations. Patients were also taking other mood stabilizer medications, and other covariates (e.g., age, weight, CYP2D6 status – PM, IM, EM) were included in the analysis. Carbamazepine was reported to significantly influence both risperidone and 9-OH-R clearance, while CYP status did not be impact overall drug clearances.

The development for the dosing strategies for paliperidone LAI involved the application of Pop PK [102]. Data was obtained from the clinical trials and pharmacokinetic data from the phase I, II, and III studies. A one-compartment model with first-order elimination that included application of the "flip-flop" model absorption rate constant (Ka) for depot agents (dual absorption zero/first order) was used. The following covariates were reported to have significant influence on paliperidone disposition – sex, body mass index (BMI), age, injection site (deltoid over gluteal for the first two injections), and needle length. Paliperidone clearance was found to be related to creatinine clearance and Vd related to BMI and sex. Further application of Pop PK analysis of depot paliperidone was developed to make dosing and switching recommendations from other oral and depot antipsychotic agents. Treatment recommendations for missed doses of paliperidone LAI from the second dose on day 8 and during the monthly maintenance doses were also developed for clinicians. Finally, options for the dosing day variability of administration for the second paliperidone LAI dose on day 8 and the subsequent monthly dosing days were determined as ±4 days for the second dose and ±7 days for the monthly maintenance dose [103].

7.3 Clinical Pharmacodynamics

Pharmacodynamic (PD) effects of antipsychotics, like many central nervous system drugs, are categorized into therapeutic effects and adverse side effects. The relationship between these two effects can be dose and/or concentration dependent and pharmacologic receptor mediated. Please note that a patient can have a therapeutic benefit from an antipsychotic and also experience an adverse effect but tolerated the medication overall. The recommended plasma concentrations for therapeutic effects for the different antipsychotics are listed in Table 7.1 [104–106]. For some agents, the plasma concentration range remains to be identified either through clinical trials, through fixed-dose design, or from routine therapeutic drug monitoring (TDM) programs. Active metabolites for some agents have been incorporated with the parent drug plasma concentrations (total drug concentration) in determining the suggested therapeutic range. Blood samples were generally obtained at "trough" conditions at least 12 h post-evening dose and prior to the morning dose for oral agents and prior to the next scheduled administration for LAIs under steady-state conditions unless otherwise specified. This section will only discuss agents where extensive studies support the suggested therapeutic range with key studies. Each agent will be divided into typical and atypical antipsychotics and presented in alphabetical order.

Clinical rating scales form the basis of patient evaluation for efficacy and adverse side effects in neuropsychiatry. In patients with schizophrenia, the two most common rating scales for therapeutic response are the Brief Psychiatric Rating Scale (BPRS) and the Positive and Negative Syndrome Scale (PANSS). The BPRS was used in early studies prior to the 1990s and afterward; the PANSS evaluation has become the "gold standard" for antipsychotic drug development. A reduction of 30–50 % for the BPRS and 20–30 % for the PANSS from baseline to an end point of 4–6 weeks in an acute trial has been established to define therapeutic improvement. To evaluate potential extrapyramidal side effects (EPS), a variety of scales are employed: the Abnormal Involuntary Movement Scales (AIMS), Simpson-Angus Scale (SAS), and the Barnes Akathisia Scale (BAS). Other adverse side effects such as anticholinergic effects are determined by the clinician's assessment of the patient. Efficacy and adverse side effect assessments are usually conducted at baseline and weekly for 4–8 weeks with the change in baseline to the study's end points that establish the drug's profile [107]. Clinicians have accepted the use of antipsychotic plasma concentrations in the overall aspects associated with patient management [108].

7.3.1 Serum or Plasma Concentration Relationships

Typical Antipsychotics: Fluphenazine (FPZ) Various clinical studies have reported a therapeutic range for FPZ between 0.5 and 2.0 ng/mL as shown in Table 7.1. Using a fixed-dose design of 5, 10, and 20 mg per day, these clinical studies reported that patients did not display significant improvement when plasma FPZ concentrations were below 0.2 ng/mL or greater than 2.8 ng/mL [109]. An "optimal" benefit was noted with FPZ concentrations between 0.13 and 0.70 ng/mL with levels greater than 2.4 ng/mL with associated less benefit [110]. Patients with FPZ concentration greater than 4.2 ng/mL reported improvements but experienced significantly more adverse side effects which can limit higher dose usage in patients [111]. A logistic regression modeling approach reported an optimal therapeutic benefit-to-risk ratio with FPZ concentrations up to 2.72 ng/mL with disabling side effects that occurred at higher levels [112]. A higher fixed-dose study with FPZ 10, 20, and 30 mg per day and an optimal threshold response with FPZ plasma concentration around 1.0 ng/mL was reported [113]. A modest correlation was found between FPZ levels and akathisia with higher drug concentrations above 2.0 ng/mL, but some patients tended to also show clinical improvement. A recommended FPZ plasma level of 0.6–0.8 ng/mL for patients sensitive to EPS and a higher a range of 1.0–1.2 ng/mL for acute and maintenance treatment was suggested. A few patients might require FPZ concentrations >1.5 ng/mL for efficacy while balancing the side effects. This study used FPZ doses higher than what would be used today. However, these results confirm higher doses can lead to increased incidences of adverse effects with minimal to modest therapeutic benefit for most patients.

Haloperidol (HAL) Haloperidol has been extensively studied and continues to be studied in examining correlations between therapeutic response, adverse side effects, and plasma concentrations [2]. From the various studies from the past 20 years, Table 7.1 reports the recommended HAL therapeutic plasma concentration range between 5 and 17 ng/mL.[4, 19, 104]. Like FPZ, early studies used higher HAL doses >20 mg/day, and a logistic regression model analysis reported that the incidence of adverse effects tended to increase when plasma HAL concentration was beyond 20 ng/mL. A threshold analysis found that 50 % of disabling EPS effects occurred more frequently when HAL plasma concentration approached 9 ng/mL and increased to 60 % at 12 ng/mL [114]. Although an "upper" therapeutic limit remains to be elucidated with HAL, these studies verify that higher drug doses/ plasma concentrations that exceeded a certain juncture are unlikely to produce added clinical benefits.

The HAL metabolite, reduced HAL (RHAL), was examined to determine its potential role in therapeutic response. At RHAL plasma concentrations of about 25 ng/mL, below this level there appears a linear relationship with HAL plasma levels, whereas above this concentration, a nonlinear relationship was reported [115]. A RHAL/HAL ratio of greater than 1.0 was suggested to be associated with a decreased response to HAL, but this finding was not confirmed [116, 117]. Another interesting aspect is that RHAL/HAL ratios > 1.0 were associated with an increased incidence of EPS [118]. However, this outcome has not been observed by other investigators [19]. Another HAL metabolite, pyridinium, was suggested to be related to EPS occurrence, but the assay for this compound is unavailable from commercial laboratories [119].

Perphenazine (PPZ) Plasma concentrations of PPZ and its dealkylated metabolite did not found to significantly correlate with therapeutic response, but a lower threshold of 0.8 ng/mL (about 2.0 mmol/L) for improvement was suggested [104]. A possible explanation for the lack of response to plasma concentrations to clinical response could be due to the short study time period of 10 days. Even though drug concentrations would have reached steady-state conditions, the time period for this study is considerably shorter than the typical 4–8 weeks for antipsychotics. An early pilot study showed that BPRS scores improved in patients with PPZ concentrations greater than 1.5 ng/mL, but that EPS occurred with levels greater than 3.0 ng/mL [120]. A larger study reported a PPZ therapeutic range of 2–6 mmol/L with a higher EPS incidence when drug levels were from 4 to 6 mmol/L [121].

Thioridazine (TM) and Mesoridazine (MES) TM and MES plasma concentrations were measured during a 3–7-week study open-label study and a flexible-dose design study with thioridazine [122]. A significant correlation between TM concentrations and clinical response was found (0.7–2.0 mmol/L (250–1250 ng/mL)). For patients aged 18–40 years, it was suggested that a TM + MES total concentration of at least 2.0 mmol/L has been achieved as these "younger" patients may be more likely to tolerate potential side effects. The study also reported that higher plasma concentrations significantly correlated with tremors and dry mouth but not with sedation or EPS. Schizophrenic patients who did not respond to chlorpromazine (500–600 ng/mL) were transitioned to TM [123]. Although the chlorpromazine plasma concentrations were greater than the suggested therapeutic range, adverse effects were not reported with patients at the upper therapeutic range of 300 ng/mL prior to the dosage increase. When switched to TM, plasma TM + MES was measured with significant improvement in BPRS scores ($p < 0.02$) when total drug concentrations were from 500 to 1100 ng/mL.

Atypical Antipsychotics: Aripiprazole (APZ) APZ and its dehydroaripiprazole (DHAPZ) metabolite plasma concentrations were measured during various TDM programs in patients with different psychiatric conditions that included adults, children, and adolescents populations [106]. A threshold APZ plasma concentration of 150 ng/mL was suggested, and only one study reported plasma levels up to 420 ng/

mL with higher APZ doses of 30 mg/day [124]. Total drug concentrations (APZ + DHAPZ) were reported in some studies, but the general findings showed that an upper level of about 300 ng/mL was found. A fixed-dose 6-week study was reported in patients with schizophrenia and assessed with the PANSS scale [125]. Clinical response was defined as a PANSS score reduction by 20 % at 6 weeks. Mean daily APZ doses did not significantly differ between responders and nonresponders (15.0 ± 5.9 versus 12.9 ± 6.9, $p = 0.203$). Responders had a trend toward a higher mean APZ plasma concentration than nonresponders (234.4 ± 156.7 ng/mL versus 163.5 ± 77.2 ng/mL, $p = 0.117$) and a significantly higher mean DHAPZ plasma concentration (101.6 ± 58.0 ng/mL versus 66.0 ± 48.4 ng/mL, $p = 0.023$). Since the nonresponding patients had APZ plasma concentrations at the lower suggested therapeutic range, it would be interesting to determine if increasing the APZ dose to achieve higher plasma levels would lead to improvement. However, fixed-dose designs do not allow for flexible dosing to address this possibility.

Clozapine (CLZ) Obtaining CLZ plasma concentrations has been widely accepted by many clinicians to assist in patient management compared to the other atypical agents shown in Table 7.1 [50, 104]. The pivotal studies were conducted in patients with schizophrenia and refractory schizophrenics. These studies dependably reported a threshold of 350 ng/mL for therapeutic response [125] with one study adding the N-desmethylclozapine plasma concentrations for a total drug concentration of 450 ng/mL [126]. An upper therapeutic limit of 600–700 ng/mL was suggested since patients tended to benefits less with these higher concentrations [127, 128].

Olanzapine (OLZ) OLZ plasma concentrations and clinical response have been extensively studied with a suggested therapeutic range of 20–80 ng/mL presented in Table 7.1, describing the overall findings from clinical trial studies to TDM programs [104]. The initial study was a fixed-dose method with OLZ 1–10 mg/day for 6 weeks using the BPRS scale for clinical response [129]. Only 13 % of the patients with OLZ plasma concentrations below 9.3 ng/mL had improved, whereas 45 % of the patients showed improvement with levels greater than 9.3 ng/mL. This study did demonstrate a possible lower threshold of clinical response with modest OLZ doses. A large fixed-dose study with OLZ 10 mg, 20 mg, and 40 mg per day reported a wide interpatient variability in OLZ plasma concentrations (mean 19.7 ± 11.4 ng/mL – 10 mg, mean 37.9 ± 22.8 ng/mL – 20 mg, mean 74.5 ± 43.7 ng/mL – 40 mg/day) which did not show any significant correlations with clinical response using the PANSS scale [130]. However, in studies from the routine TDM programs combined with the fixed-dose studies, the OLZ therapeutic range of 20–80 ng/mL was recommended [131, 132]. A review article examined a dose-response relationship for OLZ and reported that 10–15 mg/day achieves optimal therapeutic response and higher doses can be considered if plasma concentrations were less than 20 ng/mL [133].

Quetiapine (QTP) Various TDM studies have measured QTP plasma concentrations in psychiatric patients presented in Table 7.1 [94]. A lower threshold of QTP plasma level of 77 ng/mL was reported using the Clinical Global Impression (CGI).

Another study reported significantly higher EPS effects in female patients when median QTP plasma concentrations were greater than 210 ng/mL [11]. A 2-year study with hospitalized patients defined a 40 % improvement in the BPRS scores as a responder, and 57 % of that patient population had QTP serum concentrations between 70 and 170 ng/mL [134, 135]. Correlations between serum concentrations and EPS, sedation, weight gain, and cardiovascular effects were not found.

Paliperidone (PAL) and Risperidone (RIS) RIS is metabolized to 9-hydroxyrisperidone (9-OHRIS) which has been developed as an antipsychotic agent – PAL. Clinical response and plasma or serum concentration studies with RIS have combined RIS + 9-OHRIS together as a total drug concentration. As these two agents are so similar, grouping the two drugs into one category is appropriate. From a TDM program using the CGI scores for clinical response, it was reported that the recommended therapeutic concentration range for RIS (total concentration) and PAL was 20–52 ng/mL and 20–60 ng/mL, respectively [106]. These plasma concentration ranges can apply to the oral and LAIs formulation of both products [136]. Although some studies failed to demonstrate a significant relationship between plasma concentrations and clinical response [137], the AGNP-TDM consensus panel has recommended these two plasma concentration ranges for PAL and RIS [104].

Ziprasidone (ZIP) A pilot study with ZIP monotherapy (mean dose 123.1 ± 30.4 mg/day) for 8 weeks showed that plasma ZIP levels from 20 to 160 ng/mL (Mean 75.8 ng/mL) had significant clinical improvement with noted benefit with negative symptoms [138]. In a large analysis of ZIP plasma concentrations with patients with schizophrenia, schizoaffective, and affective disorders, clinical improvement measured by the CGI scale reported that concentrations between 50 and 130 ng/mL were found [139]. The range can be applied to either serum or plasma interchangeably. Correlations with adverse side effects were not found with plasma ZIP concentrations.

7.4 Central Nervous System (CNS) and Peripheral Effect Relationships

Antipsychotics exert their pharmacodynamic therapeutic actions and adverse effects in the CNS and periphery by binding to the various receptors. The recommended therapeutic plasma concentrations for antipsychotics provide a basis for CNS and peripheral pharmacologic activity. For antipsychotics to bind to CNS receptors, adequate drug concentrations are needed, as lower CSF concentrations are generally found compared to the plasma or serum concentrations (see Sect. 7.2.4). However, a strong correlation exists between antipsychotic plasma or serum and CSF concentrations [140]. Patients can have plasma drug concentrations within the therapeutic range and also possibly experience tolerable or intolerable adverse effects. When plasma drug concentrations reach the upper therapeutic range and beyond, adverse effects predominate which diminishes any therapeutic benefits. High drug concentrations in the periphery also contribute toward pharmacologic receptor activity potentially leading to clinical adverse effects. Pharmacokinetic variables (e.g., CYP metabolism) and drug transporters contribute to the wide interpatient variability in plasma concentrations that must be taken into consideration when interpreting antipsychotic actions. The pharmacologic profile of the antipsychotics is presented in Table 7.2 with the interpretation of each agent based upon in vitro published data [141–145]. Receptor occupancy at the dopamine receptor subtype 2 (D2) is related to therapeutic effects and extrapyramidal side effects (EPS). Serotonin receptor

Table 7.2 Summary of the antipsychotics receptor pharmacology and pharmacodynamics [140–145]

Drug	D2	5HT2A	M	H1	Alpha −1	PET D2 receptor @65–85 %
Reference compound						
Spiperone	++++	–	–	–	–	–
Ketanserin	–	++++	–	–	–	–
3-Quinuclidinyl-4-iodobenzilate (QNB)	–	–	++++	–	–	–
Pyrilamine	–	–	–	++++	–	–
Prazosin	–	–	–	–	++++	–
First-generation typical antipsychotics						
Chlorpromazine	+++	++	++	+++	+++	100 mg [146]
Fluphenazine	++++	++	+	++	++	N.R.
Haloperidol	+++	++	±	+	+	4 mg [146]
Loxapine	+++	++	+	++	++	10–50 mg [147]
Mesoridazine	+++	+++	+	+++	++	N.R.
Perphenazine	++++	+++	±	+++	++	4 mg [146]
Thioridazine	+++	+++	++	++	+++	100 mg [146]
Second-generation atypical antipsychotics						
Aripiprazole	++++	+++	±	++	+	10–30 mg [104]
Asenapine	+++	+++	±	++	+++	See text
Clozapine	+	++++	+++	++++	++	300 mg [146]
Iloperidone	+++	++++	±	++	++++	N.R.
Lurasidone	+++	+++	±	±	+	40–80 mg [148]
Olanzapine	++	+++	++	++++	+	12 mg [133]
Paliperidone	+++	+++	±	+++	++	6–9 mg [147]
Quetiapine	+	++	±	++	++	300–600 mg (XR) [134] See text
Risperidone	+++	++++	±	+++	+++	3–6 mg [149, 150]
Ziprasidone	+++	++++	±	++	+	120 mg [157]

± negligible, + low, ++ moderate, +++ moderate high, ++++ high, reference compound, *D2* dopamine receptor subtype 2, *5HT2A* serotonergic receptor subtype 2A, *M* muscarinic receptor, *H1* histamine receptor subtype 1, *Alpha-1* alpha adrenergic receptor subtype 1, *PET D2 Receptor @ 65–85 %* positron emission tomography dopamine receptor subtype 2 at 65–85 % occupancy, *XR* extended-release product, *N.R.* not reported subtype 2A (5HT2A) has several possible actions that include improvement in negative symptoms, mitigation of EPS, and improvement in depression and anxiety. Histamine receptor subtype 1 (H1) activity can be related to sedation and weight gain [151]. A therapeutic benefit of alpha-1 adrenergic receptor subtype 1 has not been identified, but postural hypotension, dizziness, and reflex tachycardia are related.

7.4.1 Positron Emission Tomography (PET) Studies

PET technology has been incorporated into CNS drug discovery and development for various agents beyond antipsychotics [151]. However, PET applications can be limited due to small sample sizes, studies in healthy volunteers versus patients with the medical conditions, drug dose, and expense. A basic question to reflect upon is "Is receptor occupancy data useful in dosing guidelines and is that the right question?" [152]. Antipsychotic pharmacodynamics utilizing PET technology have examined three main brain regions – putamen, striatum, and caudate, which have focused mainly on D2 receptor occupancy and its effects in balancing therapeutic efficacy and EPS effects. The mathematical models of PET applications are presented in Chap. 3– that typically follows a hyperbolic relationship between receptor occupancy and plasma drug concentrations shown in Fig. 7.2.

PET studies with antipsychotics originated over 25 years ago, and it is widely accepted that blockade of central D2 receptors is related to antipsychotic efficacy in the positive symptoms of schizophrenia (e.g., hallucinations). Although 5HT2A or other serotonin receptors have been studied, this chapter will examine only the D2 receptor actions with the antipsychotics. Initial work with typical antipsychotics and clozapine reported that therapeutic doses given to patients that had D2 receptor occupancy ranged between 65 and 85 % [146]. This range has been used for subsequent PET studies with antipsychotic drugs where about 65 % receptor occupancy achieves the minimal threshold for efficacy and above 85 % occupancy associated with adverse effects. A review article of PET studies reported that mean D2 receptor occupancy was significantly higher in patients with EPS (77 ± 9 % versus 63 ± 17 %, $p = 0.011$). Using a reduction in total PANSS or BPRS scores by 25 % defined as efficacy, a strong trend was found in patients with improvement when a mean threshold D2 receptor occupancy of 66 % was achieved (66 ± 14 % versus 58 ± 19 %, $p = 0.054$) [153]. This section will present the findings from various PET studies and the antipsychotic drug doses or plasma concentrations that reach the D2 receptor occupancy within this range (see Table 7.2). Presently, PET applications with iloperidone have not yet been reported, and only a few older typical antipsychotics have been studied.

The D2 receptor occupancy for typical antipsychotic loxapine in patients with schizophrenia ($N = 10$) was reported. Loxapine doses were between 10 and 50 mg/day for eight patients, while the other patients had higher doses of 75 mg/day and 100 mg/day [154]. The D2 receptor occupancy of about 65 % was achieved in one

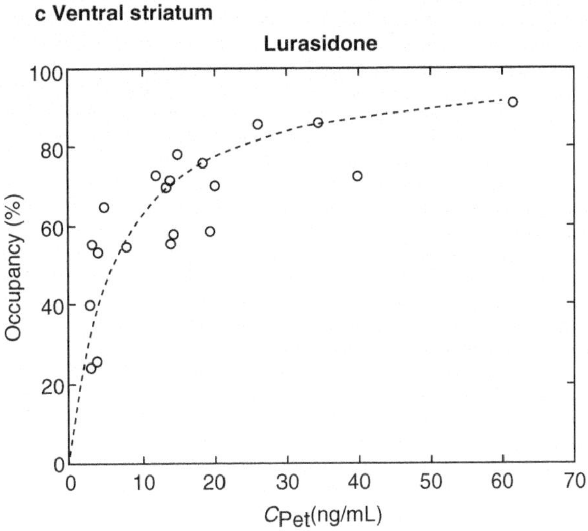

Fig. 7.2 Plot of D2 receptor occupancy versus mean serum concentration (C_{PET}) of lurasidone with the regression line (With permission from Wong et al. [148], p. 250)

patient at 10 mg (out of four patients) and up to 85 % at 20–50 mg/day. The other two patients had D2 receptor occupancy at 90 % without any reported adverse side effects. Aripiprazole 10 mg/day and 30 mg/day achieved a mean D2 receptor occupancy of 85 % and 91 %, respectively [104]. During asenapine's early development, a 100 μg dose given to three healthy subjects reported a very low D2 receptor occupancy of 12–23 % but demonstrated that this agent did possess dopamine receptor activity [147]. Lurasidone 40 mg and 80 mg given to healthy subjects ($N=20$) achieved mean D2 receptor occupancies of 66.7 ± 3.2 % and 75.3 ± 13.0 %, respectively. Lurasidone doses at 20 mg/day and below had mean D2 receptor occupancy at 50 % or less [148]. A threshold for olanzapine that reached 65 % D2 receptor occupancy was reported with a dose of about 12 mg/day. An OLZ mean plasma concentration of 22.7 ng/mL had a mean D2 receptor occupancy of 50 % [133]. Risperidone 6 mg/day was given to patients with schizophrenia ($N=8$) that produced a mean total drug concentration of 34.8 ng/mL (range 27.4–42.6 ng/mL) and a mean D2 receptor occupancy of 82 % (range 79–85 %). Doses >6 mg/day were suggested to lead to an increased incidence of EPS [149]. A subsequent study in patients also reported similar findings with risperidone doses 2–6 mg/day. Patients with the highest D2 receptor occupancy of >80 % ($N=9$) had mild EPS [150]. The pivotal clinical risperidone trial ($N=388$) used daily doses of 2 mg, 6 mg, 10 mg, and 16 mg versus haloperidol 20 mg [155]. The EPS incidence for risperidone 2 mg (7.9 %) and 6 mg (10.9 %) was below or equal to the placebo group with a slightly higher frequency for the 12 mg dose (12.3 % versus 10.6 % placebo). The EPS occurrence for risperidone 16 mg and haloperidol 20 mg was 25.0 % and 25.8 %, respectively, which was significantly greater than the placebo group ($p<0.05$). Paliperidone doses of 6–9 mg in patients ($N=13$) had a reported D2 receptor occupancy of 70–80 % [156].

Quetiapine studies have reported interesting results, that is, the 300–600 mg doses of the extended-release formulation achieves the recommended therapeutic concentrations [104], but have a low D2 receptor occupancy of <15 % [133]. Significant differences were found when samples were obtained within several hours of drug administration versus at trough times. Quetiapine sampling time may be the key variable with its elimination half-life and different D2 receptor-binding affinity [157]. A fixed-dose study with ziprasidone 40, 80, 120, and 160 mg/day in patients ($N = 16$) showed that the mean D2 receptor occupancy was 56 % (S.D. = 18 %), the mean plasma concentration was 53.4 ng/mL (S.D. = 16.0), and the optimal effective dose was 120 mg/day [158]. Each of these studies reported a hyperbolic relationship between the recommended therapeutic drug concentration ranges and D2 receptor occupancy except for clozapine and haloperidol [159]. Clozapine exhibited wide interpatient variability, and as a result, individual patient monitoring is the only accurate method for patient assessment. Haloperidol displayed a very sharp hyperbolic curve with a therapeutic range of 5–17 ng/mL for D2 receptor occupancy. LAIs agents and D2 receptor occupancy had similar results to their oral agents when taken at the end of their dosing interval 28 days, except for risperidone LAI obtained at 14 days [158]. Whether or not sustained D2 receptor occupancy is required for maintaining therapeutic benefit has not been verified and continues to be evaluated [160].

7.4.2 Pharmacogenetic Relationships to Therapeutic or Adverse Effects

Several review articles have been recently published examining the various pharmacogenetic aspects with antipsychotics [161–163]. Most of these pharmacogenetic studies have included risperidone, olanzapine, and clozapine that analyze both efficacy and adverse effects. The CYP2D6 metabolizer phenotype has significant dosing implications for aripiprazole, iloperidone, and risperidone [162]. Various pharmacogenetic variants have been identified including dopamine D3 receptor polymorphisms, the TaglA1 allele of the DRD2 gene, serotonin 5HT2C-759C/T polymorphism, and the leptin gene variant 2548-G/A (possible weight gain) [161, 162]. Other genetic biomarkers may be indentified with further research. This section presents a selected review of the atypical agents. Few studies have been conducted with the typical agents. For example, the incidence of EPS was reported with HAL, which is partially related to CYP2D6 genotype and HAL metabolism, while another study reported an association between EPS and the SLC6A3 VNTR and COMT Val158Met polymorphisms [164, 165].

Clozapine (CLZ) Clozapine metabolism is influenced by several CYPs (see Table 7.1). However, CYP1A2-163C>A polymorphism *1F/*1F was found to be associated with seizures in patients [166]. A dose-dependent relationship between seizures and clozapine has been established [50]; however, CLZ doses ≥650 mg/day was found not to be significant ($p = 0.723$) [166]. Elevated serum clozapine concentrations above 750 ng/mL were reported to have an increased risk of seizures with an odds ratio of 5.15 ($p=0.03$) [167]. Case reports of CLZ-induced seizures due to high CLZ plasma concentrations have been reported [50]. An upper threshold for CLZ has been questioned as there are very few studies with antipsychotics at their higher doses to determine safety and tolerability [167, 168]. CLZ-induced agranulocytosis in Ashkenazi Jews was associated with the haplotype HLA-B38, HLA-DR4, and HLA-DQ3 [163].

Olanzapine (OLZ) Although some adverse effects of OLZ were reported to be related to CYP2C9, TPMT1, UGT1A1, MDR1, and 5HT2A polymorphisms, the increased risk of adverse effects with these genetic factors remains to be established [169].

Risperidone (RIS) RIS disposition has been correlated with CYP2D6 status but not CYP3A5 and ABCB1 genotypes [170]. While some trends were between with increased adverse effects in CYP2D6 PMs status, the therapeutic outcomes were reported not to be significant and routine genotyping not recommended [171]. Higher total PANSS scores were found in patients who were MDR1 3435C>T carriers and CYP2D6 PMs status [172], thereby suggesting that more than one genotype can be involved with RIS pharmacodynamics. A large number of other genotypes have been reported to be associated with an increased RIS adverse effect profile which include 5HT2A, 5HT2C, 5HT6, DRD2, DRD3, BDNF, and NR1/2 (coding for the pregnane X receptor). However, evidence supporting routine screening for these genotypes in clinical practice is presently insufficient [86, 173].

7.4.2.1 QT/QTc Interval Pharmacodynamics

Several antipsychotics have been associated with QTc prolongation, and this assessment has become a required element for the pharmaceutical industry during antipsychotic drug development. The FDA cites a QTc interval greater than 500 ms as a clinically significant parameter. Increased QTc prolongation is associated with the risk of torsades de pointes and possibly linked to elevated plasma antipsychotic concentrations [174]. Case reports of torsades de pointes are published with intravenous haloperidol [175, 176]. The patient package insert for thioridazine and mesoridazine includes a "black box" warning for QTc prolongation. Thioridazine and QTc effects were compared with other antipsychotics (ziprasidone, risperidone, olanzapine, quetiapine, and haloperidol) where thioridazine exhibited the largest mean increase from baseline of 28 ms. Ziprasidone produced a modest QTc effect with a mean increase of 20.3 ms, followed by quetiapine at 14.5 ms. Concurrent use of CYP inhibitors ketoconazole and paroxetine added to the antipsychotics produced similar results on QTc prolongation [177]. Loxapine was recently reported not to produce QTc prolongation with the inhalation product [178].

QTc prolongation with iloperidone was compared to quetiapine and ziprasidone with and without concomitant CYP2D6 and CYP3A4 inhibitors [179]. Iloperidone caused a mean increase in the QTc interval of 8.5 ms which was similar to ziprasidone

(9.6 ms) and higher than quetiapine (1.6 ms). Addition of CYP inhibitors did not lead to further QTc prolongation, and no subjects had QTc intervals ≥ 500 ms. The QTc interval change was assessed in healthy volunteers who were genotyped as CYP2D6 PMs, and EMs were given a single 10 mg HAL dose [180]. Although haloperidol clearance and elimination half-life were significantly reduced in PMs versus EMs, these differences did not translate to marked QTc changes. The ABCB1 C3435T genotype CT and TT alleles were reported to be possibly involved with QTc prolongation and not CYP2D6 alleles with risperidone [181]. Investigations of potential pharmacogenetic sources for antipsychotic-induced QTc prolongation are at an early stage of investigations.

7.4.3 Other Pharmacodynamic Effects

Antipsychotics produce prolactin (PRL) elevations that can be possibly associated with sexual dysfunction and hyperprolactemia (HPRL); these effects have been linked to D2 receptor antipsychotic actions at the anterior pituitary [141–144]. The highest HPRL rates have been reported with risperidone and paliperidone. The newer agents asenapine and iloperidone are comparable to clozapine. Lurasidone PRL elevation is similar to olanzapine. PRL profiles in children and adolescents receiving antipsychotics are comparable to those observed in adults. Clinicians need to match patient symptoms with PRL elevations and monitor PRL levels based upon individual patient response [182]. Thioridazine still remains the only antipsychotic drug that has a clear dose limit of 800 mg/day due to the pigment retinopathy described since 1960 in four patients treated with 2 g for 30–50 days [183]. A dose-dependent and time-dependent relationship was described, as long-term treatment with doses >800 mg became the most important factors leading to retinopathy [184]. Whereas case reports of retinopathy also occurred at lower thioridazine doses, thus, clinicians are advised to have patients undergo annual eye evaluations with the slit-lamp procedure especially if the patient is also taking another antipsychotic like chlorpromazine [185, 186].

7.4.4 Integrating Pharmacokinetics (PK) and Pharmacodynamics (PD) of Antipsychotics

The kinetics of pharmacologic response has been described over 30 years ago examining the mathematical approaches to the dose-effect relationship using the direct and indirect link. Modeling PK with different PD models used the fixed effects, linear, and log-linear regression analyses [187]. The advent of population pharmacokinetics provided a foundational mathematical tactic to incorporate both PK and PD aspects from routine clinical data in patient care [188, 189]. The next step in utilizing population PK studies from clinical data examined the effects of different covariates such as sex, body weight, laboratory assessments, and comedications on plasma antipsychotic concentrations [95–101]. Subsequent additional factors were included to expand the overall PK-PD model. For example, smoking is a major factor among psychiatric patients that can also effect plasma concentrations of some antipsychotics [190]. Pharmacogenetic information was added and found to be a significant variable for antipsychotics metabolized by CYP2D6 [191]. Antipsychotic serum or plasma concentrations shown in Table 7.1 were added to the PK-PD models to examine the recommended therapeutic ranges [192].

The population pharmacokinetic approach has been extended to incorporate patient clinical response data. Patients with schizophrenia participating in clinical trials during drug development were assessed with the Positive and Negative Syndrome Scale (PANSS) that included 1436 patients from 16 trials from 1989 to 2009 [193]. Using different models, the Weibull model and the indirect response model adequately described the PANSS data. The following covariates were found to be important predictors for the placebo effect: disease condition, geographic regions, and drug administration route. Study duration and trial phase were reported to be predictors for the high dropout rates. Antipsychotic response with PANSS data (positive, negative, and general subscales) was evaluated among five different antipsychotics using the PK-PD method that incorporated the log-linear Emax model for maximum drug effect. Improvement (defined as 30 % decrease in PANSS score) occurred with antipsychotics when D2 receptor occupancy was greater than 65 % [194]. PK-PD modeling of EPS with seven different antipsychotics using the Markov elements reported that agents with greater than an 80 % D2 receptor occupancy were likely to experience these adverse side effects [194].

Interestingly, when assimilating plasma antipsychotic concentrations to D2 receptor occupancy and clinical response, the steady-state effective concentration (Effective Css) for the antipsychotics was discovered to be below the recommended therapeutic plasma concentrations except for ziprasidone (63.1 ng/mL) shown in Table 7.1 [104, 195]. For example, the Effective Css for haloperidol was 2.7 ng/mL, and the recommended oral dose was 5.6 mg/day [196]. Despite the implementation of these sophisticated PK-PD models, the lack of "fit" between antipsychotic plasma concentrations and D2 receptor occupancy reflects upon the complex nature of antipsychotic drugs and various psychiatric disorders. The absence of association between these two variables leads to an apparent discrepancy. However, current limitations in science and technology may be the most likely reasons as PET utilization to determine clinical efficacy may not be a sufficient quantitative biomarker when dealing with complex psychiatric diseases such as schizophrenia [152].

7.5 Conclusions and Future Directions

Antipsychotics are foundational therapeutic agents to treat various psychiatric disorders where psychotic symptoms occur. Drug development for antipsychotics has grown to include PK and PD applications. Antipsychotic pharmacokinetics can be determined using various analytical assay methods that accurately measure minute drug quantities in plasma or serum samples. Routine TDM programs for antipsychotics have been implemented successfully in European countries but have found limited applications in other countries due to their wide interpatient variability in PK and PD. Pharmacogenetic findings partially account for the interpatient variability. Data analysis combining PK and PD models has been developed to identify the many diverse factors that impact antipsychotic pharmacotherapeutics. Although specific quantitative biomarkers for complex psychiatric diseases remain to be ascertained, technology continues to progress, with the goal of maximizing antipsychotic therapy. Antipsychotic drug development has incorporated PK and PD strategies to enhance patient care, minimize adverse side effects, and optimize research and developmental costs.

References

1. Perel JM, Jann MW (2006) Antipsychotics. In: Burton ME, Shaw LM, Schentag JJ, Evans WE (eds). Applied pharmacokinetics and pharmacodynamics – principles of therapeutic drug monitoring, 4th ed. Philadelphia, Lippincott Williams and Wilkins. pp 813–838
2. Jorgensen A (1986) Metabolism and pharmacokinetics of antipsychotics. In: Bridges JW, Chasseaud LF (eds) Progress in drug metabolism, vol 9. Taylor, and Francis, London, pp 111–174
3. Moons T, de Roo M, Clees S, Dom G (2011) Relationship between P-glycoprotein and second generation antipsychotics. Pharmacogenomics 12:1193–1211
4. Mauri MC, Volonteri LS, Colasanti A, Fiorentino A, De Gaspari IF, Bareggi SR (2007) Clinical pharmacokinetics of atypical antipsychotics. Clin Pharmacokinet 46:359–388
5. Sheehan JJ, Sliwa JK, Amatniek JC, Grinspan A, Canuso CM (2010) Atypical antipsychotic metabolism and excretion. Curr Drug Metab 11:516–525
6. Bartlett JA, Maarschalk KV (2012) Understanding the oral mucosal absorption and resulting clinical pharmacokinetics of asenapine. AAPS PharmSciTech 13:1110–1115
7. Weber J, McCormack PL (2009) Asenapine. CNS Drugs 23:781–792
8. Figueroa C, Brecher M, Hamer-Maansson JE, Winter H (2009) Pharmacokinetic profiles of extended release quetiapine fumarate compared with quetiapine immediate release. Prog Neuropsychopharmacol Biol Psychiatry 33:199–204
9. Yang LP, Polsker GL (2007) Paliperidone extended release. CNS Drugs 21:417–425
10. Citrome L (2009) Using oral ziprasidone effectively: the food effect and dose–response. Adv Ther 26:739–748
11. DeVane CL, Nemeroff CB (2001) Clinical pharmacokinetics of quetiapine. Clin Pharmacokinet 40:509–522
12. Preskorn S, Ereshefsky L, Chiu YY, Poola N, Loebel A (2013) Effect of food on the pharmacokinetics of lurasidone: results of two randomized, open-label, crossover studies. Hum Psychopharmacol Clin Exp 28:495–505
13. Cohen LJ (1994) Risperidone. Pharmacotherapy 14:253–265
14. Spyker DA, Munzar P, Cassella JV (2010) Pharmacokinetics of loxapine following inhalation of a thermally generated aerosol in healthy volunteers. J Clin Pharmacol 50:169–179
15. Simpson GM, Cooper TM, Lee JH, Young M (1978) Clinical and plasma level characteristics of intramuscular and oral loxapine. Psychopharmacol 56:225–227
16. Milton GV, Jann MW (1995) Emergency treatment of psychotic symptoms. Clin Pharmacokinet 28:494–504

63. Soderberg MM, Dahl ML (2013) Pharmacogenetics of olanzapine metabolism. Pharmacogenomics 14:1319–1336
64. Zhou SF (2009) Polymorphism of human cytochrome P450 2D6 and its clinical significance. Part II. Clin Pharmacokinet 48:761–804
65. Dahl ML, Llerena A, Bondesson U et al (1994) Disposition of clozapine in man: lack of association with debrisoquine and S-mephenytoin hydroxylation polymorphisms. Br J Clin Pharmacol 37:71–74
66. Olesen OV, Linnet K (2000) Identification of the human cytochrome P450 isoforms mediating in vitro N-dealkylation of perphenazine. Br J Clin Pharmacol 50:563–571
67. Dahl-Puustinen ML, Liden A, Alm C et al (1989) Disposition of perphenazine is related to polymorphic debrisoquine hydroxylation in human beings. Clin Pharmacol Ther 46:78–81
68. Linnet K, Wilborg O (1996) Steady-state serum concentrations of the neuroleptic perphenazine in relation to CYP2D6 genetic polymorphism. Clin Pharmacol Ther 60:41–47
69. Jerling M, Dahl ML, Aberg-Wistedt A et al (1996) The CYP2D6 genotype predicts the oral clearance of neuroleptic agents perphenazine and zuclopenthixol. Clin Pharmacol Ther 59:423–428
70. Berecz R, de la Rubia A, Dorado P et al (2003) Thioridazine steady-state plasma concentrations are influenced by tobacco smoking and CYP2D6, but not by the CYP2C9 genotype. Eur J Clin Pharmacol 59:45–50
71. Von Bahr C, Movin G, Nordin C et al (1991) Plasma levels of thioridazine and metabolites are influenced by the debrisoquine hydroxylation phenotype. Clin Pharmacol Ther 49:234–240
72. Dorado P, Penas-Lledo EM, de la Rubia A, Llerena A (2009) Relevance of CYP2D6 –1584C>G polymorphism for thioridazine: mesoridazine plasma concentration ratio in psychiatric patients. Pharmacogenomics 10:1083–1089
73. Gershon S, Sakalis G, Bowers PA (1981) Mesoridazine – a pharmacodynamics and pharmacokinetic profile. J Clin Psychiatry 42:463–469
74. Gottschalk LA, Dinovo E, Bierner R (1975) Plasma levels of mesoridazine and its metabolites and clinical response in acute schizophrenia after a single intramuscular drug dose. Psychopharmacol Bull 11:33–34
75. Llerena A, Berecz R, de la Rubia A et al (2001) Effect of thioridazine dosage on debrisoquine hydroxylation phenotype in psychiatric patients with different CYP2D6 genotypes. Ther Drug Monit 23:616–620
76. Luo JP, Vasishtha SC, Hawes EM et al (2011) In vitro identification of the human cytochrome p450 enzymes involved in the oxidative metabolism of loxapine. Biopharm Drug Dispos 32:398–407
77. Cohen BM, Harris PQ, Altesman RI, Cole J (1982) Amoxapine: neuroleptic as well as antidepressant. Am J Psychiatry 139:1165–1167
78. Reed A, Huie K, Perloff ES, Cassella JV, Takahashi LH (2012) Loxapine p-glycoprotein interactions in vitro. Drug Metab Lett 6:26–32
79. Llerena A, Alm C, Dahl ML et al (1992) Haloperidol disposition is dependent on debrisoquine hydroxylation phenotype. Ther Drug Monit 14:92–97
80. Lane HY, Hu OYP, Jann MW et al (1997) Dextromethorphan phenotyping and haloperidol disposition in schizophrenic patients. Psychiatry Res 69:105–111
81. Ohnuma T, Shibata N, Matsubara Y, Arai H (2003) Haloperidol plasma concentration in Japanese psychiatric subjects with gene duplication of CYP2D6. Br J Clin Pharmacol 56:315–320
82. Panagiotidis G, Arthur HW, Kindh JD, Dahl ML, Sjoqvist F (2007) Depot haloperidol treatment in outpatients with schizophrenia on monotherapy: impact of CYP2D6 polymorphism on pharmacokinetics and treatment outcome. Ther Drug Monit 29:417–422
83. Llerena A, ed la Rubia A, Berecz R, Dorado P (2004) Relationship between haloperidol plasma concentration, debrisoquine metabolic ration, CYP2D6 and CYP2C9 genotypes in psychiatric patients. Pharmacopsychiatry 37:69–73

84. Hendset M, Molden E, Refsum H, Hermann M (2009) Impact of CYP2D6 genotype on steady-state serum concentrations of risperidone and 9-hydroxyrisperidone in patients using long-acting injectable risperidone. J Clin Psychopharmacol 29:537–541
85. Hendset H, Molden E, Kanpe M, Hermann M (2014) Serum concentrations of risperidone and aripiprazole in subgroups encoding CYP2D6 intermediate metabolizer phenotype. Ther Drug Monit 36:80–85
86. Llerena A, Berecz R, Penas-Lledo E, Suveges A, Farinas H (2013) Pharmacogenetics of clinical response to risperidone. Pharmacogenomics 14:177–194
87. Croxtall JD (2012) Aripiprazole: a review of its use in the management of schizophrenia in adults. CNS Drugs 26:155–183
88. Kubo M, Koue T, Maune H, Fukuda T, Azuma J (2007) Pharmacokinetics of aripiprazole, a new antipsychotic, following oral dosing in healthy adult Japanese volunteers: influence of CYP2D6 polymorphism. Drug Metab Pharmacokinet 22:358–366
89. Suzuki T, Mihara K, Nakamura A et al (2011) Effects of the CYP2D6*10 allele on the steady-state plasma concentrations of aripiprazole and its active metabolite, dehydroaripiprazole, in Japanese patients with schizophrenia. Ther Drug Monit 33:21–24
90. Suzuki T, Mihara K, Nakamura A et al (2014) Effects of genetic polymorphism of CYP2D6, CYP3A5, and ABCB1 on the steady-state plasma concentrations of aripiprazole and its active metabolite dehydroaripiprazole, in Japanese patients with schizophrenia. Ther Drug Monit 36(5):651–655
91. Haag S, Spigset O, Lakso HA et al (2001) Olanzapine disposition in humans is unrelated to CYP1A2 and CYP2D6 phenotypes. Eur J Clin Pharmacol 57:493–497
92. Shirley KL, Hon YY, Penzak SR et al (2003) Correlation of cytochrome P450 (CYP) 1A2 activity with olanzapine disposition in healthy volunteers. Neuropsychopharmacol. TBD 28:961–966
93. Perera V, Gross AS, Polasek TM et al (2013) Considering CYP1A2 phenotype and genotype for optimizing the dose of olanzapine in the management of schizophrenia. Expert Opin Drug Metab Toxicol 9:1115–1137
94. Bertilsson L, Carillo JA, Dahl ML et al (1994) Clozapine disposition covaries with CYP1A2 activity determined by a caffeine test. Br J Clin Pharmacol 37:471–473
95. Jann MW, Ludden TM, Ereshefsky L, Saklad SR, Richards AL (1985) Preliminary analysis of haloperidol population kinetics in schizophrenics. Clin Pharmacol Ther 37:203
96. Yukawa E, Hokazono T, Funakoshi A et al (2000) Epidemiologic investigation of the relative clearance of haloperidol by mixed-effect modeling using routine clinical pharmacokinetic data in Japanese patients. J Clin Psychopharmacol 20:685–690
97. Uchida H, Mamo DC, Pollock BG et al (2012) Predicting plasma concentrating of risperidone associated with dosage change: a population pharmacokinetic study. Ther Drug Monit 34:182–187
98. Botts S, Diaz FJ, Santoro V et al (2008) Estimating the effects of co-medications on plasma olanzapine concentrations by using a mixed model. Prog Neuropsychopharmacol Biol Psychiatry 32:1453–1458
99. Kim JR, Seo HB, Cho JY et al (2008) Population pharmacokinetic modelling of aripiprazole and its active metabolite dehydroaripiprazole in psychiatric patients. Br J Clin Pharmacol 66:802–810
100. Ng W, Uchida H, Ismail Z et al (2009) Clozapine exposure and the impact of smoking and gender: a population pharmacokinetic study. Ther Drug Monit 31:360–366
101. Vermeulen A, Piotrovsky V, Ludwig EA (2007) Population pharmacokinetics of risperidone and 9-hydroxyrisperidone in patients with acute episodes associated with bipolar I disorder. J Pharmacokinet Pharmacodyn 34:183–206
102. Samtani M, Vermeulen A, Stuyckens K (2009) Population pharmacokinetics of intramuscular paliperidone palmitate in patients with schizophrenia. Clin Pharmacokinet 48:585–600
103. Gopal S, Gassmann-Mayer C, Palumbo J, Samtani MN, Shiwach R, Alphs L (2010) Practical guidance for dosing and switching paliperidone palmitate treatment in patients with schizophrenia. Curr Med Res Opin 26:377–387

104. Baumann P, Hiemke C, Ulrich S et al (2004) The AGNP-TDM expert group consensus guidelines: therapeutic drug monitoring in psychiatry. Pharmacopsychiatry 37:243–265
105. Nazirizadeh Y, Vogel F, Bader W et al (2010) Serum concentrations of paliperidone versus risperidone and clinical effects. Eur J Clin Pharmacol 66:797–803
106. Sparshatt A, Taylor D, Patel MX, Kapur S (2010) A systematic review of aripiprazole – dose, plasma concentration, receptor occupancy, and response: implications for therapeutic drug monitoring. J Clin Psychiatry 71:1447–1456
107. Lopez LV, Kane JM (2013) Plasma levels of second-generation antipsychotics and clinical response in acute psychosis: a review of the literature. Schizophr Res 147:368–374
108. Best-Shaw L, Gudbrandsen M, Nagar J, Rose D, David AS, Patel MX (2014) Psychiatrists' perspectives on antipsychotic dose and the role of plasma concentration therapeutic drug monitoring. Ther Drug Monit 36(4):486–493
109. Dysken MW, Javaid JL, Chang SS et al (1981) Fluphenazine pharmacokinetics and therapeutic response. Psychopharmacol 73:205–210
110. Mavroidis ML, Kanter DR, Hirschowitz J et al (1984) Fluphenazine plasma levels and clinical response. J Clin Psychiatry 45:370–373
111. Van Putten T, Avavagri M, Marder SR et al (1991) Plasma fluphenazine levels and newly admitted schizophrenic patients. Psychopharmacol Bull 27:91–96
112. Koreen AR, Lieberman J, Alvir J et al (1994) Relationship of plasma fluphenazine levels to treatment response and extrapyramidal side effects in first-episode schizophrenic patients. Am J Psychiatry 151:35–39
113. Levinson D, Simpson G, Lo ES et al (1995) Fluphenazine plasma levels, dosage, efficacy, and side effects. Am J Psychiatry 152:756–771
114. Van Putten T, Marder SR, Wirshing WC et al (1991) Neuroleptic plasma levels. Psychopharmacol Bull 17:197–216
115. Jann MW, Chang WH, Lam YWF et al (1992) Comparative analysis of haloperidol and reduced haloperidol in different ethnic populations. Prog Neuropsychopharmacol Biol Psychiatry 16:193–202
116. Jann MW, Chang WH, Davis CM et al (1989) Haloperidol and reduced haloperidol plasma levels in Chinese and non-Chinese psychiatric patients. Psychiatry Res 30:45–52
117. Conley R, An Nguyen J, Tamminga C (1991) Haloperidol kinetics and clinical response. Schizophr Res 4:287 (Abstract)
118. Lane HY, Lin HY, OYP H et al (1997) Blood levels of reduced haloperidol versus clinical effects and extrapyramidal side effects of haloperidol. Prog Neuropsychopharmacol Biol Psychiatry 21:299–311
119. Crowley JJ, Ashraf-Khorassani M, Castagnoli N, Sullivan PF (2013) Brain levels of the neurotoxic pyridinium metabolite HPP+ and extrapyramidal symptoms in haloperidol-treated mice. Neurotoxic 39:153–157
120. Hansen LB, Larsen NE, Vastergard P (1981) Plasma levels of perphenazine (Trilafon) related to development of extrapyramidal side effects. Psychopharmacol 74:306–309
121. Hansen LB, Larsen NE, Gulmann N (1982) Dose-dependent response relationship of perphenazine in the treatment of acute psychoses. Psychopharmacol 78:112–115
122. Axelsson R, Martensson E (1983) Clinical effects related to the serum concentrations of thioridazine and its metabolites. In: Gram LF et al (eds) Clinical pharmacology in psychiatry. McMillan, London, pp 165–174
123. Vtial-Herne J, Gerbino L, Kay SR et al (1986) Mesoridazine and thioridazine: clinical effects and blood levels in refractory schizophrenics. J Clin Psychiatry 47:375–379
124. Molden E, Lunde H, Lunder N et al (2006) Pharmacokinetic variability of aripiprazole and the active metabolite dehydroaripiprazole in psychiatric patients. Ther Drug Monit 28:744–749
125. Lin SK, Chen CK, Liu YL (2011) Aripiprazole and dehydroaripiprazole plasma concentrations and clinical responses in patients with schizophrenia. J Clin Psychopharmacol 31:758–762

126. Perry PJ, Miller DD, Arndt SV et al (1991) Clozapine and norclozapine plasma concentrations and clinical response in treatment-refractory schizophrenics. Am J Psychiatry 48:231–235
127. Perry PJ (2000) Therapeutic monitoring of atypical antipsychotics: is it of potential clinical value? CNS Drugs 13:167–171
128. Liu HC, Chang WH, Wei FC et al (1996) Monitoring of plasma clozapine levels and its metabolites in refractory schizophrenics. Ther Drug Monit 18:200–207
129. Perry PJ, Sanger T, Beasley C (1997) Olanzapine plasma concentrations and clinical response in acutely ill schizophrenic patients. J Clin Psychopharmacol 17:472–477
130. Perry PJ, Lund BC, Sanger T, Beasley C (2001) Olanzapine plasma concentrations and clinical response: acute phase results of the North American Olanzapine Trial. J Clin Psychopharmacol 21:14–20
131. Citrome L, Stauffer VL, Chen L et al (2009) Olanzapine plasma concentrations after treatment with 10, 20, and 40 mg/d in patients with schizophrenia. J Clin Psychopharmacol 29:278–283
132. Skogh E, Reis M, Dahl ML, Lundmark J, Bengtsson F (2002) Therapeutic drug monitoring data on olanzapine and its N-desmethyl metabolite in the naturalistic clinical setting. Ther Drug Monit 24:518–526
133. Bishara D, Olofinjana O, Sparshatt A, Kapur S, Taylor D, Patel MX (2013) Olanzapine: a systematic review and meta-regression of the relationships between dose, plasma concentration, receptor occupancy and response. J Clin Psychopharmacol 33:329–335
134. Sparshatt A, Talyor D, Patel MX, Kapur S (2011) Relationship between daily dose, plasma concentrations, dopamine receptor occupancy, and clinical response to quetiapine: a review. J Clin Psychiatry 72:1108–1123
135. Gerlach M, Hunnerkopf R, Rothenhofer S et al (2007) Therapeutic drug monitoring of quetiapine and adolescents with psychotic disorders. Pharmacopsychiatry 40:72–76
136. Bowskill SV, Handley SA, Fsher DS, Flanagan RJ, Patel MX (2012) Risperidone and total 9-hydroxyrisperidone in relation to prescribed dose and other factors: data from a therapeutic drug monitoring service, 2002–2010. Ther Drug Monit 34:349–355
137. Seto K, Dumontet J, Enson MHH (2011) Risperidone in schizophrenia: is there a role for therapeutic drug monitoring? Ther Drug Monit 33:275–283
138. Mauri MC, Colasanti A, Rossattini M et al (2007) Ziprasidone outcome and tolerability: a practical clinical trial with plasma drug levels. Pharmacopsychiatry 40:89–92
139. Vogel F, Gansmuller R, Leiblein T et al (2009) The use of ziprasidone in clinical practice: analysis of pharmacokinetic and pharmacodynamics aspects from the data of a drug monitoring survey. Eur Psychiatry 24:143–148
140. Van Strien AM, van den Tweel AVW, van den Heuvel ML, di Biase M, van den Brule AJC, van Marum RJ (2014) Correlation of haloperidol concentration in blood and cerebrospinal fluid. J Clin Psychopharmacol 34:516–517
141. Richelson E (1999) Receptor pharmacology of neuroleptics: relation to clinical effects. J Clin Psychiatry 60(suppl 10):5–14
142. Richelson E, Sounder T (2000) Binding of antipsychotic drugs to human brain receptors – focus on newer generation compounds. Life Sci 68:29–39
143. Richelson E (2010) New antipsychotic drugs: how do their receptor-binding profiles compare? J Clin Psychiatry 71:1243–1244
144. Crismon ML, Argo TR, Buckley PF (2014) Chapter 50: Schizophrenia. In: DiPiro JT, Talbert RL, Yee GC et al (eds) Pharmacotherapy – a pathophysiologic approach, 9th edn. McGraw Hill, New York, pp 1019–1045
145. Kroeze WK, Hufeisen SJ, Popadak BA et al (2003) H1 histamine receptor affinity predicts short-term weight gain for typical and atypical antipsychotic drugs. Neuropsychopharmacol 28:519–526

146. Farde L, Wiessel FA, Halldin C, Sedvall G (1988) Central D2-dopamine receptor occupancy in schizophrenic patients treated with antipsychotic drugs. Arch Gen Psychiatry 45:71–76
147. Andree B, Halldin C, Vries MZ, Farde L (1997) Central 5Ht2A and D2 dopamine receptor occupancy after sublingual administration of ORG 5222 in healthy men. Psychopharmacol 131:339–345
148. Wong DF, Kuwabara H, Brasic JB et al (2013) Determination of dopamine D2 receptor occupancy by lurasidone using positron emission tomography in healthy male subjects. Psychopharmacol 229:245–252
149. Nyberg S, Eriksson B, Oxenstierna G, Halldin C, Farde L (1999) Suggested minimal effective doses of risperidone based on PET-measured D2 and 5HT2A receptor occupancy in schizophrenic patients. Am J Psychiatry 156:869–875
150. Kapur S, Remington G, Zipursky RB, Wilson AA, Houle S (1995) The D2 dopamine receptor occupancy of risperidone and its relationship to extrapyramidal symptoms: A PET study. Life Sci 57:L103–L107
151. Varnas K, Varrone A, Farde L (2013) Modeling of PET data in CNS drug discovery and development. J Pharmacokinet Pharmacodyn 40:267–279
152. Barrett JS, McGuire J, Vezina H, Spitsin S, Douglas SD (2013) PET measurement of receptor occupancy as a tool to guide dose selection in neuropharmacology: are we asking the right questions? J Clin Psychopharmacol 33:725–728
153. Uchida H, Takeuchi H, Graff-Guerro A et al (2011) Dopamine D2 receptor occupancy and clinical effects. J Clin Psychopharmacol 31:497–502
154. Kapur S, Zipursky R, Remington G, Jones C, McKay G, Houle S (1997) PET evidence that loxapine is an equipotent blocker of 5HT2 and D2 receptors: implications for the therapeutics in schizophrenia. Am J Psychiatry 154:1525–1529
155. Arakawa R, Ito H, Takano A et al (2008) Dose-finding study of paliperidone ER based on striatal and extrastriatal dopamine D2 receptor occupancy in patients with schizophrenia. Psychopharmacol 197:229–235
156. Tauscher-Wisiewski S, Kapur S, Tauscher T et al (2002) Quetiapine: an effective antipsychotics in first-episode schizophrenia despite only transiently high dopamine-2 receptor blockade. J Clin Psychiatry 63:992–997
157. Mamo D, Kapur S, Shammi CM et al (2004) A PET study of dopamine D2 and serotonin 5-Ht2 receptor occupancy in patients with schizophrenia treated with therapeutic doses of ziprasidone. Am J Psychiatry 161:818–825
158. Uchida H, Suzuki T (2014) Dose and dosing frequency of long-acting injectable antipsychotics. J Clin Psychopharmacol. [Epub ahead]
159. Uchida H, Takeuchi H, Graff-Guerrero A et al (2011) Predicting dopamine D2 receptor occupancy from plasma levels of antipsychotic drugs a systematic review of pooled analysis. J Clin Psychopharmacol 31:318–325
160. Moriguchi S, Bies RR, Remington G et al (2013) Estimated dopamine D2 receptor occupancy and remission in schizophrenia: analysis of the CATIE data. J Clin Psychopharmacol 33:682–685
161. Arranz MJ, Rivera M, Munro JC (2011) Pharmacogenetics of response to antipsychotics in patients with schizophrenia. CNS Drugs 25:933–969
162. Brennan MD (2014) Pharmacogenetics of second-generation antipsychotics. Pharmacogenomics 15:869–884
163. Zhang JP, Malhostra AK (2013) Pharmacogenetics of antipsychotics: recent progress and methodological issues. Expert Opin Drug Metab Toxicol 9:183–191
164. Gasso P, Papagianni K, Mas S et al (2013) Relationship between CYP2D6 genotype and haloperidol pharmacokinetics and extrapyramidal symptoms in healthy volunteers. Pharmacogenomic 14:1551–1563

165. Zivkovic M, Mihaljevic-Peles A, Bozina M et al (2013) The association study of polymorphisms in DAT, DRD2, and COMT genes and acute extrapyramidal adverse events in male schizophrenic patients treated with haloperidol. J Clin Psychopharmacol 33:593–599
166. Rajkumar AP, Poonkuzhali B, Kuruvilla A, Jacob M, Jacob KS (2013) Clinical predictors of serum clozapine levels in patients with treatment-resistant schizophrenia. Int Clin Psychopharmacol 28:50–56
167. Remington G, Agid O, Foussias G, Ferguson L, McDonald K, Powell V (2013) Clozapine and therapeutic drug monitoring: is there sufficient evidence for an upper threshold? Psychopharmacol 225:505–518
168. Coppola D, Liu Y, Gopal S et al (2012) A one-year prospective study of the safety, tolerability and pharmacokinetics of the highest available dose of paliperidone palmitate in patients with schizophrenia. BMC Psychiatry 12:26
169. Cabaleiro T, Lopez-Rodriguez RL, Ochoa D, Roman M, NovLBOS J, Abad-Santos F (2013) Polymorphisms influencing olanzapine metabolism and adverse effects in healthy subjects. Hum Psychopharmacol Clin Exp 28:205–214
170. Mas S, Gasso P, Alvarez S et al (2012) Intuitive pharmacogenetics: spontaneous risperidone dosage is related to CYP2D6, CYP3A5, and ABCB1 genotypes. Pharmacogenomics J 12:255–259
171. Cartwright AL, Wilby KJ, Corrgian S, Enson MHH (2013) Pharmacogenetics of risperidone: a systematic review of the clinical effects of CYP2D6 polymorphisms. Ann Pharmacther 47:350–360
172. Almoguera B, Riveiro-Alvarez R, Lopez-Castroman J et al (2013) CYP2D6 poor metabolizer status might be associated with better response to risperidone treatment. Pharmacogenet Genomics 23:627–630. V
173. Choong E, Polari A, Kamdem RH et al (2013) Pharmacogenetic study on risperidone long-acting injection: influence of cytochrome P450 2D6 and pregnane X receptor on risperidone exposure and drug-induced side-effects. J Clin Psychopharmacol 33:289–298
174. Buckley NA, Sanders P (2000) Cardiovascular adverse effects of antipsychotic drugs. Drug Safe 23:215–228
175. Hatta K, Takahashi T, Nakamura H et al (2001) The association between intravenous haloperidol and prolonged QT interval. J Clin Psychopharmacol 21:257–261
176. Tisdale JE, Rasty S, Padhi ID et al (2001) The effect of intravenous haloperidol on QT interval dispersion in critically ill patients: comparison with QT interval prolongation and assessment of risk of Torsades de Pointes. J Clin Pharmacol 41:1310–1318
177. Glassman AH, Bigger JT (2001) Antipsychotic drugs: prolonged QTc interval, Torsades de Pointes, and sudden death. Am J Psychiatry 158:1774–1782
178. Spyker DA, Voloshko P, Heyman ER, Cassella JV (2014) Loxapine delivered as a thermally generated aerosol does not prolong QTc in a through QT/QTc study in healthy subjects. J Clin Pharmacol 54:665–674
179. Potkin SG, Preskorn S, Hochfeld M, Meng X (2013) A thorough QTc study of 3 doses of iloperidone including metabolic inhibition via CYP2D6 and/or CYP3A4 and a comparison to quetiapine and ziprasidone. J Clin Psychopharmacol 33;3–10
180. Desai M, Tanus-Santos JE, Li L et al (2003) Pharmacokinetics and QT interval pharmacodynamics of oral haloperidol in poor and extensive metabolizers of CYP2D6. Pharmacogenomics J 3:105–113
181. Suzuki Y, Tsuneyama N, Kukui N et al (2014) Effect of risperidone metabolism and P-glycoprotein gene polymorphism on QT interval in patients with schizophrenia. Pharmacogenomics J 4:1–5
182. Peuskens J, Pani L, Detraux J, De Hert M (2014) The effects of novel and newly approved antipsychotics on serum prolactin levels: a comprehensive review. CNS Drugs 28:421–453
183. Cameron ME, Lawrence JM, Olrich JG (1972) Thioridazine (Mellaril retinopathy). Br J Opthal 56:131–134
184. Hamilton JD (1985) Thioridazine retinopathy within the upper dosage limit. Psychosomatics 26:823–824

for the treatment of bipolar disorder [6]. Despite this, the specific mechanisms by which lithium exerts its mood-stabilizing effects remain elusive. Lithium is a potentially toxic drug and has a narrow therapeutic range. Adverse effects are believed to be a direct consequence of the distribution of lithium to compartments in which it concentrates such as the brain, kidney, or thyroid [7]. Lithium dosage needs to be individualized, primarily by the use of serum/plasma lithium concentrations. Knowledge of the clinical pharmacokinetics and pharmacodynamics of lithium is a prerequisite for safe and effective prescription of this drug.

8.2.2 *Clinical Pharmacokinetics*

Lithium, a naturally occurring ion, is administered as a salt in the form of lithium carbonate, lithium citrate, lithium chloride, or lithium sulfate. Lithium is available in both standard- and slow-release preparations. Sustained-release formulations have been proposed as a means of diminishing post-dose variation in serum concentrations and associated adverse effects. The pharmacokinetics of lithium have been investigated by a number of studies in healthy volunteers and using carbonate salts administered in both standard-release and sustained-release dosage formulations [8–12]. Mean pharmacokinetic parameters of lithium are summarized in Table 8.1.

8.2.2.1 Absorption

Water-soluble salts, such as chloride and sulfate, are rapidly and almost completely absorbed from the upper gastrointestinal tract, while the less soluble carbonate salt is absorbed more slowly. Gastrointestinal absorption of lithium carbonate tablets or capsules appears to be virtually complete (95–100 %). The absorption of sustained-release lithium products is more variable and ranges from 60 to 90 %. The absorption half-lives were found to be 0.78 ± 0.05 h and 3.73 ± 0.37 h for standard- and sustained-release forms of lithium carbonate, respectively [10]. After a single dose of lithium carbonate, peak plasma concentration is reached at 1–2 h for standard-release dosage forms and at 4–5 h for sustained-release forms. Concomitant ingestion of food tends to increase lithium absorption. Although the extent of absorption is generally not altered in elderly subjects, delayed gastric emptying and intestinal transit times may increase the risk of gastrointestinal adverse effects in this patient population.

8.2.2.2 Distribution

Lithium is not bound to plasma proteins. Although the volume of distribution of lithium is approximately equal to that of body water (0.7–1.0 L/kg), lithium concentrations in various intra-compartmental spaces equilibrate very slowly with the extracellular fluid volume. Distribution of lithium across the blood–brain barrier is

Table 8.1 Summary of the mean pharmacokinetic parameters of mood stabilizers

	Bioavailability (%)	Protein binding (%)	Volume of distribution (L/kg)	Clearance (L/h)	Half-life (h)	Metabolism (%)	Active metabolites
Lithium	95–100[a] 60–90[b]	0	0.7–1	0.6–2.4	18–24		
Carbamazepine	75–85	75	0.8–2	1.1–3.6	5–26	75 – CYP3A4, CYP2C8, CYP1A2 15 – UGT	Carbamazepine epoxide
Valproic acid	>90	70–95	0.13–0.19	0.36–1.20	9–18	10 – CYP2C9, CYP2A6, CYP2B6 40 – UGT1A3, UGT2B7 35 – β-oxidation	
Lamotrigine	>95	55	0-9–1.5	1.6–2.6	15–35	80 – UGT1A4, UGT2B7	

[a]Standard formulations

[b]Sustained-release formulations

slow, and peak concentration in the brain is reached about 24 h after ingestion. Brain lithium concentrations, evaluated by using ^{7}Li magnetic resonance spectroscopy, were found to be approximately half those in serum, occasionally increasing to 75–80 % [13]. As lithium distributes to erythrocytes, it was occasionally suggested that lithium concentrations in red blood cells may more closely reflect brain concentrations and therefore be more predictive of lithium neurotoxicity, than serum concentrations [14]. However, the clinical relevance of measurement of red blood cell lithium concentrations appears to be poorly substantiated [15].

8.2.2.3 Elimination

Lithium is not metabolized and is almost completely excreted (>95 %) via the kidney as a free cation. Negligible amounts (less than 5 % the administered dose) are lost through feces, saliva, and sweat. Similarly to sodium, lithium is able to freely cross the glomerular membrane. Eighty percent of lithium is reabsorbed by passive diffusion in the proximal tubules. A small proportion is reabsorbed more distally via the epithelial sodium channel. The renal tubular reabsorption of lithium is very closely linked with sodium reabsorption and is influenced by changes in the renal clearance of sodium. Lithium clearance varies from 0.6 to 2.4 L/h with high interindividual variability and is closely associated with creatinine clearance, averaging about 20 % of glomerular filtration rate. The plasma half-life of lithium is 18–24 h in subjects with normal renal function.

8.2.2.4 Factors Affecting Lithium Pharmacokinetics

Excessive sweating, vomiting, diarrhea, inadequate fluid intake, and low sodium diet are potential causes of dehydration that may lead to compensatory increases in lithium reabsorption in the proximal tubule with subsequent decreased lithium clearance. Concomitant administration of other medications including thiazide diuretics, nonsteroidal anti-inflammatory drugs, and angiotensin-converting enzyme inhibitors may decrease lithium elimination potentially leading to toxic effects [16, 17].

With increasing age, a reduction in lithium clearance occurs in association with a decrease in creatinine clearance [18]. Thus, elderly patients usually require lower lithium dosages to achieve a target serum lithium concentration.

During the last months of pregnancy, lithium clearance increases by 30–50 %, in association with the progressive increase in plasma volume and glomerular filtration rate [19]. Therefore, lithium dose needs to be increased to maintain therapeutic lithium levels.

Lithium clearance is decreased in patients with abnormal renal function, and, therefore, the risk of lithium intoxication is considerably increased [12]. The use of lithium is contraindicated in cases of severe renal insufficiency, while in patients with mild or moderate reduction in renal function, dosages must be adapted accordingly to prevent lithium toxicity.

8.2.3 *Clinical Pharmacodynamics*

Lithium has been shown to exert a variety of pharmacological actions [20, 21]. However, the precise mechanisms by which lithium achieves its therapeutic benefits are not yet fully understood. This is partly related to the complex, underlying pathophysiology of bipolar disorder, involving many interacting neurotransmitters and neuronal circuits within the brain [2]. Moreover, many studies investigating the potential mechanism of action of lithium were performed at the preclinical level, in vitro or in vivo, by using concentrations of lithium much higher than those that are used therapeutically. Therefore, many findings from these investigations cannot be easily translated for application in human studies, especially as appropriate animal models of bipolar disorder have not yet been established.

Research into the mechanisms of action of lithium has been conducted at multiple levels, ranging from macroscopic changes in brain structure to microscopic alterations at the cellular, intracellular, and molecular levels [20]. Macroscopically, lithium can alter brain structure. In particular, it appears to preserve or increase the volume of certain brain regions primarily implicated in bipolar disorder such as the prefrontal cortex, hippocampus, and amygdala, possibly reflecting its neuroprotective effects. At the neuronal level, lithium acts both pre- and postsynaptically to modulate neurotransmission. In particular, lithium modulates neuronal function by decreasing excitatory neurotransmission through glutamate and dopamine and increasing inhibitory neurotransmission via gamma-aminobutyric acid (GABA). At the intracellular and molecular levels, lithium alters the second messenger systems that operate within neurons such as the adenyl cyclase (AC) and cyclic adenosine monophosphate (cAMP) system, the phosphoinositide cycle ("inositol depletion hypothesis"), protein kinase C (PKC), myristoylated alanine-rich C-kinase substrate (MARCKS), and intracellular calcium, which ultimately alter neurotransmission and promote cellular viability. These processes are complex and often interrelated and involve a number of different proteins. As bipolar disorder is increasingly recognized as a degenerative disease, it has also been proposed that the neuroprotective effects of lithium may mediate its therapeutic actions [22]. In this regard, lithium has been shown to reduce the oxidative stress caused by multiple episodes of mania and depression. Further, it promotes neuroprotective pathways facilitating the actions of protective proteins such as brain-derived neurotrophic factor (BDNF) and B-cell lymphoma 2 (Bcl-2), and reduces apoptotic processes through inhibition of glycogen synthase kinase 3β (GSK3β) and autophagy. Recent experimental evidence indicates that lithium decreases the brain arachidonic acid cascade, another signaling pathway possibly involved in the pathophysiology of bipolar disorder [23].

8.2.3.1 Serum or Plasma Concentration Relationship

A number of pharmacodynamic studies have investigated the relationship between serum/plasma lithium concentrations and therapeutic response and adverse effects. Overall, there seems to be a correlation between lithium concentrations and clinical effect, and therapeutic ranges for the acute and prophylactic treatment of bipolar disorder have been identified. However, several issues may complicate the clinical interpretation of these studies [24]. Some factors are related to the serum lithium concentrations and include the timing of blood sampling relative to the last dose, the daily lithium dosage schedule, and the lithium formulation. In this respect, substantial variations in lithium levels usually occur over a 24 h period, depending on the time, interval, dose, and formulation. Due to this, it is generally accepted that lithium dosage should be adjusted on the basis of the concentrations in serum drawn (optimally) 12 h (security interval 10–14 h) after the last dose [8]. Another important aspect that has to be considered when evaluating studies on the relationship between concentrations and therapeutic effect is the definition of response. As bipolar disorder is an episodic illness, relapse rates are commonly used, particularly in the prophylactic treatment. On the other hand, efficacy studies in the acute treatment may use measures of morbidity severity such as clinical rating scales. In patients with bipolar disorder, the most common rating scales for therapeutic response are the Young Mania Rating Scale (YMRS) or the Bech–Rafaelsen Mania Rating Scale (BRMS). Depressive symptoms are usually evaluated by the Hamilton Rating Scale for Depression (HRSD) or the Montgomery–Åsberg Depression Rating Scale (MADRS).

Early efficacy trials of lithium in the treatment of acute manic episodes found that most patients had an increased chance of responding at serum lithium concentrations above 0.8 mmol/L, although individual patients responded at lower concentrations [25, 26]. A study specifically designed to evaluate the relationship between lithium dose/concentration and treatment response in acute mania found an increasing response as lithium concentrations increased from 0.8 to 2 mmol/L [25]. Prien et al. [26] documented that manic patients required lithium concentrations between 0.9 and 1.4 mmol/L. Conversely, Takahashi et al. [27] reported that there was no significant correlation between serum lithium concentration and the degree of improvement in 80 Japanese patients with acute mania. There have been no studies that have specifically evaluated the relationship between serum lithium concentrations and clinical response in the treatment of bipolar depression.

The optimal serum lithium concentration for preventing mania and depression in maintenance treatment is far from well established. Typically, it has been considered that lithium concentrations should be maintained between 0.6 and 1.0 mmol/L [28], but some authors still favor 0.8–1.2 mmol/L [29]. After examining potentially relevant parameters for the prophylactic antidepressant efficacy of lithium in recent randomized controlled trials, Severus et al. [30] concluded that lithium efficacy against manic relapse/recurrence appears rather robust at plasma concentrations between 0.8 and 1.2 mmol/L but may be more modest against depressive relapse/recurrence and dependent on whether a response during the preceding acute episode was achieved by lithium treatment. Concentrations below 0.6 mmol/L have been shown in controlled trials to be less effective in preventing relapses [31]. A systematic review of controlled studies, reporting on the long-term treatment of mood disorders in bipolar patients who were assigned to specific target lithium concentration ranges [32], concluded that 0.4 mmol/L is the minimum efficacious serum lithium concentration and that optimal response is achieved at serum concentrations between 0.6 and 0.75 mmol/L. Higher concentrations may be useful for patients with predominantly manic symptoms but are associated with increased incidence of adverse events and decreased adherence.

In conclusion, plasma lithium concentrations should be optimized to the individual symptom and tolerability profile of patients. Bipolar patients likely to develop depressive episodes may benefit from prophylactic levels of 0.4–0.8 mmol/L, whereas in those more likely to develop mania, levels of 0.6–1.0 mmol/L may be more effective [33–35].

8.2.3.2 CNS Effect Relationship

After demonstration of the feasibility of ^{7}Li magnetic resonance spectroscopy (MRS) to measure human brain tissue lithium concentrations in vivo, some studies have characterized the brain pharmacokinetics of lithium in patients with bipolar disorder [13]. Preliminary investigations have examined the possible relationship between brain lithium levels and therapeutic response, with suggestions that lithium brain levels may be of clinical significance [36, 37]. In a study of 14 patients with bipolar disorder, Kato et al. [36] found that improvement in manic symptoms correlated with brain lithium concentrations ($r=0.65$, $p<0.05$), but not with serum lithium concentrations ($r=0.33$). On the other hand, Sachs et al. [37] did not find a correlation between lithium brain levels and outcomes for 25 patients with bipolar disorder during maintenance treatment. Because the relationship between lithium brain concentrations and response has only been investigated in small patient samples, more comprehensive studies are needed to evaluate the potential clinical relevance of these techniques.

8.2.3.3 Adverse Events Relationships

Lithium is associated with both acute and chronic adverse effects that can limit tolerability [5]. Most are determined by treatment dose and duration and patient characteristics, but some are idiosyncratic. Common acute adverse effects of lithium include nausea, vomiting, diarrhea, fine hand tremor, fatigue, headache, polydipsia, and polyuria. These adverse effects are usually transient and are often associated rapid increases in plasma lithium concentration and, therefore, can also occur when the dose of lithium is raised. However, serious adverse effects can develop with long-term treatment, including hypothyroidism, renal insufficiency, diabetes insipidus, and changes in cardiac function and cognition. These chronic adverse effects are relatively uncommon and usually occur after many years of treatment with lithium.

Lithium toxicity may arise as a consequence of an accidental or intentional intake of excessive amounts of lithium or may be due to accumulative high levels during ongoing chronic therapy [21]. The most common symptoms and signs of acute toxicity are gastrointestinal (nausea, vomiting, and diarrhea), neurological (tremor, ataxia, dysarthria, nystagmus, confusion, seizures, and coma), renal (polyuria and renal failure), and cardiovascular (ECG changes in the form of prolonged QT interval and T-wave inversion, conduction disturbances, and arrhythmias). These manifestations of toxicity occur when the serum concentration exceeds 1.5 mmol/L [38]. Serum levels of more than 2.5 mmol/L could be fatal, and such individuals should therefore be promptly treated immediately after stopping lithium treatment [39, 40]. The symptoms of lithium intoxication vary according to concentrations: with 1.5–2 mmol/L, gastrointestinal complaints and tremor; with 2–2.5 mmol/L, confusion and somnolence; and with >2.5 mmol/L, seizures and death. Chronic toxicity usually develops when renal function decreases, resulting in lithium accumulation. Symptoms may even occur in patients with lithium concentrations within the therapeutic range [38, 41]. Chronic intoxication primarily presents as neurotoxicity, but toxic effects may also involve the kidney, heart, and gut. The gradual accumulation of lithium within the brain is accentuated by the fact that the half-life of lithium is longer in neural tissue than in plasma [38, 41]. Furthermore, lithium excretion via the kidneys has an upper limit, and once this is reached lithium accumulation becomes rapid [12].

8.2.3.4 Integrating Clinical Pharmacokinetics and Pharmacodynamics: Dosing Regimen

As lithium has a relatively narrow therapeutic index, monitoring of serum/plasma lithium concentrations is the basis for optimal use and dosing of lithium. This requires achieving a balance between therapeutic benefits and adverse effects. Patients are usually initiated on low, divided doses of lithium, which are then adjusted until the desired concentration is reached. In this respect, different dosing methods, mainly based on pharmacokinetic principles, have been described, and a direct proportionality between the renal clearance of lithium and the dosage required to reach a certain serum lithium concentration is well established [7]. It is generally recommended to prescribe lithium in a two- or three-times daily regimen. Such multiple daily schedules are thought to be advantageous in maintaining more constant plasma lithium concentrations than single daily regimens, which are associated with significant fluctuations throughout the day, possibly resulting in adverse effects or breakthrough symptoms. However, single daily or alternate daily schedules have been recently suggested as useful options for lithium administration [42]. With regard to this, in clinical practice, no significant differences have been demonstrated in adverse effect profile or control of manic symptoms between either dosing regimen [43]. Moreover, a single daily regimen may have additional potential benefits in terms of increasing compliance and reducing the risk of long-term renal damage. The administration of lithium every alternate day as opposed to a daily single dose has been reported to reduce the risk of adverse effects while increasing the relapse rate [44, 45].

8.2.4 *Conclusions and Future Directions*

Although the pharmacological treatment of bipolar disorder has evolved rapidly during the last decade, lithium is still a suitable first-line treatment option in the management of this condition. Monitoring of serum/plasma lithium concentrations, in association with clinical judgment, still represents the best guide for dosage individualization and for safe and effective prescription of this drug. The optimum lithium serum concentrations for the treatment of bipolar disorder and those associated with the risk of toxicity and relapse are shown in Fig. 8.1 [46]. With the advances in pharmacogenomics and in understanding the mechanism of action, a further development of personalized lithium therapy will presumably be reached.

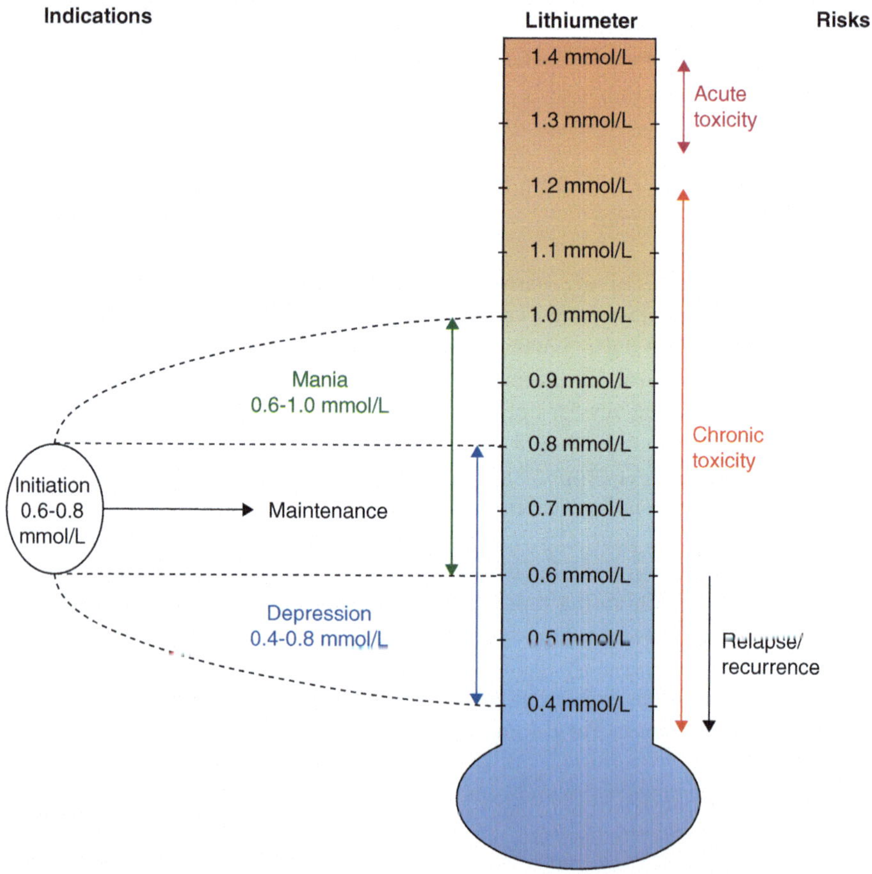

Fig. 8.1 The optimum lithium serum concentrations for the treatment of bipolar disorder and those associated with the risk of toxicity and relapse (From Mahli and Berk [46], with permission)

8.3 Antiepileptics

8.3.1 Introduction

In addition to the treatment of epilepsy, antiepileptics are extensively prescribed for the management of a variety of nonepileptic neurological conditions, such as neuropathic pain, migraine, and essential tremor, and psychiatric disorders, such as bipolar disorder and anxiety [3, 47]. This presumably reflects their complex mechanism of action involving a wide range of pharmacological effects on different neurotransmitter systems and ion channels.

Antiepileptics began to be studied as mood stabilizers in the late 1970s when a logical parallel was drawn between affective and seizure disorders, based on the theory that mania may "kindle" further episodes of mania [48]. Since the first compounds tested, namely, carbamazepine and valproic acid, proved effective in treating the manic phase of bipolar disorder, it was hypothesized that any anticonvulsant would be a mood stabilizer, especially for mania.

Three antiepileptic agents, namely, carbamazepine, valproic acid, and lamotrigine, are currently approved for the treatment of various aspects of bipolar disorder in most countries [49]. Large-scale, randomized, double-blind, well-controlled studies have documented that carbamazepine and valproic acid are highly effective in the treatment of acute mania [48, 50]. On the other hand, neither carbamazepine nor valproic acid has robust evidence supporting their efficacy in the treatment of acute bipolar depression. Valproic acid and, to a lesser extent, carbamazepine appear to be effective in the prophylactic treatment of many bipolar patients, including those refractory or intolerant to lithium. Lamotrigine is approved for maintenance treatment of bipolar I disorder [51, 52]. Differently from valproic acid and carbamazepine which are predominantly antimanics, lamotrigine is most effective for preventing the recurrent depressive episodes of bipolar disorder. The effectiveness of lamotrigine in the acute treatment of mood episodes has not been established. In recent years, several other antiepileptic drugs, including gabapentin, topiramate oxcarbazepine, levetiracetam, tiagabine, or zonisamide, have been investigated for their potential mood-stabilizing properties with diverging or inconclusive results [53].

8.3.2 Clinical Pharmacokinetics

Pharmacokinetic parameters of carbamazepine, valproic acid, and lamotrigine are summarized in Table 8.1.

8.3.2.1 Carbamazepine

Carbamazepine is an iminodibenzyl derivative structurally related to the tricyclic antidepressants. It is commercially available as immediate-release tablets, chewable tablets, controlled-release tablets, sustained-release formulations, suspensions, and suppositories. The pharmacokinetics of carbamazepine in humans have been extensively investigated [54, 55].

Absorption of carbamazepine from the gastrointestinal tract is rather slow and extremely variable, probably due to its slow dissolution in the gastrointestinal fluid and/or to its anticholinergic properties [54, 55]. Peak plasma carbamazepine concentrations usually occur between 4 and 8 h after administration of single oral doses of the immediate-release tablets but may be considerably longer depending on the formulation employed. Oral suspensions of carbamazepine are absorbed more rapidly and produce higher peak concentrations than tablets. Conversely, sustained-release formulations are absorbed more slowly than immediate-release tablets and produce more stable serum drug concentrations during the dosage interval. Food has not been shown to significantly affect the gastrointestinal absorption of carbamazepine. Because of the lack of an injectable formulation, the absolute bioavailability of carbamazepine in humans has not been determined. However, based on the recovery of radiolabeled carbamazepine in urine and feces after single-dose administration of ^{14}C-labeled carbamazepine in a gelatin capsule, the oral bioavailability has been estimated to range from 75 to 85 % [54, 55]. The bioavailability of carbamazepine is similar whether given as immediate-release or chewable tablets, solutions, suspensions, or syrups. The bioavailability of many sustained-release formulations, however, is about 15–35 % lower than that of immediate-release formulations, resulting in lower serum concentrations at steady state when patients are switched from immediate- to sustained-release dosage forms.

Carbamazepine is highly bound (75–80 %) to plasma proteins, including albumin and α_1-acid glycoprotein. The protein binding is independent of total plasma concentrations over the therapeutic range but may be reduced at supratherapeutic levels. The binding of carbamazepine to plasma proteins shows very little interindividual variation, suggesting that there is no need to monitor free rather than total plasma concentrations. The plasma protein binding of the active metabolite carbamazepine-10,11-epoxide is about 50 %. Carbamazepine is a neutral and lipophilic compound that distributes rapidly to various organs and tissues. The apparent volume of distribution of carbamazepine ranges between 0.8 and 2.0 L/kg in human adults. These values have been calculated assuming complete bioavailability of the drug, and the real volumes therefore might be slightly lower and less variable. Both carbamazepine and its epoxide metabolite readily pass into the central nervous system (CNS), and their concentrations in cerebrospinal fluid reflect the free fraction of the drug. Transport of carbamazepine at the blood–brain barrier is presumably mediated by drug efflux transporters such as P-glycoprotein (P-gp) [56, 57]. The ratio between brain and plasma concentrations has been reported to range from 0.8 to 1.6 for carbamazepine and from 0.5 to 1.5 for carbamazepine epoxide [54]. Salivary concentrations of carbamazepine and carbamazepine epoxide in humans are similar to the unbound concentrations in plasma and have been reported to range from 20 to 30 % of plasma concentrations for parent drug and from 30 to 40 % for the metabolite. Determination of salivary carbamazepine concentrations may represent a useful and easy tool for measuring unbound drug. Carbamazepine penetrates the placenta extensively and rapidly and distributes to different tissues and organs of the fetus homogeneously. Fetal plasma concentrations of carbamazepine, determined in the human umbilical cord, were found to range between 50 and 80 % of maternal levels. Carbamazepine is transferred to breast milk where its concentrations of carbamazepine in breast milk have been reported to be approximately 30–40 % of those in maternal plasma.

Carbamazepine is extensively metabolized in the liver, with less than 2 % of an oral dose excreted unchanged in urine. The major pathways of carbamazepine biotransformation include the epoxide–diol pathway, aromatic hydroxylation, and conjugation reactions [54, 55]. The epoxide–diol pathway is quantitatively the most important and results in the formation of carbamazepine-10,11-epoxide. This metabolite is pharmacologically active and accumulates in serum at clinically relevant concentrations, contributing to both therapeutic and adverse effects. The epoxidation reaction is catalyzed by CYP3A4 and, to a lesser extent, CYP2C8. The epoxide metabolite is subsequently hydrolyzed to an inactive diol metabolite by a microsomal epoxide hydrolase and then excreted in urine. An additional, but quantitatively less important, pathway of carbamazepine metabolism is represented by aromatic hydroxylation, mediated by CYP1A2 and resulting in the formation of four possible phenolic products, 1-, 2-, 3-, and 4-hydroxycarbamazepine. Conjugation reactions of carbamazepine and its metabolites are usually regarded as the third most important route of biotransformation and include glucuronidation and sulfuration. The glucuronidation reactions are catalyzed by uridine diphosphate glucuronosyltransferases (UGTs). The specific UGT isoform responsible for these reactions is yet unidentified.

Carbamazepine metabolism follows first-order kinetics and may vary considerably across subjects, resulting in a poor correlation between dose and serum concentration of both parent drug and its metabolites. It is well documented that carbamazepine induces its own metabolism during long-term therapy (autoinduction). The autoinduction process involves the epoxide–diol pathway, and it has been demonstrated that both the carbamazepine epoxidation and the subsequent epoxide hydrolysis are induced, although the latter reaction to a lesser extent. The course of the autoinduction process appears to be complex, discontinuous, and prolonged [58]. There is evidence that it may start within 24 h of first exposure to carbamazepine and seems to be complete within 1–5 weeks of treatment. Autoinduction of carbamazepine is dose dependent, so each increase in dose will result in further autoinduction. Carbamazepine metabolism is also subject to heteroinduction by concomitant administration of enzyme-inducing antiepileptic drugs (e.g., phenytoin or phenobarbital) [54, 55]. Like other first-generation antiepileptics such as phenobarbital and phenytoin, carbamazepine is potent and a broad-spectrum inducer of several metabolic enzymes including CYPs (CYP1A2, CYP2A6, CYP2B6, CYP2C9, CYP2C19, and CYP3A4), UGTs, and microsomal epoxide hydrolase [59].

After a single dose, the half-life of carbamazepine varies between 20 and 65 h, but after autoinduction is completed (about 20–30 days after starting treatment), half-lives are in the range of 5–26 h [54]. The clearance of carbamazepine appears to be age dependent, with higher clearance reported in younger children and lower clearances reported in older patients. Carbamazepine is cleared more rapidly in the third trimester of pregnancy. Patients with significant liver disease may have a decreased clearance of carbamazepine. Renal disease and dialysis do not alter the clearance of carbamazepine.

Carbamazepine is eliminated by biotransformation followed by urinary and biliary excretion of the parent drug and the formed metabolites. After administration of a single oral dose of ^{14}C-labeled carbamazepine, 72 % of the radioactivity was excreted in the urine, and the remaining 28 % was recovered in feces [54].

8.3.2.2 Valproic Acid

Valproic acid is structurally related to free fatty acids and differs from all other known antiepileptics. Three different chemical forms of valproic acid are commonly used: the free acid, the sodium salt (sodium valproate), and valproate semisodium or divalproex, which is composed of equal parts of valproic acid and sodium valproate. Several formulations are available including a syrup, a gelatin capsule, uncoated tablets, enteric-coated (delayed-release) tablets, and extended- or sustained-release tablets. Different reviews are available on the pharmacokinetics of valproic acid in man [60–62].

When administered as uncoated tablets containing the sodium salt, valproate dissociates rapidly in the stomach to the corresponding acid. Valproic acid is well absorbed from all the oral dosage forms. The oral bioavailability of standard formulations (including enteric-coated and the sustained-release formulations) is almost complete. On the other hand, the rate of absorption is quite variable, depending on the oral formulation. Peak concentrations usually occur within 2–3 h for syrup, capsules, and uncoated tablets, between 3 and 5 h for enteric-coated tablets, and between 5 and 10 h for sustained-release formulations. Maximum concentrations are considerably lower with sustained-release formulations, which ensure a reduced fluctuation in plasma drug concentration during the dosing interval. When enteric-coated tablets are used, concomitant intake with food may result in retention of the tablet in the stomach for up to several hours, with a consequent delay in drug absorption; however, when the tablet reaches the intestine, dissolution of the active principle occurs rapidly and unhindered.

Valproic acid is highly (≥90 %) bound to plasma proteins, primarily albumin. Protein binding is saturable at therapeutic concentrations. Accordingly, the extent of binding decreases with increasing valproate concentration, resulting in an increase in the percent free or unbound drug. As a consequence of the high binding to plasma proteins, valproic acid is subject to displacement interactions with other drugs [59]. The apparent volume of distribution of valproic acid is relatively small and appears to range from 0.13 to 0.19 L/kg. Despite its hydrophilic nature, valproic acid enters the CNS rapidly. The processes governing the passage of the drug across the blood–brain barrier involve both passive diffusion and a bidirectional carrier-mediated transport, presumably involving P-gp. The brain to plasma concentration ratios based on the total and unbound plasma concentration are on average around 0.1 and 0.5, respectively, with considerable interindividual variability. The ratio between the cerebrospinal fluid concentration and the unbound concentration in plasma ranges between 0.6 and 1.0. Valproic acid distributes to a variety of other tissues such as the liver, kidney, bones, and intestines.

The elimination of valproic acid occurs virtually entirely by metabolism. Only a minor fraction of the administered dose of valproic acid is excreted unchanged in the urine. The biotransformation of valproic acid involves a variety of processes including direct glucuronide conjugation (40 %), mediated by UGT (UGT1A3, UGT2B7), mitochondrial β-oxidation (35 %), and minor CYP-dependent oxidation (10 %), mainly mediated by CYP2C9, but also CYP2A6 and CYP2B6. Valproic acid glucuronide and 3-oxo-valproic acid are by far the most abundant metabolites, representing about 40 % and 33 %, respectively, of the urinary excretion of valproic acid dose. Two desaturated metabolites of valproic acid, 2-ene-valproic acid and 4-ene-valproic acid, retain anticonvulsant activity, but their serum and brain concentrations are probably too low to contribute significantly to therapeutic activity. The 4-ene-valproic acid metabolite has been associated with liver toxicity. As formation of this hepatotoxic metabolite is mediated by CYP enzymes, concomitant administration of valproic acid with enzyme-inducing antiepileptics such as phenobarbital, phenytoin, and carbamazepine may increase the risk of hepatotoxicity. However, elevation of 4-ene-valproic acid levels has not been clearly documented in patients with valproic acid hepatotoxicity. Valproic acid is considered to be a broad-spectrum inhibitor of various drug-metabolizing enzymes as it inhibits different CYPs including CYP2C9 and, to a lesser extent, CYP2C19 and CYP3A4; some UGTs, namely, UGT1A4 and UGT2B7; and epoxide hydrolase [59].

The half-life of valproic acid is in the order of 9–18 h, but shorter values (5–12 h) are observed in patients taking enzyme-inducing comedication. The elimination is slower in newborns, especially those born prematurely. On the other hand, children eliminate the drug at a faster rate compared with adults and therefore require larger dosages per unit of body weight to achieve plasma drug concentrations comparable with those observed in adults. Although total plasma valproic acid concentrations in the elderly are similar to those found in the young, unbound drug concentrations are increased in the elderly (as a result of an age-related decrease in intrinsic metabolic clearance, in the presence of a reduced plasma protein binding), and, therefore, the possibility of a reduction in dose requirements should be contemplated in these patients. Alterations in the pharmacokinetics of valproic acid are also observed in pregnancy, with a progressive decrease in total concentration and little or no change in unbound concentration.

8.3.2.3 Lamotrigine

Lamotrigine is a phenyltriazine chemically unrelated to other anticonvulsants. Lamotrigine is available as a conventional tablet and a chewable/dispersible tablet. The pharmacokinetic profile of lamotrigine has been extensively reviewed [63–66].

Lamotrigine is rapidly and completely absorbed after oral administration, with negligible first-pass metabolism and an absolute bioavailability of ≥95 %. Peak

synaptic plasticity. Valproic acid shares with lithium other effects on downstream signal transduction cascades, such as inhibition of protein kinase C (PKC) and myristoylated alanine-rich C-kinase substrate (MARKCS). Valproic acid and lamotrigine also inhibit glycogen synthase kinase 3β (GSK3β), an enzyme that contributes to many cellular functions including apoptosis, whereas carbamazepine does not. Other common effects of lithium and valproic acid are to increase the activity of the extracellular signal-regulated kinase (ERK) pathway, resulting in enhanced transcription of neurogenesis and cell survival factors, such as antiapoptotic protein Bcl-2 and BDNF. Valproic acid may also regulate gene expression and transcription by acting as histone deacetylase inhibitor. Another intracellular pathway recently involved in the mechanism of action of mood stabilizers is the brain arachidonic acid cascade. Chronic administration of mood stabilizers, such as lithium, valproic acid, carbamazepine, and lamotrigine, has been reported to decrease the turnover of brain arachidonic acid [23].

8.3.4 *Relationship Between Serum or Plasma Concentrations and Clinical Effects*

8.3.4.1 Carbamazepine

Several studies have investigated the relationship between plasma carbamazepine concentrations and clinical effects in patients with epilepsy, and a therapeutic range has been estimated at 4–12 μg/mL [73]. However, both the lower and the upper limit of the therapeutic range are poorly defined.

A limited number of studies have assessed the relationship between plasma carbamazepine levels and clinical response in bipolar patients, and results have been somewhat controversial. Some early investigations suggested that plasma carbamazepine level could be used as a predicting marker of therapeutic effect in patients with bipolar disorder [74]. In this respect, Ballenger and Post [75] reported that carbamazepine levels of 7–12 μg/mL should be recommended for use in affective disorders, while Okuma et al. [74, 76] found that 7 μg/mL of carbamazepine plasma concentration would be sufficient to exert antimanic and prophylactic effects in Japanese patients. Vasudev et al. [77] reported that 3–9 μg/mL of carbamazepine levels with an average of 6.0 ± 2.4 μg/mL may represent the therapeutic range in favorable responders. By contrast, other studies documented that carbamazepine levels in plasma or cerebrospinal fluid were not related to the degree of antidepressant or antimanic response [78, 79]. Concerning the role of carbamazepine epoxide, it was suggested that this metabolite might contribute to overall clinical efficacy of carbamazepine in bipolar patients [77]. In this respect, Petit et al. [80] reported a significant correlation found between carbamazepine-10,11-epoxide and the clinical response in affective disorders. Chbili et al. [81] have recently assessed the relationship between plasma levels of carbamazepine and its active epoxide metabolite and the therapeutic response in 13 patients with bipolar disease kept on a fixed individual dose of carbamazepine for 19 weeks. The psychopathologic state, evaluated by the Brief Psychiatric Rating Scale (BPRS), did not correlate with the plasma levels of carbamazepine, whereas both mean plasma levels of carbamazepine-10,11-epoxide concentrations and carbamazepine-10,11-epoxide to plasma carbamazepine ratio were closely correlated with mean values of BPRS scores ($r=0.80$, $p<0.01$, $r=-0.89$, $p<0.01$, respectively). Optimum therapeutic response was observed among patients who had a plasma metabolite level of 1.4 μg/mL and a plasma carbamazepine concentration of 7 μg/mL simultaneously. These results suggest that both plasma carbamazepine and carbamazepine-10,11-epoxide levels must be fixed to achieve optimum therapeutic response.

The most common adverse effects of carbamazepine include diplopia, dizziness, headache, vomiting, sedation, and lethargy and appear to be related to the peak serum concentrations. Although side effects have been reported to occur over a wide range of carbamazepine concentrations, they are more likely to appear at concentrations exceeding 10–12 μg/mL [73]. In massive CBZ poisoning, plasma concentrations above 40 μg/mL have been associated with an increased risk of coma, seizures, respiratory failure, and cardiac conduction defects [82]. Weaver et al. [83] described four clinical stages of carbamazepine intoxication: (a) coma and seizures (serum concentrations >25 μg/mL); (b) moderate stupor, combativeness, hallucinations, and choreiform movements (concentrations 15–25 μg/mL); (c) drowsiness and ataxia (concentrations 11–15 μg/mL); and (d) mild ataxia, but otherwise normal neurological examination (concentrations <11 μg/mL).

Carbamazepine may occasionally cause cardiovascular adverse effects such as sinus bradycardia and varying degrees of atrioventricular conduction disturbances, decreased bone mineral density, and endocrinological effects such as an antidiuretic hormone-like effect, resulting in water retention and hyponatremia. The risk of hyponatremia increases with increasing carbamazepine dosages and concentrations and is generally more common in elderly subjects. Carbamazepine is rarely associated with potentially lethal adverse effects including agranulocytosis, aplastic anemia, toxic hepatitis, and severe cutaneous rashes such as Stevens–Johnson syndrome and toxic epidermal necrolysis. These reactions are generally considered idiosyncratic and unpredictable irrespective of dosage. A strong association has been documented between the human leukocyte antigen *HLA–B*1502* and Stevens–Johnson syndrome/toxic epidermal necrolysis induced by carbamazepine in Han Chinese [84]. FDA recognized this allele as a valid pharmacogenomic biomarker, and screening should be performed for patients with Asian ancestry before starting carbamazepine.

8.3.4.2 Valproic Acid

Many studies have evaluated the correlation between plasma concentration of valproic acid and therapeutic/toxic response in patients with epilepsy. Concentrations of 50 μg/mL and higher are required for therapeutic effects, whereas concentrations exceeding 100 μg/mL have been associated with toxicity [73]. As a consequence, therapeutic monitoring of plasma levels of valproic acid is well established in the treatment of epilepsy.

Available studies on the relationship between valproic acid concentrations and response in bipolar disorder produced conflicting results [85, 86]. A target concentration range for the mood-stabilizing action of valproic acid has not yet been established, but a concentration of at least 50 μg/mL was required in most studies. In a study of 65 acutely manic patients, Bowden et al. [87] found that patients with valproate serum concentrations between 45 and 100–125 μg/mL were much more likely to have efficacious and well-tolerated responses that those with lower or higher levels. In another investigation involving 30 patients with manic disorder, Vasudev et al. [77] reported that valproic acid responders (>50 % reduction in YMRS) had mean levels of 67.6 ± 12.0 μg/mL, although sampling time was unclear. A modest but significant correlation between increasing valproic acid levels and reductions in YMRS was evident at week 2 ($r=0.64$, $p<0.05$), but not maintained thereafter. Allen et al. [88] performed a post hoc analysis of pooled intent-to-treat data from three randomized, placebo-controlled studies of divalproex treatment for acute mania involving 374 patients to test a hypothesized linear relationship between serum concentration and response and to determine optimal blood levels for treatment of acute mania. The results of this study suggested that the best response in acute mania is seen at valproate levels >94 μg/ml. In general, most of these trials used fixed-dose scheduling and did not measure valproic acid concentration as an outcome measure. Moreover, they shared a number of methodological limitations including retrospective nature or open-label and uncontrolled design, unclear methods or lack of details regarding specific assay used, administration of the rating scales, and blood sampling.

In summary, evidence from the literature suggests that correlations between serum or plasma concentrations of valproic acid and effects are weak, and attempts to define therapeutic cutoffs are presently unclear. However, even in the absence of a well-established correlation between plasma concentrations and clinical effects in patients with bipolar disorder, therapeutic monitoring of valproic acid may still prove useful as a measure of compliance, as a means to monitor drug interactions, and in special patient populations [85, 86].

The association between plasma concentrations of valproic acid and adverse effects is unclear. Nausea and vomiting, lethargy, dizziness, and tremor have all been reported already at levels >60 μg/mL [77]. However, nausea, vomiting, and sedation were otherwise reported as more common in patients with levels >125 mg/L, but dizziness frequently first reported at levels even <25 μg/mL [87]. Increased weight gain has occurred at levels >125 μg/mL, while reductions in white blood cells and platelets weakly correlated to valproic acid concentrations [89]. Although valproic acid is known to cause elevated serum ammonia levels and rarely induce hyperammonemic encephalopathy, correlations with drug concentrations are poor [90–93]. Carbamazepine is rarely associated with potentially lethal adverse effects such as aplastic anemia, hepatotoxicity, and pancreatitis. These reactions are unpredictable irrespective of dosage and do not appear to be related to valproic acid concentrations, dose, or treatment duration [94, 95].

8.3.4.3 Lamotrigine

Studies in patients with epilepsy have documented that no clear-cut relationship exists between clinical response and serum lamotrigine concentrations [73, 96]. In most studies a considerable overlap in the serum concentrations of lamotrigine between responders and nonresponders or between patients with or without adverse effects has been reported [96–98]. Patients treated with therapeutic doses have serum lamotrigine concentrations in the order of 2.5–15 μg/mL. Morris et al. [99] suggested that an appropriate reference range of serum concentrations for lamotrigine would be 3–14 μg/mL in patients with refractory epilepsy.

To the best of our knowledge, no study has so far evaluated the relationship between plasma concentrations of lamotrigine and therapeutic and/or toxic effects in the maintenance treatment of bipolar disorder. On the other hand, an open-label, prospective study has recently investigated the possible correlation between plasma concentrations of lamotrigine and its therapeutic effects in 34 inpatients with treatment-resistant depressive disorder during an 8-week treatment of lamotrigine augmentation [100]. The subjects were depressed patients who had already shown insufficient response to at least three psychotropics, including antidepressants, mood stabilizers, and atypical antipsychotics. The diagnoses were major depressive disorder ($n = 12$), bipolar I disorder ($n = 7$), and bipolar II disorder ($n = 15$). The final doses of lamotrigine were 100 mg/day for 18 subjects who were not taking valproate and 75 mg/day for 16 subjects taking valproate. There was a significant linear relationship between the plasma concentrations of lamotrigine and percentage of depressive symptom improvements, as evaluated by the MADRS, at week 8 ($r = 0.418$, $p < 0.05$). The receiver operating characteristics analysis indicated that a plasma lamotrigine concentration of 12.7 mmol/L or greater was significantly ($p < 0.001$) predictive of response (50 % or more reduction in the MADRS score). The present study suggests that an early therapeutic response to lamotrigine is dependent on its plasma concentration and that a plasma lamotrigine concentration of 12.7 μmol/L (corresponding to 3 μg/mL) may be a threshold for a good therapeutic response in treatment-resistant depressive disorder.

Lamotrigine is generally well tolerated. The most common side effects are dose dependent and include headache, nausea, insomnia, vomiting, dizziness, diplopia, ataxia, and tremor. According to a retrospective survey in patients with epilepsy, the incidence of lamotrigine toxicity was found to increase significantly with concentrations >15 μg/mL [99]. Skin rash complicates the initial treatment with lamotrigine. The incidence of skin rash is increased by large initial doses, rapid dosage titration, and concurrent use of valproic acid. As a consequence, rashes caused by lamotrigine can be minimized by very slow up-titration of drug during initiation of therapy and by avoiding or managing drug interaction with valproic acid. Skin rash occurs more frequently in children. Severe Stevens–Johnson syndrome/toxic epidermal necrolysis rarely develops during lamotrigine treatment.

8.3.5 Conclusions and Future Directions

The pharmacokinetic properties of the three antiepileptics currently approved as mood stabilizers are relatively complex, and their mechanism of action in bipolar disorder is largely unknown. While therapeutic monitoring of plasma levels of carbamazepine, valproic acid, and, to a lesser extent, lamotrigine is well recognized in the management of epilepsy, this practice is less frequently used to optimize the treatment of bipolar disorder. This is partly related to the lack of a clear-cut correlation between plasma concentrations of these agents and therapeutic response, as documented by the available studies in patients with bipolar disorder. However, several characteristics of these antiepileptics, such as the large interindividual pharmacokinetic variability, the narrow therapeutic range, and the high potential for drug interactions, suggest that their effective use may be facilitated by application of therapeutic drug monitoring, as strongly recommended by recent consensus guidelines [101]. With the expanding role of these mood stabilizers in the management of bipolar disorder, further investigation of the correlation between serum concentrations and efficacy is warranted to maximize clinical benefit and/or avoid adverse events and nonadherence.

References

1. Goodwin GM, Mahli GS (2007) What is a mood stabilizer? Psychol Med 35:609–614
2. Bowden CL (2008) Bipolar pathophysiology and development of improved treatments. Brain Res 1235:92–97
3. Bialer M (2012) Why are antiepileptic drugs used for nonepileptic conditions? Epilepsia 53(Suppl 7):26–33
4. Malhi GS, Adams D, Cahill CM, Dodd S, Berk M (2009) The management of individuals with bipolar disorder: a review of the evidence and its integration into clinical practice. Drugs 69:2063–2101
5. Mahli GS, Tanious M, Das P, Berk M (2012) The science and practice of lithium therapy. Aust N Z J Psychiatry 46:192–211
6. Cipriani A, Hawton K, Stockton S, Geddes JR (2013) Lithium in the prevention of suicide in mood disorders: updated systematic review and meta-analysis. BMJ 346:f3646
7. Bettinger TL, Crismon ML (2006) Lithium. In: Burton ME, Shaw LM, Schentag JJ, Evans WE (eds) Applied pharmacokinetics & pharmacodynamics, 4th edn. Lippincott Williams & Wilkins, Philadelphia, pp 798–812
8. Amidsen A (1977) Serum level monitoring and clinical pharmacokinetics of lithium. Clin Pharmacokinet 2:73–92
9. Cooper TB, Simpson GM, Lee JH, Bergner PE (1978) Evaluation of a slow-release lithium carbonate formulation. Am J Psychiatry 135:917–922
10. Thornhill DP (1978) Pharmacokinetics of ordinary and sustained release lithium carbonate in manic patients after acute dosage. Eur J Clin Pharmacol 14:267–271
11. Ward ME, Musa MN, Bailey L (1994) Clinical pharmacokinetics of lithium. J Clin Pharmacol 34:280–285
12. Grandjean EM, Aubry JM (2009) Lithium: updated human knowledge using a evidence-based approach. Part II: clinical pharmacology and therapeutic monitoring. CNS Drugs 23:331–349

13. Soares JC, Boada F, Keshavan MS (2000) Brain lithium measurements with ^{7}Li magnetic resonance spectroscopy (MRS): a literature review. Eur Neuropsychopharmacol 10:151–158
14. Camus M, Henneré G, Baron G, Peytavin G, Massias L, Mentré F, Farinotti R (2003) Comparison of lithium concentrations in red blood cells and plasma in samples collected for TDM, acute toxicity, or acute-on-chronic toxicity. Eur J Clin Pharmacol 59:583–587
15. El Balkhi S, Megarbane B, Poupon J, Baud FJ, Galliot-Guilley M (2009) Lithium poisoning: is determination of the red blood cell lithium concentration useful? Clin Toxicol 47:8–13
16. Finley PR, Warner MD, Peabody CA (1995) Clinical relevance of drug interactions with lithium. Clin Pharmacokinet 29:172–191
17. Dunner DL (2003) Drug interactions of lithium and other antimanic/mood-stabilizing medications. J Clin Psychiatry 64(Suppl 5):38–43
18. Sproule BA, Hardy BG, Shulman KI (2000) Differential pharmacokinetics of lithium in elderly patients. Drugs Aging 16:165–177
19. Schou M (1990) Lithium treatment during pregnancy, delivery, and lactation: an update. J Clin Psychiatry 51:410–413
20. Malhi GS, Tanious M, Das P, Coulston CM, Berk M (2013) Potential mechanisms of action of lithium in bipolar disorder: current understanding. CNS Drugs 27:135–153
21. Oruch R, Elderbi MA, Khattab HA, Pryme IF, Lund A (2014) Lithium: a review of pharmacology, clinical uses, and toxicity. Eur J Pharmacol 740:464–473
22. Machado-Vieira R, Manji HK, Zarate CA Jr (2009) The role of lithium in the treatment of bipolar disorder: convergent evidence for neurotrophic effects as a unifying hypothesis. Bipolar Disord 11(Suppl 2):92–109
23. Rao JS, Rapoport SI (2009) Mood-stabilizers target the brain arachidonic acid cascade. Curr Mol Pharmacol 2:207–214
24. Sproule B (2002) Lithium in bipolar disorder: can drug concentrations predict therapeutic effect? Clin Pharmacokinet 41:639–660
25. Stokes PE, Kocsis JH, Arcuni OJ (1976) Relationship of lithium chloride dose to treatment response in acute mania. Arch Gen Psychiatry 33:1080–1084
26. Prien RF, Caffey EM, Klett CJ (1972) Comparison of lithium carbonate and chlorpromazine in the treatment of mania. Arch Gen Psychiatry 26:146–153
27. Takahashi R, Sakuma A, Itoh K, Itoh H, Kurihara M (1975) Comparison of efficacy of lithium carbonate and chlorpromazine in mania: report of collaborative study group on treatment of mania in Japan. Arch Gen Psychiatry 32:1310–1318
28. Hopkins HS, Gelenberg AJ (2000) Serum lithium levels and the outcome of maintenance therapy of bipolar disorder. Bipolar Disord 2(3 Pt 1):174–179
29. Chen ST, Altshuler LL, Melnyk KA, Erhart SM, Miller E, Mintz J (1999) Efficacy of lithium vs. valproate in the treatment of mania in the elderly: a retrospective study. J Clin Psychiatry 60:181–186
30. Severus WE, Grunze H, Kleindienst N, Frangou S, Moeller HJ (2005) Is the prophylactic antidepressant efficacy of lithium in bipolar I disorder dependent on study design and lithium level? J Clin Psychopharmacol 25:457–462
31. Gelenberg AJ, Kane JM, Keller MB, Lavori P, Rosenbaum JF, Cole K, Lavelle J (1989) Comparison of standard and low serum levels of lithium for maintenance treatment of bipolar disorder. N Engl J Med 321:1489–1493
32. Severus WE, Kleindienst N, Seemuller F, Frangou S, Möller HJ, Greil W (2008) What is the optimal serum lithium level in the long-term treatment of bipolar disorder: a review? Bipolar Disord 10:231–237
33. Kleindienst N, Severus WE, Greil W (2007) Are serum lithium levels related to the polarity of recurrence in bipolar disorders? Evidence from a multi-center trial. Int Clin Psychopharmacol 22:125–131
34. Kleindienst N, Severus WE, Moller HJ, Greil W (2005) Is polarity of recurrence related to serum lithium level in patients with bipolar disease? Eur Arch Psychiatr Clin Neurosci 255:72–74

35. Severus WE, Kleindienst N, Evoniuk G, Bowden C, Möller HJ, Bohus M, Frangou S, Greil W, Calabrese JR (2009) Is the polarity of relapse/recurrence in bipolar-I disorder patients related to serum lithium levels? Results from an empirical study. J Affect Disord 115:466–470
36. Kato T, Inubushi T, Takahashi S (1994) Relationship of lithium concentrations in the brain measured by lithium-7 magnetic resonance spectroscopy to treatment response in mania. J Clin Psychopharmacol 14:330–335
37. Sachs GS, Renshaw PF, Lafer B, Stoll AL, Guimarães AR, Rosenbaum JF, Gonzalez RG (1995) Variability of brain lithium levels during maintenance treatment: a magnetic resonance spectroscopy study. Biol Psychiatry 38:422–428
38. Chen KP, Shen WW, Lu ML (2004) Implication of serum concentration monitoring in patients with lithium intoxication. Psychiatry Clin Neurosci 58:25–29
39. Gadallah MF, Feinstein EI, Massry SG (1988) Lithium intoxication: clinical course and therapeutic considerations. Miner Electrolyte Metab 14:146–149
40. Simard M, Gumbiner B, Lee A, Lewis H, Norman D (1989) Lithium carbonate intoxication: a case report and review of the literature. Arch Intern Med 149:36–46
41. Oakley PW, Whyte IM, Carter GL (2001) Lithium toxicity: an iatrogenic problem in susceptible individuals. Aust N Z J Psychiatry 35:833–840
42. Malhi GS, Tanious M (2011) Optimal frequency of lithium administration in the treatment of bipolar disorder clinical and dosing considerations. CNS Drugs 25:289–298
43. Ljubicic D, Letica-Crepulja M, Vitezic D, Bistrovic IL, Ljubicic R (2008) Lithium treatments: single and multiple daily dosing. Can J Psychiatry 53:323–331
44. Jensen HV, Davidsen K, Toftegaard L, Mellerup ET, Plenge P, Aggernaes H, Bjorum N (1996) Double-blind comparison of the side-effect profiles of daily versus alternate day dosing schedules in lithium maintenance treatment of manic-depressive disorder. J Affect Disord 36:89–93
45. Plenge P, Amin M, Agarwal AK, Greil W, Kim MJ, Panteleyeva G, Park JM, Prilipko L, Rayushkin V, Sharma M, Mellerup E (1999) Prophylactic efficacy of lithium administered every second day: a WHO multicentre study. Bipolar Disord 1:109–116
46. Mahli GS, Berk M (2012) Is the safety of lithium no longer in the balance? Lancet 379:690–692
47. Johannessen Landmark C (2008) Antiepileptic drugs in non-epilepsy disorders: relations between mechanisms of action and clinical efficacy. CNS Drugs 22:27–47
48. Post RM, Ketter TA, Uhde T, Ballenger JC (2007) Thirty years of clinical experience with carbamazepine in the treatment of bipolar illness: principles and practice. CNS Drugs 21:47–71
49. Weisler RH, Cutler AJ, Ballenger JC, Post RM, Ketter TA (2006) The use of antiepileptic drugs in bipolar disorders: a review based on evidence from controlled trials. CNS Spectr 11:788–799
50. Haddad PM, Das A, Ashfaq M, Wieck A (2009) A review of valproate in psychiatric practice. Exp Opin Drug Metab Toxicol 5:539–551
51. Weisler RH, Calabrese JR, Bowden CL, Ascher JA, De Veaugh-Geiss J, Evoniuk G (2008) Discovery and development of lamotrigine for bipolar disorder: a story of serendipity, clinical observations, risk taking, and persistence. J Affect Dis 108:1–9
52. Bowden CL, Singh V (2012) Lamotrigine (Lamictal IR) for the treatment of bipolar disorder. Exp Opin Pharmacother 13:2565–2571
53. Grunze H (2010) Anticonvulsants in bipolar disorder. J Ment Health 19:127–141
54. Spina E (2002) Carbamazepine: chemistry, biotransformation, and pharmacokinetics. In: Levy RH, Mattson RH, Meldrum BS, Perucca E (eds) Antiepileptic drugs, 5th edn. Lippincott Williams & Wilkins, Philadelphia, pp 236–246
55. Sillanpaa M, Haataja L, Tomson T, Johannesen S (2009) Carbamazepine. In: Shorvon S, Perucca E, Engel J (eds) Treatment of epilepsy, 3rd edn. Wiley-Blackwell Publishing Ltd, Oxford, pp 459–474
56. Luna-Tortos C, Fedrowitz M, Löscher W (2008) Several major antiepileptic drugs are substrates for human P-glycoprotein. Neuropharmacology 55:1364–1375

57. Zhang C, Kwan P, Zuo Z, Baum L (2012) The transport of antiepileptic drugs by P-glycoprotein. Adv Drug Deliv Rev 64:930–942
58. Anderson GD (1998) A mechanistic approach to antiepileptic drug interactions. Ann Pharmacother 32:554–563
59. Perucca E (2005) Clinically relevant drug interactions with antiepileptic drugs. Br J Clin Pharmacol 61:246–255
60. Levy RH, Shen DD, Abbott FS, Riggs W, Hachad H (2002) Valproic acid: chemistry, biotransformation, and pharmacokinetics. In: Levy RH, Mattson RH, Meldrum BS, Perucca E (eds) Antiepileptic drugs, 5th edn. Lippincott Williams & Wilkins, Philadelphia, pp 780–800
61. Perucca E (2002) Pharmacological ad therapeutic properties of valproate: a summary after 35 years of clinical experience. CNS Drugs 16:695–714
62. Bourgeois BFD (2009) Valproate. In: Shorvon S, Perucca E, Engel J (eds) Treatment of Epilepsy, 3rd edn. Wiley-Blackwell Publishing Ltd, Oxford, pp 685–698
63. Dickins M, Chen C (2002) Lamotrigine: chemistry, biotransformation, and pharmacokinetics. In: Levy RH, Mattson RH, Meldrum BS, Perucca E, Levy RH, Mattson RH, Meldrum BS, Perucca E (eds) Antiepileptic drugs, 5th edn. Lippincott Williams & Wilkins, Philadelphia, pp 370–379
64. Goldsmith DR, Wagstaff AJ, Ibbotson T, Perry CM (2003) Lamotrigine: a review of its use in bipolar disorder. Drugs 63:2029–2050
65. Biton V (2006) Pharmacokinetics, toxicology and safety of lamotrigine in epilepsy. Exp Opin Drug Metab Toxicol 2:1009–1018
66. Matsuo F, Riaz A (2009) Lamotrigine. In: Shorvon S, Perucca E, Engel J (eds) Treatment of epilepsy, 3rd edn. Wiley-Blackwell Publishing Ltd, Oxford, pp 535–558
67. Hussein Z, Posner J (1997) Population pharmacokinetics of lamotrigine monotherapy in patients with epilepsy: retrospective analysis of routine monitoring data. Br J Clin Pharmacol 43:457–464
68. Chen C, Casale EJ, Duncan B, Culverhouse EH, Gilman J (1999) Pharmacokinetics of lamotrigine in children in the absence of other antiepileptic drugs. Pharmacotherapy 19:437–441
69. Ohman I, Vitols S, Tomson T (2000) Lamotrigine in pregnancy: pharmacokinetics during the delivery, in the neonate, and during lactation. Epilepsia 41:709–713
70. Stahl SM (2013) Mood stabilizers. In: Stahl SM (ed) Stahl's essential psychopharmacology, 4th edn. Cambridge University Press, New York, pp 370–387
71. Rogawski MA, Loscher W (2004) The neurobiology of antiepileptic drugs for the treatment of nonepileptic conditions. Nat Med 10:685–692
72. Schloesser RJ, Martinowich K, Manji HK (2012) Mood-stabilizing drugs: mechanism of action. Trends Neurosci 35:36–46
73. Patsalos PN, Berry DJ, Bourgeois BFD, Cloyd JC, Glauser TA, Johannessen SI, Leppik IE, Tomson T, Perucca E (2008) Antiepileptic drugs – best practice guidelines for therapeutic drug monitoring: a position paper by the subcommission on therapeutic drug monitoring, ILAE Commission on Therapeutic Strategies. Epilepsia 49:1239–1276
74. Okuma T, Yamashita I, Takahashi R, Itoh H, Otsuki S, Watanabe S, Sarai K, Hazama H, Inanaga K (1990) Comparison of the antimanic efficacy of carbamazepine and lithium carbonate by double-blind controlled study. Pharmacopsychiatry 23:143–150
75. Ballenger JC, Post RM (1980) Carbamazepine in manic depressive illness: a new treatment. Am J Psychiatry 137:782–790
76. Okuma T, Inanaga K, Otsuki S, Sarai K, Takahashi R, Hazama H, Mori A, Watanabe M (1979) Comparison of the antimanic efficacy of carbamazepine and chlorpromazine: a double-blind controlled study. Psychopharmacology (Berl) 66:211–217
77. Vasudev K, Goswami U, Kohli K (2000) Carbamazepine and valproate monotherapy: feasibility, relative safety and efficacy, and therapeutic drug monitoring in manic disorder. Psychopharmacology (Berl) 150:15–23
78. Post RM, Uhde TW, Ballenger JC, Chatterji DC, Greene RF, Bunney WE Jr (1983) Carbamazepine and its -10,11-epoxide metabolite in plasma and CSF. Relationship to antidepressant response. Arch Gen Psychiatry 40:673–676

79. Post RM, Uhde TW, Wolff EA (1984) Profile of clinical efficacy and side effect of carbamazepine in psychiatric illness: relationship to blood and CSF levels of carbamazepine and its -10,11-epoxide metabolite. Acta Psychiatr Scand 313(Suppl):104–120
80. Petit P, Lonjon R, Cociglio M (1991) Carbamazepine and its 10,11-epoxide metabolite in acute mania: clinical and pharmacokinetic correlates. Eur J Clin Pharmacol 41:541–546
81. Chbili C, Bannour S, Khlifi S, Ben Hadj Ali B, Saguem S (2014) Relationships between pharmacokinetic parameters of carbamazepine and therapeutic response in patients with bipolar disease. Ann Biol Clin 72:453–459
82. Hojer J, Malmlund HO, Berg A (1993) Clinical features of 28 consecutive cases of laboratory confirmed massive poisoning with carbamazepine alone. J Toxicol Clin Toxicol 31:449–458
83. Weaver DF, Camfield P, Fraser A (1988) Massive carbamazepine overdose: clinical and pharmacological observations in five episodes. Neurology 38:755–759
84. Chung WH, Hung SI, Hong HS, Hsih MS, Yang LC, Ho HC, Wu JY, Chen YT (2004) Medical genetics: a marker for Stevens-Johnson syndrome. Nature 428:486
85. Fleming J, Chetty M (2006) Therapeutic drug monitoring of valproate in psychiatry. how far we progressed? Clin Neuropharmacol 29:350–359
86. Haymond J, Ensom MHH (2010) Does valproic acid warrant therapeutic drug monitoring in bipolar affective disorder? Ther Drug Monit 32:19–29
87. Bowden CL, Janicak PG, Orsulak P, Swann AC, Davis JM, Calabrese JR, Goodnick P, Small JG, Rush AJ, Kimmel SE, Risch SC, Morris DD (1996) Relation of serum valproate concentration to response in mania. Am J Psychiatry 153:765–770
88. Allen MH, Hirschfeld RM, Wozniak PJ, Baker JD, Bowden CL (2006) Linear relationship of valproate serum concentration to response and optimal serum levels for acute mania. Am J Psychiatry 163:272–275
89. Bowden CL, Calabrese JR, McElroy SL, Gyulai L, Wassef A, Petty F, Pope HG Jr, Chou JC, Keck PE Jr, Rhodes LJ, Swann AC, Hirschfeld RM, Wozniak PJ (2000) A randomized, placebo-controlled 12-month trial of divalproex and lithium in treatment of outpatients with bipolar I disorder. Arch Gen Psychiatry 57:481–489
90. Haidukewych D, John G, Zielinski JJ, Rodin EA (1985) Chronic valproic acid therapy and incidence of increases in venous plasma ammonia. Ther Drug Monit 7:290–294
91. Ratnaike RN, Schapel GJ, Purdie G, Rischbieth RH, Hoffmann S (1986) Hyperammonaemia and hepatotoxicity during chronic valproate therapy: enhancement by combination with other antiepileptic drugs. Br J Clin Pharmacol 22:100–103
92. Kugoh T, Yamamoto M, Hosokawa K (1986) Blood ammonia level during valproic acid therapy. Jpn J Psychiatry Neurol 40:663–668
93. Dealberto MJ (2007) Valproate-induced hyperammonaemic encephalopathy: review of 14 cases in the psychiatric setting. Int Clin Psychopharmacol 22:330–337
94. Chapman SA, Wacksman GP, Patterson BD (2001) Pancreatitis associated with valproic acid: a review of the literature. Pharmacotherapy 21:1550–1560
95. Werlin SL, Fish DL (2006) The spectrum of valproic acid-associated pancreatitis. Pediatrics 118:1660–1663
96. Bartoli A, Guerrini R, Belmonte A, Alessandri MG, Gatti G, Perucca E (1997) The influence of dosage, age, and comedication on steady state plasma lamotrigine concentrations in epileptic children: a prospective study with preliminary assessment of correlations with clinical response. Ther Drug Monit 19:252–260
97. Johannessen SI, Tomson T (2006) Pharmacokinetic variability of newer antiepileptic drugs: when is monitoring needed? Clin Pharmacokinet 45:1061–1075
98. Kilpatrick ES, Forrest G, Brodie MJ (1996) Concentration-effect and concentration-toxicity relationships with lamotrigine: a prospective study. Epilepsia 37:534–538
99. Morris RG, Black AB, Harris AL, Batty AB, Sallustio BC (1998) Lamotrigine and therapeutic drug monitoring: retrospective survey following the introduction of a routine service. Br J Clin Pharmacol 46:547–551

100. Kagawa S, Mihara K, Nakamura A, Nemoto K, Suzuki T, Nagai G, Kondo T (2014) Relationship between plasma concentrations of lamotrigine and its early therapeutic effect of lamotrigine augmentation therapy in treatment-resistant depressive disorder. Ther Drug Monit 36:730–733
101. Hiemke C, Baumann P, Bergemann N, Conca A, Dietmaier O, Egberts K, Fric M, Gerlach M, Greiner C, Gründer G, Haen E, Havemann-Reinecke U, Jaquenoud Sirot E, Kirchherr H, Laux G, Lutz UC, Messer T, Müller MJ, Pfuhlmann B, Rambeck B, Riederer P, Schoppek B, Stingl J, Uhr M, Ulrich S, Waschgler R, Zernig G (2011) AGNP consensus guidelines for therapeutic drug monitoring in psychiatry: update 2011. Pharmacopsychiatry 44:195–235

Chapter 9
Antidepressants

Patrick R. Finley, Jennifer Le, and Kelly C. Lee

Abstract Antidepressants have made major contributions towards the treatment of anxiety and mood disorders. A variety of pharmacologic classes of these agents emerged since the 1960s. Tricyclics and monoamine oxidase inhibitors were early agents developed and remain in use today. Plasma concentration monitoring for therapeutic effects were initiated with the tricyclic agents. However, safety concerns persisted with these agents and the selective serotonin reuptake inhibitors (SSRIs) arose. Since the introduction of the SSRIs, these agents became the foremost prescribed medications for depression and anxiety disorders. The SSRIs have also expanded the understanding of cytochrome P450 (CYP) metabolism, drug transporters, and drug-drug interaction mechanisms. Serotonin norepinephrine reuptake inhibitors (SNRIs) joined the SSRIs but with a dual pharmacologic mechanism of action. Various other pharmacologic types of antidepressants have been fostered such as bupropion, vilazodone, mirtazapine, and vortioxetine. Persons with polymorphic CYP metabolism (e.g., poor or ultrarapid metabolizers) may explain the occurrence of adverse events despite modest drug dosages or the lack of efficacy regardless of the appropriate doses. Pharmacokinetic and pharmacodynamics studies have been conducted for all the antidepressants, exploring the potential association of plasma concentrations with therapeutic outcomes (efficacy and toxicity) but routine therapeutic drug monitoring (TDM) is only recommended for a few agents. There is reason to believe, however, that the incorporation of pharmacogenetic information with TDM practices may ultimately lead to enhanced efficacy, reduced toxicity, and minimized risk for drug interactions.

P.R. Finley, PharmD (✉)
Department of Clinical Pharmacy, School of Pharmacy, University of California, San Francisco, CA, USA
e-mail: patrick.finley@ucsf.edu

J. Le, PharmD, MAS • K.C. Lee, PharmD
Department of Clinical Pharmacy, Skaggs School of Pharmacy and Pharmaceutical Sciences, University of California San Diego, San Diego, CA, USA
e-mail: jenle@ucsd.edu; kellylee@uncsd.edu

M. Jann et al. (eds.), *Applied Clinical Pharmacokinetics and Pharmacodynamics of Psychopharmacological Agents*,
DOI 10.1007/978-3-319-27883-4_9

Keywords Tricyclics • Selective serotonin reuptake inhibitors • Serotonin norepinephrine reuptake inhibitors • Monoamine oxidase inhibitors • Miscellaneous agents • CYP metabolism • Serum concentrations • Pharmacogenomics

9.1 Introduction

Antidepressants are one of the most commonly prescribed classes of medications in healthcare today. The major classifications of antidepressants include selective serotonin reuptake inhibitors (SSRI), serotonin-norepinephrine reuptake inhibitors (SNRI), norepinephrine reuptake inhibitors (NRI), tricyclic and tetracyclic antidepressants (TCA), and monoamine oxidase inhibitors (MAOI). The clinical flexibility of antidepressants offer these medications utility in effectively treating a broad spectrum of mental illnesses, encompassing depression, anxiety disorders, insomnia, obsessive-compulsive disorder, and post-traumatic stress disorder.

While the older classes of antidepressants have been utilized clinically for nearly three decades, the successful development and release of fluoxetine in 1988 represented a seminal event, not only in the treatment of depressive illness but also in the age of modern pharmaceutics. Fluoxetine's introduction was met with almost immediate commercial success and three other medications from this same antidepressant class (SSRI) were released within the next decade. New medications or formulations from other antidepressant classes soon hit the market as well, including SNRI and NRI. Together, these newer antidepressant medications greatly expanded the pharmacological armamentarium for depression and anxiety disorders, and their popularity continued to soar through the intervening years. In 2011, the Department of Health and Human Services reported that one in ten adults older than 12 years of age had received a prescription for an antidepressant within the past year.

The burgeoning popularity of antidepressants can be attributed to many factors, including extensive marketing, a growing awareness of the high prevalence of mood disorders, or the common perception that newer agents are better tolerated than older compounds. With time, we came to realize that, while these medications represent a significant scientific breakthrough in the management of mental illness, they are also quite complex from a pharmacological perspective. They are fully capable of inducing serious toxicities and a wide variety of drug interactions which are often overlooked by clinicians. Given the ubiquity of antidepressant prescribing, it is imperative that health professionals have an excellent understanding of how these medications can be safely and effectively administered.

In this chapter, we have provided a summary of the current medical literature describing the pharmacokinetic and pharmacodynamic characteristics of antidepressants with an emphasis on the clinical relevance of their respective actions. While the evidence supporting routine therapeutic monitoring for these medications is rather limited, the pharmacokinetic disposition and pharmacological activity of all antidepressants is highly relevant in consideration of drug interaction potential, adverse effects, withdrawal phenomenon, toxic exposures, and other therapeutic misadventures.

9.2 Clinical Pharmacokinetics

9.2.1 Selective Serotonin Reuptake Inhibitors (SSRI)

At the present time, there are six members of the SSRI class that have been released in the United States. Collectively, they have been approved and marketed for a relative broad array of indications primarily relating to depression and anxiety disorders. While they all have the same basic pharmacological propensity for blocking the presynaptic reuptake of serotonin, they are remarkably different in regard to basic chemical structure and pharmacokinetic disposition.

Fluoxetine is formulated as a racemic mixture, with the S isomer of the parent compound having an affinity for the serotonin transporter (SERT) which is 1.5 times greater than the R isomer [1]. This difference is even greater with the stereoselective species of the demethylated active metabolite, where S-norfluoxetine has a SERT affinity which is 20 times greater than R-norfluoxetine. Fluoxetine is slowly absorbed from the gastrointestinal (GI) tract with peak concentrations achieved approximately 6–8 h after oral administration of the immediate-release preparations and 7–10 h later with the weekly formulation [2]. The rate of absorption is delayed slightly (e.g., maximum concentration achieved 1–2 h later) by coadministration with food, which is clinically relevant as patients often are instructed to take fluoxetine with meals to minimize GI upset. Approximately 80 % of fluoxetine is ultimately absorbed (i.e., bioavailability) and this is not affected by food (Table 9.1) [30]. Fluoxetine, like all other SSRI, is quite lipophilic and has a large volume of distribution once it is absorbed. It readily crosses the blood-brain barrier where CNS concentrations are greater than those found in the periphery [31]. It is also highly protein bound with 94.5 % of the drug bound to plasma proteins in peripheral circulation.

Owing to the stereoselective nature of fluoxetine, its metabolic fate is quite complex. It appears that the parent compound is metabolized primarily by the CYP2D6 and CYP2C9 isoenzymes, and pharmacokinetic studies of the dose/concentration relationship indicate that this is a nonlinear process [32]. CYP2D6 isoenzymes are responsible for demethylating the S and R isomers, while CYP2C9 metabolizes the R species. Pharmacogenetic studies also reveal that concentrations vary considerably with CYP2D6 phenotypes as poor metabolizers were found to have fluoxetine levels that were four times greater than ultra-rapid metabolizers [33]. In spite of this, the Clinical Pharmacogenetics Implementation Consortium (CPIC) did not endorse a change in dosing recommendation based on CYP2D6 phenotypes due to the fact that the combination of fluoxetine and norfluoxetine is responsible for therapeutic

Table 9.1 Pharmacokinetic parameters for antidepressants [3–6]

Drug	Bioavailability (%)[a]	Clearance (L/h)[b]	Volume of distribution (L/kg)	Half-life (h)	Active metabolite
Amitriptyline [7–9]	30–60	19–72	6–36	9–46	Yes
Amoxapine [10]	46–82	42–73[c]	8–14	6–16	Yes
Bupropion [11, 12]	N/A	126–140	19	18	Yes
Citalopram [13]	80	23–38	14	26–36	No
Clomipramine [14–16]	36–62	23–122	9–25	15–62	Yes
Desipramine [17]	33–51	78–168	24–60	12–28	No
Desvenlafaxine	80	210	3–5	9–15	No
Doxepin [18]	13–45	41–61	9–33	8–25	Yes
Duloxetine	43–50	114	20	10–12	No
Escitalopram	80	36	12–26	27–33	No
Fluoxetine [19]	80	5–42	12–42	26–220	Yes
Fluvoxamine [13]	53	33–320	25	32	No
Imipramine [20, 21]	30–70	32–102	9–23	6–28	Yes
Ketamine	16	58	3	2.5	No
Levomilnacipran	92	21–29	6	12	No
Maprotiline [22]	70–90	17–34	16–32	27–50	No
Mirtazapine [13]	50	[c]	4.5	13–34	No
Nortriptyline [23, 24]	46–70	17–79	15–32	18–56	No
Paroxetine	50–64	15–92	2–12	18–21	No
Phenelzine	[c]	[c]	[c]	1.5–4.0	No
Selegiline transdermal	25–30	16	[c]	18–25	No
Sertraline	>44	96	>20	26	No
Tranylcypromine	[c]	[c]	1.1–5.7	1.5–3.5	No
Trazodone [25, 26]	70–90	7–12	1–2	3–14	No
Trimipramine [27]	18–63	40–105	17–48	16–40	Yes
Venlafaxine [13]	13–45	40–129	5	4–5	Yes
Vilazodone [28]	75	32.7	28	66	No
Vortioxetine [29]	72 (with food)	70	37	25	No

Adapted from Finley PR. Antidepressants (AHFS 28:16.04)
[a]Values are low due to extensive presystemic elimination
[b]Values approach or exceed hepatic blood flow due to an inherent artifact in calculating clearance from oral dose data
[c]Reliable values are not available in the literature
N/A = data are not available

activity and the total concentration of these two species may not vary with gene status [34]. The elimination half-life for fluoxetine is 4–6 days in multiple-dose studies, and the half-life of the active metabolite is 4–16 days, suggesting that steady-state dynamics may not be achieved for as long as 1 month in some subjects.

Pharmacokinetic drug interactions are a major concern with fluoxetine. Both fluoxetine and norfluoxetine are potent inhibitors of CYP2D6 activity, with the

S-norfluoxetine species exhibiting CYP2D6 inhibition that is fivefold higher than R-norfluoxetine [35]. Fluoxetine is also a potent inhibitor of CYP2C19 activity, and possibly CYP2C9, but the in vivo effects of the parent compound and metabolite on CYP3A4 substrates are moderate at most [36]. Fluoxetine does not appear to be a substrate for p-glycoprotein (Pgp), but in vitro evidence suggests that it is an intermediate inhibitor of this important CNS transport protein [37].

The pharmacokinetic disposition of fluoxetine may be quite different in certain populations. For example, the half-life of both fluoxetine and its active metabolite are prolonged substantially in patients with significant liver impairment, but renal compromise did not appear to affect plasma concentrations [38]. Results from studies of elderly subjects do not suggest that there is a marked difference in fluoxetine concentrations (vs younger controls), but comparisons of pharmacokinetic disposition in children versus adolescents indicate that the former population has concentrations that are twofold higher, when adjusted for total body weight [2].

Sertraline was the second SSRI released in the United States, but in comparison to other antidepressants, the pharmacokinetic disposition has not been well characterized. It is slowly absorbed from the upper GI tract, with maximum concentrations achieved between 4 and 8 h after oral administration [39, 40]. The bioavailability has been reported to be >44 %, but this value has not been confirmed or quantified more precisely with comparative oral and intravenous study data. The absorption of sertraline appears to increase with food, as maximum concentrations were 25 % higher and achieved 2.5 h earlier (vs fasting controls) but the clinical significance of this finding is unclear [41]. Sertraline is highly bound to plasma proteins (98 %) and has a large volume of distribution but the precise value has not been published.

Sertraline is metabolized primarily by the CYP2C19 enzyme and genetic polymorphisms have been demonstrated to have a significant effect on plasma concentrations [42]. As a result, CPIC guidelines recommend a 50 % decrease in daily dose when initiating treatment in CYP2C19 poor metabolizers [43]. Sertraline appears to exhibit linear pharmacokinetics in daily doses up to 400 mg with an average terminal half-life of 26 h reported with multiple-dose regimens [44]. Desmethyl-sertraline is the primary product of sertraline metabolism and it has demonstrated an in vitro affinity for serotonin reuptake which is only 5–10 % as potent as the parent compound [45]. Desmethyl-sertraline has a considerably longer half-life, however, and plasma concentrations are threefold higher than sertraline at steady state [46].

Early in vitro studies suggested that sertraline and its primary metabolite had high inhibitory potential for the CYP2D6 isoenzyme [47]. Subsequent prospective studies with CYP2D6 substrates revealed that sertraline had minimal effects on plasma concentrations [48]. Research conducted more recently suggests that sertraline may have more significant CYP2D6 inhibitory potential among extensive metabolizers [49]. Sertraline has demonstrated potent inhibitory properties in regard to Pgp activity, but pharmacokinetic studies examining this action on relevant substrates have not been published at the present time [37].

Sertraline's metabolism appears to be quite sensitive to hepatic function. In a study of subjects diagnosed with mild liver impairment, sertraline's terminal half-life was significantly prolonged (52 h vs 22 h in controls). Renal disease did not appear to alter sertraline's disposition to an appreciable extent. The clearance of sertraline in the elderly has been reported to decrease by 40 % (vs younger subjects) and the corresponding half-life was determined to be 37 h (vs 22 h). No significant differences in sertraline pharmacokinetics have been found when comparing plasma concentrations in pediatric subjects versus adult controls.

Paroxetine is slowly absorbed from the GI tract, with maximum plasma concentrations occurring 5–6 h after oral dosing [50]. Peak concentrations of the controlled preparation range from 6 to 10 h after administration [50]. Food does not appear to affect the rate or extent of absorption. Paroxetine undergoes extensive first-pass metabolism, and bioavailability estimates range from 50 % with single dose administration to 64 % with multiple dosing, reflecting the partial saturability (or nonlinearity) of its pharmacokinetic disposition [51, 52]. Paroxetine is highly protein bound (95 %) and achieves much higher concentrations in the CNS than peripheral circulation. Reported values for the volume of distribution range from 2 to 12 L/kg [48].

Paroxetine is converted via the CYP2D6 system into an unstable catechol intermediate before becoming methylated, most likely via catechol-O-methyltransferase (COMT). There is indirect evidence that CYP3A4 may also play a role in paroxetine degradation, as carbamazepine has been shown to induce metabolism. This metabolic process is saturable at doses considered to be within the therapeutic range, resulting in a nonlinear increase in plasma concentrations with repeated or escalating exposures. Paroxetine metabolites are not believed to contribute significantly to therapeutic effects or side effects. The terminal half-life is approximately 18 h at steady state with daily doses of 20 mg and 21 h with 30 mg [53]. Pharmacogenetic investigations have demonstrated a strong influence of CYP2D6 phenotypic variations on plasma levels, with ultra-rapid metabolizers experiencing very low or undetectable concentrations of paroxetine. As a result, CPIC guidelines recommend that clinicians avoid paroxetine in patients who have demonstrated this CYP2D6 phenotype.

Studies designed to investigate differences in paroxetine pharmacokinetics in special populations have been hampered by the comparatively large range in plasma concentrations. This is true of studies comparing elderly subjects to younger controls, as well as for investigations conducted among patients with hepatic disease. Of note is that paroxetine's pharmacokinetic disposition is significantly affected by severe renal disease (creatinine clearance < 30 ml/min) where a fourfold increase in plasma concentrations has been reported. Mild renal disease did not appear to have an effect [50, 54].

Paroxetine has demonstrated the highest in vitro affinity for inhibiting CYP2D6 activity among the SSRI, and this pattern has been evident in controlled investigations of CYP2D6 substrates as well [55]. This appears to be a dose-dependent phenomenon, and CYP2D6 is the only enzyme in the P450 family that paroxetine effects. It is also, however, a potent inhibitor of Pgp activity [37].

Citalopram hydrobromide is manufactured as a racemic mixture of S and R enantiomers, with the S moiety (escitalopram) commercially available as a separate formulation. Citalopram is more rapidly absorbed than other SSRI with peak concentrations occurring 1–4 h after administration [56]. Bioavailability has been reported to be 80 % in comparison to intravenous formulations, and food did not appear to affect the absorption process [57, 58]. In the peripheral circulation, 80 % of citalopram can be found bound to plasma proteins.

Citalopram is metabolized by CYP2C19 to N-desmethylcitalopram. This species also exists in a racemic mixture, and S-desmethylcitalopram has been demonstrated to have an affinity for serotonin reuptake which is comparable to S-citalopram. Research characterizing the disposition of this metabolite indicates that it does not readily penetrate the blood-brain barrier, and CNS concentrations are low or undetectable. In vitro evidence suggests that citalopram may also be a substrate for the CYP3A4 isoenzyme, but controlled studies examining the impact of potent CYP3A4 inhibitors (e.g., ketoconazole) and inducers (carbamazepine) yielded conflicting results [48]. Subsequent demethylation of these metabolites by CYP2D6 produces a didesmethylcitalopram species which is believed to be responsible for QT prolongation in susceptible patients. The relationship of citalopram dose to plasma concentration appears to be linear, and the terminal half-life has been reported to range from 26 to 36 h [56, 59]. Because CYP2C19 is the primary metabolic pathway for citalopram conversion, the FDA has recommended that patients who have the poor metabolizer phenotype should receive an initial dose of citalopram that is 50 % lower than normal.

The pharmacokinetic parameters for citalopram can differ widely among special populations. Liver impairment has a significant effect on disposition, with an average half-life of 83 h reported in patients with cirrhosis (vs 37 h in controls). Moderate renal disease also prolonged half-life, from 37 to 49 h. Elderly subjects had clearance values that were approximately 30 % lower than younger controls.

Citalopram is considered to be a weak inhibitor of CYP2D6 metabolism. The R-desmethylcitalopram species has a more potent effect on this metabolic pathway than the S enantiomer [60]. Citalopram is a substrate for Pgp but has demonstrated only weak inhibitory effects on the transporter [37].

The absorption of escitalopram is very similar to citalopram's, with peak concentrations occurring 3–4 h after oral administration and bioavailability estimates of 80 %. Absorption is not affected by the presence of food in the GI tract [61]. Plasma protein binding of escitalopram is considerably less than citalopram's, averaging approximately 56 % [62, 63]. CYP2C19 is also the principle metabolic enzyme for escitalopram, and the dose/concentration relationship is also linear. The terminal half-life for escitalopram averages 27–33 h after multiple-dose administration [64]. Elderly subjects, as well as those suffering from liver or kidney disease, appear to have prolonged terminal half-lives that are similar in magnitude to those reported for citalopram.

In vitro affinity for CYP2D6 isoenzyme is considered weak for escitalopram, just as it is for the racemic parent compound. In spite of this, studies with CYP2D6 substrates such as desipramine and metoprolol have reported that escitalopram increases the AUC for these medications by 100 % and 82 %, respectively [61]. An explanation for this discrepancy is not forthcoming.

Fluvoxamine was actually the first SSRI introduced in Europe but it has not been FDA approved for depression in the United States, where the only current indication is obsessive-compulsive disorder. As a result, it is not widely prescribed in the United States. The absorption process is relatively slow but complete, with maximum concentrations reported as 2–8 h after oral doses of tablets and capsules and 4–12 h for the enteric-coated preparation [65]. The bioavailability has been reported to be only 53 % due to first-pass effects, and the volume of distribution estimates are very large (25 L/kg) [66]. Approximately 80 % of fluvoxamine is bound to plasma proteins.

Fluvoxamine exhibits nonlinear pharmacokinetics, with a half-life of 32 h evident after continued administration of 200 mg daily doses (divided). Both CYP2D6 and CYP1A2 are believed to be the metabolic enzymes primarily responsible for its degradation [48]. Substantial changes in fluvoxamine pharmacokinetics have been observed in special populations. In elderly subjects, the terminal half-life was reported to be prolonged by 63 %, and pediatric patients exhibited a doubling of their AUC (vs adult controls) [67]. Liver disease has also been associated with a significant decrease in clearance but renal disease does not appear to influence its disposition.

Fluvoxamine has been demonstrated to exert broad and potent inhibitory effects on several CYP isoenzymes. In vitro and in vivo evidence supports strong inhibition of CYP1A2, CYP2C9, CYP2C19, and CYP3A4 but not CYP2D6 [48]. Inhibitory effects on Pgp have been determined to be intermediate [37].

9.2.2 *Serotonin Norepinephrine Reuptake Inhibitors (SNRI)*

Venlafaxine was the first SNRI approved for the treatment of major depression in the United States, followed by duloxetine, desvenlafaxine (the active metabolite of venlafaxine), and levomilnacipran (the active isomer of milnacipran, a racemic compound approved for fibromyalgia in the United States and depression in Europe).

Venlafaxine exists as a racemic mixture of R and S isomers but the stereoselective properties of this compound do not appear to be clinically relevant in human models. It is commercially available as both an immediate-release formulation (IR) and an extended-release product (XR), with the latter medication much more commonly prescribed in the clinical setting. Venlafaxine is rapidly absorbed, with peak concentrations observed approximately 2 h after oral ingestion of the IR formulation and 6–8 h for the XR product [68]. Food has not been documented to alter the absorption process. Following absorption, venlafaxine exhibits a high first-pass effect with the majority of the medication not reaching the general circulation as the parent compound. Reported values for venlafaxine bioavailability range from 12.6 to 45 % [69]. Venlafaxine distributes widely throughout the body with a volume of distribution of approximately 5 L/kg and only 27 % of the drug is bound to plasma proteins [70].

Venlafaxine is rapidly metabolized by the liver to several chemical species, most notably through o-demethylation to form the desmethyl metabolite. This metabolite, available commercially as Pristiq, is present in steady-state concentrations that are three times higher than the parent compound and is believed to contribute substantially to therapeutic effects [70]. The N-desmethyl metabolite is also active in in vitro models but in vivo effects are much less significant. Venlafaxine is primarily metabolized via the CYP2D6 isoenzyme, and the plasma half-life of venlafaxine and desmethylvenlafaxine are 3.6–4.2 h and 10 h, respectively [70]. Genotypic variations in CYP2D6 status appear to influence the plasma half-life of venlafaxine but not the active metabolite, with values of 8 h reported for extensive metabolizers and 15 h for poor metabolizers [68]. As the therapeutic effects of venlafaxine are due to the combination of parent compound and active metabolite, the clinical relevance of this finding is unclear. Venlafaxine appears to exhibit nonlinear pharmacokinetics when individual doses exceed 225 mg.

The pharmacokinetic disposition of venlafaxine can vary in special populations. For individuals with liver disease, mild to moderate impairments have resulted in observed half-lives that are 30–60 % longer than controls, and this effect is even more substantial with severe impairment [71]. Renal compromise only appears to be clinically relevant with end-stage disease, where a 50 % decrease in clearance values has been reported [72]. Metabolism is not affected to a great extent by age or gender [73]. Venlafaxine is only a weak substrate for Pgp transporters, but it has been demonstrated to induce Pgp activity in human models [74].

When administered as an oral formulation, desvenlafaxine is slowly absorbed with a peak concentration achieved after 7–8 h [75]. Food does not appear to influence the absorption process, and the bioavailability is approximately 80 % [76, 77]. Plasma protein binding is low (30 %) and the volume of distribution ranges from 3.4 to 5 L/kg [70, 76]. The elimination of desvenlafaxine occurs primarily via glucuronidation (via UDP glucuronyltransferase) and, to a lesser extent, the CYP3A4 isoenzyme [70]. Desvenlafaxine exhibits linear pharmacokinetics and the terminal half-life has been reported to range from 9 to 11 h [75]. Hepatic impairment has only been demonstrated to have a modest effect on desvenlafaxine disposition, with a 35 % increase in AUC values found with severe disease [78]. The elimination of desvenlafaxine is much more sensitive to renal compromise as mild, moderate, and severe impairments have been reported to increase AUC by 42 %, 46 %, and 108 %, respectively [76, 79]. Similar declines in clearance values have been reported with elderly subjects in a manner consistent with anticipated declines in renal function.

Desvenlafaxine is considered to be a mild inhibitor of the CYP2D6 isoenzyme as coadministration with the substrate desipramine resulted in a 36 % increase in TCA concentrations [80]. Conversely, potent CYP3A4 inhibitors such as ketoconazole have been reported to increase desvenlafaxine's AUC by 43 % [81].

Duloxetine is slowly absorbed from the GI tract, with peak concentrations occurring 6 h after oral administration, and this process is not affected substantially by coadministration with food [82]. The reported bioavailability for duloxetine is low, ranging from 43 to 50 % [83]. In the circulation, duloxetine is highly protein bound (>90 %) and possesses a very large volume of distribution of approximately 20 L/kg [82, 84].

Duloxetine is converted to inactive metabolites by both the CYP1A2 and CYP2D6 isoenzymes. Drug interaction studies suggest that CYP1A2 is the major metabolic pathway, as potent 1A2 inhibitors such as fluvoxamine have a much greater impact on duloxetine concentrations than CYP2D6 inhibitors (e.g., paroxetine) [83, 85]. The terminal half-life for duloxetine has been reported to range from 10 to 12 h but it is not clear if duloxetine exhibits nonlinear metabolism as conflicting results have been published in the literature [83, 86]. Liver disease has been reported to have a profound impact on duloxetine metabolism and dosage adjustments are recommended for even mild impairment. One comparative study found that duloxetine clearance decreased from a value of 160 L/h in controls with normal liver function to 24 L/h in those with moderate hepatic impairment (based on Child-Pugh definitions) and corresponding half-lives were reported to be 13 h and 48 h, respectively [87]. There were no significant pharmacokinetic differences found in duloxetine disposition based on age, gender, or mild to moderate renal impairment. Drug interactions are an important consideration with duloxetine administration due to the fact that it appears to be a potent CYP2D6 inhibitor. Research with the CYP2D6 substrate desipramine indicates that plasma concentrations increased by nearly 300 % following duloxetine coadministration [85].

Levomilnacipran is the more pharmacologically active isomer derived from the racemic compound milnacipran. The only preparation of levomilnacipran that is currently marketed is extended release capsules. It is slowly but completely absorbed from the GI tract, with peak plasma concentrations occurring 6–8 h after oral administration [88, 89]. Food does not significantly impact the absorption process for levomilnacipran and bioavailability is reported to be 92 %. In the general circulation, levomilnacipran is not highly protein bound (22 %) and the volume of distribution is approximately 6 L/kg. Renal elimination has been reported to account for 58 % of levomilnacipran clearance, but metabolic conversion occurs as well, as evidenced by a 60 % increase in concentrations following the introduction of the CYP3A4 inhibitor, ketoconazole. The terminal half-life for levomilnacipran is approximately 12 h in the plasma. Renal impairment appears to have a more dramatic effect on levomilnacipran disposition than liver disease. Individuals with moderate renal impairment (creatinine clearance values of 30–50 ml/min) had a doubling of plasma concentrations, and severe impairment (creatinine clearance < 30 ml/min) resulted in levomilnacipran levels that increased threefold [PI].

The time to peak plasma concentration is approximately 2 h after the oral dose and is independent of the dose. Food can slow the rate of absorption but does not affect the extent of the absorption; dose adjustment is not required when administered with food [88]. Steady-state plasma concentrations are achieved within 5 days and the elimination half-life of mirtazapine after oral administration is approximately 20–40 h [115].

Mirtazapine is extensively metabolized and eliminated in the urine (75 %) and feces (25 %). Mirtazapine's major metabolic pathways include demethylation and oxidation followed by conjugation. The 8-hydroxy metabolite of mirtazapine is formed by CYP2D6 and CYP1A2, while the N-desmethyl and N-oxide metabolite are formed by CYP3A [116–118]. The desmethyl metabolite is pharmacologically active and has a similar pharmacokinetic prolife as the parent compound. The (R)– enantiomer has an elimination half-life that is approximately twice as long and has plasma levels that are three times higher than the (S)+ enantiomer. Mirtazapine is highly protein bound (85 %) over concentrations of 10–1000 ng/mL. Mirtazapine binds more tightly to human liver proteins (2.8 times) than human plasma proteins [115].

In a study of 14 Japanese patients, the metabolic clearance of mirtazapine and mirtazapine 8-hydroxylation activities were significantly lower in CYP2D6 intermediate metabolizers and poor metabolizers than extensive metabolizers ($p<0.05$) [119]. Trough plasma concentration/dose ratios of mirtazapine were significantly higher in CYP2D6 intermediate metabolizer/poor metabolizer group than extensive metabolizer group and higher in the CYP3A5 poor-expressor group (*3/*3) than expressor group (*1/*1 and *1/*3) ($p<0.05$). Mirtazapine 8-hydroxylation and N-demethylation activities were also inhibited by quinidine and ketoconazole, respectively. CYP2D6 intermediate metabolizers and poor metabolizers showed significantly lower mirtazapine 8-hydroxylation activities ($p<0.001$) and metabolic clearance ($p<0.05$) than extensive metabolizers. Trough concentrations were significantly higher in the CYP2D6 intermediate metabolizer group than extensive metabolizer group ($p<0.05$). Mirtazapine metabolism was not affected by risperidone or duloxetine alone but was affected when given concomitantly [119].

In patients older than 55 years, the clearance of mirtazapine was reduced by as much as 40 % compared to the younger group [115]. The greatest reduction in clearance was seen in elderly females. In general, females had significantly longer elimination half-lives compared to males (37 h vs 26 h, respectively). Despite these differences, no specific dose adjustment is recommended based on gender due to significant overlap in individual AUCs and half-lives between groups [115].

The elimination half-life of mirtazapine was increased by 40 % in mild to moderate hepatic impairment compared to those with normal hepatic function at a daily dose of 15 mg. The increased half-life resulted in 57 % increase in AUC and 33 % decrease in clearance of mirtazapine. In those with moderate and severe renal impairment, there were significant decrease in the clearance of mirtazapine and increase in AUC (54 % and 215 % for moderate and severe renal impairment, respectively). Peak plasma levels of mirtazapine were also doubled in those with severe renal impairment and the drug should be used cautiously in these individuals [115].

Vortioxetine (1-[2-(2,4-dimethyl-phenylsulfanyl)-phenyl]-piperazine, hydrobromide) is the first antidepressant in a class of multimodal antidepressants [120]. While the specific antidepressant mechanism of action is not fully understood, vortioxetine appears to exert its effect by inhibiting the reuptake of serotonin. The main pharmacological activity of vortioxetine is due to the parent drug. Steady-state mean Cmax are 9, 18, and 33 ng/mL within 7–11 h (Tmax) of administration of 5, 10, and 20 mg/day, respectively. The mean terminal half-life is approximately 66 h and steady-state plasma concentrations are achieved within 2 weeks of dosing. The absolute bioavailability of vortioxetine is 75 % and food does not affect the pharmacokinetics. Vortioxetine is extensively distributed with an apparent volume of distribution estimated at 2600 L. It is highly protein bound (98 %) and there was no effect on protein binding in those with hepatic or renal impairment [120]. There were no differences in plasma concentrations between men or women [121].

Vortioxetine is extensively metabolized via oxidation (CYP2D6, CYP3A4/5, CYP2C19, CYP2C9, CYP2A6, CYP2C8, and CYP2B6 enzymes) and glucuronidation [122, 123]. CYP2D6 is the primary enzyme responsible for metabolizing vortioxetine, resulting in an inactive carboxylic acid metabolite. Poor metabolizers of CYP2D6 have approximately twice the plasma concentration of vortioxetine compared to extensive metabolizers. Vortioxetine also lacks any inhibitory or inducing property for CYP450 enzymes [124]. Approximately 59 % and 26 % of the drug is eliminated in the urine and feces, respectively, as metabolites. Hepatic or renal impairment (mild, moderate, severe) does not affect the clearance of vortioxetine [120].

Ketamine is a noncompetitive N-methyl-D-aspartate (NMDA) receptor antagonist that was discovered in 1962 as an anesthetic [125]. It is a racemic compound similar to the psychomimetic drug, phencyclidine (PCP), but is much less potent and has a shorter duration of action than PCP. Ketamine has been associated with illicit use, but in the last 15 years, the drug has been clinically investigated and found to have robust and rapid antidepressant activities. The (R)– and (S)+ enantiomers of ketamine have differential affinity for the NMDA receptor with (S)+ having a fourfold greater binding affinity for the PCP site of the NMDA receptor [126]. Ketamine is also a μ-opioid receptor agonist in the CNS and spinal cord at anesthetic doses [127].

Ketamine is administered parenterally when used for therapeutic purposes. The peak plasma concentration of ketamine occurs within 1 min after an intravenous administration, and the half-life, which corresponds to the anesthetic effect of the drug, lasts approximately 10–15 min [125]. The elimination half-life is 2 h for the parent drug and 4 h for the metabolite, norketamine. The bioavailability for the intramuscular, intranasal, and oral route is 93 %, 25–50 %, and 16 %, respectively. The oral route results in lower peak plasma concentrations of the parent drug, ketamine, and higher levels of norketamine and dehydronorketamine [125].

Ketamine is extensively metabolized by hepatic enzymes, CYP2B6 and CYP3A4, to norketamine [125]. The metabolites are excreted renally (90 %) and fecally (5 %) and 4 % of the drug is excreted unchanged in the urine.

9.3 Clinical Pharmacodynamics

The precise mechanism of pharmacological action mediating the therapeutic effects of currently available antidepressants continues to elude researchers. For many years now, it has been assumed that depression was precipitated by a deficiency of biogenic amines in the central nervous system (e.g., serotonin, norepinephrine, and dopamine). While there are many lines of evidence lending credence to this hypothesis, the most compelling argument in support may simply reside in the fact that all of the effective antidepressants approved to date have been demonstrated to enhance the activity of at least one of these neurotransmitters [128].

There is now ample reason to believe, however, that this theory is not entirely correct and that antidepressant activity may be attenuated by other means [128]. For example, the putative actions of SSRI in the synapse – to bind to the presynaptic serotonin transporter (5HTT) and increase local serotonin concentrations – has been demonstrated to occur within hours of administration yet clinical benefits are not typically apparent for several days or weeks [55, 129, 130]. Furthermore, while all SSRI share the same strong affinity for blocking the 5HTT site, they are not therapeutically interchangeable and individuals who fail to respond to one member of the class may have a robust and complete therapeutic response to another [131].

Evidence has also accumulated in recent years that antidepressants have other pharmacological actions, particularly in regard to addressing the stress diathesis model of mood disorders. These mechanisms include alterations in glutaminergic transmission, promotion of neurogenesis, and anti-inflammatory properties [128, 132, 133]. Indeed, recent investigations demonstrating the rapid and profound antidepressant effects of medications lacking any appreciable effects on monoamine transmission strongly suggest that other pharmacodynamic properties of antidepressants may be associated with therapeutic activity [134].

In spite of the uncertainties encountered with the biogenic amine hypothesis, it is certainly instructive to review the pharmacodynamics actions of the different antidepressant agents within the context of adverse effects as well as therapeutic effects. In the section below, we have summarized the pharmacodynamics actions of antidepressants, highlighting the chemical properties and pharmacological differences that may be of clinical relevance.

9.3.1 Selective Serotonin Reuptake Inhibitors (SSRI)

All of the members of the SSRI class have demonstrated a strong affinity for binding to and effectively blocking the 5HTT in vitro. This affinity is greatest for paroxetine, followed closely by sertraline. Genetic polymorphisms have been identified for this receptor but the clinical significance of this finding remains unclear [135]. Clinical studies employing PET technology have suggested that chronic administration of SSRI requires 5HTT occupancy of at least 80 % to exert therapeutic effects.

With higher doses, the occupancy of this receptor was observed to plateau at approximately 85 %, indicating that therapeutic effects are not enhanced by dose escalation but the incidence and severity of adverse effects may increase [136].

At the present time, there is no convincing evidence that SSRI either inhibit the breakdown or promote the synthesis of serotonin. Instead, it has long been postulated that blockade of the 5HTT receptor would lead to an increase in synaptic concentrations of serotonin. This increase has not always been found to be particularly robust or sustained in investigations, and it is now believed that the therapeutic effects seen with chronic administration are due to a desensitization of the presynaptic 5HT1a autoreceptor. This effect may also initiate a decrease in glutamatergic firing.

The high affinity that SSRI have exhibited for the 5HTT is not observed with any other neurotransmitter receptors, which is why this class of antidepressants was originally termed "selective." It is not accurate to assume, however, that the SSRI do not have direct pharmacological effects on other neurotransmitters. Sertraline is believed to possess at least mild effects on blocking dopamine reuptake, as in vitro studies have demonstrated Ki values that are 2–3 orders of magnitude smaller than other SSRI (i.e., sertraline has higher affinity than others). Paroxetine has exhibited a similar affinity, quantitatively, for the muscarinic receptor, which may explain the higher risk of anticholinergic side effects reported with this SSRI in clinical trials. A comparison of affinities for the norepinephrine transporter (relative to serotonin) suggests that fluoxetine would be most likely to exert noradrenergic effects, which may be responsible for the comparatively high incidence of onset insomnia reported with this SSRI.

As mentioned previously, it is quite possible that antidepressant properties are mediated via pharmacological actions not necessarily involving the direct effects of biogenic amines. With SSRI, there have been several investigations which have reported anti-inflammatory properties for various agents, including inhibition of lymphocyte proliferation, decreases in inflammatory cytokines such as tumor necrosis factor (TNF-alpha), and increases in anti-inflammatory cytokines such as interleukin-10 (IL-10) [128].

9.3.2 Serotonin Norepinephrine Reuptake Inhibitors (SNRI)

Members of the SNRI class exhibit a high affinity for blocking norepinephrine as well as serotonin reuptake but it remains unclear if this multimodal effect confers therapeutic superiority over SSRI [131, 137–139]. Although all four members of this class share this pharmacological portfolio, there are substantial differences among them in regard to relative selectivity and dose-dependent effects.

Venlafaxine possesses an affinity for blocking serotonin reuptake which is nearly 30 times higher than norepinephrine in in vitro human models [140]. The affinity for norepinephrine reuptake inhibition with venlafaxine is considerably less than with secondary tricyclic agents and comparable to Ki values reported for sertraline and fluoxetine. However, venlafaxine's pharmacological profile is dose dependent and noradrenergic effects become more prominent at higher doses [141]. Furthermore, venlafaxine is rapidly metabolized to an active species (o-desmethylvenlafaxine) which is present in higher concentrations that are 2–3 times greater than the parent compound at steady state, contributing to venlafaxine's overall effects. Desvenlafaxine's pharmacological properties are similar to venlafaxine's, with an affinity for serotonin reuptake inhibition which is considerably greater than norepinephrine. Desvenlafaxine is also similar to venlafaxine in the sense that it has a low affinity for dopamine reuptake, and affinities for other neurotransmitter systems are minimal [140, 142].

The pharmacodynamics profile for duloxetine is also similar to venlafaxine's, with in vitro affinity for the serotonin transporter overshadowing that of norepinephrine. Duloxetine's clinical effects were originally attributed solely to serotonin reuptake inhibition, but subsequent research has revealed that it has relatively balanced neurotransmitter effects, with potent physiological activity mediated by both serotonin and norepinephrine at doses prescribed within the therapeutic range [143, 144]. Duloxetine has a low affinity for blocking dopamine reuptake and virtually no affinity for other neurotransmitters.

Levomilnacipran has a distinct pharmacological profile from other SNRI as it has demonstrated a higher affinity for blocking norepinephrine reuptake than serotonin but the clinical ramification of this property is uncertain. Noradrenergic effects of levomilnacipran appear to increase in a dose-dependent manner as evidenced by increases in diastolic blood pressure and heart rate with escalating doses. However, the serotonergic effects also become comparatively greater with higher doses and the relative contribution of these two neurotransmitters to pharmacological activity becomes comparable as doses approach 120 mg daily (i.e., maximum recommended dose) [145]. Levomilnacipran exhibits virtually no affinity for any other neurotransmitter systems in in vitro investigations.

9.3.3 Norepinephrine Reuptake Inhibitors (NRI)

From a structural or pharmacological standpoint, bupropion is actually quite similar to the classic stimulant medications, though it lacks their reinforcing or abuse potential. Bupropion has exhibited minimal direct effects on serotonin homeostasis and it is widely believed that its antidepressant properties are due to alterations in dopaminergic or noradrenergic transmission, though there continues to be considerable controversy in this regard [95]. Bupropion itself is only a weak inhibitor of reuptake blockade for dopamine or norepinephrine in vitro but in vivo effects are more pronounced, most likely due to the fact that the active metabolite, hydroxyl-bupropion, has more potent effects at these transporters and plasma concentrations are much greater than the parent compound at steady state [146].

Bupropion has also been found to be a potent antagonist for certain nicotinic acetylcholinergic receptors. This may explain the beneficial effects observed with bupropion for smoking cessation, and this pharmacological action may also contribute indirectly to the firing rate of noradrenergic neurons [95].

In animal models, bupropion appears to decrease noradrenergic activity in the locus coeruleus, suggesting possible anxiolytic effects [147]. However, bupropion has also been demonstrated to increase aggressive behaviors in mice with such tendencies, suggesting that the effects on anxiety levels may be state dependent [148].

9.3.4 *Tricyclic and Tetracyclic Antidepressants (TCA)*

TCA therapeutically modulate mood by inhibiting the reuptake of neurotransmitters, specifically norepinephrine and serotonin, to increase their activity at postsynaptic receptors; however, the receptor binding affinity of these neurotransmitters differs between each TCA. TCA possess a common core 3-ring structure with an amine side chain – either secondary or tertiary [149]. Secondary amines (including desipramine [active, demethylated metabolite of imipramine], nortriptyline [active metabolite of amitriptyline], protriptyline, and maprotiline) preferentially block norepinephrine reuptake, whereas tertiary amines (including amitriptyline, clomipramine, doxepin, imipramine, and trimipramine) inhibit serotonin reuptake.

TCA display moderate affinity to α_1-, some α_2-, and no β-adrenergic receptors [106]. The blockade of α_1 contributes to the hypotensive effect that may occur with initial administration of TCA. Sensitivity of α_1 receptors increases over weeks of treatment, resulting in the desired antidepressant effect. In contrast, the initial inhibition of the α_2 autoreceptor wanes with long-term exposure. TCA affect other neurotransmitters, directly and indirectly. They inhibit the transport of dopamine into noradrenergic terminals in the cerebral cortex and decrease the activity of D_2 dopamine autoreceptors [106]. They also inhibit the muscarinic cholinergic and histamine H_1 receptors. Lastly, TCA bind to glutathione S-transferase-pi that allows these drugs to pass through placenta to accumulate in utero and potentially cause congenital malformations [150]. As such, TCA should be used cautiously during pregnancy.

9.3.5 *Monoamine Oxidase Inhibitors (MAOI)*

While MAO-A and MAO-B enzymes reside in the mitochondrial membranes that are widely distributed throughout the body, including the central nervous system, the inhibition of MAO-A, specifically, is more directly associated with treating depression [106]. Hepatic MAO-A inactivates the monoamine tyramine. Tyramine exerts sympathomimetic effects and is a naturally occurring compound present in certain foods (e.g., pickled, aged, smoked, or processed meats [except cured ham], chocolate, alcoholic beverages, fermented cheeses, sour cream, yogurt, sauces, miso soup, kimchi, beans, peas, and peanuts).

9.3.6 Miscellaneous Agents

Vilazodone binds tightly to serotonin reuptake site (Ki = 0.1 nM) but does not have high affinity to the norepinephrine (Ki = 56 nM) or dopamine (Ki = 37 nM) reuptake sites [62]. Vilazodone is a potent reuptake inhibitor of serotonin (IC50 = 1.6 nM) and binds selectively to 5HT1A receptors (IC50 = 2.1 nM) as a partial agonist. 5HT1A receptors, when activated, increase potassium conductance and reduce the firing rate of serotonergic neurons in the cortex and hippocampus [151]. This negative feedback mechanism appears to be responsible for the delayed onset of therapeutic response to serotonergic antidepressants such as SSRI [152].

In one PET study, 6 h after a single 40 mg dose of vilazodone, occupancy effects at the 5HT1A receptor were found in only three out of four human subjects. At lower dose of 20 mg, 5HT1A receptor occupancy could not be demonstrated [153]. It is possible that repeated doses of vilazodone could result in consistent receptor occupancy. In addition, it appears that vilazodone preferentially occupies the autoreceptor versus the postsynaptic receptor, which has been theorized to accelerate and augment the clinical effects of SSRI [153, 154].

Mirtazapine exerts its antidepressant effects by enhancing central serotonergic and noradrenergic activity. Mirtazapine is also a potent antagonist at 5HT2 and 5HT3 receptors, which may be responsible for the decreased rate of nausea/vomiting, insomnia, and anxiety [115]. Due to mirtazapine's activity at the 5HT3 receptors, it has been often compared to ondansetron, an agent solely used as antiemetic. The interaction between ondansetron and mirtazapine, when given concomitantly, has been reported [155, 156]. Due to both drugs competing for CYP1A2, CYP2D6, and CYP3A4, the therapeutic effects of ondansetron may be inhibited by mirtazapine, and therefore, cessation of one of the drugs is recommended. Mirtazapine does not have any direct effect on 5HT1A and 5HT1B receptors. Mirtazapine has potent antagonist properties at the H1 receptor which is responsible for the sedative effect and potentially weight gain effects due to increased appetite [115]. Mirtazapine is also a moderate peripheral $\alpha 1$ adrenergic antagonist, which may explain its orthostatic hypotensive properties. In vitro and in vivo studies have shown that mirtazapine has virtually no anticholinergic activity and has been confirmed in clinical trials which show very low incidence of anticholinergic side effects.

The antidepressant activity of mirtazapine can be attributed to the parent drug, (S)+ enantiomer or (R)− enantiomer, depending on the test used to measure antidepressant effect [115]. Desmethyl mirtazapine was shown to have anti-anxiety activity in rats but less antidepressant effect per rat EEG profile compared to the parent compound. The metabolite is also less active in $\alpha 2$, 5HT2, and H1 antagonistic activity compared to the parent compound.

In two double-blind, placebo-controlled trials in children aged 7–18 years, mirtazapine failed to show any differences in primary or secondary endpoints compared to placebo. Significant weight gain (48.8 % vs 5.7 %), urticarial rash (11.8 % vs 6.8 %), and hypertriglyceridemia (2.9 % vs 0 %) were commonly observed. Mirtazapine is not indicated for use in patients less than 18 years old.

Vortioxetine has high affinity to human serotonin transporter (Ki = 1.6 nM) but not to norepinephrine (Ki = 113 nM) or dopamine (Ki > 1000 nM) transporters [120]. It potently and selectively inhibits reuptake of serotonin receptors. It is also an antagonist at 5HT3A (Ki = 3.7 nM), 5HT1D (Ki = 54 nM), and 5HT7 (Ki = 19 nM) receptors, a partial agonist at 5HT1B (Ki = 33 nM) receptor, and agonist at 5HT1A (Ki = 15 nM) receptor [157–159]. Vortioxetine appears to exert its antidepressant effect primarily through its activity at 5HT receptors and SERT inhibition.

In two PET studies using 5HTT ligands, the mean 5HT transporter occupancy was approximately 50 % at 5 mg/day, 65 % at 10 mg/day, and 80 % at 20 mg/day [160, 161]. In rat EEG studies, vortioxetine did not produce changes in wake, REM, slow-wave sleep [162]. It did, however, increase vigilance (measured as time awake) in a dose-dependent manner [162]. Due to the multimodal mechanism of vortioxetine, the drug appears to increase frontal cortical activity in a pattern that differs from SSRI and SNRI. One of the areas of intense investigation and clinical utility for vortioxetine is in the areas of cognitive function and attention as a result of these findings [163].

Ketamine is a synthetic derivative of PCP and the biological mechanisms for its antidepressant effects remain largely unknown. Ketamine binds to the PCP site within the ion channel and at rest. Mg2+ blocks the influx of Ca2+ and Na+. Upon depolarization and in the presence of co-agonists glutamate and glycine, Ca2+ and Na+ enter the cell [164]. Studies indicate that the NMDA receptor blockade leads to upregulation in AMPA receptor expression and activation of the mammalian target of rapamycin (mTOR) intracellular cascade that is required for the antidepressant activity of ketamine [165]. In addition, the brain-derived neurotrophic factor (BDNF) that plays a role in neuroplasticity may serve as a biomarker for ketamine's antidepressant activity. One of the key desirable features of ketamine is its rapid onset of antidepressant effects. Antidepressant effects have been observed within hours of a single intravenous infusion, which offers significant advantage over traditional antidepressants that may take weeks to see beneficial effect. Studies have also implicated the use of ketamine for suicidal ideation and bipolar depression [166, 167].

Unfortunately, the magnitude and persistence of the response are unpredictable and variable depending on the route of administration and frequency of doses [168, 169]. In addition, the long-term benefits and toxicity of ketamine including risk for dependence remain unclear.

9.4 Plasma Concentration Relationships

Therapeutic drug monitoring (TDM) has proven to be invaluable for many medications which possess a strong association between plasma concentrations and therapeutic response and/or adverse effects. For most available antidepressants, however, the benefits of routine TDM have not been forthcoming and these practices are not considered to be the standard of care for any antidepressants at the present time [48].

This may be due to the inherent difficulties encountered in sampling drug concentrations from the effective compartment (i.e., the central nervous system). Attempts at extrapolating CNS concentrations from peripheral concentrations have not been particularly successful due to the multitude of variables influencing the homeostasis of medication in the brain (e.g., transport proteins, synaptic metabolism, receptor binding). Recent attempts at correlating plasma concentrations with PET scans quantifying receptor occupancy have been intriguing but await further exploration. Below is a summary of the research evidence which has examined the statistical association of plasma concentrations with patient response for the various antidepressant classes.

9.4.1 Selective Serotonin Reuptake Inhibitors (SSRI)

Many researcher groups have analyzed the steady-state concentrations of the SSRI in an attempt to identify a therapeutic range to optimize efficacy and minimize toxicity, but the majority of these efforts have not been particularly insightful or clinically relevant [48, 66]. More often than not, the plasma concentration range that researchers reported was quite broad, leading clinicians to question if the cost and inconvenience of serum sampling were worth the benefit. In addition to the difficulties previously mentioned with TDM practices for antidepressants, research efforts with SSRI in particular have also been hampered by the fact that several of the compounds have active metabolites, racemic mixtures, nonlinear pharmacokinetics, or relatively high first-pass effects. Such factors have rendered the practice of predicting plasma concentrations to be quite challenging (i.e., poor correlation between daily dosages and steady-state concentrations) as well as contributing to the methodological complexity of plasma sampling, modeling, and data interpretation. In spite of these variables, a recent review of the benefits of TDM for psychiatric drugs concluded that there was Level 2 evidence supporting plasma concentration monitoring for all of the SSRI and their respective metabolites, with Level 2 defined as sufficient evidence to recommend monitoring levels for the purposes of dose titration, special indications, or problem solving [48]. These recommended therapeutic ranges can be found in Table 9.2. Preliminary research utilizing PET scans to investigate correlations between plasma concentrations of SSRI and occupancy of the serotonin transporter receptors has revealed that most SSRI require at least 80 % occupancy to improve the likelihood of therapeutic benefit [136, 170]. It is hoped that this revelation will stimulate further research and improve TDM practices with SSRI in the future.

9.4.2 Serotonin Norepinephrine Reuptake Inhibitors (SNRI)

The SNRI suffer from many of the same pharmacokinetic hindrances as SSRI and, as a result, routine plasma concentration monitoring is not recommended. In addition, most of the SNRI tend to have shorter plasma half-lives than SSRI,

Table 9.2 Therapeutic drug monitoring of antidepressants

Drug	Usual daily dose (mg)	Recommended plasma concentration (ng/mL)	Level of evidence to support therapeutic drug monitoring[a]
Amitriptyline [7–9] (+ nortriptyline)	100–300	80–200	4
Bupropion [11, 12] (+ hydroxybupropion)	200–450	225–1500	3
Citalopram [13]	10–40	50–110	2
Clomipramine [14] (+ norclomipramine)	75–250	230–450	1
Desipramine [17]	100–300	100–300	2
Desvenlafaxine	50–100	100–400	2
Doxepin [18] (+ nordoxepin)	100–300	50–150	2
Duloxetine	60–120	30–120	2
Escitalopram	5–20	15–80	2
Fluoxetine [18] (+ norfluoxetine)	10–40	120–500	2
Fluvoxamine [13]	100–300	60–230	2
Imipramine [20, 21] (+ desipramine)	100–300	175–300	1
Maprotiline [22]	75–225	75–130	2
Mirtazapine [13]	15–45	30–80	2
Nortriptyline [23, 24]	50–150	70–170	1
Paroxetine	10–40	30–120	3
Phenelzine	30–60	N/A	N/A
Selegiline transdermal	6–12	N/A	N/A
Sertraline	25–200	10–150	2
Tranylcypromine	15–60	N/A	N/A
Trazodone [25, 26]	150–600	700–1000	2
Venlafaxine [13] (+ desvenlafaxine)	150–300	100–400	2
Vilazodone [28]	20–40	N/A	N/A
Vortioxetine [29]	10–20	N/A	N/A

Adapted from Hiemke et al. [48]
[a]Levels of recommendations (definitions):
1 – *strongly recommended* for dosage titration and special indications
2 – *recommended* for dosage titration and special indications
3 – *useful* for special indications
4 – *potentially useful* for special indications

so the timing of serum sampling becomes problematic as well. In spite of these complexities, recent TDM guidelines published by the European Expert Panel AGNP concluded that there is Level 2 evidence supporting the use of SNRI in certain circumstances. In studies analyzing receptor occupancy, the SNRI have been found to have a fairly high occupancy rate for both 5HT and NE receptors, generally in the range of 40–60 %, after administration of therapeutic doses [171].

9.4.3 *Norepinephrine Reuptake Inhibitors (NRI)*

Plasma concentrations have also been studied for the safety and efficacy of the NRI, bupropion, with some interesting findings. For example, early research examining the concentrations of bupropion and its three active metabolites demonstrated that a superior therapeutic response was found with higher concentrations of the parent compound but not the metabolites [11].

In contrast, researchers explored the association of the active metabolite 4-OH bupropion with therapeutic response and found that concentrations exceeding 860 ng/ml were associated with a much higher likelihood of marked improvement in depressive symptoms [172]. Unfortunately, they were unable to quantify plasma concentrations of the parent drug due to its instability at room temperature in plasma. Also, it should be noted that the sample size was relatively small and that 90 % of the study subjects were taking other psychoactive medications. It is interesting to note, however, that this threshold of 860 ng/ml is considerably higher than that endorsed in the AGNP guidelines (225 ng/ml), where bupropion was concluded to have Level 2 evidence of support for TDM practices.

9.4.4 *Tricyclic and Tetracyclic Antidepressants (TCA)*

The benefits of TDM have been well studied and are clearly evident for most TCA, especially due to their narrow therapeutic index and an extremely poor safety profile with chronic use and acute intoxication [173–175]. A meta-analysis of 45 studies validated the importance of performing TDM for amitriptyline, particularly in a controlled and randomized environment, to achieve the antidepressant response [176]. The therapeutic reference ranges for TCA are defined for the treatment of depression and access to the assays that measure drug concentrations are readily available (Table 9.2). TDM of TCA appears to be cost-effective and implementing early within the first 3 weeks of the initiation of therapy for depression has been associated with improved clinical response and reduced central nervous system and cardiovascular side effects [174, 175]. The penetration of drugs into the brain is critical for therapeutic effects, and animal studies reveal a linear relationship between steady-state plasma and brain concentrations of TCA [177]. As such, plasma or serum (instead of whole blood), steady state concentrations are used in the TDM practice to optimize response to TCA therapy. Plasma concentrations are usually measured after 1 week of therapy once steady state is achieved, unless in the presence of significant toxicity when immediate TDM may be necessary. Mid-interval concentrations (e.g., 12 h after the most recent oral dose of TCA administered at 24-h intervals) are used for its convenience and provide a good estimate of average concentrations [105].

Based on systematic reviews and meta-analyses, a strong concentration-therapeutic response relationship is observed for nortriptyline, imipramine, and desipramine [48, 173]. Clinical response to nortriptyline appears to correlate well to the total serum, rather than free, drug concentrations [178, 179]. For nortriptyline and other TCA, total serum drug concentrations are used in the TDM process. Furthermore, some TCA (including imipramine, amitriptyline, clomipramine, and maprotiline) require the monitoring of total drug concentrations that should incorporate both parent drug and active metabolites since they contribute inclusively to the clinical effectiveness. The lower limits of the TCA's therapeutic ranges should always be targeted for clinical response, as concluded in studies of imipramine, due to the narrow therapeutic index [176, 180].

The concentration-response relationship for imipramine is linear, where increasing the concentration augments the probability of achieving a therapeutic response. However, nortriptyline, desipramine, and amitriptyline display a curvilinear relationship, denoting amelioration of antidepressant response when concentrations exceed the therapeutic range [175]. This unique pharmacodynamic relationship was observed for nortriptyline in the first study on TDM in psychiatry [178]. Furthermore, free concentrations of nortriptyline exceeding 10 ng/ml inhibit clinical response [179]. The most plausible explanation for this curvilinear relationship is the occurrence of side effects that limits the clinical utility of TCA at high concentrations. As such, most serious adverse effects are associated with high drug concentrations; therefore, the occurrence of side effects generally defines the upper limit of the therapeutic range [181, 182].

Serious cardiotoxicity, including sinus tachycardia and prolongation of cardiac conduction that may lead to arrhythmias, is associated with high drug concentrations that are usually observed during acute intoxication [106]. Because of the severity of these cardiac effects, TCA should be avoided in patients with a history of cardiac disease, including myocardial infarction, congestive heart failure, and arrhythmias. Even in patients without any cardiac disease, orthostatic hypotension, which can be significant enough to precipitate falls and injuries, may occur due to the TCA's potent antagonistic α_1 activity. Compared to other TCA, nortriptyline is least likely to cause postural hypotension. In addition to cardiovascular effects, significant adverse effects on the central nervous system, including weakness, fatigue, confusion, and seizures, may occur with TCA therapy due to its antagonistic effects on histamine receptors. TCA should be used cautiously in pediatric patients due to their potential to induce seizures and cardiotoxicity.

TCA exhibit potent anticholinergic effects that include dry mouth, altered taste, epigastric distress, constipation, dizziness, tachycardia, blurred vision, and urinary retention. The correlation between drug concentrations and these anticholinergic effects appears to vary with the type of TCA. For example, decreased saliva production and dry mouth (except drowsiness) are strongly associated with plasma amitriptyline concentrations, yet the correlation is absent for nortriptyline [183]. TCA should be used cautiously in geriatric patients due to their cardiovascular and anticholinergic effects.

There are inherent challenges within the practice of TDM for TCA, despite its availability for many decades. In fact, one study demonstrated the need to improve TDM for TCA (including maprotiline, clomipramine, imipramine, desipramine, nortriptyline, and amitriptyline) in hospitals since 20 % of therapeutic adjustments were considered inappropriate [184]. The presence of active metabolites for some TCA requires the measurement of both parent drug and active metabolites, and the potential for altered protein binding also contributes to the complexity of TDM for TCA [185]. In addition, TCA share common hepatic metabolic pathways with other medications; therefore, drug-drug interactions may unpredictably alter concentrations of TCA. Furthermore, the targeted steady-state concentrations that optimize therapeutic response and minimize toxicity, particularly for use in the actual clinical settings, may differ from established ranges that were developed in a controlled environment, especially for amitriptyline and clomipramine [176, 186].

In light of the complexity of TDM for TCA, an interdisciplinary approach that integrates efforts of physicians, pharmacists, and laboratory personnel should be employed to optimize TDM of antidepressants [187]. When robust data are available, TDM should be combined with pharmacogenetic tests to personalize therapy [48, 173]. Pharmacogenetic tests that incorporate genotype or phenotype information may be invaluable in characterizing genetic polymorphisms that contribute to adverse drug reactions and drug-drug interactions [181]. Recently, dried blood spot, which is a sampling technique that utilizes an ultralow volume, was evaluated for amitriptyline, nortriptyline, imipramine, desipramine, and clomipramine, in a robust liquid chromatography-tandem mass spectrometry (LC-MS/MS) method that efficiently runs within 5 min [188]. Dried blood spot eliminates the need for centrifugation or freezing of samples and measures drug concentration in whole blood. The concentrations from dried blood spot samples are usually 15 % lower than plasma. Future studies should explore and validate this sampling strategy in the clinical setting.

9.4.5 Monoamine Oxidase Inhibitors (MAOI)

Monitoring plasma concentrations is not recommended based on the dearth of data on the TDM of MAOI. However, special precautions should be made when initiating or discontinuing MAOI, including the transdermal selegiline patch. The long terminal half-lives produce a delayed onset of antidepressant effect (e.g., 1–2 weeks), which may persist for as long as 2 weeks after drug discontinuation [189]. As such, to prevent a hypertensive reaction or the serotonin syndrome, a washout period of 2 weeks is recommended after discontinuing tranylcypromine, phenelzine, or selegiline and before initiating another antidepressant. Furthermore, other antidepressants should be discontinued 2 weeks before to initiating MAOI.

Concurrent consumption of MAOI and tyramine-rich foods (>6 mg per day) may induce a hypertensive crisis. At low doses, ingestion of selegiline does not require dietary restrictions because it lacks inhibition of MAO-A; however, at high doses (i.e., >10 mg per day) that are may be used therapeutically for depression, it inhibits both MAO-A and MAO-B. Especially if administered orally, dietary restrictions to prevent hypertensive reactions are required. Furthermore, with the prolonged effect of MAOI, a diet limiting typramine-rich food should continue until 2 weeks after discontinuing MAOI. The dose of the transdermal patch at 6 mg per 24 h may not require dietary restrictions. Incremental dose increase of 3 mg per 24 h at 2 week intervals (up to a maximum dose of 12 mg per 24 h) may be warranted, although the clinical effectiveness of doses exceeding 6 mg per 24 h is uncertain.

9.4.6 *Miscellaneous Agents*

While therapeutic drug monitoring is not routinely conducted for antidepressants other than TCA, there are reference ranges that have been established for some antidepressants. The recommended therapeutic range for mirtazapine, for example, is 30–80 ng/mL with toxic levels estimated at 160 ng/mL [190–192]. However, the AGNP consensus guideline does point out that significant relationship between drug concentration and therapeutic outcome is lacking for mirtazapine [48].

The expected plasma levels for vilazodone is 20–50 ng/mL and 5–15 ng/mL for the M10 and M17 metabolites. There is insufficient data on the expected plasma levels for vortioxetine and ketamine.

9.5 Pharmacogenetic Relationships

9.5.1 *Therapeutic Effects*

Despite the number of antidepressants available, 30–50 % of patients do not respond to the first antidepressant medication and only 30 % of patients achieve remission of symptoms [139, 193, 194]. In the last decade, pharmacogenomics or "personalized medicine" has been successfully used to optimize selection of medications, avoid adverse effects, or optimize drug doses [195, 196]. It has been estimated that up to 42 % of the variance in antidepressant response is associated with genetic variations [197].

Therapeutic effects of SSRI have been attributed to genetic variants of the serotonin transporter gene (5HTTLPR, rs4795541) [195, 198]. Based on the presence of either a long (*l*) or short (*s*) allele, patients may have varying response to SSRI; patients with the long (*l*) allele, with twice the expression of the serotonin transporter, have been shown to have improved response to SSRI. It has been estimated that 50–60 % of Caucasians and 25–40 % of Asians are carriers of the *l* allele and therefore ethnicity may play a critical role in selection of antidepressants [195, 199, 200].

Variation in COMT enzyme, responsible for degradation of dopamine and norepinephrine, was also shown to be associated with duloxetine response in major depressive disorder as measured by the 17-item Hamilton Rating Scale for Depression (HAM-D-17) [201].

In addition to acute response to antidepressants, disease remission from major depressive disorder has been a major focus of pharmacogenomic studies. In a meta-analysis of 33 candidate gene association (CGA) studies between 5HTTLPR and antidepressant response, those with *l* allele had a 28 % increased odds of achieving disease remission with SSRI than those with *s* allele [198]. In another CGA, calcium/calmodulin-dependent protein kinases (CaMK) single nucleotide polymorphisms (SNP) were significantly associated with remission from depression among Chinese patients [202]. The CaMK pathway appears to be important for neuroplasticity which may be one potential mechanism of antidepressants [203, 204]. As an additional evidence for the importance of ethnicity in selection of antidepressants, Asians who were homozygote carriers for the serotonin transporter (SLC6A4 STin2)/*l*allele had a fourfold greater response to SSRI than *s* carriers [205].

Multiple genes/alleles are involved in determining response to antidepressants including brain-derived neurotrophic factor (BDNF), serotonin receptors (HTR1A, HTR2A, HTR5), and tryptophan hydroxylase [205], some which may not have been discovered.

9.5.2 Toxic Effects

It is estimated that 30 % of patients discontinue antidepressants within the first 6 weeks of starting antidepressant treatment [206]. Pharmacogenomic studies evaluating the toxic effects of antidepressants have been primarily focused on cytochrome P450 enzymes, most notably CYP2C19 and CYP2D6 enzymes that are involved in metabolism of most currently marketed antidepressants [207]. Variants of the CYP2D6 enzyme can predispose individuals to being classified as ultra-rapid metabolizers, extensive metabolizers, intermediate metabolizers, or poor metabolizers of drugs that undergo metabolism by CYP2D6 [208–210]. In one study, patients identified as poor metabolizers who received antidepressants and antipsychotics influenced by CYP2D6 isoenzyme had significantly more moderate or marked side effects compared to individuals identified as UMs [211]. The impact of side effects was notable and associated with significantly longer hospitalization stays compared to patients with other metabolizer status [212].

In a recent Genome-Based Therapeutic Drugs for Depression (GENDEP) study report, CYP2C19 and CYP2D6 genotype variants predicted serum concentrations of escitalopram and nortriptyline and their metabolites; however, genotype nor serum concentrations did not predict treatment response [213]. These results provide further evidence that measurement of antidepressant response is complex and identifying a specific predictable biomarker will be challenging. While there are no standard testing recommendations for genotyping patients who are prescribed these drugs, the CPIC provides recommendations on dosing of amitriptyline and nortriptyline based on patients' genotype (ultra-rapid, extensive, and poor metabolizer) for CYP2D6 and CYP2C19 isoenzymes [214, 215].

Vilazodone, during development, was investigated specifically for its genetic biomarkers that may indicate therapeutic response to the drug. Patients who were identified as positive for the M1 biomarker (M1+) was found to have a significantly better response to vilazodone as measured by Montgomery-Asberg Depression Rating Scale (MADRS) score compared to those taking placebo [216]. Remission rates were also higher in the M1+ group as well. Patients who were M2+ were also associated with having higher likelihood of gastrointestinal adverse effects (e.g., nausea, vomiting) compared to M2−. Despite these early findings, there is no recommendation in the prescribing information that advocates for routine testing of the M1 biomarker.

Based on significant volume of scientific evidence, genetic variants appear to play a role in determining response and remission to antidepressants and development or worsening of adverse effects. There is also increasing evidence that gene-environment interactions play a role in treatment response and disease remission but methodological challenges exist to study such interactions [217, 218]. The utility of pharmacogenetic testing in routine psychiatric practice is unclear, and currently, there is no recommendation to conduct testing prior to initiating antidepressant treatment [219]. Significant barriers exist in clinical implementation of pharmacogenomic testing and the reality of personalized medicine such as cost of testing, clinical decision support for prescribers, and availability of trained healthcare providers to educate patients. There are legal and ethical dilemmas that exist for prescribers, patients, family members, and society as a whole. Before widespread use of pharmacogenomic testing for patients who are about to initiate or have initiated treatment with antidepressants, these barriers must be overcome.

9.6 Conclusion

The high prevalence of depressive illness has hastened the development and release of a wide range of therapeutic agents, with several unique compounds released within the past 3 years. While early exploration of useful antidepressants was heavily influenced by the monoamine hypothesis, the discovery of agents with more novel and complex pharmacological actions has broadened therapeutic options considerably. Overall, the pharmacokinetic properties of antidepressants are quite diverse, including clinically relevant differences in half-lives, active metabolites, stereoselectivity, and inhibitory effects on liver enzymes. Even though routine TDM practices have not been implemented for most commonly prescribed antidepressants, clinicians are well advised to familiarize themselves with the pharmacokinetic disposition of these agents to maximize efficacy, minimize toxicity, and avoid potential drug interactions. Preliminary investigations exploring the merits of pharmacogenetic testing for antidepressants have been promising but remain inconclusive at the present time and await further study before empiric testing can be justified.

References

1. Gram L (1994) Fluoxetine. N Engl J Med 331(20):1354–1361
2. Prozac (fluoxetine capsules) (2014) Prescribing information. Eli Lilly and Company, Inc., Indianapolis
3. DeVane CL, Jarecke R (1992) Cyclic antidepressants. In: Evans WE, Schentag JJ, Jusko WJ (eds) Applied pharmacokinetics, principles of therapeutic drug monitoring, 3rd edn. Applied Therapeutics, Vancouver
4. Preskorn SH, Dorey RC, Jerkovich GS (1988) Therapeutic drug monitoring of tricyclic antidepressants. Clin Chem 34(5):822–828
5. DeVane CL (1999) Metabolism and pharmacokinetics of selective serotonin reuptake inhibitors. Cell Mol Neurobiol 19(4):443–466
6. Rudorfer MV, Potter WZ (1999) Metabolism of tricyclic antidepressants. Cell Mol Neurobiol 19(3):373–409
7. Young RC (1991) Hydroxylated metabolites of antidepressants. Psychopharmacol Bull 27(4):521–532
8. Kupfer DJ, Hanin I, Spiker DG, Grau T, Coble P (1977) Amitriptyline plasma levels and clinical response in primary depression. Clin Pharmacol Ther 22(6):904–911
9. Ziegler VE, Co BT, Taylor JR, Clayton PJ, Biggs JT (1976) Amitriptyline plasma levels and therapeutic response. Clin Pharmacol Ther 19(6):795–801
10. Takeuchi H, Yokota S, Shimada S, Ohtani Y, Miura S, Kubo H (1993) Pharmacokinetics of amoxapine and its active metabolites in healthy subjects. Curr Ther Res 53:427–434
11. Golden RN, De Vane CL, Laizure SC, Rudorfer MV, Sherer MA, Potter WZ (1988) Bupropion in depression. II. The role of metabolites in clinical outcome. Arch Gen Psychiatry 45(2):145–149
12. Preskorn SH (1991) Should bupropion dosage be adjusted based upon therapeutic drug monitoring? Psychopharmacol Bull 27(4):637–643
13. Mendlewicz J (2001) Optimising antidepressant use in clinical practice: towards criteria for antidepressant selection. Br J Psychiatry Suppl 42:S1–S3
14. Reisby N, Gram LF, Bech P et al (1979) Clomipramine: plasma levels and clinical effects. Commun Psychopharmacol 3(5):341–351
15. Traskman L, Asberg M, Bertilsson L et al (1979) Plasma levels of chlorimipramine and its demethyl metabolite during treatment of depression. Clin Pharmacol Ther 26(5):600–610
16. Stern RS, Marks IM, Mawson D, Luscombe DK (1980) Clomipramine and exposure for compulsive rituals: II. Plasma levels, side effects and outcome. Br J Psychiatry 136:161–166
17. Nelson JC, Jatlow P, Quinlan DM, Bowers MB Jr (1982) Desipramine plasma concentration and antidepressant response. Arch Gen Psychiatry 39(12):1419–1422
18. Linnoila M, Seppala T, Mattila MJ, Vihko R, Pakarinen A, Skinner T 3rd (1980) Clomipramine and doxepin in depressive neurosis. Plasma levels and therapeutic response. Arch Gen Psychiatry 37(11):1295–1299
19. Lundmark J, Reis M, Bengtsson F (2000) Therapeutic drug monitoring of sertraline: variability factors as displayed in a clinical setting. Ther Drug Monit 22(4):446–454
20. Reisby N, Gram LF, Bech P et al (1977) Imipramine: clinical effects and pharmacokinetic variability. Psychopharmacology (Berl) 54(3):263–272
21. Glassman AH, Perel JM, Shostak M, Kantor SJ, Fleiss JL (1977) Clinical implications of imipramine plasma levels for depressive illness. Arch Gen Psychiatry 34(2):197–204
22. Gwirtsman HE, Ahles S, Halaris A, DeMet E, Hill MA (1983) Therapeutic superiority of maprotiline versus doxepin in geriatric depression. J Clin Psychiatry 44(12):449–453
23. Glassman AH (1985) Tricyclic antidepressants – blood level measurements and clinical outcome – an APA-Task-Force report. Am J Psychiat 142(2):155–162

24. Montgomery S, Braithwaite R, Dawling S, Mcauley R (1978) High plasma nortriptyline levels in treatment of depression. 1. Clin Pharmacol Ther 23(3):309–314
25. Putzolu S, Pecknold JC, Baiocchi L (1976) Proceedings: Trazodone: clinical and biochemical studies II. Blood levels and therapeutic responsiveness. Psychopharmacol Bull 12(1):40–41
26. Mann JJ, Georgotas A, Newton R, Gershon S (1981) A controlled study of trazodone, imipramine, and placebo in outpatients with endogenous depression. J Clin Psychopharmacol 1(2):75–80
27. Suckow RF, Cooper TB (1984) Determination of trimipramine and metabolites in plasma by liquid chromatography with electrochemical detection. J Pharm Sci 73(12):1745–1748
28. Mika J, Jurga AM, Starnowska J et al (2015) Effects of chronic doxepin and amitriptyline administration in naive mice and in neuropathic pain mice model. Neuroscience 294:38–50
29. Wang YQ, Takata Y, Li R et al (2015) Doxepin and diphenhydramine increased non-rapid eye movement sleep through blockade of histamine H1 receptors. Pharmacol Biochem Behav 129:56–64
30. Bergstrom RF, Lemberger L, Farid NA, Wolen RL (1988) Clinical pharmacology and pharmacokinetics of fluoxetine: a review. Br J Psychiatry Suppl 3:47–50
31. Strauss WL, Layton ME, Hayes CE, Dager SR (1997) 19F magnetic resonance spectroscopy investigation in vivo of acute and steady-state brain fluvoxamine levels in obsessive-compulsive disorder. Am J Psychiatry 154(4):516–522
32. von Moltke LL, Greenblatt DJ, Duan SX et al (1997) Human cytochromes mediating N-demethylation of fluoxetine in vitro. Psychopharmacology (Berl) 132(4):402–407
33. Walden M, Carrier CT (2003) Sleeping beauties: the impact of sedation on neonatal development. J Obstet Gynecol Neonatal Nurs (JOGNN/NAACOG) 32(3):393–401
34. Hicks JK, Bishop JR, Sangkuhl K et al (2015) Clinical Pharmacogenetics Implementation Consortium (CPIC) guideline for CYP2D6 and CYP2C19 genotypes and dosing of selective serotonin reuptake inhibitors. Clin Pharmacol Ther 98(2):127–134
35. Stevens JC, Wrighton SA (1993) Interaction of the enantiomers of fluoxetine and norfluoxetine with human liver cytochromes P450. J Pharmacol Exp Ther 266(2):964–971
36. Sager JE, Lutz JD, Foti RS, Davis C, Kunze KL, Isoherranen N (2014) Fluoxetine- and norfluoxetine-mediated complex drug-drug interactions: in vitro to in vivo correlation of effects on CYP2D6, CYP2C19, and CYP3A4. Clin Pharmacol Ther 95(6):653–662
37. Weiss J, Dormann SM, Martin-Facklam M, Kerpen CJ, Ketabi-Kiyanvash N, Haefeli WE (2003) Inhibition of P-glycoprotein by newer antidepressants. J Pharmacol Exp Ther 305(1):197–204
38. Altamura AC, Moro AR, Percudani M (1994) Clinical pharmacokinetics of fluoxetine. Clin Pharmacokinet 26(3):201–214
39. Hughes ZA, Starr KR, Langmead CJ et al (2005) Neurochemical evaluation of the novel 5-HT1A receptor partial agonist/serotonin reuptake inhibitor, vilazodone. Eur J Pharmacol 510(1–2):49–57
40. Zoloft (sertraline) (2014) Prescribing information. Pfizer, Inc., New York
41. Ronfeld RA, Tremaine LM, Wilner KD (1997) Pharmacokinetics of sertraline and its N-demethyl metabolite in elderly and young male and female volunteers. Clin Pharmacokinet 32(Suppl 1):22–30
42. Wang JH, Liu ZQ, Wang W et al (2001) Pharmacokinetics of sertraline in relation to genetic polymorphism of CYP2C19. Clin Pharmacol Ther 70(1):42–47
43. Hicks JK, Bishop JR, Sangkuhl K et al (2015) Clinical Pharmacogenetics Implementation Consortium (CPIC) guideline for CYP2D6 and CYP2C19 genotypes and dosing of selective serotonin reuptake inhibitors. Clin Pharmacol Ther. doi:10.1002/cpt.147, [Epub ahead of print]
44. Warrington SJ (1992) Clinical implications of the pharmacology of serotonin reuptake inhibitors. Int Clin Psychopharmacol 7(Suppl 2):13–19
45. Owens MJ, Morgan WN, Plott SJ, Nemeroff CB (1997) Neurotransmitter receptor and transporter binding profile of antidepressants and their metabolites. J Pharmacol Exp Ther 283(3):1305–1322

46. Rogowsky D, Marr M, Long G, Moore C (1994) Determination of sertraline and desmethylsertraline in human serum using copolymeric bonded-phase extraction, liquid chromatography and gas chromatography-mass spectrometry. J Chromatogr B Biomed Appl 655(1):138–141
47. Crewe HK, Lennard MS, Tucker GT, Woods FR, Haddock RE (1992) The effect of selective serotonin re-uptake inhibitors on cytochrome P4502D6 (CYP2D6) activity in human liver microsomes. Br J Clin Pharmacol 34(3):262–265
48. Hiemke C, Baumann P, Bergemann N et al (2011) AGNP consensus guidelines for therapeutic drug monitoring in psychiatry: update 2011. Pharmacopsychiatry 44(6):195–235
49. Alfaro CL, Lam YW, Simpson J, Ereshefsky L (1999) CYP2D6 status of extensive metabolizers after multiple-dose fluoxetine, fluvoxamine, paroxetine, or sertraline. J Clin Psychopharmacol 19(2):155–163
50. Paxil (paroxetine hydrochloride) (2003) Prescribing information. GlaxoSmithKline, Research Triangle Park
51. Dechant KL, Clissold SP (1991) Paroxetine. A review of its pharmacodynamic and pharmacokinetic properties, and therapeutic potential in depressive illness. Drugs 41(2):225–253
52. Lund J, Christensen JA, Bechgaard E, Molander L, Larsson H (1979) Pharmacokinetics of femoxetine in man. Acta Pharmacol Toxicol (Copenh) 44(3):177–184
53. Kaye CM, Haddock RE, Langley PF et al (1989) A review of the metabolism and pharmacokinetics of paroxetine in man. Acta Psychiatr Scand Suppl 350:60–75
54. Bartoszyk GD, Hegenbart R, Ziegler H (1997) EMD 68843, a serotonin reuptake inhibitor with selective presynaptic 5-HT1A receptor agonistic properties. Eur J Pharmacol 322(2-3):147–153
55. Nemeroff CB, DeVane CL, Pollock BG (1996) Newer antidepressants and the cytochrome P450 system. Am J Psychiatry 153(3):311–320
56. Sangkuhl K, Klein TE, Altman RB (2011) PharmGKB summary: citalopram pharmacokinetics pathway. Pharmacogenet Genomics 21(11):769–772
57. Page ME, Cryan JF, Sullivan A et al (2002) Behavioral and neurochemical effects of 5-(4-[4-(5-Cyano-3-indolyl)-butyl)-butyl]-1-piperazinyl)-benzofuran-2-carboxamide (EMD 68843): a combined selective inhibitor of serotonin reuptake and 5-hydroxytryptamine(1A) receptor partial agonist. J Pharmacol Exp Ther 302(3):1220–1227
58. Celexa (citalopram hydrobromide) (2014) Prescribing information. Forest Phamaceuticals, Inc., St. Louis
59. Kragh-Sorensen P, Overo KF, Petersen OL, Jensen K, Parnas W (1981) The kinetics of citalopram: single and multiple dose studies in man. Acta Pharmacol Toxicol (Copenh) 48(1):53–60
60. Caccia S (2004) Metabolism of the newest antidepressants: comparisons with related predecessors. IDrugs (The Investigational Drugs Journal) 7(2):143–150
61. Rao N (2007) The clinical pharmacokinetics of escitalopram. Clin Pharmacokinet 46(4):281–290
62. Viibryd (vilazodone hydrochloride) (2011–2015) Prescribing information. Forest Pharmaceuticals, Inc. Subsidiary of Forest Laboratories, LLC, Cincinnati
63. Lexapro (escitalopram oxalate) (2009) Prescribing information. Forest Pharmaceuticals, Inc., St Louis
64. Sogaard B, Mengel H, Rao N, Larsen F (2005) The pharmacokinetics of escitalopram after oral and intravenous administration of single and multiple doses to healthy subjects. J Clin Pharmacol 45(12):1400–1406
65. van Harten J (1995) Overview of the pharmacokinetics of fluvoxamine. Clin Pharmacokinet 29(Suppl 1):1–9
66. Mandrioli R, Mercolini L, Saracino MA, Raggi MA (2012) Selective serotonin reuptake inhibitors (SSRIs): therapeutic drug monitoring and pharmacological interactions. Curr Med Chem 19(12):1846–1863

67. Orlando R, De Martin S, Andrighetto L, Floreani M, Palatini P (2010) Fluvoxamine pharmacokinetics in healthy elderly subjects and elderly patients with chronic heart failure. Br J Clin Pharmacol 69(3):279–286
68. Nichols AI, Focht K, Jiang Q, Preskorn SH, Kane CP (2011) Pharmacokinetics of venlafaxine extended release 75 mg and desvenlafaxine 50 mg in healthy CYP2D6 extensive and poor metabolizers: a randomized, open-label, two-period, parallel-group, crossover study. Clin Drug Investig 31(3):155–167
69. Schweizer E, Feighner J, Mandos LA, Rickels K (1994) Comparison of venlafaxine and imipramine in the acute treatment of major depression in outpatients. J Clin Psychiatry 55(3):104–108
70. Klamerus KJ, Maloney K, Rudolph RL, Sisenwine SF, Jusko WJ, Chiang ST (1992) Introduction of a composite parameter to the pharmacokinetics of venlafaxine and its active O-desmethyl metabolite. J Clin Pharmacol 32(8):716–724
71. Effexor (venlafaxine hydrochloride) (2004) Prescribing information. Wyeth Pharmaceuticals, Philadelphia
72. Troy SM, Schultz RW, Parker VD, Chiang ST, Blum RA (1994) The effect of renal disease on the disposition of venlafaxine. Clin Pharmacol Ther 56(1):14–21
73. Klamerus KJ, Parker VD, Rudolph RL, Derivan AT, Chiang ST (1996) Effects of age and gender on venlafaxine and O-desmethylvenlafaxine pharmacokinetics. Pharmacotherapy 16(5):915–923
74. Ehret MJ, Levin GM, Narasimhan M, Rathinavelu A (2007) Venlafaxine induces P-glycoprotein in human Caco-2 cells. Hum Psychopharmacol 22(1):49–53
75. Nichols AI, Abell M, Chen Y, Behrle JA, Frick G, Paul J (2013) Effects of desvenlafaxine on the pharmacokinetics of desipramine in healthy adults. Int Clin Psychopharmacol 28(2):99–105
76. Pristiq (desvenlafaxine) (2014) Prescribing information. Wyeth Pharmaceuticals Inc., Subsidiary of Pfizer Inc., New York
77. Parker GB, Brotchie HL, Hyett M (2011) Tolerance to desvenlafaxine in rapid metabolizing depressed patients. Int Clin Psychopharmacol 26(2):84–87
78. Baird-Bellaire S, Behrle JA, Parker VD, Patat A, Paul J, Nichols AI (2013) An open-label, single-dose, parallel-group study of the effects of chronic hepatic impairment on the safety and pharmacokinetics of desvenlafaxine. Clin Ther 35(6):782–794
79. Boinpally R, Henry D, Gupta S, Edwards J, Longstreth J, Periclou A (2014) Pharmacokinetics and safety of vilazodone in hepatic impairment. Am J Ther 22(4):269–277
80. Patroneva A, Connolly SM, Fatato P et al (2008) An assessment of drug-drug interactions: the effect of desvenlafaxine and duloxetine on the pharmacokinetics of the CYP2D6 probe desipramine in healthy subjects. Drug Metab Dispos 36(12):2484–2491
81. Patat A, Baird-Bellaire S, Behrle J et al (2007) Lack of clinically relevant effect of pharmacokinetic interaction between ketoconazole on desvenlafaxine-SR pharmacokinetics. Clin Pharmacol Ther 81(Suppl 1):64–71
82. Cymbalta (duloxetine hydrochloride) (2004) Prescribing information. Eli Lilly and Company, Indianapolis
83. Lobo ED, Bergstrom RF, Reddy S et al (2008) In vitro and in vivo evaluations of cytochrome P450 1A2 interactions with duloxetine. Clin Pharmacokinet 47(3):191–202
84. Boinpally R, Gad N, Gupta S, Periclou A (2014) Influence of CYP3A4 induction/inhibition on the pharmacokinetics of vilazodone in healthy subjects. Clin Ther 36(11):1638–1649
85. Skinner MH, Kuan HY, Pan A et al (2003) Duloxetine is both an inhibitor and a substrate of cytochrome P4502D6 in healthy volunteers. Clin Pharmacol Ther 73(3):170–177
86. Tianmei S, Knadler MP, Lim MT et al (2007) Pharmacokinetics and tolerability of duloxetine following oral administration to healthy Chinese subjects. Clin Pharmacokinet 46(9):767–775
87. Suri A, Reddy S, Gonzales C, Knadler MP, Branch RA, Skinner MH (2005) Duloxetine pharmacokinetics in cirrhotics compared with healthy subjects. Int J Clin Pharmacol Ther 43(2):78–84

88. Remeron (mirtazapine) tablets (2015) Prescribing information. Merck & Co, Inc., Whitehouse Station
89. Fetzima (levomilnacipran) (2014) Prescribing information. Forest Phamaceuticals, Inc., St. Louis
90. Chen L, Boinpally R, Greenberg WM, Wangsa J, Periclou A, Ghahramani P (2014) Effect of hepatic impairment on the pharmacokinetics of levomilnacipran following a single oral dose of a levomilnacipran extended-release capsule in human participants. Clin Drug Investig 34(5):351–359
91. Findlay JW, Van Wyck FJ, Smith PG et al (1981) Pharmacokinetics of bupropion, a novel antidepressant agent, following oral administration to healthy subjects. Eur J Clin Pharmacol 21(2):127–135
92. Wellbutrin SR (bupropion hydrochloride) (2015) Prescribing information. GlaxoSmithKline, LLC, Research Triangle Park
93. Wellbutrin XL (bupropion hydrochloride) (2015) Prescribing information. GlaxoSmithKline, LLC, Research Triangle Park
94. Schroeder DH (1983) Metabolism and kinetics of bupropion. J Clin Psychiatry 44(5 Pt 2):79–81
95. Dwoskin LP, Rauhut AS, King-Pospisil KA, Bardo MT (2006) Review of the pharmacology and clinical profile of bupropion, an antidepressant and tobacco use cessation agent. CNS Drug Rev 12(3-4):178–207
96. Laizure SC, DeVane CL, Stewart JT, Dommisse CS, Lai AA (1985) Pharmacokinetics of bupropion and its major basic metabolites in normal subjects after a single dose. Clin Pharmacol Ther 38(5):586–589
97. Pollock BG, Sweet RA, Kirshner M, Reynolds CF 3rd (1996) Bupropion plasma levels and CYP2D6 phenotype. Ther Drug Monit 18(5):581–585
98. Zhu AZ, Zhou Q, Cox LS, Ahluwalia JS, Benowitz NL, Tyndale RF (2014) Gene variants in CYP2C19 are associated with altered in vivo bupropion pharmacokinetics but not bupropion-assisted smoking cessation outcomes. Drug Metab Dispos 42(11):1971–1977
99. Hsyu PH, Singh A, Giargiari TD, Dunn JA, Ascher JA, Johnston JA (1997) Pharmacokinetics of bupropion and its metabolites in cigarette smokers versus nonsmokers. J Clin Pharmacol 37(8):737–743
100. Worrall SP, Almond MK, Dhillon S (2004) Pharmacokinetics of bupropion and its metabolites in haemodialysis patients who smoke. A single dose study. Nephron Clin Pract 97(3):c83–c89
101. Hesse LM, Venkatakrishnan K, Court MH et al (2000) CYP2B6 mediates the in vitro hydroxylation of bupropion: potential drug interactions with other antidepressants. Drug Metab Dispos 28(10):1176–1183
102. Jefferson JW, Pradko JF, Muir KT (2005) Bupropion for major depressive disorder: pharmacokinetic and formulation considerations. Clin Ther 27(11):1685–1695
103. Kotlyar M, Brauer LH, Tracy TS et al (2005) Inhibition of CYP2D6 activity by bupropion. J Clin Psychopharmacol 25(3):226–229
104. Reese MJ, Wurm RM, Muir KT, Generaux GT, St John-Williams L, McConn DJ (2008) An in vitro mechanistic study to elucidate the desipramine/bupropion clinical drug-drug interaction. Drug Metab Dispos 36(7):1198 1201
105. Watanabe MD, Winter ME (2004) Tricyclic antidepressants: amitriptyline, despiramine, imipramine, and nortriptyline. In: Winter ME (ed) Basic clinical pharmacokinetics, 4th edn. Lippincott Williams and Wilkins, Baltimore, pp 423–437
106. Baldessarini RJ (2006) Drug therapy of depression and anxiety disorders. In: Brunton LL, Lazo JS, Parker KL (eds) Goodman and Gilman's the pharmacologic basis of therapeutics, 11th edn. McGraw-Hill Medical Publishing Division, New York, pp 429–459
107. Piafsky KM, Borga O (1977) Plasma protein binding of basic drugs. II. Importance of alpha 1-acid glycoprotein for interindividual variation. Clin Pharmacol Ther 22(5 Pt 1):545–549
108. Freilich DI, Giardina EG (1984) Imipramine binding to alpha-1-acid glycoprotein in normal subjects and cardiac patients. Clin Pharmacol Ther 35(5):670–674

109. Emsam (selegiline transdermal patch) (2015) Prescribing Information. Mylan Specialty L.P, Basking Ridge
110. Reynolds GP, Elsworth JD, Blau K, Sandler M, Lees AJ, Stern GM (1978) Deprenyl is metabolized to methamphetamine and amphetamine in man. Br J Clin Pharmacol 6(6):542–544
111. Nickel B, Schulze G, Szelenyi I (1990) Effect of enantiomers of deprenyl (selegiline) and amphetamine on physical abuse liability and cortical electrical activity in rats. Neuropharmacology 29(11):983–992
112. Roberts C, Hagan JJ, Bartoszyk GD, Kew JN (2005) Effect of vilazodone on 5-HT efflux and re-uptake in the guinea-pig dorsal raphe nucleus. Eur J Pharmacol 517(1–2):59–63
113. Khan A (2009) Vilazodone, a novel dual-acting serotonergic antidepressant for managing major depression. Expert Opin Investig Drugs 18(11):1753–1764
114. Boinpally R, Alcorn H, Adams MH, Longstreth J, Edwards J (2013) Pharmacokinetics of vilazodone in patients with mild or moderate renal impairment. Clin Drug Investig 33(3):199–206
115. Welch LP, Leader WG, Chandler MH (1993) Predicting vancomycin pharmacokinetics by using aminoglycoside pharmacokinetics. Clin Pharm 12(12):909–913
116. Kelder J, Funke C, De Boer T, Delbressine L, Leysen D, Nickolson V (1997) A comparison of the physicochemical and biological properties of mirtazapine and mianserin. J Pharm Pharmacol 49(4):403–411
117. Delbressine LP, Moonen ME, Kaspersen FM et al (1998) Pharmacokinetics and biotransformation of mirtazapine in human volunteers. Clin Drug Investig 15(1):45–55
118. Stormer E, von Moltke LL, Shader RI, Greenblatt DJ (2000) Metabolism of the antidepressant mirtazapine in vitro: contribution of cytochromes P-450 1A2, 2D6, and 3A4. Drug Metab Dispos 28(10):1168–1175
119. Okubo M, Murayama N, Miura J, Chiba Y, Yamazaki H (2015) Effects of cytochrome P450 2D6 and 3A5 genotypes and possible coadministered medicines on the metabolic clearance of antidepressant mirtazapine in Japanese patients. Biochem Pharmacol 93(1):104–109
120. Liang J, Liu X, Zheng J, Yu S (2013) Effect of amitriptyline on tetrodotoxin-resistant Nav1.9 currents in nociceptive trigeminal neurons. Mol Pain 9:31
121. Areberg J, Luntang-Jensen M, Sogaard B, Nilausen DO (2012) Occupancy of the serotonin transporter after administration of Lu AA21004 and its relation to plasma concentration in healthy subjects. Basic Clin Pharmacol Toxicol 110(4):401–404
122. Uldam HK, Juhl M, Pedersen H, Dalgaard L (2011) Biosynthesis and identification of an N-oxide/N-glucuronide metabolite and first synthesis of an N-O-glucuronide metabolite of Lu AA21004. Drug Metab Dispos 39(12):2264–2274
123. Hvenegaard MG, Bang-Andersen B, Pedersen H, Jorgensen M, Puschl A, Dalgaard L (2012) Identification of the cytochrome P450 and other enzymes involved in the in vitro oxidative metabolism of a novel antidepressant, Lu AA21004. Drug Metab Dispos 40(7):1357–1365
124. Chen G, Lee R, Hojer AM, Buchbjerg JK, Serenko M, Zhao Z (2013) Pharmacokinetic drug interactions involving vortioxetine (Lu AA21004), a multimodal antidepressant. Clin Drug Investig 33(10):727–736
125. Kulaksiz-Erkmen G, Dalmizrak O, Dincsoy-Tuna G, Dogan A, Ogus IH, Ozer N (2013) Amitriptyline may have a supportive role in cancer treatment by inhibiting glutathione S-transferase pi (GST-pi) and alpha (GST-alpha). J Enzyme Inhib Med Chem 28(1):131–136
126. White PF, Ham J, Way WL, Trevor AJ (1980) Pharmacology of ketamine isomers in surgical patients. Anesthesiology 52(3):231–239
127. Bergman SA (1999) Ketamine: review of its pharmacology and its use in pediatric anesthesia. Anesth Prog 46(1):10–20
128. Walker FR (2013) A critical review of the mechanism of action for the selective serotonin reuptake inhibitors: do these drugs possess anti-inflammatory properties and how relevant is this in the treatment of depression? Neuropharmacology 67:304–317

129. Andrews JM, Nemeroff CB (1994) Contemporary management of depression. Am J Med 97(6A):24S–32S
130. Auerbach SB, Lundberg JF, Hjorth S (1995) Differential inhibition of serotonin release by 5-HT and NA reuptake blockers after systemic administration. Neuropharmacology 34(1):89–96
131. Rush AJ, Trivedi MH, Wisniewski SR et al (2006) Bupropion-SR, sertraline, or venlafaxine-XR after failure of SSRIs for depression. N Engl J Med 354(12):1231–1242
132. Stahl SM (2013) Mechanism of action of ketamine. CNS Spectr 18(4):171–174
133. Wolkowitz OM, Wolf J, Shelly W et al (2011) Serum BDNF levels before treatment predict SSRI response in depression. Prog Neuropsychopharmacol Biol Psychiatry 35(7):1623–1630
134. Iadarola ND, Niciu MJ, Richards EM et al (2015) Ketamine and other N-methyl-D-aspartate receptor antagonists in the treatment of depression: a perspective review. Ther Adv Chronic Dis 6(3):97–114
135. Kroeze Y, Zhou H, Homberg JR (2012) The genetics of selective serotonin reuptake inhibitors. Pharmacol Ther 136(3):375–400
136. Meyer JH (2007) Imaging the serotonin transporter during major depressive disorder and antidepressant treatment. J Psychiatry Neurosci 32(2):86–102
137. Cipriani A, Furukawa TA, Salanti G et al (2009) Comparative efficacy and acceptability of 12 new-generation antidepressants: a multiple-treatments meta-analysis. Lancet 373(9665): 746–758
138. Papakostas GI, Thase ME, Fava M, Nelson JC, Shelton RC (2007) Are antidepressant drugs that combine serotonergic and noradrenergic mechanisms of action more effective than the selective serotonin reuptake inhibitors in treating major depressive disorder? A meta-analysis of studies of newer agents. Biol Psychiatry 62(11):1217–1227
139. Thase ME (2003) Effectiveness of antidepressants: comparative remission rates. J Clin Psychiatry 64(Suppl 2):3–7
140. Richelson E (2001) Pharmacology of antidepressants. Mayo Clin Proc 76(5):511–527
141. Debonnel G, Saint-Andre E, Hebert C, de Montigny C, Lavoie N, Blier P (2007) Differential physiological effects of a low dose and high doses of venlafaxine in major depression. Int J Neuropsychopharmacol 10(1):51–61
142. Deecher DC, Beyer CE, Johnston G et al (2006) Desvenlafaxine succinate: a new serotonin and norepinephrine reuptake inhibitor. J Pharmacol Exp Ther 318(2):657–665
143. Hunziker ME, Suehs BT, Bettinger TL, Crismon ML (2005) Duloxetine hydrochloride: a new dual-acting medication for the treatment of major depressive disorder. Clin Ther 27(8):1126–1143
144. Trivedi MH, Desaiah D, Ossanna MJ, Pritchett YL, Brannan SK, Detke MJ (2008) Clinical evidence for serotonin and norepinephrine reuptake inhibition of duloxetine. Int Clin Psychopharmacol 23(3):161–169
145. Asnis GM, Henderson MA (2015) Levomilnacipran for the treatment of major depressive disorder: a review. Neuropsychiatr Dis Treat 11:125–135
146. Learned-Coughlin SM, Bergstrom M, Savitcheva I, Ascher J, Schmith VD, Langstrom B (2003) In vivo activity of bupropion at the human dopamine transporter as measured by positron emission tomography. Biol Psychiatry 54(8):800–805
147. Dong J, Blier P (2001) Modification of norepinephrine and serotonin, but not dopamine, neuron firing by sustained bupropion treatment. Psychopharmacology (Berl) 155(1):52–57
148. Redolat R, Gomez MC, Vicens P, Carrasco MC (2005) Bupropion effects on aggressiveness and anxiety in OF1 male mice. Psychopharmacology (Berl) 177(4):418–427
149. Birmaher B, Brent D, Issues AWGoQ et al (2007) Practice parameter for the assessment and treatment of children and adolescents with depressive disorders. J Am Acad Child Adolesc Psychiatry 46(11):1503–1526
150. Dalmizrak O, Kulaksiz-Erkmen G, Ozer N (2011) The inhibition characteristics of human placental glutathione S-transferase-pi by tricyclic antidepressants: amitriptyline and clomipramine. Mol Cell Biochem 355(1–2):223–231

151. Araneda R, Andrade R (1991) 5-Hydroxytryptamine2 and 5-hydroxytryptamine 1A receptors mediate opposing responses on membrane excitability in rat association cortex. Neuroscience 40(2):399–412
152. Celada P, Puig M, Amargos-Bosch M, Adell A, Artigas F (2004) The therapeutic role of 5-HT1A and 5-HT2A receptors in depression. J Psychiatry Neurosci 29(4):252–265
153. Rabiner EA, Gunn RN, Wilkins MR et al (2000) Drug action at the 5-HT(1A) receptor in vivo: autoreceptor and postsynaptic receptor occupancy examined with PET and [carbonyl-(11)C]WAY-100635. Nucl Med Biol 27(5):509–513
154. Artigas F, Celada P, Laruelle M, Adell A (2001) How does pindolol improve antidepressant action? Trends Pharmacol Sci 22(5):224–228
155. Koch H, Nanev D (2012) Important interaction between mirtazapine and ondansetron. Afr J Psychiatry (Johannesbg) 15(3):160
156. Lozano R (2013) Mirtazapine and ondansetron: a dual pharmacodynamic and pharmacokinetic interaction. Afr J Psychiatry (Johannesbg) 16(1):56
157. Bang-Andersen B, Ruhland T, Jorgensen M et al (2011) Discovery of 1-[2-(2,4-dimethylphenylsulfanyl)phenyl]piperazine (Lu AA21004): a novel multimodal compound for the treatment of major depressive disorder. J Med Chem 54(9):3206–3221
158. Mork A, Pehrson A, Brennum LT et al (2012) Pharmacological effects of Lu AA21004: a novel multimodal compound for the treatment of major depressive disorder. J Pharmacol Exp Ther 340(3):666–675
159. Westrich L, Haddjeri N, Dkhissi-Benyahya O, Sanchez C (2015) Involvement of 5-HT(7) receptors in vortioxetine's modulation of circadian rhythms and episodic memory in rodents. Neuropharmacology 89:382–390
160. Areberg J, Sogaard B, Hojer AM (2012) The clinical pharmacokinetics of Lu AA21004 and its major metabolite in healthy young volunteers. Basic Clin Pharmacol Toxicol 111(3):198–205
161. Stenkrona P, Halldin C, Lundberg J (2013) 5-HTT and 5-HT(1A) receptor occupancy of the novel substance vortioxetine (Lu AA21004). A PET study in control subjects. Eur Neuropsychopharmacol 23(10):1190–1198
162. Pehrson AL, Leiser SC, Gulinello M et al (2015) Treatment of cognitive dysfunction in major depressive disorder–a review of the preclinical evidence for efficacy of selective serotonin reuptake inhibitors, serotonin-norepinephrine reuptake inhibitors and the multimodal-acting antidepressant vortioxetine. Eur J Pharmacol 753:19–31
163. Sanchez C, Asin KE, Artigas F (2015) Vortioxetine, a novel antidepressant with multimodal activity: review of preclinical and clinical data. Pharmacol Ther 145:43–57
164. Traynelis SF, Wollmuth LP, McBain CJ et al (2010) Glutamate receptor ion channels: structure, regulation, and function. Pharmacol Rev 62(3):405–496
165. Li N, Lee B, Liu RJ et al (2010) mTOR-dependent synapse formation underlies the rapid antidepressant effects of NMDA antagonists. Science 329(5994):959–964
166. Price RB, Iosifescu DV, Murrough JW et al (2014) Effects of ketamine on explicit and implicit suicidal cognition: a randomized controlled trial in treatment-resistant depression. Depress Anxiety 31(4):335–343
167. Xu AJ, Niciu MJ, Lundin NB et al (2015) Lithium and valproate levels do not correlate with Ketamine's antidepressant efficacy in treatment-resistant bipolar depression. Neural Plast 2015:858251
168. Zarate CA Jr, Singh JB, Carlson PJ et al (2006) A randomized trial of an N-methyl-D-aspartate antagonist in treatment-resistant major depression. Arch Gen Psychiatry 63(8):856–864
169. Murrough JW, Perez AM, Pillemer S et al (2013) Rapid and longer-term antidepressant effects of repeated ketamine infusions in treatment-resistant major depression. Biol Psychiatry 74(4):250–256
170. Meyer JH, Wilson AA, Sagrati S et al (2004) Serotonin transporter occupancy of five selective serotonin reuptake inhibitors at different doses: an [11C]DASB positron emission tomography study. Am J Psychiatry 161(5):826–835

171. Nogami T, Takano H, Arakawa R et al (2013) Occupancy of serotonin and norepinephrine transporter by milnacipran in patients with major depressive disorder: a positron emission tomography study with [(11)C]DASB and (S, S)-[(18)F]FMeNER-D(2). Int J Neuropsychopharmacol 16(5):937–943
172. Laib AK, Brunen S, Pfeifer P, Vincent P, Hiemke C (2014) Serum concentrations of hydroxybupropion for dose optimization of depressed patients treated with bupropion. Ther Drug Monit 36(4):473–479
173. Baumann P, Hiemke C, Ulrich S et al (2004) The AGNP-TDM expert group consensus guidelines: therapeutic drug monitoring in psychiatry. Pharmacopsychiatry 37(6):243–265
174. Muller MJ, Dragicevic A, Fric M et al (2003) Therapeutic drug monitoring of tricyclic antidepressants: how does it work under clinical conditions? Pharmacopsychiatry 36(3):98–104
175. Preskorn SH, Fast GA (1991) Therapeutic drug monitoring for antidepressants: efficacy, safety, and cost effectiveness. J Clin Psychiatry 52(Suppl):23–33
176. Ulrich S, Lauter J (2002) Comprehensive survey of the relationship between serum concentration and therapeutic effect of amitriptyline in depression. Clin Pharmacokinet 41(11):853–876
177. Glotzbach RK, Preskorn SH (1982) Brain concentrations of tricyclic antidepressants: single-dose kinetics and relationship to plasma concentrations in chronically dosed rats. Psychopharmacology (Berl) 78(1):25–27
178. Asberg M, Cronholm B, Sjoqvist F, Tuck D (1971) Relationship between plasma level and therapeutic effect of nortriptyline. Br Med J 3(5770):331–334
179. Perry PJ, Browne JL, Alexander B et al (1985) Relationship of free nortriptyline levels to therapeutic response. Acta Psychiatr Scand 72(2):120–125
180. Bruijn JA, Moleman P, Mulder PG et al (1996) A double-blind, fixed blood-level study comparing mirtazapine with imipramine in depressed in-patients. Psychopharmacology (Berl) 127(3):231–237
181. Jaquenoud Sirot E, van der Velden JW, Rentsch K, Eap CB, Baumann P (2006) Therapeutic drug monitoring and pharmacogenetic tests as tools in pharmacovigilance. Drug Saf 29(9):735–768
182. Dawling S (1982) Monitoring of tricyclic antidepressant therapy. Clin Biochem 15(1):56–61
183. Gupta SK, Shah JC, Hwang SS (1999) Pharmacokinetic and pharmacodynamic characterization of OROS and immediate-release amitriptyline. Br J Clin Pharmacol 48(1):71–78
184. Vuille F, Amey M, Baumann P (1991) Use of plasma level monitoring of antidepressants in clinical practice. Towards an analysis of clinical utility. Pharmacopsychiatry 24(6):190–195
185. Riant P, Urien S, Albengres E, Renouard A, Tillement JP (1988) Effects of the binding of imipramine to erythrocytes and plasma proteins on its transport through the rat blood-brain barrier. J Neurochem 51(2):421–425
186. Pfuhlmann B, Gerlach M, Burger R et al (2007) Therapeutic drug monitoring of tricyclic antidepressants in everyday clinical practice. J Neural Transm Suppl 72:287–296
187. Baumann P, Ulrich S, Eckermann G et al (2005) The AGNP-TDM Expert Group Consensus Guidelines: focus on therapeutic monitoring of antidepressants. Dialogues Clin Neurosci 7(3):231–247
188. Berm EJ, Paardekooper J, Brummel-Mulder E, Hak E, Wilffert B, Maring JG (2015) A simple dried blood spot method for therapeutic drug monitoring of the tricyclic antidepressants amitriptyline, nortriptyline, imipramine, clomipramine, and their active metabolites using LC-MS/MS. Talanta 134:165–172
189. Finley PR (2005) Antidepressants. In: Murphy JE (ed) Clinical pharmacokinetics, 5th edn. American Society of Health-System Pharmacists, Inc., Baltimore, pp 119–134
190. Meineke I, Kress I, Poser W, Ruther E, Brockmoller J (2004) Therapeutic drug monitoring of mirtazapine and its metabolite desmethylmirtazapine by HPLC with fluorescence detection. Ther Drug Monit 26(3):277–283
191. Reis M, Prochazka J, Sitsen A, Ahlner J, Bengtsson F (2005) Inter- and intraindividual pharmacokinetic variations of mirtazapine and its N-demethyl metabolite in patients treated for major depressive disorder: a 6-month therapeutic drug monitoring study. Ther Drug Monit 27(4):469–477

192. Shams M, Hiemke C, Hartter S (2004) Therapeutic drug monitoring of the antidepressant mirtazapine and its N-demethylated metabolite in human serum. Ther Drug Monit 26(1):78–84
193. Rush AJ, Trivedi MH, Wisniewski SR et al (2006) Acute and longer-term outcomes in depressed outpatients requiring one or several treatment steps: a STAR*D report. Am J Psychiatry 163(11):1905–1917
194. Trivedi MH, Rush AJ, Wisniewski SR et al (2006) Evaluation of outcomes with citalopram for depression using measurement-based care in STAR*D: implications for clinical practice. Am J Psychiatry 163(1):28–40
195. Kirchheiner J, Seeringer A, Viviani R (2010) Pharmacogenetics in psychiatry–a useful clinical tool or wishful thinking for the future? Curr Pharm Des 16(2):136–144
196. Lee KC, Ma JD, Kuo GM (2010) Pharmacogenomics: bridging the gap between science and practice. J Am Pharm Assoc (2003) 50(1):e1–e14; quiz e5–7
197. Tansey KE, Guipponi M, Hu X et al (2013) Contribution of common genetic variants to antidepressant response. Biol Psychiatry 73(7):679–682
198. Porcelli S, Fabbri C, Serretti A (2012) Meta-analysis of serotonin transporter gene promoter polymorphism (5-HTTLPR) association with antidepressant efficacy. Eur Neuropsychopharmacol 22(4):239–258
199. Risch N, Herrell R, Lehner T et al (2009) Interaction between the serotonin transporter gene (5-HTTLPR), stressful life events, and risk of depression: a meta-analysis. JAMA 301(23):2462–2471
200. Yoshida K, Ito K, Sato K et al (2002) Influence of the serotonin transporter gene-linked polymorphic region on the antidepressant response to fluvoxamine in Japanese depressed patients. Prog Neuropsychopharmacol Biol Psychiatry 26(2):383–386
201. Houston JP, Kohler J, Ostbye KM, Heinloth A, Perlis RH (2011) Association of catechol-O-methyltransferase variants with duloxetine response in major depressive disorder. Psychiatry Res 189(3):475–477
202. Shi Y, Yuan Y, Xu Z et al (2012) Genetic variation in the calcium/calmodulin-dependent protein kinase (CaMK) pathway is associated with antidepressant response in females. J Affect Disord 136(3):558–566
203. Montminy M (1997) Transcriptional regulation by cyclic AMP. Annu Rev Biochem 66:807–822
204. Pilar-Cuellar F, Vidal R, Diaz A et al (2013) Neural plasticity and proliferation in the generation of antidepressant effects: hippocampal implication. Neural Plast 2013:537265
205. Niitsu T, Fabbri C, Bentini F, Serretti A (2013) Pharmacogenetics in major depression: a comprehensive meta-analysis. Prog Neuropsychopharmacol Biol Psychiatry 45:183–194
206. Maddox JC, Levi M, Thompson C (1994) The compliance with antidepressants in general practice. J Psychopharmacol 8(1):48–52
207. Ereshefsky L, Riesenman C, Lam YW (1996) Serotonin selective reuptake inhibitor drug interactions and the cytochrome P450 system. J Clin Psychiatry 57(Suppl 8):17–24; discussion 5
208. Kirchheiner J, Schmidt H, Tzvetkov M et al (2007) Pharmacokinetics of codeine and its metabolite morphine in ultra-rapid metabolizers due to CYP2D6 duplication. Pharmacogenomics J 7(4):257–265
209. Gaedigk A, Gotschall RR, Forbes NS, Simon SD, Kearns GL, Leeder JS (1999) Optimization of cytochrome P4502D6 (CYP2D6) phenotype assignment using a genotyping algorithm based on allele frequency data. Pharmacogenetics 9(6):669–682
210. Gaedigk A, Simon SD, Pearce RE, Bradford LD, Kennedy MJ, Leeder JS (2008) The CYP2D6 activity score: translating genotype information into a qualitative measure of phenotype. Clin Pharmacol Ther 83(2):234–242
211. Laika B, Leucht S, Heres S, Steimer W (2009) Intermediate metabolizer: increased side effects in psychoactive drug therapy. The key to cost-effectiveness of pretreatment CYP2D6 screening? Pharmacogenomics J 9(6):395–403

212. Ruano G, Szarek BL, Villagra D et al (2013) Length of psychiatric hospitalization is correlated with CYP2D6 functional status in inpatients with major depressive disorder. Biomark Med 7(3):429–439
213. Hodgson K, Tansey K, Dernovsek MZ et al (2014) Genetic differences in cytochrome P450 enzymes and antidepressant treatment response. J Psychopharmacol 28(2):133–141
214. Hicks JK, Swen JJ, Thorn CF et al (2013) Clinical Pharmacogenetics Implementation Consortium guideline for CYP2D6 and CYP2C19 genotypes and dosing of tricyclic antidepressants. Clin Pharmacol Ther 93(5):402–408
215. Leckband SG, Kelsoe JR, Dunnenberger HM et al (2013) Clinical Pharmacogenetics Implementation Consortium guidelines for HLA-B genotype and carbamazepine dosing. Clin Pharmacol Ther 94(3):324–328
216. Rickels K, Athanasiou M, Robinson DS, Gibertini M, Whalen H, Reed CR (2009) Evidence for efficacy and tolerability of vilazodone in the treatment of major depressive disorder: a randomized, double-blind, placebo-controlled trial. J Clin Psychiatry 70(3):326–333
217. Musil R, Zill P, Seemuller F et al (2013) Genetics of emergent suicidality during antidepressive treatment–data from a naturalistic study on a large sample of inpatients with a major depressive episode. Eur Neuropsychopharmacol 23(7):663–674
218. Hall-Flavin DK, Winner JG, Allen JD et al (2013) Utility of integrated pharmacogenomic testing to support the treatment of major depressive disorder in a psychiatric outpatient setting. Pharmacogenet Genomics 23(10):535–548
219. Evaluation of Genomic Applications in Practice and Prevention (EGAPP) Working Group (2007) Recommendations from the EGAPP Working Group: testing for cytochrome P450 polymorphisms in adults with nonpsychotic depression treated with selective serotonin reuptake inhibitors. Genet Med 9(12):819–825

Chapter 10
Clinical Pharmacokinetics and Pharmacodynamics of Anxiolytics and Sedative/Hypnotics

C. Lindsay DeVane

Abstract Medications to promote sedation and reduce anxiety and its associated symptoms have been sought since recorded history. The development of the benzodiazepines represented a major therapeutic endeavor due to their safety profile especially when taken in overdose situations compared to the barbiturates and early non-barbiturates such as meprobamate. Benzodiazepines continue to be one of the most commonly prescribed agents available in a variety of dosage formulations used for all age groups. Their pharmacokinetic (PK) and pharmacodynamic (PD) profiles have been extensively studied in adult healthy volunteers, the elderly, and patients with hepatic and renal impairment. Most benzodiazepines are metabolized by the phase I oxidative CYP enzyme system and the remaining agents by the phase II glucuronidation. Many long-acting benzodiazepines are metabolized to an active metabolite desmethyldiazepam. Alprazolam and buspirone were FDA approved for panic and generalized anxiety disorders, respectively. Various sedative-hypnotic non-benzodiazepine agents have been developed that are agonists of the alpha-1 GABA-A subreceptor site and the melatonin receptors type 1 and 2. All of these agents produce common PD effects such as sedation and psychomotor impairment. Benzodiazepines also produce antiepileptic actions, muscle relaxation, and anterograde amnesia. PK-PD modeling has been conducted for benzodiazepines and non-benzodiazepines that mainly focus on sedation and psychomotor impairment. The elderly have more pronounced sedative and psychomotor impairment from these agents compared to the adult population. Gender can be another significant factor as females were found to have significantly higher zolpidem plasma concentrations than males and when given comparative doses also displayed more pronounced psychomotor impairment which led to the FDA recommendation of lower doses prescribed.

Keywords GABA-A receptor • Melatonin receptors • Orexin receptor • CYP metabolism • Benzodiazepines • Diazepam • Desmethyldiazepam • Alprazolam • Buspirone • Zolpidem • Eszopiclone • Zaleplon • Suvorexant • Ramelteon • Tasimelteon

---

C.L. DeVane, PharmD
Department of Psychiatry and Behavioral Sciences, Medical University of South Carolina, Charleston, SC 29425, USA
e-mail: devaneL@musc.edu

M. Jann et al. (eds.), *Applied Clinical Pharmacokinetics and Pharmacodynamics of Psychopharmacological Agents*,
DOI 10.1007/978-3-319-27883-4_10

10.1 Introduction

Drugs used to reduce or relieve the symptoms of anxiety and induce a calmer and more relaxed anticipation of future events are known as anxiolytics. Drugs used to induce, prolong, or improve the quality of sleep, or produce a partial anesthesia, are known as sedative-hypnotics. Often the designation of a drug as having one or more of these therapeutic effects is a function of dosage and differences in the degree of their pharmacodynamic (PD) effects. Evidence suggests that humans have used various plant preparations beginning before recorded history for the purpose of producing antianxiety effects and inducing sleep [1]. Organized drug development over the past century has resulted in the synthesis of thousands of molecules for potential development as safe and effective anxiolytics and sedative-hypnotics. A few have found a place in contemporary therapeutics. The key milestones in this drug development process are listed in Table 10.1 [2].

This chapter will focus on the marketed anxiolytics and sedative/hypnotics that are currently in widespread clinical use. Most of these compounds belong to the benzodiazepine class of drugs. Their disposition has been thoroughly studied and summaries of this voluminous literature are readily available [3, 4]. This discussion will emphasize data that have proven useful in drug selection and dosage regimen design for individual patients [5]. The characteristics of the prototype compounds are summarized and references provided for more detailed discussion of the less widely used drugs.

Table 10.1 Time line for development of sedative-hypnotics and anxiolytics

Prerecorded history	
Hieroglyphics and pottery artifacts document wine from grape cultivation	
Alcohol in various fermented beverages appears in many cultures	
500 BC	
Opium plant products are smoked or taken orally	
1721	London Pharmacopoeia describes products made from opium with camphor similar to paregoric
1800s	Alcohol derivatives are synthesized including paraldehyde and chloral hydrate
1800s	Barbiturates (>2500 derivatives) are synthesized; some become enduring products: amobarbital, butabarbital, pentobarbital, and secobarbital
1950s	Nonbarbiturate sedative-hypnotics are introduced: meprobamate, methaqualone, methyprylon; glutethimide; ethchlorvynol
1955	Synthesis of the first benzodiazepine, chlordiazepoxide; eventual synthesis of hundreds of derivatives
1960	Marketing of chlordiazepoxide
1963	Marketing of diazepam
1963–1980s	Marketing of multiple benzodiazepines with expanding indications
1980s	Non-benzodiazepine benzodiazepine receptor agonists are introduced
2005	Ramelteon approved in the USA as a melatonin receptor agonist for treatment of insomnia

From: Allen et al. [12], Ban [1], Strang et al. [6], Wick [2]

10.2 Historical Development of Anxiolytics and Sedative-Hypnotics

Alcohol may have the most extensive history of drugs being consumed for sedative properties. The history begins with beer-like beverages, or mead, being consumed in China and the Middle East as early as 6000 BC [1]. By 2000 BC, the production of wine from fermented grapes was wide spread. Natural products were cultivated and processed to specifically produce behavioral effects. Opium consumption was proliferating as early as 500 BC [6]. For several subsequent centuries, alcohol and opium preparations were the only available sedative-hypnotics. Drug development during this time was essentially stagnant until solutions of bromide salts appeared in the eighteenth century followed by the availability of paraldehyde and chloral hydrate in the late part of the nineteenth century [7]. In 1864, von Baeyer synthesized malonylurea (barbituric acid) from which thousands of derivatives were synthesized in the twentieth century [8]. Some of these compounds were developed for clinical use and became the barbiturate class of drugs.

Several barbiturates are still widely used. Sodium thiopental is a rapid-onset general anesthetic of the barbiturate class that has been used extensively in surgical practice. It recently drew public attention as a primary component of lethal injections. When shortages of drug supply appeared, its manufacturer became reluctant to continue production [9]. Butabarbital, amobarbital, secobarbital, and pentobarbital as sedative-hypnotics became widely prescribed in medical practice in various oral formulations. A hangover effect of excessive daytime drowsiness is a common problem with barbiturate use for sedation. Solid dosage forms of barbiturates are relatively inexpensive and are used extensively in some countries, especially in Eastern Europe and South America.

Phenobarbital was the first modern anxiolytic and is the prototype barbiturate. It is still widely used in human and veterinary medicine as an antiepileptic compound. It possesses a broad central nervous system (CNS) depressive ability and is capable of producing anxiolytic effects at relatively low dosages. A problem with phenobarbital common to many barbiturates is hepatic enzyme induction resulting in numerous potential drug-drug interactions. Increasingly profound CNS depression occurs with increasing dosage that can ultimately produce anesthesia, coma, respiratory depression, and death [10]. Combining a barbiturate and alcohol produces a synergistic pharmacodynamic depressive effect on the CNS. Numerous accidental deaths have been attributed to normal doses of secobarbital or amobarbital when taken with alcohol [11]. The barbiturate's multiple disadvantages stimulated a search for more effective and less dangerous drugs.

Development of non-barbiturates with a goal of producing similar antianxiety and sedative effects as the barbiturates resulted in marketing of several drugs with diverse structures, some of which remain in limited production. Meprobamate, used since 1955 as an antianxiety drug [12], along with methaqualone, ethchlorvynol, and glutethimide, as sedative-hypnotics, had similar or more profound liabilities than the barbiturates. They were extensively prescribed in the decade preceding the marketing of the benzodiazepines despite increasing recognition of their lethality. Overdosage with meprobamate proved notoriously difficult to treat [13]. Methaqualone obtained cult status for its ability to produce a dysphoric and disinhibitory emotional state that led to its abuse as a date-rape drug that enabled unwanted sexual assaults [14]. It was removed from the US market by 1985. Other compounds were also removed or production was discontinued due to low sales volume and recognition of their toxicity. These drugs are not discussed further as the benzodiazepines and subsequently developed compounds are far better alternatives.

The availability of efficacious anxiolytics with predictable dose effects was a highly desirable goal of drug development in the middle twentieth century. The discovery of the benzodiazepines was the result of the accidental synthesis of chlordiazepoxide in 1955 by Leo Sternbach at Hoffmann-La Roche [2]. In 1960, it was marketed for agitation associated with acute alcohol withdrawal and was quickly followed by diazepam in 1963. The chemical classification of the benzodiazepines derives from the basic structure of a benzene ring adjacent to a 7-membered diazepam ring. The marketed drugs are designated as having a 1,4 or a 1,5 benzodiazepine structure according to the placement of a nitrogen atom at these two sites on the diazepam ring [15].

Hundreds of benzodiazepines have been synthesized and several developed between1960 and 1980 have had enduring commercial success. The popularity of the benzodiazepines derives from their broad utility and safety. These drugs can be prescribed with more impunity from overdose toxicity than any previously available anxiolytics and sedative-hypnotics and so have become the preferred treatment for most patients. For example, the dose that is lethal for 50 % of the animals in toxicology studies (LD_{50}) requires at least ten times the exposure to diazepam as to secobarbital [16]. The selective serotonin reuptake inhibitors (SSRI) have emerged as effective anxiolytics in the 1990s and are discussed elsewhere in this text.

The World Health Organization (WHO) lists four benzodiazepines on its current biannual List of Essential Medicines [17]. These include midazolam as a preoperative medication and sedative for short-term procedures and lorazepam and diazepam as anticonvulsants. Diazepam is also listed as a medicine for anxiety disorders and under the category of medicines for common symptoms in palliative care. The same three drugs are also regarded as essential drugs for children. A small number of alternatives to the benzodiazepines for use as sedative-hypnotics became available but have not displaced the essential role of benzodiazepines to any substantial degree.

With usage driven by availability in multiple formulations, low toxicity, efficacy in a wide variety of conditions, both medical and psychological, the benzodiazepines are the principle anxiolytics used worldwide. Benzodiazepines have multiple uses outside of their FDA-approved indications and are listed in Table 10.2. The dependence-producing properties and propensity for producing withdrawal syndromes in some patients, discussed below, have limited further widespread use of the benzodiazepines and related drugs. While most anxiety disorders can be managed with a benzodiazepine alone, the antidepressants, discussed elsewhere, are often combined with a benzodiazepine to treat various anxiety disorders.

Table 10.2 Major indications of benzodiazepines

Indications and additional uses	Drugs of choice/suitable alternatives
Anxiety disorders	
Generalized anxiety disorder	Diazepam, lorazepam, alprazolam, chlordiazepoxide, oxazepam
Panic disorder	Alprazolam, lorazepam, clonazepam
Social phobia	Diazepam, alprazolam
Other anxious conditions	
Preoperative anxiety	Diazepam
Conscious anesthesia	Midazolam (IV), diazepam (IV)
Critical care ventilation maintenance	Diazepam
Delirious states	Diazepam, lorazepam
Alcohol withdrawal	Chlordiazepoxide, lorazepam
Seizures	Clonazepam (as daily anticonvulsant; diazepam (IV for status epilepticus)
Nausea and vomiting (chemotherapy-related and various etiologies)	Diazepam; any of the medium to longer-acting benzodiazepines
Insomnia	Choice dictated by specific complaint of difficulty falling asleep; difficulty maintaining sleep or early morning awakening; approved benzodiazepines include flurazepam, estazolam, quazepam, temazepam, and triazolam
Akathisia from antipsychotic use	Diazepam

10.3 Pharmacokinetic Properties of Anxiolytics and Sedative-Hypnotics

The benzodiazepines are similar in many physiochemical, pharmacokinetic, and pharmacodynamic characteristics. The drugs are highly lipid soluble with good oral absorption profiles. Most are extensively bound to plasma proteins but this characteristic has not proven to be of major importance for drug selection. Distribution of benzodiazepines is extensive in the body as is expected from drugs that produce CNS effects [18]. This characteristic can occasionally be problematic, for example, for infants of women breast-feeding and receiving high doses of diazepam [19].

The benzodiazepines can be distinguished by different metabolic pathways involved in their metabolism. One group of benzodiazepines is primarily oxidized by phase I enzymes, predominantly the cytochrome P450 enzymes, resulting in demethylated or hydroxylated metabolites. These by-products often possess pharmacological activity. The metabolites are further conjugated by phase II metabolic reactions to glucuronidated metabolites that are inactive and excreted in the urine. A second group of drugs undergoes conjugation reactions as the primary means of elimination from the body. Drugs in the first category include chlordiazepoxide, diazepam, and flurazepam. Drugs in the second category undergoing glucuronidation as their primary route of elimination include oxazepam, lorazepam, and midazolam. These metabolic characteristics are displayed in Fig. 19.1.

The PD effects of benzodiazepines are the result of enhancing gamma-aminobutyric acid (GABA) neurotransmission [20]. GABA is the main inhibitory neurotransmitter in the CNS. It has three types of receptors but most drug binding involves GABA-A receptors and its various subunits. As a class of drugs with mechanisms of action involving GABA, the benzodiazepines are considered to possess anxiolytic, anticonvulsant, sedative, hypnotic, and skeletal muscle relaxant properties. This complex pharmacology has been the subject of extensive investigation [21]. The drugs decrease the subjective experience of anxiety and, according to the dose, produce a mild sedation that can be increased to the level of anesthesia with sufficient drug administration. An amnestic effect can be produced that is characterized by an anterograde memory impairment [22]. This is an often cited advantage for certain surgical or dental procedures to minimize recall of pain. Some studies have claimed a more favorable anticonvulsant effect with drugs belonging to the 1,5-benzodiazepine structural class. However, effective anticonvulsants have been developed from both the 1,4 (diazepam) and 1,5 (clobazam) categories of benzodiazepines [23].

The choice of a specific drug often involves matching the agent's elimination half-life with the therapeutic PD effects as needed for acute or chronic anxiolytic treatment. A choice can be made to allow dosing just once daily and requiring little tapering upon discontinuation to avoid a return of baseline or rebound symptoms. Further considerations pertaining to individual drugs are given below. A summary of the major benzodiazepine pharmacokinetic properties and clinical pharmacokinetic data of value in clinical practice are presented in Table 19.1.

10.4 Specific Benzodiazepine Anxiolytics

Alprazolam This (1,4)-benzodiazepine in 1981 was the first drug FDA approved specifically for panic disorder. Randomized controlled trials using placebo, tricyclic antidepressants, and monoamine oxidase inhibitors had established its efficacy to reduce the number of panic attacks and also lessen the symptoms of agoraphobia [24]. Experience has shown that the onset of its anxiolytic effects is rapid, within 2 h following oral administration, but the drug demonstrates a fairly limited period of pharmacodynamic effects due to an intermediate elimination half-life. Its development paralleled the increase in public awareness of the dysfunctionality associated with panic disorder [25]. The effective daily dosage is generally higher than that needed to treat generalized anxiety disorder, the FDA-approved indication for most anxiolytic benzodiazepines. Total daily dosage of alprazolam in clinical practice often exceeds 4 mg per day with an occasional patient requiring over 8 mg daily. Unfortunately, this dosage increases the risk and severity of dependence. This is evident by the difficulty some patients experienced in decreasing or discontinuing treatment. Fortunately, evidence for the development of tolerance to the antipanic effects with long-term administration is lacking [26].

Alprazolam quickly became the most widely prescribed benzodiazepine shortly after its marketing. Given its success in treating panic symptoms, other benzodiazepines were tested in clinical trials and several have since received FDA approval. Notably, patients requiring long-term treatment for periods longer than 4–6 months are often switched to clonazepam allowing a reduction in number of doses per day to a single administration [27]. This benefit reflects the longer elimination half-life (range 18–50 h) and slower clearance of clonazepam.

The gastrointestinal absorption rate of alprazolam is rapid, with peak plasma concentrations occurring within 1–4 h after administration so its antianxiety effects are felt almost immediately. Alprazolam was shown to be well absorbed from the buccal mucosa so that patients in stressful situations, when liquids to facilitate oral administration are unavailable, can still obtain anxiolytic effects by placing the drug dose under the tongue for sublingual absorption. Alprazolam has been marketed in multiple formulations and dosage strengths but only for oral administration. Alprazolam can be administered via the sublingual route with similar absorption properties as the oral route [28].

As a CYP3A4 substrate, alprazolam is subject to drug-drug interactions from multiple metabolic inducers or inhibitors to increase or decrease clearance [29]. It has an intermediate elimination half-life in adults, and treatment of panic disorder often requires the drug to be administered two to three times a day in order to maintain relatively stable plasma drug concentrations. Once-daily dosing may create a situation of excessive drowsiness for a short period of time after drug administration with breakthrough anxiety occurring near the end of an 8–12 h dosage interval. Clinical trials that established the efficacy of alprazolam in panic disorder showed that 6–12 mg/day in treatment-resistant patients could reduce multiple daily panic attacks to a frequency of only a few attacks a week.

Plasma concentration ranges have not been defined that serve as guidelines for target dosing. Adjustment of daily dosing to achieve the optimal efficacy is empirical, allowing enough time for a new steady state to occur between adjustments to evaluate therapeutic effects. A problem that became apparent with alprazolam after several years of experience was the difficulty in withdrawing some patients from high daily dosing regimens when a reduction in dosage or discontinuation was desired [30].

General guidelines that have become widely accepted to reduce the total daily dose include a recommendation to reduce no faster than one-fourth of the total dose each week. With this approach, a patient desiring to eliminate alprazolam would reduce a 4 mg/day dosing regimen by 1 mg per day for 1 week, followed by a second reduction of an addition mg to 2 mg/day the second week and continuing until a satisfactory goal was reached or until breakthrough anxiety and panic attacks defined the minimum maintenance dose. Alternatively, many patients can be switched to a benzodiazepine with a longer elimination half-life to prevent or minimize a withdrawal syndrome. Clonazepam has been a favorite choice [31].

Alprazolam was briefly investigated in clinical trials during the 1980s for antidepressant effects as its safety in overdosage is far superior to the tricyclic antidepressants, the other drug category used for the treatment of panic disorder during this time. This would be an advantage in suicidal patients [32]. However, evidence for antidepressant effects has not been convincing and subsequently tested benzodiazepines such as adinazolam were not found to be any better for depression.

Chlordiazepoxide As previously described, chlordiazepoxide was the first compound synthesized in the benzodiazepine class and the first marketed, initially with a primary indication for use in alcohol withdrawal. Chlordiazepoxide and diazepam were further differentiated by their manufacturer, Hoffmann-La Roche, by marketing in different formulations. Chlordiazepoxide was formulated into capsules while diazepam was formulated in tablets. The latter eventually became available in sustained-release capsules, oral solution, parenteral form, and suppository form for rectal administration. Chlordiazepoxide became part of the standard of care for alcohol withdrawal and has retained this recommendation [33]. Intramuscular (IM) injection of 25–100 mg every 8 h has been the recommended dose to minimize agitation, promote sleep, and suppress epileptiform withdrawal seizures. An advantage of chlordiazepoxide is its relatively long elimination half-life so that it contributes to a smooth course of alcohol withdrawal. Oral doses may be similar on a daily basis divided into several administrations. A pharmacokinetic study demonstrated oral absorption was reasonably rapid and complete suggesting that oral administration could be as useful as IM dosing [34].

With an elimination half-life of medium duration, chlordiazepoxide is a versatile drug for anxiety if immediate relief of symptoms is not needed due to its relative slow absorption profile. It has multiple pathways of elimination that do not produce pharmacologic active metabolites.

Also, use in liver disease, old age, and situations where CYP induction/inhibition would be problematic, chlordiazepoxide is an advantageous choice [35].

Clobazam This (1, 5)-benzodiazepine has been marketed since the mid-1970s in many countries outside the USA for the treatment of epilepsy. It is only available orally and has the claimed advantage of producing less sedation than clonazepam [36, 37]. Such differences may be due to affinity for two different subunits of the GABA-A receptor complex [38]. However, tolerance to its anticonvulsant effects has been a disadvantage, and animal studies showed it to be more susceptible to development of tolerance than clonazepam [39]. Tolerance to the anticonvulsant effects develops more quickly to both clobazam and clonazepam than to valproate which may account for a lack of popularity of the benzodiazepines for this use.

Clonazepam An anticonvulsant effect is a characteristic common to several benzodiazepines, notably diazepam in addition to clonazepam and clobazam. Clonazepam has found a role in substituting for alprazolam when a longer-acting antipanic effect is desired, and diazepam has the advantage as an anticonvulsant in being available in parenteral dosage forms. This becomes important when an anticonvulsant effect is needed urgently for indications such as status epilepticus.

Clorazepate This orally administered drug is rapidly converted to desmethyldiazepam, the same molecular entity that is the long-acting metabolite of diazepam.

Lacking any intrinsic pharmacological activity, clorazepate is a prodrug for desmethyldiazepam and should be expected to have many of the same qualities as this metabolite with a long elimination half-life of 20–179 h.

Diazepam Diazepam is the prototype 1,4-benzodiazepine. Early in its development, it was found to be more potent than chlordiazepoxide as a sedative, anticonvulsant, and muscle relaxant [40]. However, the pharmacologic effects of the benzodiazepines are quite similar across drugs and what often determines their preferred use has been differences in dosage, their pharmacokinetic characteristics in the intended population, and the availability of evidence for efficacy. The anxiolytic effects are mediated by alpha-2 GABA-A receptors, while the sedative effects and antiepileptic effects appear to involve alpha-1 GABA-A receptors [20]. Myorelaxant actions of diazepam appear to arise from actions at alpha-2 or alpha-3 GABA-A receptors. Diazepam, in comparison to chlordiazepoxide, was developed more extensively by Hoffmann-La Roche for multiple indications that covered the entire life span. These included anxiety during labor and delivery, childhood epilepsy, and symptoms of anxiety in adult and elderly patients with both acute and chronic symptoms. Diazepam became the most prescribed drug in the USA from 1969 to 1982 [41].

The benzodiazepines have physiochemical properties of lipid solubility and pKa values corresponding to non-ionization at physiological pH suggesting absorption should be relatively unhindered by physiological barriers. Diazepam has a rapid absorption through the gut wall and then through the cerebral capillaries, producing a potent CNS drug concentration within minutes after oral absorption. This rapid distribution results in immediate pharmacodynamic effects. However, the same physiological chemical properties that lead to an immediate pharmacologic effect also contribute to a rapid distribution throughout the body that effectively reduces the CNS concentration in favor of increasing drug concentrations in other tissues. As this process continues, hepatic metabolism of diazepam is forming desmethyldiazepam (DMD), a metabolite with similar pharmacological activity. As DMD increases in the body, pharmacodynamic effects are prolonged due to the slow elimination half-life of DMD.

Diazepam is the prototype benzodiazepine and likely the most important drug of its class due to its historical significance. The oral bioavailability is nearly complete. Depending upon the patient's previous experience with the drug, the initial perception of pharmacodynamic effects after oral administration may be felt as a diminution of anxiety, a slight sedative effect, or a slight dysphoric effect. The metabolism of diazepam is by CYP2C19 and CYP3A. Upon dosing to steady state, the DMD metabolite eventually assumes a higher plasma concentration than the parent drug. The metabolite is eliminated much more slowly with an average half-life of 36–96 h. For forensic investigations, the presence of DMD in the plasma is consistent with the patient having taken a diazepam dose sometime in the past 3–4 days.

When plasma albumin concentration is low, as often occurs in elderly patients, usual daily doses of diazepam can produce exaggerated pharmacologic effects and adverse events [42]. Standard dosage increases should proceed cautiously in the elderly with low albumin to avoid increased drug intolerance. Whenever diazepam is discontinued, the possibility of withdrawal symptoms should be kept in mind. The sudden loss of receptor occupancy can result in a return or relapse of symptoms and occasional rebound of anxiety more intense than that originally experienced before treatment. This situation requires that drug withdrawal occur slowly, sometimes over weeks or months, to avoid any withdrawal syndrome.

Lorazepam Lorazepam has the distinction of being a benzodiazepine available in both oral and parenteral dosage forms and being metabolized by phase II glucuronidation. These characteristics contribute to its versatile anxiolytic and antiepileptic actions with low concern for use in patients with hepatic diseases. Lorazepam is used extensively by intramuscular, intravenous, and oral administration.

Midazolam Midazolam is well absorbed by various routes of administration but is only available in the USA in a parenteral formulation. It has proven to be useful for producing a state called "conscious anesthesia" allowing procedures such as endoscopy to be performed without pain and limited recall memory for the actual procedure. The level of vital sign monitoring usually provided by anesthesiologists in surgical settings is often unnecessary. Other uses include maintenance of mechanical ventilation, treatment of intractable seizures, and palliative sedation [43]. The drug's clinical utility is facilitated by a pharmacokinetic profile of a short elimination half-life and a lack of active metabolites. Midazolam is subject to numerous drug-drug interactions from induction or inhibition of CYP3A4 [44].

Oxazepam Oxazepam is a metabolite of diazepam that was developed as a separate drug. Following diazepam administration, oxazepam is usually formed to such a minor extent that it is not quantifiable in plasma and likely contributes minimally to the therapeutic effects of diazepam. It is further metabolized to a glucuronide conjugate and excreted in the urine. By developing the drug separately as a preformed product, a major distinguishing feature of both oxazepam and lorazepam is that they are metabolized by phase II enzymes to glucuronides and then largely renally excreted as highly water-soluble compounds. This route of elimination and the characteristics of lower lipid solubility confer several major differences between the drugs. Metabolism by phase II enzymes typically means less susceptibility to drug interactions compared to drugs metabolized by phase I oxidative enzymes such as CYP3A4. Oxazepam is available in oral form. Lorazepam or oxazepam may be preferred in elderly patients or those with coexisting hepatic dysfunction as their metabolism is less affected by age and liver disease due to a metabolic profile that mostly involves glucuronidation by liver enzymes [35, 45].

10.5 Non-benzodiazepine Anxiolytics

Buspirone This drug was introduced into clinical practice in 1986 to treat generalized anxiety disorder and quickly became widely prescribed as the first non-dependence-producing anxiolytic with comparative efficacy to the benzodiazepines

[46]. The FDA approval was for generalized anxiety disorder and the drug was shown to be ineffective for panic disorder. The initial impression of its effectiveness was not sustained as it appeared that patients who were benzodiazepine naive responded better than those who were switched from a benzodiazepine to avoid an adverse drug event (drowsiness, dependence). The elimination half-life of buspirone is only about 2 h which is short for use in treating chronic anxiety and therefore the drug must be dosed multiple times per day. The drug has found other uses including reduction of marijuana use dependence and in reducing tobacco smoking. Because it lacks a perceptible antianxiety effect upon immediate administration, patients and clinicians must wait for several weeks to fully evaluate its benefits in chronic anxiety disorders. Unlike the benzodiazepines, there is less concern for pharmacodynamic interactions with dependence-producing drugs. Buspirone is often used as an alternative anxiolytic in patients who are at risk to escalate dosage and become dependent. However, this population, sometimes with an extensive history of benzodiazepine use, has reported that the therapeutic effects of buspirone are disappointing or nonexistent. For this reason, buspirone may be a good choice for patients with mild anxiety who are benzodiazepine naive.

The usual daily dose is divided into two dosage intervals using a total dose of 10–15 mg initially and not exceeding 60 mg daily. Several weeks of continuous therapy may be needed to produce full benefits at a given dosage level. Buspirone's clearance is subject to inhibition by CYP3A4 inhibition so interactions with strong inhibitors of this enzyme should be anticipated or avoided. Studies of buspirone's plasma concentration in relation to clinical effects have not found drug concentration ranges that serve as biomarkers of effect, i.e., dosage is titrated according to clinical effects. It is possible that a therapeutic plasma concentration range exists, but plasma concentrations from usual doses of buspirone are generally in the low ng/ml range, making it difficult to conduct well-designed concentration versus effect studies.

10.6 Benzodiazepine Sedative-Hypnotics

Estazolam This (1,4)-benzodiazepine was developed in the 1970s for oral administration as a sedative-hypnotic with a relatively long elimination half-life (range 8–31 h, mean of 19 h [47]. Because of this characteristic, estazolam has a liability for producing a hangover effect the morning after administration [48]. Thus, it has not been as well received as similar drugs without the carryover effect.

Flurazepam This benzodiazepine was the first specifically marketed for insomnia and was therefore highly successful, especially when considered against the major sedative-hypnotics available in the 1970s (glutethimide, ethchlorvynol, methaqualone). Flurazepam is rapidly absorbed from the gastrointestinal tract producing its maximum concentration in plasma within 30–60 min. It behaves similarly to diazepam with plasma drug concentration rapidly rising and then falling to be replaced by active metabolites that sustain and prolong the sedative effects of the parent drug. The elimination half-life of flurazepam is short, less than 2 h, but its active metabolites, *N*-1-hydroxyethylflurazepam and desalkylflurazepam have half-lives of 2–4 h and 36–100 h, respectively. The overall pharmacodynamic profile becomes one of rapid sedative effects with an intermediate metabolite to sustain sleep and a long-acting metabolite that minimizes or prevents any early morning awakening. While this profile sounds ideal, for many patients, including most elderly patients, the slow accumulate of the desalkyl metabolites causes a morning after cognitive impairment. Patients can awaken with difficulty arising due to an excessive sedation.

Temazepam Temazepam, like oxazepam, is another minor metabolite of diazepam that has been developed as a separate drug [49]. However, it has no pharmacologically active metabolites so the pharmacodynamic effects theoretically relate to only the parent drug concentration in the CNS. An initial formulation for oral administration released the drug too slowly to be effective at reducing the time to sleep onset, but this deficit was corrected to take advantage of the drug's rapid absorption in subsequent formulations [50]. Following rapid absorption, temazepam undergoes conjugation with a minor degree of demethylation giving the drug an overall elimination half-life of 3–15 h. It's clinical trial data support efficacy for both promoting sleep onset and prolonging total sleep time [51].

Triazolam This benzodiazepine is characterized by a short half-life, approximately 1.5 h, like flurazepam, but it doesn't possess long-acting metabolites. This gives it a unique profile of being able to hasten sleep onset but not provide effective sedation during the night for patients who either have middle of the night awakening or need to prolong total sleep time. This is an advantage for situations such as jet lag when only a brief treatment of insomnia is needed but presents problems if the patient must take the drug for more than a few days. Problems include development of tolerance, rebound insomnia, and dependence [52, 53]. In addition, some patients have reported a disinhibition and amnestic effect from taking triazolam. For patients naive to this drug, it is advisable to try a test dose at home or under familiar circumstances before taking a dose to induce sleep while flying or in an unfamiliar setting where awakening with disorientation may be hazardous. As triazolam is metabolized by CYP3A4, inhibitory drug-drug interactions are potential hazardous [54].

Quazepam Like other (1, 4)-benzodiazepines, quazepam was developed in the 1970s as a sedative-hypnotic. It has multiple metabolites that produce a combined pharmacodynamic profile of rapid-onset and sustained effects [55]. It is partially metabolized to desalkylflurazepam which creates a potential disadvantage of accumulation upon chronic dosing to contribute to daytime sedation [56]. This characteristic can be undesirable for some patients, especially the elderly [57]. Thus, its commercial value has been less successful than other sedative-hypnotics. Nevertheless, it has a useful profile that should be applicable to many patients. In a sleep laboratory study comparing quazepam to triazolam [58], both drugs increased total sleep time but withdrawal favored quazepam which produced less rebound insomnia. Similar to the non-benzodiazepines (zolpidem), its onset of sedative effects can be significantly impaired or eliminated if taken with food which decreases both the rate and extent of absorption [59].

10.7 Non-benzodiazepine Sedative-Hypnotics

The pharmacokinetic properties of these agents are presented in Table 10.3. Overall, these agents are rapidly absorbed with a T_{max} of under 2.0 h and possess an elimination half-life less than 3 h except for eszopiclone and suvorexant which are about 6 h and 12 h, respectively.

Eszopiclone Three similar drugs, zolpidem, zopiclone, and eszopiclone, were all marketed after the benzodiazepines and are all specific agonists at the benzodiazepine GABA-A alpha-1 subreceptor site. This confers the sedative-hypnotic properties but not anticonvulsant effects from GABA-A affinity. These drugs are all short acting and used exclusively as sedative-hypnotics. The S-enantiomer of zopiclone, eszopiclone, has about 50 times the affinity at the GABA-A receptor-binding complex than the racemic compound. It is highly metabolized, producing several active metabolites from biotransformation mediated by CYP3A4 and CYP2E1 [60]. It is well absorbed orally, but when taken with food, its absorption rate slows and is mirrored by a lesser effect on deceasing sleep onset. The dosage recommended is between 1 and 2 mg at bedtime [61].

Ramelteon This is the first successful melatonin receptor agonist to be marketed for the treatment of insomnia in 2005. While melatonin had been discovered in the early part of the twentieth century, its receptor was not cloned until the 1990s [62]. Multiple receptors are found in the central nervous system with some in the suprachiasmatic nucleus involved in circadian rhythm and sleep [62]. Ramelteon has been especially recommended for its effects on decreasing the time to sleep onset. Ramelteon is primarily metabolized by the CYP1A2 and to a minor extent, CYP2C

Table 10.3 Pharmacokinetic properties of the non-benzodiazepine sedative-hypnotics [60, 64, 67, 68–70]

Drug	T_{max} (h)	Metabolism	*V/F* (L)	T1/2 β (h)
Eszopiclone	1.6	CYP3A4, CYP2E1	132	6.0
Ramelteon	1.6	CYP1A2	N.R.	1.3
Suvorexant	2.0	CYP3A4, CYP2C19	49	12
Tasimelteon	2.0	CYP1A2, CYP3A4	56–126	1.3–3.7
Zaleplon	1.4	Aldehyde oxidase	285	1.0
Zolpidem	1.4	CYP3A4	70	2.1

T_{max} time to maximum plasma concentration, *CYP* cytochrome P450, *V/F* distribution, *L* liters, *T1/2* β elimination half-life and CYP3A4. The recommended dosage is 8 mg about 30 min before the desired bedtime [63]. Age but gender was reported to significantly affect drug clearance as the elderly had a much lower ramelteon mean clearance (384 ± 84 ml/min/kg vs. 883 ± 175 ml/min/kg, $p < 0.01$) [64].

Suvorexant This agent is the first in class as a distinct pharmacologic for the treatment of insomnia. Suvorexant is an orexin receptor antagonist where orexin neurons have been located in the lateral hypothalamus. Receptor antagonism is suggested to promote sleep by blocking the brain's orexin-mediated wake system, enabling transition to sleep [65]. Suvorexant pharmacokinetic properties are shown in Table 10.3. The FDA recommended cautious dose escalation in obese females with a noted increase in suvorexant area under the plasma concentration time curve (AUC) and C_{max} by 46 % and 25 %, respectively [66]. Suvorexant 40 and 150 mg lacked significant effects on respiration during sleep as measured by oxygen saturation and promoted sleep efficiency [65].

Tasimelteon A slight change in the structure of ramelteon results in tasimelteon. This drug is a melatonin receptor MT1 and MT2 agonist specifically recommended for a diagnosis of disturbances in the sleep-wake cycle [67]. This agent is available only in a 20 mg capsule and is metabolized extensively by CYP1A2 and CYP3A4 and prone to many significantly drug-drug interactions. When taken with a high-fat meal, the agent's T_{max} and C_{max} was increased by and reduced by 1.75 h and 44 %, respectively. Therefore, tasimelteon is recommended to be taken without food [66]. Hepatic or renal impairment was shown not to significantly alter tasimelteon disposition, and dosage adjustments were not suggested [68].

Zaleplon With a biological half-life of only 1–1.5 h, zaleplon is used primarily to reduce difficulty in falling asleep. It can be expected to be less effective or not effective at eliminating early morning awakening or prolonging sleep time. Zaleplon is metabolized by the aldehyde oxidase and CYP3A4 [70]. Its potency and rapid onset of effects are reasons to use lower doses in the elderly and only administer for bedtime use [61].

Zolpidem With a biological half-life of 2–3 h, zolpidem should be nearly as effective as zaleplon at reducing sleep latency but also provide some degree of benefit for middle of the night awakening. Zolpidem is metabolized by CYP3A4 and other CYP enzymes [71]. Like triazolam, zolpidem has numerous anecdotal reports of causing disinhibition reactions and loss of memory for the time around drug administration. These problems seem to be present in a greater degree in women and in the elderly [72]. Females were found to have zolpidem concentrations significantly greater than males C_{max}/dose ($p < 0.001$) and AUC/dose ($p < 0.001$), but weight-normalized clearance and elimination half-life did not reach significance [72]. A lower dosage recommendation for females was FDA approved.

10.8 Clinical Pharmacodynamic Modeling

Benzodiazepines produce these PD effects of antiepileptic and anxiolytic actions, muscle relaxation, and sedation [61]. Benzodiazepines also can cause anterograde amnesia but each benzodiazepine may produce different dose-dependent effects on various memory parameters such as immediate versus delayed recall [22]. Benzodiazepines also produce physical dependence, tolerance, and withdrawal symptoms [73]. Non-benzodiazepine sedative-hypnotics are designed for sleep disorders such as insomnia and non-24 h sleep-wake disorder. Except for physical dependence and antiepileptic activity, benzodiazepines and non-benzodiazepine agents have been extensively modeled for their PD effects.

The kinetics of a PD response has been previously described as a link from a drug's pharmacokinetic properties where the E_{max} and sigmoidal E_{max} models evolved with hysteresis loops for drug efficacy and tolerance developed [74]. Diazepam free plasma concentrations were correlated to the digit symbol substitution test (DSST), and wheel tracking indicated a tolerance hysteresis loop development which matches its memory impairment and sedative action [75]. A further extensive study reported that alprazolam and diazepam but not lorazepam showed development of acute tolerance that was related to the drug concentrations [76]. Alprazolam single doses of 2, 4, 8, and 10 mg were given to healthy volunteers and the medication displayed linear pharmacokinetic properties. Alprazolam's PD effects reported a concentration-effect curve to a clockwise hysteresis loop related to the distribution rate into the systemic circulation [77]. Pharmacokinetic and PD models have been evaluated with various benzodiazepines [78–80]. Lorazepam PD was reported to have significant effects on memory impairment in the elderly without significant actions on mood, sedation, or anxiety [81]. Benzodiazepines, when used in the elderly, should be prudently prescribed with a careful assessment of their risks and benefits.

Both zaleplon and zolpidem were found to have dose and concentration-dependent PD effects on the DSST scores and other psychomotor actions in adult healthy volunteers [82]. Zaleplon, zolpidem, and eszopiclone were reported to have a lesser effect than the benzodiazepines on memory impairment [70]. Significantly greater zolpidem concentrations were reported for elderly males and females compared to adult healthy volunteers (AUC 40 %, elderly females and 31 % elderly males, $p<0.01$) [83]. A recent survey in emergency departments reported that persons >65 years taking zolpidem had the highest rates of adverse events when evaluated in the emergency room [84]. As previously indicated, adult females also had significantly higher zolpidem serum concentrations than adult males [72]. The PD effects were assessed by the DSST, reaction times, and memory tests. Zolpidem doses of 1, 1.75, and 3.5 mg led to dose-dependent impairment in all PD effects, and these enhanced PD actions (e.g., reduced DSST scores) were more pronounced in the female group compared to the male group. Based upon the pharmacokinetic and PD effects of zolpidem on females, the FDA recommended that lower doses be prescribed in the package insert. Therefore, both age and gender play a significant role in zolpidem disposition and PD actions. Careful patient monitoring is needed for these agents when used in females and the elderly population.

10.9 Conclusions and Future Directions

The value of pharmacokinetics and PD are often conceived as deriving from knowing a desired plasma drug concentration range is a target for designing drug dosage regimens. This is particularly useful when linearity of metabolism is maintained with increasing total amount of daily dose. Substantial experimental evidence exists for linear pharmacokinetics of benzodiazepines across the usual daily dose range. Under these conditions, if half the desired plasma concentration is produced from a given dose, then the target concentration should be achieved by doubling the dose. However, for the anxiolytics and sedative-hypnotics, the results of plasma concentration versus PD effect studies have not identified rigorous target concentration ranges associated with optimal therapeutic effects.

However, there remains value in knowing the general characteristics of a drug's pharmacokinetics. Knowledge of metabolic pathways and a drug's affinity for inhibiting or inducing drug-metabolizing enzymes can be valuable in avoiding drug-drug interactions. The elimination half-life is especially useful in guiding the time between dosage adjustments that are necessary for the patient to reach a new steady state following either an increase or decrease in daily drug dosage.

The necessity of sleep for maintenance of health appears to be an absolute requirement in all members of the animal kingdom. The variability in the temporal patterns of sleep is broad, from quick naps to hibernation. The species variability can be astounding. What appears to be a universal characteristic is that deprivation of sleep eventually leads to a deterioration of the organism's functioning and if maintained for a sufficient period, can even lead to death. However, the ability to go for long periods without sleep is beneficial for the survival of many organisms, but eventually sleep must occur. During the past two centuries, humans have been drawn to and have exploited chemical means of both increasing and decreasing sleep, usually for the purpose of improving performance or promoting health.

The use of prescription and nonprescription drugs to treat sleep disorders is extensive in the USA and most countries around the world. As the FDA requires that new drugs introduced into the market in the USA be safe and effective, then a substantial research effort is expended to develop these compounds. The proper use of these drugs requires an extensive knowledge of pharmacology, physiology, medicine, and other aspects of health that are influenced by the ingestion of the sedative-hypnotics. They are certainly not without potential harm and have been a favorite for suicide attempts by drug overdose historically.

The specific indications for use of benzodiazepine drugs shown in Table 10.2 have developed as a result of specific marketing efforts by manufacturers in a desire to differentiate products when more than one benzodiazepine were developed by the same company. Other influences included the period of time in the development of the drug class when a new molecule appeared and the desire to expand the market with new drugs for new indications rather than repurposing existing drugs for additional uses. The specificity has also been guided to some extent by the differences in metabolism of a few drugs. For example, flurazepam and oxazepam which are glucuronidated after absorption as their major pathway for disposition from the body confers some stability in the range of clearance for patients with hepatic disease, advanced alcohol abuse, or aging. Also, the presence of pharmacologically active metabolites has served as a basis for choosing one drug over another. Finally, the inherent rate at which some drugs are absorbed from the gastrointestinal tract may be faster than others thus conferring a more desirable profile as a sedative-hypnotic.

Although the benzodiazepines' dominance of the market for conditions requiring antianxiety effects or sedation has been overwhelming, a few compounds have been developed that have found a place in pharmacotherapy. These include buspirone as an oral anxioloytic and suvorexant, ramelteon, and tasimelteon for sedation. The "Z" drugs, eszopiclone, zaleplon, and zolpidem, have gained wide acceptance for their use in the treatment of acute and chronic insomnia.

References

1. Ban TA (2001) Pharmacotherapy of mental illness. A historical analysis. Prog Neuropsychopharmacol Biol Psychiatry 25:709–727
2. Wick JY (2013) The history of benzodiazepines. Consult Pharm 28:538–548
3. Greenblatt DJ, Shader RI, Divoll M, Harmatz JS (1981) Benzodiazepines: a summary of pharmacokinetic properties. Br J Clin Pharmacol 11(suppl):11–16
4. Garzone PD, Kroboth PD (1989) Pharmacokinetics of the newer benzodiazepines. Clin Pharmacokinet 16:337–364
5. Wang JS, DeVane CL (2003) Pharmacokinetics and drug interactions of the sedative hypnotics. Psychopharmacol Bull 37:10–29
6. Strang J, Griffiths P, Gossop M (1997) Heroin smoking by chasing the dragon: origins and history. Addiction 92:673–684
7. Sourkes TL (1992) Early clinical neurochemistry of CNS-active drugs Chloral hydrate. Mol Chem Neuropathol 17:21–30
8. Lopez-Munoz F, Ucha-Udabe R, Alamo C (2005) The history of barbiturates a century after their clinical introduction. Neuropsychiatr Dis Treat 1(4):329–343
9. Welsh-Huggins A. Key death penalty drug discontinued by US maker. NBC News, 21 Jan 2011. www.nbcnews.com/id/41196734. Accessed 20 Aug 2015
10. Morselli PL, Franco-Morselli R (1980) Clinical pharmacokinetics of antiepileptic drugs in adults. Pharmacol Ther 10:65–101
11. Solomon F, White CC, Parron DL et al (1979) Sleeping pills, insomnia and medical practice. N Engl J Med 300:803–808
12. Allen MD, Greenblatt DJ, Noel BJ (1977) Meprobamate overdosage: a continuing problem. Clin Toxicol 11:501–515
13. Powell LW, Mann GT, Kaye S (1958) Acute meprobamate poisoning. N Eng J Med 259:716–718

14. Elsohly MA, Salamone SJ (1999) Prevalence of drugs used in cases of alleged sexual assault. J Anal Toxicol 23:141–146
15. Tietz EL, Rosenberg HC, Chiu TH (1969) A comparison of the anticonvulsant effects of 1,4- and 1,5-benzodiazepines in the amygdala-kindled rats and their effects on motor function. Epilepsy Res 3:31–43
16. Gable RS (1993) Toward a comparative overview of dependence potential and acute toxicity of psychoactive substances used nonmedically. Am J Drug Alcohol Abuse 19:263–281
17. World Health Organization, Essential medicines. Accessed 123 May 2015. http://www.who.int/medicines/publications/essentialmedicines/en/index.html
18. DeVane CL (2008) Principles of pharmacokinetics and pharmacodynamics. In: Schatzberg AF, Nemeroff CB (eds) Textbook of psychopharmacology, 4th ed. American Psychiatric Publishing, Inc, Washington DC.
19. Dusci LJ, Good SM, Hall RW, Iiett KF (1990) Excretion of diazepam and its metabolites in human milk during withdrawal from combination high dose diazepam and oxazepam. Br J Clin Pharmacol 29:123–126
20. Squires RF, Braestrup C (1977) Benzodiazepine receptors in rat brain. Nature 266:732–734
21. Johnstone GA (1996) GABA-A receptor pharmacology. Pharmacol Ther 69:173–198
22. Schraf MB, Fletcher K, Graham JP (1988) Comparative amnestic effects of benzodiazepine hypnotic agents. J Clin Psychiatry 49:134–137
23. Laurijssens BE, Greenblatt DJ (1996) Pharmacokinetic-pharmacodynamic relationships for benzodiazepines. Clin Pharmacokinet 30:52–76
24. Ballenger JC, Burrows GD, DuPont RL Jr et al (1988) Alprazolam in panic disorder and agoraphobia: results from a multicenter trial. Arch Gen Psychiatry 45:413–422
25. Sheehan DV, Sheehan KH, Raj BA (2007) The speed of onset of action of alprazolam-XR compared to alprazolam-CT in panic disorder. Psychopharmacol Bull 40:63–81
26. Dupont RI, Swinson RP, Ballenger JC et al (1992) Discontinuation of alprazolam after long-term treatment of panic-related disorders. J Clin Psychiatry 12:352–354
27. Tesar GE, Rosenbaum JF, Pollack MH et al (1991) Double-blind, placebo-controlled comparison of clonazepam and alprazolam for panic disorder. J Clin Psychiatry 52:69–76
28. Scavone JM, Greenblatt DJ, Shader RI (1987) Alprazolam kinetics following sublingual and oral administration. J Clin Psychopharmacol 7:332–334
29. Greenblatt DJ, Wright CE (1993) Clinical pharmacokinetics of alprazolam. Therapeutic implications. Clin Pharmacokinet 24:453–471
30. Fyer AJ, Liebowitz MR, Gorman JM, Campeas R et al (1987) Discontinuation of alprazolam treatment in panic patients. Am J Psychiatry 144:303–308
31. DeVane CL, Ware MR, Lydiard RB (1991) Pharmacokinetics, pharmacodynamics, and treatment issues of benzodiazepines: alprazolam, adinazolam, and clonazepam. Psychopharmacol Bull 27:463–473
32. Rickels K, Feighner JP, Smith WT (1985) Alprazolam, amitriptyline, doxepin, and placebo in the treatment of depression. JAMA Psychiatry 42:134–141
33. McKeon A, Frye MA, Delanty N (2008) The alcohol withdrawal syndrome. J Neurol Neurosurg Psychiatry 79:854–862
34. Greenblatt DJ, Shader RI, MacLeod SM, Sellers EM, Franke K, Giles HG (1978) Absorption of oral and intramuscular chlordiazepoxide. Eur J Clin Pharmacol 13:267–274
35. Wilkinson GR (1978) The effects of liver disease and aging on the disposition of diazepam, chlordiazepoxide, oxazepam and lorazepam in man. Acta Psychiatr Scand 58(Suppl274):56–74
36. Conry JA, Ng YT, Paolicchi JM et al (2009) Clobazam in the treatment of Lennox-Gastaut syndrome. Epilepsia 50:1158–1166
37. Wildin JD, Pleuvry BJ, Mawer GE, Onon T, Millington L (1990) Respiratory and sedative effects of clobazam and clonazepam in volunteers. Br J Clin Pharmacol 29:169–177
38. McKernan RM, Rosahl TW, Reynolds DS et al (2000) Sedative but not anxiolytic properties of benzodiazepines are mediated by the GABA-A receptor alpha1 subtype. Nat Neurosci 3(6):587–592

39. Vajda FJ, Lewis SJ, Harris QL, Jarsrott B, Young NA (1987) Tolerance to the anticonvulsant effects of clonazepam and clobazam in the amygdaloid kindled rat. Clin Exp Neurol 23:155–164
40. Crestani F, Low K, Keist R, Mandelli MJ et al (2001) Molecular targets for the myorelaxant action of diazepam. Mol Pharmacol 59:442–445
41. Jick H, Miettinen OS, Shapiro S, Lewis GP et al (1970) Comprehensive drug surveillance. JAMA 213:1455–1460
42. Greenblatt DJ, Shader RI (1974) Benzodiazepines. N Engl J Med 291:1011–1015
43. Reves JG, Fragen RJ, Vinik HR, Greenblatt DG (1985) Midazolam: pharmacology and uses. Anesthesiology 62:310–324
44. Spina SP, Ensom MH (2007) Clinical pharmacokinetic monitoring of midazolam in critically ill patients. Pharmacotherapy 27:389–398
45. Salzman C, Shader RI, Greenblatt DJ, Harmatz JS (1983) Long v short half-life benzodiazepines in the elderly: kinetics and clinical effects of diazepam and oxazepam. Arch Gen Psychiatry 40:294–297
46. Jann MW (1988) Buspirone: an update on a unique anxiolytic agent. Pharamacotherapy 8:100–116
47. Allen MD, Greenblatt DJ, Arnold JD (1979) Single and multiple dose kinetics of estazolam, a triazolo benzodiazepine. Psychopharmacology 66:267–274
48. Roehrs T, Zorick F, Lord N et al (1983) Dose related effects of estazolam on sleep of patients with insomnia. J Clin Psychopharmacol 3:152–156
49. DeVane CL (1981) Temazepam evaluation. Pharmacotherapy 1:12
50. Fuccella LM (1979) Bioavailability of temazepam in soft gelatin capsules. Br J Clin Pharmacol 8:31S–35S
51. Bixler EO, Kales A, Soldatos CR, SAcharf MB et al (1978) Effectiveness of temazepam with short-intermediate, and long-term use sleep laboratory evaluation. J Clin Pharmacol 18:110–118
52. Kales A, Scharf MB, Kales JD, Soldatos CR (1979) Rebound insomnia. A potential hazard following withdrawal of certain benzodiazepines. JAMA 241:1692–1695
53. Griffiths RR, Johnson MW (2005) Relative abuse liability of hypnotic drugs: a conceptual framework and algorithm for differentiating among compounds. J Clin Psychiatry 66(Suppl 9):31–41
54. Varhe A, Olkkola KT, Neuvoven PJ (1994) Oral triazolam is potentially hazardous to patients receiving systemic antimycotics ketoconazole or itraconazole. Clin Pharmacol Ther 56:601–607
55. Kales A, Sharf M, Bixler EO et al (1981) Dose response studies with quazepam. Clin Pharmacol Ther 30:194–200
56. Chung M, Hilbertt JM, Gural RP, Radwanski E et al (1984) Multi-dose quazepam kinetics. Clin Pharmacol Ther 35:520–524
57. Roth TG, Roehrs TA, Koshorek GL, Greenblatt DJ, Rosenthal LD (1997) Hypnotic effects of low doses of quazepam in older insomniacs. J Clin Psychopharmacol 17:401–406
58. Mamelak M, Csima A, Price V (1984) A comparative 25 night sleep laboratory study on the effects of quazepam and triazolam on chronic insomniacs. J Clin Pharmacol 24:65–75
59. Yasui-Furukori N, Takahata T, Kondo T et al (2004) Time effects of food intake on the pharmacokinetics and pharmacodynamics of quazepam. Br J Clin Pharmacol 55:382–388
60. Najib J (2006) Eszopiclone, a nonbenzodiazepine sedative-hypnotic agent for the treatment of transient and chronic insomnia. Clin Ther 28:491–516
61. Dopp JM, Phillips BG et al (2014) Sleep disorders. In: DiPiro JT, Talbert RL, Yee GC (eds) Pharmacotherapy: a pathophysiologic approach, 9th edn. McGraw Hill, New York, pp 1115–1126
62. De Bodinat C, Guardiola-Lemaitre B, Mocaer E, Renard P et al (2010) Agomelatine, the first melatonergic antidepressant discovery, characterization and development. Nat Rev Drug Discov 9:628–642

63. Rajaratnam SMW, Cohen DA, Rogers NL (2009) Melatonin and melatonin analogues. Sleep Med Clin 4:179–193
64. Karim A, Tolbert D, Cao C (2006) Disposition kinetics and tolerance of escalating single doses of ramelton, a high-affinity MT1 and MT2 melatonin receptor agonist indicated for insomnia. J Clin Pharmacol 46:140–148
65. Greenblatt DJ, Harmatz JS, Karim A (2007) Age and gender effects on the pharmacokinetics and pharmacodynamics of ramelton, a hypnotic agent acting via melatonin receptors MT1 and MT2. J Clin Pharmacol 47:485–496
66. Uemura N, McCrea J, Sun H et al (2015) Effects of orexin receptor antagonist suvorexant on respiration during sleep in healthy subjects. J Clin Pharmacol 55:1093–1100
67. Patel KV, Aspesi AV, Evoy KE (2015) Suvorexant: a dual orexin receptor antagonist for the treatment of sleep onset and sleep maintenance insomnia. Ann Pharmacother 49:477–483
68. Bonacci JM, Venci JV, Gandhi MA (2015) Tasimelteon (Hetlioz™): a new melatonin receptor agonist for the treatment of non-24-hour sleep wake disorder. J Pharm Pract 28:473–478
69. Torres R, Kramer WG, Baroldi P (2015) Pharmacokinetics of the dual melatonin receptor agonist tasimelteon in subjects with hepatic or renal impairment. J Clin Pharmacol 55:525–533
70. Drover DR (2004) Comparative pharmacokinetics and pharmacodynamics of short-acting hypnosedatives – zaleplon, zolpidem, and zopiclone. Clin Pharmacokinet 43:227–238
71. Von Moltke LL, Greenblatt DJ, Granda BW et al (1999) Zolpidem metabolism in vitro: responsible cytochromes, chemical inhibitors, and in vivo correlations. Br J Clin Pharmacol 48:89–97
72. Greenblatt DJ, Harmatz JS, Singh NN et al (2013) Gender differences in pharmacokinetics and pharmacodynamics of zolpidem following sublingual administration. J Clin Pharmacol 54:282–290
73. Wolf B, Griffiths RR (1991) Physicial dependence on benzodiazepines: differences within the class. Drug Alcohol Depend 29:153–156
74. Holford NHG, Sheiner LB (1982) Kinetics of pharmacologic response. Pharmacol Ther 16:143–166
75. Ellinwood EH, Nikaido A, Heatherly D (1984) Diazepam: prediction of pharmacodynamics from pharmacokinetics. Psychopharmacology 83:297–298
76. Ellinwwod EH, Heatherly DGH, Nikaido AM et al (1985) Comparative pharmacokinetics and pharmacodynamics of lorazepam, alprazolam, and diazepam. Psychopharmacology 86:392–399
77. Wright CE, Sisson TL, Fleishaker JG, Antal EJ (1997) Pharmacokinetics and psychomotor performance of alprazolam: concentration-effect relationship. J Clin Pharmacol 37:321–329
78. Gupta SK, Ellinwood EH, Nikaido AM, Heatherly DG (1990) Simultaneous modeling of the pharmacokinetic and pharmacodynamic properties of benzodiazepines. I Lorazepam. J Pharmacokinet Biopharm 18:89–102
79. Gupta SK, Ellinwood EH, Nikaido AM, Heatherly DG (1990) Simultaneous modeling of the pharmacokinetic and pharmacodynamic properties of benzodiazepines. II Triazolam. Pharm Res 7:570–576
80. Dos Santos FM, Goncalves JC, Caminta R et al (2009) Pharmacokinetic/pharmacodynamics modeling of psychomotor impairment induced by oral clonazepam in healthy volunteers. Ther Drug Monit 31:566–574
81. Pomara N, Lee SH, Bruno D et al (2015) Adverse performance effects of acute lorazepam administration in elderly long-term users: pharmacokinetic and clinical predictors. Prog Neuropsychopharmacol Biol Psychiatry 56:129–135
82. Greenblatt DJ, Harmatz JS, von Moltke LL et al (1998) Comparative kinetics and dynamics of zaleplon, zolpidem, and placebo. Clin Pharmacol Ther 64:553–561
83. Greenblatt DJ, Harmatz JS, Singh NN et al (2014) Pharmacokinetics of zolpidem from sublingual zolpidem tartrate tablets in healthy elderly versus non-elderly subjects. Drugs Aging 31:731–736
84. Hampton LM, Daubresse M, Chang H-Y, Alexander GC, Budnitz DS (2015) Surveillance of advertise psychiatric medication events. JAMA Psychiatry 313:1256–1257

Chapter 11
Opioid Analgesics

Sally K. Guthrie and Christian Teter

Abstract Opioid analgesics represent a major therapeutic approach to pain management but challenge clinicians and healthcare systems for appropriate usage and long-term patient benefits. Opioids can be full agonists and partial agonists–antagonists for therapeutic effects that involve the mu, kappa, and delta opioid receptors. Opioids can be administered by different routes that include intravenous, intramuscular, oral, sublingual, transdermal, nasal spray, and rectal suppositories. Opioids can be short-acting and medium-acting agents based upon their elimination half-life that requires multiple daily dosing regimens. Sustained-release formulations have been developed for several opioids. The transdermal formulation allows for once-daily application. Some opioids are metabolized by the CYP enzyme system, while other opioids are primarily metabolized via glucuronidation. Depending upon the opioid, these agents are metabolized to active metabolites that possess analgesic effects that can be greater than, equal to, or less than the parent drug. Morphine has been the prototypical opioid analgesic agent and its pharmacokinetic and pharmacodynamic profile extensively studied in various patient populations. Besides their therapeutic analgesic effects, opioids can produce a variety of adverse effects related to their pharmacokinetic and pharmacodynamic actions that includes physical dependence, tolerance, respiratory depression, cardiovascular effects, sedation, cognitive impairment, gastrointestinal effects, histamine effects, and miosis. An integrated pharmacokinetic–pharmacodynamic approach to opioid treatment can lead to its optimal pharmacotherapy.

Keywords Opioid • Receptors • Short acting • Medium acting • Formulations • Analgesia • Respiratory depression • Cardiovascular effects • Tolerance • Dependence

---

S.K. Guthrie, PharmD (✉)
Department of Clinical Pharmacy, College of Pharmacy, University of Michigan, Ann Arbor, MI, USA
e-mail: salgut@med.umich.edu

C. Teter, PharmD
Department of Pharmacy Practice, University of New England, Portland, ME, USA
e-mail: cteter@une.edu

M. Jann et al. (eds.), *Applied Clinical Pharmacokinetics and Pharmacodynamics of Psychopharmacological Agents*,
DOI 10.1007/978-3-319-27883-4_11

11.1 Introduction

The term "opioids" encompasses all agents that bind to opioid receptors and includes endogenous opioids, such as met- and leu-enkephalin, and dynorphin, as well as exogenous opioids. The endogenous opioid system includes mu (μ), kappa (κ), and delta (δ) receptors, and opioids may act as agonists, partial agonists, or antagonists at any one or combination of these receptors [1, 2].

Morphine, the gold standard opioid, is derived from the opium poppy. Opium is one of the oldest known drugs, with reports of use going back to ~3400 BC when opium was cultivated in Southwest Asia (www.deamuseum.org/ccp/opium.history.html). Both morphine and codeine, as well as a third compound, thebaine, are present in the opium poppy resin collected from the seed pods of the opium poppy, *Papaver somniferum*. Additional opioids have been fashioned by slightly altering the basic morphine structure or, more recently, by designing and synthesizing drugs that are engineered to bind to the opioid receptors. Although drugs may act as agonists, antagonists, or partial agonists at the opioid receptors, this chapter will only discuss drugs that are used as analgesics and possess either agonist or partial agonist activity at the μ receptor. Opioid antagonists such as naloxone and naltrexone are presented in Chap. 14.

Many, but not all, opioids bear structural and pharmacological resemblance to morphine. Semisynthetic opioids are created by slightly altering the structure of morphine, and new synthetic opioids are designed to fit the structure of opioid receptors although the actual structure may bear little resemblance to morphine itself [2]. Semisynthetic or synthetic opioids include heroin, hydromorphone, oxymorphone, levorphanol, hydrocodone, oxycodone, meperidine, and methadone. The very short-acting synthetic opioids that are commonly used in surgical analgesia (fentanyl, sufentanil, remifentanil, and alfentanil) are presented in Chap. 15. A third group of commonly used opioids is composed of drugs that are used as analgesics and have μ agonist, partial agonist, or antagonist activity but also have activity at other opioid receptors (usually κ agonist activity), including butorphanol and buprenorphine. Lastly, there are opioid medications with activity via non-opioid mechanisms (e.g., tramadol acting at monoamine transporters) that are included in this chapter.

The first part of this chapter will focus on the opioid clinical pharmacokinetics (PK), and the second section will present the pharmacodynamics (PD), followed lastly by a discussion of PK–PD modeling.

11.2 Clinical Pharmacokinetics

11.2.1 Absorption

Opioids are administered using a variety of routes, depending on the indication for their use. While intravenous (IV) administration delivers the entire amount of drug into the venous blood, a nonparenteral route may not deliver the entire dose of drug into the system circulation but is often necessary for treatment of pain. Nonparenteral routes may include oral, rectal, sublingual, intranasal, transdermal, or pulmonary inhalation. The most commonly used and easiest nonparenteral route of administration for the opioids is the oral route.

The oral bioavailability of opioids is a major determinant for their preferred use. Agents that have higher oral bioavailability and a longer duration of action are more suitable for the management of patients with chronic pain. The clinical PK of the opioids is presented in Table 11.1. The opioids are well absorbed in the gastrointestinal tract via a passive process, but none of the opioids are 100 % bioavailable. Although some agents (morphine, methadone, fentanyl) act as substrates for the P-glycoprotein efflux pump located at the gastrointestinal wall and the blood–brain barrier, this physiological barrier decreases their absorption and entrance into the brain as these agents must cross these membranous barriers [3, 4]. The opioids undergo some degree of first-pass hepatic metabolism limiting their oral bioavailability, which ranges from <20 % up to 80 % and is a source of the large interindividual variability. The opioids that exhibit ≥60 % oral bioavailability are hydromorphone, methadone, and tramadol. The oral bioavailability is generally <60 % for codeine, dihydrocodeine, and oxymorphone and unknown for hydrocodone. However, these opioids are often orally administered, and increasing doses are used to compensate for low bioavailability. Buccal or sublingual bioavailability of buprenorphine and fentanyl is superior to the oral route of administration.

Methadone oral bioavailability shows significant intersubject variability, ranging from 36 to 100 %, but averages around 75 %. The C_{max} occurs between 2.5 and 4 h following oral administration, although a second peak may be seen in some individuals (usually at about 4 h) due to enterohepatic recirculation [5]. Oral absorption rates are comparable from tablets, quick-dissolving tablets, and liquid solution formulation [6].

Tramadol is rapidly absorbed following a single oral administration of 100 mg, with peak concentrations occurring from 1.6 to 1.9 h. While intestinal absorption is probably 100 %, first-pass metabolism in the liver reduces oral bioavailability to about 70 %. Following multiple daily 100 mg doses of tramadol, the bioavailability increases to 90–100 % (C_{max} increases by 16 % and area under the curve [AUC] increases by 36 %, compared to a single 100 mg dose), possibly due to the saturation of first-pass metabolism [7]. Tramadol bioavailability is increased following a high-fat meal, although the resulting 10 % increase in AUC is not considered clinically relevant [8].

Like tramadol, absorption pharmacokinetic parameters of oral oxycodone are altered by a high-fat meal with an increase in AUC of about 20 % accompanied by a concurrent decrease in T_{max} to approximately 47–91 % compared to the control (fasting administration) group [9].

The oral bioavailability of the short-acting opioids is quite low (fentanyl, remifentanil, alfentanil, and sufentanil) and, except for fentanyl, these drugs are always administered intravenously. Fentanyl undergoes a high degree of first-pass metabolism with bioavailability approximating ~30 % after rapid swallowing [10]. Fentanyl is available in a variety of different formulations that will be discussed later in the Alternative Formulations section of this chapter.

Table 11.1 Opioid oral bioavailability

Drug	Fraction bioavailable (F)	T_{max} (time of maximum concentration)
Medium–long acting		
Codeine	42–71 % (mean 53 %) [11]	1.3 ± 0.22 h [12]
Dihydrocodeine	20.6–19.7 % [13]	3.84–4.46 h [13]
Heroin	Negligible [14]	–
Hydrocodone	Possibly high [15]	3.5–7 h [15]
Hydromorphone	65 ± 33 % [16]	1.00 ± 0.27 h [16]
Levorphanol	–	~1.5 h [17]
Meperidine	48–63 % (mean 56 %) [18]	1.3 h [19]
Methadone	70–80 % [5]	2.5–4 h [5]
Morphine	19–47 % [20–22]	0.5–1.5 h [20, 23–25]
Oxycodone	60 ± 20 % [26]	0.5–1 h [26]
Oxymorphone	~10 % [27]	0.5 h [27]
Tramadol	70 % [28]	1.6–1.9 h [28]
Short acting		
Fentanyl	32 ± 10 % [10]	101 ± 48.8 min [10]
Partial agonist–antagonist		
Buprenorphine	~15 % or less [29]	–
Butorphanol	17 % [30]	1–1.5 h [30]

The oral bioavailability of the agonist/antagonists, buprenorphine and butorphanol, is about 10 %. Buprenorphine is widely used as a sublingual film or tablet, which displays a higher bioavailability of ~20–80 %. Both buprenorphine and butorphanol are available in nonparenteral formulations that will be discussed more in the Alternative Formulations section of this chapter.

11.2.2 Distribution

After absorption, most opioids distribute widely in the body, and distribution is affected by differences in tissue and plasma protein binding and permeability across tissue membranes [31]. Opioids are bound to plasma proteins to varying degrees, and those with the lowest plasma protein binding have volumes of distribution (V_d) in the 2–5 L/kg range. Lipophilicity is often correlated with a high degree of plasma protein binding. As seen in Table 11.2, opioids with the highest plasma protein binding are often used in surgical anesthesia where a rapid onset of effect (i.e., rapid entry into the brain) occurs.

All opioids bind to albumin, while some drugs also bind to alpha$_1$ acid glycoprotein (α_1 AGP) and to lipoproteins. While opioids display non-saturable plasma protein binding, the fraction bound to plasma proteins may vary depending on the presence of disease or other physical stress if the opioid binds to α_1 AGP (such as methadone, alfentanil, fentanyl, and sufentanil) [32]. Since α_1 AGP is an acute-phase reactant protein, the bound fraction of drug may increase in acute disease states, such as a myocardial infarction. Methadone exhibits such low plasma protein binding that any physiologic changes in plasma protein binding would cause a minimal change in the total drug concentration. Most of the opioids have low to moderate hepatic clearance. The actual free drug concentration will not be changed by alterations in the fraction of plasma protein binding. However, both fentanyl and sufentanil are high hepatic clearance drugs, and changes in plasma protein binding are associated with changes in free concentration and possibly with changes in pharmacodynamics [33].

In addition to plasma protein binding, opioid drug distribution is governed by the octanol coefficient, which is a measure of lipophilicity, and the drug's pK_a (opioids are weak bases, pK_a ranging from ~6.5 to 8.7) [34–36]. Opioids are moderately to highly lipid soluble agents and generally enter the central nervous system (CNS). Also, transport through the blood–brain barrier will be influenced for the opioids that are P-glycoprotein substrates.

The shorter-acting opioids, remifentanil (0.47 L/kg) and alfentanil (0.75 L/kg), have a smaller V_d, whereas butorphanol (12 L/kg) and levorphanol (10–13 L/kg) have a larger V_d than most of the opioids. A relatively small V_d, combined with relatively high lipid solubility, results in a rapid onset of effect for remifentanil, alfentanil, sufentanil, and alfentanil. All four drugs undergo a significant redistribution phase when the drugs move out of the blood stream and into adipose and the duration of action correlates better with the redistribution than the actual elimination phase since elimination occurs after the drugs have leeched out of the adipose reserves. Because of redistribution, the pharmacokinetic parameters differ following a short bolus injection in comparison to a longer infusion. Following a short bolus, the accumulation of drug in adipose is small, and it is difficult to accurately measure the small concentration that is present during the terminal elimination phase. Conversely, following a longer infusion, more drug will be stored in the adipose deposits, leading to an increase in the measurable V_d. Also, the drug will need to leech out of the adipose prior to elimination. Consequently, the measurable elimination $T½$ is longer following an infusion than following a bolus injection, although practically speaking, with the short-acting opioids, the duration of action is a more clinically significant parameter than the elimination $T½$. The PK parameters are reported in Table 11.2 via a bolus IV injection.

11.2.3 Metabolism

All opioids undergo hepatic metabolism prior to their elimination via both Phase I and Phase II metabolism. Table 11.2 includes opioid metabolites that are inactive, but others possess significant analgesic activity, while several agents possess significant neurotoxic activity [2].

Table 11.2 Opioid pharmacokinetic parameters

Drug	Protein binding fraction bound	Volume of distribution	Metabolites	Clearance	% Cleared renally unchanged parent compound	Elimination *T*½
Medium–long acting						
Codeine	56.1 ± 2.5 % [37]	389 ± 157 L (V_{ss}) [37] 3.97 ± 1.20 L · kg^{-1} (V_z) [38] 3.48 ± 0.18** L · kg^{-1} (V_z) [11]	Codeine 6-glucuronide Norcodeine Norcodeine 6-glucuronide Morphine* Morphine 3-glucuronide Morphine 6-glucuronide* [39]	1.8 ± 0.49 L · kg^{-1} · h^{-1} [38] 0.73 ± 0.05** L · kg^{-1} · h^{-1} [11]	4.41 ± 1.38 % [37]	3.60 ± 0.15** h [11] 1.47 ± 0.32 h [37] 2.2 ± 0.4 h [38] 2.1 ± 0.08** h [12] 2.3 ± 0.4 h [40]
Dihydrocodeine	–	1.07 ± 0.61 L · kg^{-1} (V_{dist}) IV dose 50 mg [13]	Dihydrocodeine 6-glucuronide Nordihydrocodeine 6-glucuronide Dihydromorphine Nordihydromorphine [41]	16.74 ± 0.84 L · min^{-1} [13]	~23.5 % [42]	4.4 h extensive CYP2D6 metabolizers 5.0 h poor CYP2D6 metabolizers [43] 4.46 ± 0.24**h [13] 4.3 ± 1.3 h [44]
Heroin	61–80 % [45]	37 ± 16 L (V_{ss}) [46] 29.5 L (V_1) [47]	6-acetylmorphine* Morphine* Morphine 3-glucuronide* [14] Morphine 6-glucuronide* [47]	30.8 ± 2.1 ml · kg^{-1} · min^{-1} [14] 11.6 ± 2.8 L · min^{-1} [46]	Not detected [48]	3.0 ± 1.3 min [14] 3.0 ± 1.0 min [46] 7.6 min [44]
Hydrocodone	–	–	Hydromorphone* Norhydrocodone* Hydrocodol* Hydromorphol* [49]	664 ± 214 ml · kg^{-1} · h^{-1} in extensive CYP2D6 metabolizer and 387 ± 75 ml · kg^{-1} · h^{-1} in poor CYP2D6 metabolizers [50]	10.2 ± 1.8 % CYP2D6 extensive metabolizers and 18.1 ± 4.5 % CYP2D6 poor metabolizers [50]	4.24 ± 0.99 h CYP2D6 extensive metabolizers and 6.16 ± 1.97 h CYP2D6 poor metabolizers [50]

Hydromorphone	93 % [16, 51]	1.22 ± 0.23 L · kg^{-1} (V_d) [16]	Hydromorphone 3-glucuronide* Dihydromorphine Dihydromorphine glucuronide [52]	14.64 ± 7.60 ml · kg^{-1} · min^{-1} [53]	Only a small amount [54]	2.36 ± 0.58 h [51]
Levorphanol	40 ± 2.6 % [17]	10.1–13 L · kg^{-1} (V_{ss}) [17]	Levorphanol 3-glucuronide [17]	13.0–18.4 ml · kg^{-1} · min^{-1} [17]	–	11.2–11.6 h [17]
Meperidine	64–82 % [19]	198–333 (mean 269) L (V_{ss}) [19]	Normeperidine* Normeperidinic acid Normeperidinic acid conjugates Meperidinic acid Meperidinic acid conjugates [18, 55]	0.71–1.32 (mean 1.06) L · min^{-1} [19] 684 ± 206 ml · min^{-1} [56]	~5 % – this increases up to 70 % in acidic urine and decreases to 1 % in alkaline urine [19]	3.1–4.1 (mean 3.6) h [19]
Methadone	89.4 ± 2.9 % [57]	2–5 L · kg^{-1} (V_{ss}) [5]	2-ethylidene-1,5-dimethy-3,3 diphenylpyrrolidine (EDDP) [5] 2-ethyl-5-methyl-3,3-diphenylpyraline (EMDP) [58]	6.9 ± 1.5 L · h^{-1} (Cl/F – healthy subjects) [59]	Highly dependent on urine pH – 23.8 % (urine pH ~5.8) and 13.7 % (urine pH ~6.4) [60]	12–51 h (single dose, healthy) [5] somewhat dependent on urine pH
Morphine	35.1 ± 1.8 % [61]	279.3 ± 99.5 L (V_{area}) [20]	Morphine 3-glucuronide Morphine 6-glucuronide* Morphine 3,6-glucuronide Normorphine Normorphine 6-glucuronide Morphine 3-ethereal sulfate [62]	23.8 ± 4.0** ml · kg^{-1} · min^{-1} [24]	1.3–17 % [24]	1.9 ± 0.2** h [24]

(continued)

Table 11.2 (continued)

Drug	Protein binding fraction bound	Volume of distribution	Metabolites	Clearance	% Cleared renally unchanged parent compound	Elimination *T*½
Oxycodone	55 % [63]	2.60 ± 0.52 [64]	Noroxycodone Oxymorphone* α-/β-oxymorphol Noroxymorphone α-/β-noroxymorphol α-/β-oxycodol [65]	0.78 ± 0.2 $L \cdot min^{-1}$ [26]	8.4 ± 2.7 % [26]	4.89 ± 0.77 h [26]
Oxymorphone	88–90 % [63]	–	6-hydroxyoxymorphone oxymorphone 3-glucuronide* [66]	23.53 ± 13.18 $L \cdot min^{-1}$ (Cl/F) [67]	1.9 ± 0.7 % ** [68]	7.25 ± 4.40 h [67]
Tramadol	~20 % [69]	203 ± 40 L ($V\beta$) [28]	*N*-demethyltramadol *O*-demethyltramadol* *O*-demethyltramadol conjugates [70]	467 ± 124 $ml \cdot min^{-1av}$ [28]	12.0 ± 4.8 % [71]	5.16 ± 0.81 h [28]
Short acting						
Alfentanil	88.2 ± 3.3 % [72]	226 ± 48 $ml \cdot kg^{-1}$ (V_{ss}) [73]	Noralfentanil *N*-phenylpropionamide [74]	2.65 ± 0.90 $ml \cdot kg^{-1} \cdot min^{-1}$ [73]	~1 % [75]	84 ± 13 min [73]
Fentanyl	84.4 ± 1.9 % [76]	3.39 ± 0.20** L kg^{-1} (V_d area) [77]	Norfentanyl Despropionylfentanyl Hydroxyfentanyl Hydroxynorfentanyl [78]	956 ± 65** $ml \cdot min^{-1}$ [77]	2.1 ± 0.42 % ** [79]	219 ± 10 min** [77]
Remifentanil	92 % [80]	31.8 ± 7.4 L (V_{ss}) [81]	Remifentanil carboxylic acid metabolite *N*-dealkylremifentanil [81]	2.9 ± 0.4 $L \cdot min^{-1}$ [81]	Negligible [82]	20.47 ± 13.03 min *T*½ β [83]
Sufentanil	92.5 ± 0.7 % [76]	2.86 ± 0.25** $L \cdot kg^{-1}$ [84]	Norsufentanil Also – five additional minor metabolites [85]	12.66 ± 0.78** $ml \cdot kg^{-1} \cdot min^{-1}$ [84]	0.6 % [86]	164 ± 22 min** *T*½ β [84]

Partial agonist–antagonist						
Buprenorphine	95 ± 3 % [87]	334.9 ± 116.2** L [88]	Buprenorphine conjugate Norbuprenorphine Norbuprenorphine conjugate [89]	76.8 ± 13.1** L · h^{-1} [88]	Negligible [89]	3.21 ± 1.25 h** [88]
Butorphanol	83 % [90]	791 ± 246 L (V_{ss}) [91]	Norbutorphanol Hydroxybutorphanol Norbutorphanol conjugate Hydroxybutorphanol conjugate [90]	121 ± 31 L · h^{-1} [91]	5 % [90]	5.95 ± 1.82 h [91]

Mean ± SD (except ** Mean ± SEM)

V_{ss} volume of distribution at steady state, V_z oral apparent volume of distribution, * active metabolite

11.2.3.1 Opioids Primarily Biotransformed by Deacetylation or by the Actions of Esterases or Carboxylesterases

Remifentanil, uniquely among the opioids, is largely metabolized via extrahepatic esterases to form an inactive carboxylic acid metabolite. An additional minor amount of remifentanil is *N*-dealkylated via CYP3A4 forming an inactive metabolite. Heroin is rapidly deacetylated to 6-monacetylmorphine (6-MAM) and morphine, both very potent analgesics. 6-MAM is then deacetylated to morphine, which is metabolized as stated below.

Meperidine undergoes conversion to two main metabolites. Meperidinic acid is inactive and formed by carboxylesterase. The second metabolite, normeperidine, is mainly formed from meperidine by CYP3A4, although other pathways may be involved, including CYP2B6, CYP2D6, and CYP2C19. Normeperidine is neurotoxic and is responsible for meperidine's significant adverse effects when used for long durations or in patients with renal impairment.

11.2.3.2 Opioids Primarily Conjugated

Phase II metabolism (conjugation) is the predominant metabolic pathway for morphine, hydromorphone, oxymorphone, and levorphanol. Although conjugation often inactivates many drugs, some opioid glucuronides have significant pharmacologic activity. Morphine is predominantly metabolized to two glucuronides, morphine 3-glucuronide (M3G) and morphine 6-glucuronide (M6G). About 45–60 % of morphine is converted to M3G in humans. Although this metabolite possesses little activity, animal studies suggest that it may have neuroexcitatory activity and a hyperalgesic effect. Approximately 10–15 % of morphine is conjugated to form M6G, which possesses greater pain blocking activity than morphine itself. M6G is less lipophilic than morphine and crosses more slowly into the brain than morphine [92]. When morphine is chronically administered, the analgesic effect increases over time due to the accumulation of M6G. This compound has both a slower onset of activity and a longer elimination $T½$ than morphine (4–8 vs. 1.6–4.8 h, respectively) [92]. When morphine is used for a short duration, in patients with normal renal function, effects attributed to M3G or M6G metabolites are debatable since both are renally eliminated. The Phase I metabolism of morphine is minor with formation of the inactive *N*-demethylmorphine. A very small conversion to hydromorphone occurs, although the amount generated is likely to be clinically insignificant [93].

Similar to morphine, hydromorphone is metabolized via glucuronidation to hydromorphone 3-glucuronide, which does not have analgesic potency but is neurotoxic upon accumulation in the body. While the major metabolite for hydromorphone is a 3-glucuronide, a minor amount of hydromorphone is *N*-demethylated, probably via CYP2C9 or CYP3A4, to norhydromorphone.

Oxymorphone has a ketone at the 6-position so, unlike morphine, it cannot be conjugated at this position. The major metabolite of oxymorphone is an inactive 3-glucuronide, and a small amount of drug is hydroxylated at the 6-position to form 6-hydroxymorphone, which has some analgesic activity but is present in very small amounts.

Levorphanol is the optical isomer of dextromethorphan, but unlike dextromethorphan, there is no evidence that levorphanol is metabolized via CYP450 system. It is almost entirely biotransformed to levorphanol 3-glucuronide, and the activity of this metabolite is unknown.

11.2.3.3 Opioids Primarily Biotransformed by CYP450 Enzymes

The balance of the opioids discussed in this chapter primarily undergo Phase I metabolism and Phase II conjugation. The CYP2D6 enzyme plays an important role in the metabolism of several opioids: codeine, dihydrocodeine, hydrocodone, and tramadol [94, 95]. Some opioid metabolites possess greater pharmacologic activity than their parent compound. For instance, codeine is partially metabolized to morphine. Since codeine only possesses about one-half the analgesic potency of morphine, it is possible that the analgesic effect of codeine is largely dependent on its conversion to morphine via CYP2D6. The percentage of morphine generated from a codeine dose varies from 0.3 to 0.34 % for persons who are CYP2D6 poor metabolizers, to 4–8 % for extensive metabolizers, and up to 15.3 % in ultrarapid metabolizers [96]. Since extensive metabolizers convert from 4 to 8 % of their codeine dose to morphine, metabolites generated in this group would also include M3G, M6G, codeine 6-glucuronide, norcodeine, and norcodeine 6-glucuronide. Codeine-6-glucuronide may contribute to analgesic effects, but the two norcodeine metabolites are probably inactive.

Similar to codeine, hydrocodone is *O*-demethylated via CYP2D6 to a more potent analgesic, hydromorphone. However, the fraction converted is evidently small and the analgesic potency of the parent, hydrocodone, is high enough that CYP2D6 activity is not the major determinant of the oral hydrocodone effect [97].

Dihydrocodeine is also a CYP2D6 substrate, and it is *O*-demethylated to dihydromorphine, which has greater activity than dihydrocodeine. While the majority of dihydrocodeine is excreted as dihydrocodeine-6-glucuronide, some amount is converted to dihydromorphine. CYP450 enzymes other than CYP2D6 may be capable of converting dihydrocodeine to dihydromorphine. However, such a small fraction of dihydrocodeine is converted to dihydromorphine that the CYP2D6 polymorphism is not likely a significant factor in the analgesia seen with dihydrocodeine [43].

Tramadol is a semisynthetic codeine derivative, and formation of its major metabolite (*O*-desmethyltramadol) is mediated via CYP2D6. Poor metabolizers experience less analgesic activity because most of the μ opioid activity occurs due to the tramadol *O*-desmethyl metabolite. A less active metabolite, *N*-desmethyltramadol, is also formed via CYP2B6 and CYP3A4. Tramadol still has modest analgesic activity, even in CYP2D6 poor metabolizers [8].

The CYP3A4 enzyme is responsible for the majority of metabolism of fentanyl, alfentanil, sufentanil, and oxycodone. Alfentanil is almost exclusively metabolized to two inactive metabolites, noralfentanil and *N*-phenylpropionamide. Both fentanyl and sufentanil exhibit high hepatic extraction so, when administered intravenously, clearance is more a function of liver blood flow than hepatic enzyme activity, although both drugs are extensively metabolized to *N*-dealkylated (inactive) metabolites via CYP3A4 [33].

Oxycodone is metabolized via CYP3A4 primarily by *N*-demethylation to noroxycodone, a very weak μ agonist. About 10 % is metabolized to oxymorphone via CYP2D6, which is about 14 times more potent than morphine. However, oxycodone appears to be responsible for most of the analgesic activity since it is about seven to ten times more potent than morphine, so CYP2D6 activity has less significance for oxycodone compared to codeine [65].

Buprenorphine undergoes *N*-dealkylation via CYP3A4 to norbuprenorphine, which possesses weak analgesic activity. Additionally both buprenorphine and norbuprenorphine form 3-glucuronides and neither of these metabolites are active. Butorphanol is metabolized to hydroxybutorphanol about 60–80 % and *N*-dealkylated to norbutorphanol, probably via CYP3A4. Subsequently, small amounts of these metabolites are biotransformed to inactive glucuronide conjugates. Butorphanol undergoes high hepatic extraction, so its clearance is highly dependent on liver blood flow rather than metabolic enzyme activity.

In summary, opioids are significantly metabolized by hepatic enzymes that sometimes leads to active metabolites that are more potent than the parent compound. The importance of specific enzymatic pathways varies considerably among these drugs, and a thorough understanding of the metabolic pathways is needed to optimize patient therapy.

11.2.4 Elimination

In general, the opioids are highly metabolized, and their metabolites are largely eliminated in the urine. With the exceptions of dihydrocodeine, hydrocodone, methadone, tramadol, and meperidine (dependent upon urine pH), less than 10 % of the unchanged parent opioid is cleared in the urine (as shown in Table 11.2).

A fraction of unmetabolized methadone undergoes glomerular filtration and pH-dependent tubular reabsorption in kidney tubules. The pK_a of methadone is 9.2, which indicates more ionized drug undergoes renal clearance in acidic urine (pH less than 6). Consequently, methadone elimination *T*½ is shorter when the urine is acidic versus an alkaline state (20±4 vs. 42±9 h) [60]. It is unknown if

enters the brain. Alterations in the drug's PK administered via nasal spray might occur in the presence of rhinitis, which is usually accompanied by local histamine release and arteriole dilation in the nasal epithelium. While the effect of rhinitis on fentanyl pharmacokinetics has not been evaluated, it is possible that an increase in blood flow to the nasal epithelium might decrease time to t_{max} and increase both C_{max} and bioavailability.

Butorphanol is also available as a nasal spray. Bioavailability via nasal spray is at least twice that compared to the sublingual or buccal formulations and ranges from 69 to 71 %. When optimized with buffer strength, pH, and isotonicity, the sublingual and buccal formulations were less bioavailable by 20 % and 30 %, respectively. Additionally, the T_{max} was less than 1 h for the nasal spray, compared to over 1.5 h for the sublingual formulation. A study conducted in 18 subjects with acute or allergic rhinitis found that rhinitis did not significantly affect the t_{max}, C_{max}, or bioavailability, although concomitant administration of a topical nasal decongestant (oxymetazoline) resulted in a delay in t_{max} (0.25 versus 0.75 h) and a decrease in C_{max} 3.01 versus 1.61 ng/ml. The oxymetazoline caused vasoconstriction of nasal blood vessels that slowed the delivery of drug through the nasal mucosa, but the overall bioavailability was not altered [84].

11.2.6.3 Transdermal

Skin is composed of lipophilic keratinous stratum corneum and varies in thickness depending on the anatomical site. The extent of drug absorption through the skin is optimal for drugs characterized by small molecular weight (<500), high lipophilicity ($\log P > 2$–5), and unionized drug [104]. Environmental factors can alter the transdermal absorption of drugs. For instance, heat (possibly fever) may increase transdermal absorption, as can changes in the thickness of the dermal layer, and the skin integrity (with broken skin allowing greater absorption). Transdermal drug administration allows continuous drug input. When a drug is rapidly cleared, such as fentanyl, the absorption rate through the skin becomes the rate-limiting process for achieving steady-state concentrations.

Buprenorphine and fentanyl are both available for transdermal application, but their transdermal systems differ. Transdermal administration of fentanyl used the "transdermal therapeutic system" (TTS). The TTS uses a membrane-controlled system designed for 72 h of wear. The rectangular transdermal patch for fentanyl includes an impermeable backing layer, then a drug reservoir layer, followed by a membrane that controls the rate of diffusion of drug out of the reservoir, and finally an adhesive layer to hold the patch on to the skin. To increase the drug delivery rate and amount of drug to the body, the area of the patch is increased, resulting in 12 (5.25 cm^2), 25 (10.5 cm^2), 50 (21 cm^2), 75 (31.5 cm^2), and 100(42 cm^2) μg/h systems [112]. Small amounts of skin absorption enhancers, such as alcohol, are often added to the formulation to increase delivery of the drug through the epidermis. The fentanyl concentrates in the upper skin layers and diffuses slowly through the skin. Consequently, the onset of effect of fentanyl transdermal is slow, with detectable amounts 2 h after application. Drug diffusion from the upper skin layer is slow during the first 4 h following patch application, then increases over the next 4–8 h, and remains relatively constant during the next 16 h. After a variable lag time, ranging from 12 to 24 h (less for the larger patches), a steady-state concentration is reached and that drug concentration is maintained for approximately 24 h. Drug concentrations decrease gradually over the following 48 h, possibly due to depletion of the alcohol enhancer. Fentanyl continues to diffuse from the drug reservoir in the upper skin layers even after the patch is removed from the skin. Following removal of the patch, fentanyl clearance is very close (43.3 L/h) to the intravenous administration, but the elimination *T*½ following patch removal ranges from 13 to 25 h, probably due to continued diffusion from the epidermal reservoir [107]. After use, the patches may still contain more than 50 % of the initial amount of the drug, so appropriate disposal of the patch after use is crucial for patient and public safety. Ingestion or injection of the residual fentanyl has been linked to the accidental drug overdoses [113].

The buprenorphine patch (Butrans®) can be worn for up to 7 days. Similar to the fentanyl patch, a larger dose is provided by using a larger-sized patch, and the buprenorphine transdermal patch available in the United States is marketed in five different strengths: 5 (6.25 cm^2), 7.5 (9.375 cm^2), 10 (12.5 cm^2), 15 (18.75 cm^2), and 20 (25 cm^2) μg/h. Higher-dose transdermal systems are available in other countries. The buprenorphine transdermal system is composed of an inert backing layer and an overlapping adhesive film with a well in the center. The edges of the adhesive film extend to the skin. The active drug layer is contained in the well in the adhesive film, and a drug-polymer matrix is included in the adhesive that covers the well and adheres directly to the skin [105]. Unlike the fentanyl patch, a diffusion membrane is not included; the drug is included in a polymer matrix that diffuses directly into the skin. Using the transdermal system, a steady-state drug concentration is achieved by the third day, and the absolute bioavailability of drug from the transdermal system is approximately 15 %. After removal of the patch from the skin, the drug concentration decreases by about 50 % over the first 12 h (range 10–24 h), and buprenorphine displays a terminal elimination rate of approximately 26 h. Overall bioavailability can be affected by the site of administration (greater in upper back than on chest or patella) and body habitus, with approximately 20 % lower exposure in the elderly subjects that have a lower body fat, compared to adults with normal or high body fat. Similar to the fentanyl patch, as the body temperature increases, this factor may enhance drug absorption rate [105].

11.2.6.4 Rectal

Rectal administration can be a useful alternative when vomiting is present or when medical conditions lead to situations when the oral route of administration is not possible. However, other non-oral routes have proved more popular than rectal administration possibly due to cultural or social constraints. Similar to oromucosal route, rectal administration partially bypasses first-pass hepatic metabolism. Rectal suppository formulations are available for morphine, hydromorphone, and oxymorphone. The t_{max} for hydromorphone administered rectally is later than t_{max} following oral drug (1 h vs. 1.5 h). Similarly, the t_{max} occurs later for oxymorphone and for morphine when these agents are given rectally [53, 109, 114]. Tramadol bioavailability following rectal administration is slightly higher than oral administration (77 % vs. 70 %), and t_{max} is 3.3 h. T_{max} is delayed when compared with oral dosing [110]. For all of these drugs, PK parameters vary considerably depending on the rectal placement, and absorption rate tends to be slower than with oromucosal administration.

11.2.7 Summary of Alternative Formulations

Due to the large first-pass effect combined with the slow oral absorption of most opioids, alternative routes of administration have been established. Consistent plasma concentrations can be maintained for a several days with transdermal buprenorphine or fentanyl. When a more rapid onset of effect is required, the oromucosal or nasal spray routes of administration for fentanyl, buprenorphine, and butorphanol may prove useful. Rectal opioid administration is not often used but could be helpful when the oral route of administration is not an option. Following rectal drug delivery, the rate of drug absorption is consistent with or slightly slower than oral dosing. The overall drug bioavailability following rectal administration may be higher due to partial bypass of the first-pass metabolism or a lower bioavailability depending on drug placement in the rectum.

11.3 Clinical Pharmacodynamics (PD)

11.3.1 (Opioid Mechanism of Action)

The opioids that are found naturally within the brain are termed "endogenous opioids" and include the enkephalins, endorphins, and dynorphins. Opioids from outside the body are termed "exogenous opioids" and include a long list of ligands (e.g., morphine, fentanyl, codeine, etc.). Both the endogenous and exogenous opioids act primarily via three G-protein-coupled receptors (GPCRs): mu opioid receptor (MOR), kappa opioid receptor (KOR), and the delta opioid receptor (DOR) [115]. An overview of opioid medications that act via these three opioid receptor subtypes is shown in Table 11.4 [2, 115–118]. MORs have a well-established role in pain and analgesia; however, they also have effects on the respiratory and cardiovascular systems, mood and behavior, and hormone secretion. KORs and DORs have been associated with analgesia and a wide variety of other physiologic and behavioral effects [43]. Most of the *clinically relevant analgesic opioid medications* are comparatively selective for MORs [2]. KOR agonists are associated with

Table 11.4 Opioid receptor profiles of various medications (*pharmacologically weak and strong MOR agonists included*)

Drug	Opioid receptors involved in drug actions	Miscellaneous drug actions
Full agonists (MOR)		
Codeine	MOR (full)	
Fentanyl	MOR (full), KOR (partial), DOR (full)	
Hydrocodone	MOR (full), KOR (full)	
Hydromorphone	MOR (full), KOR (full), DOR (full)	
Meperidine	MOR (full), KOR (full), DOR (full)	Serotonin-reuptake inhibition Normeperidine (*metabolite*): indirect NMDA activation
d,l-methadone	MOR (full) (*l-methadone and d-methadone each possess unique pharmacologic profiles*)	d-methadone isomer: NMDA antagonist
Morphine	MOR (full), KOR (partial), DOR (full)	Morphine-3-glucuronide (*metabolite*): indirect NMDA activation
Oxycodone	MOR (full), KOR (full), DOR (full)	
Tramadol	MOR (full)	Serotonin-reuptake inhibitor; norepinephrine-reuptake inhibitor
Partial agonists (MOR) + mixed KOR agonists/antagonists		
Buprenorphine	MOR (partial), KOR (antagonist)	
Butorphanol	MOR (partial), KOR (full)	

Table adapted from the following sources: Refs. [2, 115–118]

analgesia but also can produce dysphoric reactions and psychotomimetic effects and are generally avoided as long-term treatment options.

Any clinical differences between opioids are likely due to their relative and varied agonist and partial agonist activity at the three opioid receptor types [2]. Many effects (e.g., respiratory depression) are dose related and become more pronounced with higher doses. These concepts are discussed further within the PK/PD modeling section. As with many medication classes, selectivity for one receptor system is often lost with opioids as doses are increased. In other cases (e.g., mixed agonist–antagonist), medications may exert simultaneous effects at multiple opioid receptor types at typical therapeutic doses. Furthermore, the PD properties of opioids may be isomer dependent. For example, methadone is a mixture of R-methadone (*more potent analgesia*) and S-methadone (*an NMDA antagonist*) [2]. Therefore, opioid isomers need to be considered in terms of both clinical efficacy (e.g., analgesia) and adverse effects when attempting to assess PK and PD relationships.

Due to the pharmacologic actions on the opioid receptors, this explains the overall similar clinical profiles (despite subtle differences) among the various opioid medications [117]. The focus of this chapter is on the analgesic and associated other effects produced by opioids with MOR activity. Opioid selection is often chosen based on PK parameters, and doses of these agents can generally be standardized using equipotency conversions (i.e., morphine milligram equivalents). The primary exception is methadone, which may require special attention during dose conversions. The reader should consult one of the many available equianalgesic (morphine milligram equivalent) tables [119, 120] to help guide them with opioid dosing, including recommendations for special conversion ratios when switching to methadone from another opioid [2, 121, 122].

11.3.2 Clinical Effects

Prototypical opioids (i.e., morphine-like drugs acting at the MOR) produce a variety of clinical effects, including analgesia, respiratory depression, mood and behavioral changes (e.g., euphoria), and sedation [2, 117]. Each of these clinical effects is discussed in greater detail below, which is followed by a PK/PD modeling section that ties the PK and PD relationships into one therapeutic concept.

11.3.3 Analgesia

Opioids are highly effective for pain management as analgesic effects occur without a loss of consciousness and do not impact other somatosensory abilities (e.g., proprioception) [117]. Multiple sites of action have been put forth for opioid analgesic efficacy.

Opioid analgesic mechanism of action can partly be explained by GABA-mediated effects (please see Table 11.5 [2, 117] for a variety of physiologic responses produced by MOR–GABA interactions within the central nervous system). Specifically, activation of MORs in the central nervous system may inhibit GABA neurons, which in turn allows for activation of other brain regions. For example, increased periaqueductal gray matter (PAG) activity has been associated directly with the suppression of pain [123]. Activation of MORs within the PAG may inhibit GABAergic neurons, which in turn allows for activation of PAG outflow. The end result of this descending neuronal pathway is the increased activity of monoamine-mediated pain inhibition [117, 124]. This pathway for analgesia is consistent with medications that act specifically via monoamines to produce analgesic effects, such as tramadol and serotonin–norepinephrine reuptake inhibitors (SNRIs) [2]. Opioids with relatively significant KOR agonist activity (e.g., butorphanol) may have analgesic properties; however, KOR stimulation has been associated with adverse events such as dysesthesias, paresthesias, dysphoria, and anxiety [2, 124].

In the spinal dorsal horn, MORs are involved in both presynaptic and postsynaptic pain-reducing PD effects: (1) presynaptic MOR activation results in a blockade of voltage-sensitive Ca2+ channels on C fibers, which in turn reduces Ca2+ influx

Table 11.5 MOR activation inhibits GABAergic neurons in various regions of the CNS

Brain/spinal region effects	Physiologic outcome	Clinical outcome
PAG outflow is increased secondary to MOR-mediated inhibition of GABA activity	Results in forebrain and spinal monoamine transmission	Analgesia
MOR-mediated inhibition of GABAergic neurons within the mesocorticolimbic dopamine system in the CNS (i.e., "reward pathway").	Dopamine transmission from VTA to NAc is enhanced	Drug reward occurs via "positive reinforcement" and feelings of well-being and euphoria
Parasympathetic outflow enhanced due to MOR-mediated inhibition of GABAergic activity	Increased parasympathetic outflow	Miosis
Hippocampal pyramidal cell excitation secondary to MOR-mediated inhibition of GABAergic neurons	Increased excitatory actions	Seizure activity

Table adapted from the following sources: Refs. [2, 117]
Abbreviations: *CNS* central nervous system, *NAc* nucleus accumbens, *PAG* periaqueductal gray, *VTA* ventral tegmental area

into the neuron, and (2) postsynaptic MOR activation opens K+ channels allowing efflux of K+ from the neuron. Together, these pre- and postsynaptic effects result in decreased excitation and neuronal discharge (secondary to cell hyperpolarization) in the spinal dorsal horn [117] and a reduction in the release of pain neurotransmitters such as glutamate and substance P [2]. Opioid-induced NMDA antagonism may also play a role for opioid analgesia (i.e., among opioids with NMDA effects such as S-methadone) [2, 125].

Lastly, opioid efficacy for producing analgesia is partly explained by a lower psychological distress level reported among patients following opioid administration. Specifically, opioids may reduce the affective and/or distressing effects of pain versus the actual pain sensation itself [126]. Patients may report that the pain is present; however, they describe the pain as more tolerable following opioid administration [117]. Under normal circumstances, endogenous opioids are released during times of physical or psychological stress, likely to allow continual functioning of the organism in the face of a threat. Perhaps, opioid agonists augment this process by dampening the HPA axis as described further below.

11.3.4 Drug Reward

The rewarding properties of opioids likely involve the mesocorticolimbic dopamine system (i.e., the reward pathway) [117]. Opioid inhibition of GABA neurons within the ventral tegmental area (VTA) may allow for more intense dopaminergic transmission from the VTA to the nucleus accumbens (NAc) [2]. Hence, it is thought that activation of the "reward pathway" via opioids occurs secondary to opioid actions on GABAergic activity in this area of the brain [127] (see Table 11.5 [2, 117]).

11.3.5 Tolerance and Physical Dependence

Following chronic opioid use, tolerance and/or physical dependence (*with a drug-specific withdrawal phenomenon*) is likely to occur that depends on both the opioid dose and duration [117]. Although a thorough discussion of substance use disorders is beyond the scope of this chapter, it is imperative to recognize that tolerance and physical dependence are not necessarily synonymous with "addiction." In regard to PK/PD modeling, mechanisms for opioid-induced tolerance are described in this chapter.

Following exposure to opioids, MORs may undergo a desensitization and internalization process [117]. However, different opioid agonists appear to cause differing levels of tolerance. Some of the PD changes likely represent opioid receptor and G-protein uncoupling [117], while other PD effects are likely due to various intracellular and extracellular adaptations [128]. For example, intracellular mechanisms for opioid desensitization and tolerance include cAMP response element-binding (CREB) protein adaptations [129]. The desensitization process has also been associated with arrestin-mediated pathways [117, 128], although it has also been proposed that arrestin-mediated pathways are "not necessary" for MOR desensitization [130]. Regardless of the exact underlying mechanisms for desensitization and tolerance to opioids, these adaptations are likely to have an impact on PK–PD relationships. Clinical response to an opioid at a particular drug plasma concentration may change over time due to the tolerance mechanisms. Furthermore, some symptoms (e.g.., miosis) may not develop tolerance as quickly as others such as analgesia and sedation [117]. Finally, specific opioids such as morphine may be more likely than other agents to produce tolerance [130], which has been postulated to be related to "efficacy" at altering opioid receptor signaling [131]. All of these factors may significantly alter and complicate PK/PD models for opioid medications.

11.3.6 Respiratory System

Opioids possess a direct pharmacologic depressant effect on the intrinsic respiratory rhythm generated in the medulla [117, 132]. Another feature of opioids is the inhibition of the ventilatory response to elevated CO2, which may be partly explained by opioid-induced reduction in the excitability of chemosensory neurons (e.g., the carotid body) [2, 117, 132]. Due to the respiratory depression, opioids must be used cautiously among patients with respiratory conditions, such as obstructive sleep apnea [117]. Furthermore, these respiratory depressant effects are linked to elevated intracranial pressure and with a generally increased risk of morbidity and mortality [117]. It is crucial to note that opioid antagonists (e.g., naloxone) are very effective at reducing respiratory depression in life-threatening situations [117]. In regard to PK–PD modeling, respiration changes induced by opioids are a PD parameter that has been successfully employed in these models.

11.3.7 Cardiovascular System

Opioids can cause orthostatic hypotension secondary to multiple pharmacologic receptor effects [2, 117]. For example, opioid-induced histamine release is associated with orthostasis. Additionally, opioids may dampen the sympathetic nervous system [2] and blunt reflex vasoconstriction caused by elevated PCO2 [117]. Opioids are also associated with a reduction in oxygen consumption and cardiac work [117], and this partly explains their use in acute coronary syndrome guidelines [133]. While there are clear opioid effects on the cardiovascular system, cerebral circulation is not directly impacted by opioids. It is important to note, however, that opioid-induced respiratory depression can lead to CO2 elevation with cerebral vasodilation and increased cerebrospinal fluid pressure.

Prolonged QT interval has been associated specifically with methadone [2] and should not be used in patients at risk for prolonged QT interval (e.g., taking other medications or medical conditions known to prolong the QT interval). Furthermore, various methadone doses (e.g., 60 mg/day, 100 mg/day) have been proposed as thresholds at which increased risk for prolonged QT interval may occur and additional ECG monitoring should be implemented [2, 134]. The use of PK/PD modeling to determine who is at risk for methadone-related QT interval prolongation is briefly discussed in the PK–PD modeling section.

11.3.8 Sedation, Dysphoria, and Other Cognitive/Psychiatric Effects

Opioids cause sedation and cognitive impairment [117] and have been associated with myoclonus and seizure activity, and this effect may be secondary to opioid inhibition of GABA interneurons (shown in Table 11.5) [2, 117] Morphine-3-glucuronide (M3G) and normeperidine have been linked to seizure activity, which can occur via non-opioid mechanisms, such as indirect activation of *N*-methyl-*D*-aspartic acid (NMDA) receptors [117, 135]. Normeperidine accumulation may cause symptoms of neurotoxicity, such as tremors and seizure activity, and these effects may not be reversed with naloxone administration [2, 117, 136].

11.3.9 Neuroendocrine Effects

Opioids are known to impact the hypothalamic pituitary–adrenal (HPA) axis, by inhibition of HPA hormonal release [117]. More specifically, opioids appear to reduce circulating cortisol, as a result of blocking corticotropin-releasing hormone (CRH) [117]. A complete review of the neuroendocrine complexities associated with opioids is beyond the scope of this chapter. However, the ability of the opioids to inhibit activity of the HPA axis likely mediates some of their ability to dampen the psychological distress associated with pain.

11.3.10 Gastrointestinal and Genitourinary Systems

The opioids are well known to cause many effects within the gastrointestinal tract [117]. For example, patients treated with opioids often experience constipation [2, 117]. In fact, opioidergic drugs such as loperamide are used therapeutically as antidiarrheal medications [117]. The mechanisms that contribute to opioid-induced constipation are mediated by the enteric nervous system and include a reduction in intestinal propulsatile activity and decreased intestinal secretions [117, 137]. Opioid antagonists, such as naloxone, have been used to improve the opioid-induced constipation (see Chap. 23). Nausea and vomiting may be caused by direct opioid stimulation of the chemoreceptor trigger zone (located within the medulla) and are generally included in the side effect profile of opioid medications [2, 117]. Analogous to effects on the gastrointestinal tract, opioids cause urinary retention [2, 117]. It is important to note that tolerance can develop to opioid-induced urinary retention and may be reversed with peripheral opioid antagonists such as methylnaltrexone [117, 138].

11.3.11 Histamine Release (Particularly with Morphine and Meperidine)

Side effects associated with opioid-induced histamine release include bronchospasm, vasodilation, and hypotension. Furthermore, skin flushing may be apparent [2, 117]. Certain opioids are more likely than others to induce histamine release. For example, fentanyl is associated with less histaminergic effects and may be preferable in patients at risk for respiratory problems (e.g., patient with asthma) [117].

11.3.12 Miosis

MOR activity inhibits GABAergic interneurons, which in turn regulate parasympathetic control of the pupil (see Table 11.5 [2, 117]). By blocking these GABAergic neurons, increased parasympathetic outflow in turn causes pupillary constriction (i.e., miosis) [117]. A highly useful aspect of this "observable" effect is in the application used in PK/PD modeling.

11.3.13 PK/PD Modeling

It has been well documented that dose–response relationships for opioid analgesics demonstrate wide variability between patients and even between pain episodes within the same individual [139]. However, successful PK/PD modeling has been completed with the opioids, which has provided some insights into their clinical effects. It should be noted that a complication of PK/PD modeling for opioid analgesia is the challenge assessing opioid concentrations at one of their primary sites of action (i.e., central nervous system). Therefore, an indirect measure of drug concentrations (e.g., accessible plasma concentrations) provides the link to PD effects in studies that have been conducted. Hence, one must consider differences that may exist between plasma concentrations compared to drug levels at the "effect site" (e.g., central nervous system) [140]. Table 11.6 [140–153] provides examples of this lag time for various opioid medications. To further complicate PK/PD modeling of the opioids, it has been shown that enantiomers may possess different qualities as it pertains to PK and PD relationships [154, 155]. For example, in a PK–PD analysis of R,S-methadone, R-methadone behaved more predictably [155]. Additionally, various opioid metabolites contribute to clinical effects, which even further complicate the relationship between PK and PD variables. For example, morphine and M6G both contribute to analgesia, and therefore, plasma concentrations of both active moieties need to be considered. Lastly, sex differences may or may not contribute to the complexities found in the PK/PD modeling of opioids [156, 157]. It is important to note that various PD variables may respond differently to the same opioid concentrations [158]. Thus, the selection of PD variables must be carefully considered in model development and interpretation. Despite these many barriers, the PK/PD modeling approach has provided useful information that can be used to help guide opioid analgesic use.

As shown in Table 11.6 [140–153], PD variables that are objectively measured have been successfully employed in opioid PK/PD models. For example, electroencephalogram (EEG) and pupil size are PD parameters that are reliably measured and can be paralleled to opioid PK variables [140]. Respiration is another physiologic function for which opioid PK/PD modeling has been successful at predicting responses to opioids [132]. PD variables that are less objective include pain assessments (i.e., experimental and clinical pain) [140] and effects on mood [154, 156]. Studies have demonstrated an inverse relationship between methadone concentrations and measures of mood disturbance (e.g., items for "tension" and "vigor"), particularly as methadone concentrations approached their trough levels [154, 159]. Other more rare events (e.g., QT prolongation) have also been used in PK–PD modeling studies. A simulation study used pooled data from five clinical trials among 284 subjects who had received methadone for at least 30 days. This study assessed the PK–PD relationships between seven different methadone doses (range 80–200 mg/day), methadone concentrations, and increased QT prolongation. The study, which pooled data from trials possessing multiple methadone concentration and QT assessment time points in the same individual, identified a linear relationship between methadone concentrations and QT interval. Furthermore, the PK–PD model predicted that close to 2 % of patients would experience QT interval greater than 500 ms at doses ranging from 180 to 200 mg/day [160]. Therefore, methadone should be cautiously used at doses approaching or greater than 180 mg/day.

Regardless of the specific PD variable used in the PK/PD model, the pharmacologic effects of opioids generally appear to parallel their plasma concentrations but to varying degrees between opioid medications and depending on which PD vari-

Table 11.6 PK/PD modeling for opioid agonists (parent compounds; metabolites not included)

Opioid agonist (*partial and full*)	Measure of lag time[a] between plasma and effect site[b]	Effect site measure	References
Buprenorphine	75 min	Respiration	[153]
Buprenorphine	155 min	Antinociception	[152]
Fentanyl	Studies ranged from 4.7 to 6.6 min	Electroencephalogram (EEG)	[147–149]
Fentanyl	16.4 min	Respiration	[153]
Methadone	7.7–9 min	Analgesia	[141, 142]
Methadone	18.6 min	Sedation	[142]
Morphine	1.7 h	Postoperative analgesia (patients)	[144, 145]
Morphine	1.2 h	Respiration	[146]
Morphine	2.8–3.9 h	Pupil size	[143, 150]
Morphine	34 min (median reported)	Experimental pain (multiple methods)	[151]
Oxycodone	0 min (i.e., no lag time)	Visceral pain	[151]
Oxycodone	17 min (median reported)	Somatic pain	[151]

Table adapted from the following sources: Refs. [140–153]
[a]Calculated by half-life = $0.693/k_{e0}$ (i.e., first-order rate constant)
[b]Effect site = site of action (e.g., central nervous system)

able is chosen [140]. For example, as shown in Table 11.6 [140–153], fentanyl effects may be more closely tied to its plasma concentrations as compared to morphine, which may have a longer delay between its plasma concentration time course and clinical effects [140]. Therefore, PK/PD models may be more useful for some opioids as compared to others.

Case Study (Example)
A clinician gathers information regarding morphine and determines the morphine T_{max} to be about 1 h. When asked to estimate the expected time of "maximum effects" related to morphine administration, the clinician explains there is a "lag time" between morphine plasma concentrations and morphine effects of approximately 3 h, and this varies based upon which clinical effect is under question. Additionally, M6G is formed from morphine, and this active metabolite will contribute its own effects that must be considered. However, if this same clinician was asked the very same question about methadone, the answer would be less than one-half hour to begin observing opioid effects secondary to methadone, and this too would vary based upon the clinical effect being measured.

11.3.14 Summary

An integrated PK–PD relationship can be used to guide opioid treatment decisions, assist in drug development, and help answer important research questions pertaining to opioid pharmacotherapy. PK–PD models continue to evolve using various PD variables and by using medications with unique PK profiles (e.g., novel drug delivery systems). One of the key points from existing PK–PD models is that the lag time between measurable concentrations (i.e., typically plasma) and effect site concentrations (i.e., typically the CNS) varies widely among the opioids. Therefore, an accurate prediction of response related to dose and plasma concentration requires incorporation of lag time into model development and clinical decision making. Many other factors can complicate PK–PD modeling (e.g., metabolites, tolerance), and an understanding of how these factors may impact a particular opioid medication in PK–PD modeling is essential.

References

1. Portenoy RK, Ahmed E (2014) Principles of opioid use in cancer pain. J Clin Oncol 32(16):1662–1670
2. Trescot AM, Datta S, Lee M, Hansen H (2008) Opioid pharmacology. Pain Physician 11(2 Suppl):S133–S153
3. Lin JH, Yamazaki M (2003) Role of P-glycoprotein in pharmacokinetics: clinical implications. Clin Pharmacokinet 42(1):59–98
4. Mercer SL, Coop A (2011) Opioid analgesics and P-glycoprotein efflux transporters: a potential systems-level contribution to analgesic tolerance. Curr Top Med Chem 11(9): 1157–1164
5. Eap CB, Buclin T, Baumann P (2002) Interindividual variability of the clinical pharmacokinetics of methadone: implications for the treatment of opioid dependence. Clin Pharmacokinet 41(14):1153–1193
6. Gourevitch MN, Hartel D, Tenore P et al (1999) Three oral formulations of methadone. A clinical and pharmacodynamic comparison. J Subst Abuse Treat 17(3):237–241
7. Lee CR, McTavish D, Sorkin EM (1993) Tramadol. A preliminary review of its pharmacodynamic and pharmacokinetic properties, and therapeutic potential in acute and chronic pain states. Drugs 46(2):313–340
8. Grond S, Sablotzki A (2004) Clinical pharmacology of tramadol. Clin Pharmacokinet 43(13):879–923
9. Benziger DP, Kaiko RF, Miotto JB, Fitzmartin RD, Reder RF, Chasin M (1996) Differential effects of food on the bioavailability of controlled-release oxycodone tablets and immediate-release oxycodone solution. J Pharm Sci 85(4):407–410
10. Streisand JB, Varvel JR, Stanski DR et al (1991) Absorption and bioavailability of oral transmucosal fentanyl citrate. Anesthesiology 75(2):223–229
11. Findlay JW, Butz RF, Welch RM (1977) Codeine kinetics as determined by radioimmunoassay. Clin Pharmacol Ther 22(4):439–446
12. Kim I, Barnes AJ, Oyler JM et al (2002) Plasma and oral fluid pharmacokinetics and pharmacodynamics after oral codeine administration. Clin Chem 48(9):1486–1496
13. Rowell FJ, Seymour RA, Rawlins MD (1983) Pharmacokinetics of intravenous and oral dihydrocodeine and its acid metabolites. Eur J Clin Pharmacol 25(3):419–424

14. Inturrisi CE, Max MB, Foley KM, Schultz M, Sin S-U, Houde RW (1984) The pharmacokinetics of heroin in patients with chronic pain. N Engl J Med 310(19):1213–1217
15. Valtier S, Bebarta VS (2012) Excretion profile of hydrocodone, hydromorphone and norhydrocodone in urine following single dose administration of hydrocodone to healthy volunteers. J Anal Toxicol 36:507–514, *Jul 10:bks058*
16. Vallner JJ, Stewart JT, Kotzan JA, Kirsten EB, Honigberg IL (1981) Pharmacokinetics and bioavailability of hydromorphone following intravenous and oral administration to human subjects. J Clin Pharmacol 21(4):152–156
17. Dixon R, Crews T, Inturrisi C, Foley K (1983) Levorphanol: pharmacokinetics and steady-state plasma concentrations in patients with pain. Res Commun Chem Pathol Pharmacol 41(1):3–17
18. Edwards D, Svensson CK, Visco JP, Lalka D (1982) Clinical pharmacokinetics of pethidine: 1982. Clin Pharmacokinet 7(5):421–433
19. Mather LE, Meffin PJ (1978) Clinical pharmacokinetics pethidine. Clin Pharmacokinet 3(5):352–368
20. Osborne R, Joel S, Trew D, Sleven M (1990) Morphine and metabolite behavior after different routes of administration: demonstration of the importance of the active metabolite morphine-6-glucuronide. Clin Pharmacol Ther 47(1):12–19
21. Sawe J, Dahlstrom B, Paalzow L, Rane A (1981) Morphine kinetics in cancer patients. Clin Pharmacol Ther 30:629–635
22. Sawe J, Svensson JO, Rane A (1983) Morphine metabolism in cancer patients on increasing oral doses – no evidence for autoinduction or dose-dependence. Br J Clin Pharmacol 16(1):85–93
23. Sawe J (1986) High dose morphine and methadone in cancer patients. Clinical pharmacokinetic considerations on oral treatment. Clin Pharmacokinet 11(2):87–106
24. Hoskin PJ, Hanks GW, Aherne GW, Chapman D, Littleton P, Filshie J (1989) The bioavailability and pharmacokinetics of morphine after intravenous, oral and buccal administration in healthy volunteers. Br J Clin Pharmacol 27(4):499–505
25. Gourlay GK, Cherry DA, Cousins MJ (1986) A comparative study of the efficacy and pharmacokinetics of oral methadone and morphine in the treatment of severe pain in patients with cancer. Pain 25(3):297–312
26. Pöyhiä R, Seppälä T, Olkkola KT, Kalso E (1992) The pharmacokinetics and metabolism of oxycodone after intramuscular and oral administration to healthy subjects. Br J Clin Pharmacol 33(6):617–621
27. Smith HS (2009) Clinical pharmacology of oxymorphone. Pain Med 10(1 Suppl):S3–S10, Oxymorphone
28. Lintz W, Barth H, Osterloh G, Schmidt-Böthelt E (1986) Bioavailability of enteral tramadol formulations. 1st communication: capsules. Arzneimittel Forschung 36(8):1278–1283
29. Bullingham RES, McQuay HJ, Porter EJB, Allen MC, Moore RA (1982) Sublingual buprenorphine used postoperatively: ten hour plasma drug concentration analysis. Br J Clin Pharmacol 13(5):665–673
30. Pachter IJ, Evens RP (1985) Butrophanol. Drug Alcohol Depend 14(3):325–338
31. Inturrisi CE (2002) Clinical pharmacology of opioids for pain. Clin J Pain 18(4 Suppl):S3–S13
32. Wood M (1986) Plasma drug binding: implications for anesthesiologists. Anesth Analg 65(7):786–804
33. Lemmens HJ (1995) Pharmacokinetic-pharmacodynamic relationships for opioids in balanced anaesthesia. Clin Pharmacokinet 29(4):231–242
34. Gulaboski R, Cordeiro MN, Milhazes N et al (2007) Evaluation of the lipophilic properties of opioids, amphetamine-like drugs, and metabolites through electrochemical studies at the interface between two immiscible solutions. Anal Biochem 361(2):236–243
35. Lombardo F, Shalaeva MY, Tupper KA, Gao F (2001) ElogD(oct): a tool for lipophilicity determination in drug discovery. 2. Basic and neutral compounds. J Med Chem 44(15):2490–2497

36. Garrett ER, Chandran VR (1985) Pharmacokinetics of morphine and its surrogates VI: bioanalysis, solvolysis kinetics, solubility, pK'a values, and protein binding of buprenorphine. J Pharm Sci 74(5):515–524
37. Vree TB, Wissen CPWGMV-V (1992) Pharmacokinetics and metabolism of codeine in humans. Biopharm Drug Dispos 13(6):445–460
38. Quiding H, Anderson P, Bondesson U, Boréus LO, Hynning P-Å (1986) Plasma concentrations of codeine and its metabolite, morphine, after single and repeated oral administration. Eur J Clin Pharmacol 30(6):673–677
39. Gasche Y, Daali Y, Fathi M et al (2004) Codeine intoxication associated with ultrarapid CYP2D6 metabolism. N Engl J Med 351(27):2827–2831
40. Moolenaar F, Grasmeuer G, Visser J, Meijer DKF (1983) Rectal versus oral absorption of codeine phosphate in man. Biopharm Drug Dispos 4(2):195–199
41. Kirkwood LC, Nation RL, Somogyi AA (1997) Characterization of the human cytochrome P450 enzymes involved in the metabolism of dihydrocodeine. Br J Clin Pharmacol 44(6):549–555
42. Ammon S, Hofmann U, Griese E-U, Gugeler N, Mikus G (1999) Pharmacokinetics of dihydrocodeine and its active metabolite after single and multiple oral dosing. Br J Clin Pharmacol 48(3):317–322
43. Fromm MF, Hofmann U, Griese E-U, Mikus G (1995) Dihydrocodeine: a new opioid substrate for the polymorphic CYP2D6 in humans. Clin Pharmacol Ther 58(4):374–382
44. Davies KN, Castleden CM, McBurney A, Jagger C (1989) The effect of ageing on the pharmacokinetics of dihydrocodeine. Eur J Clin Pharmacol 37(4):375–379
45. Cohn GL, Cramer JA, McBride W, Brown RC, Kleber HD (1974) Heroin and morphine binding with human serum proteins and red blood cells. Exp Biol Med 147(3): 664–666
46. Giardin F, Rentsch KM, Schwab M-A et al (2003) Pharmacokinetics of high doses of intramuscular and oral heroin in narcotic addicts. Clin Pharmacol Ther 74(4):341–352
47. Rook EJ, Huitema ADR, van den Brink W, van Ree JM, Beijnen JH (2006) Population pharmacokinetics of heroin and its major metabolites. Clin Pharmacokinet 45(4):401–417
48. Yeh SY, Gorodetzky CR, McQuinn RL (1976) Urinary excretion of heroin and its metabolites in man. J Pharmacol Exp Ther 196(2):249–256
49. Cone EJ, Darwin WD, Gorodetzky CW, Tan T (1978) Comparative metabolism of hydrocodone in man, rat, guinea pig, rabbit, and dog. Drug Metab Dispos 6(4):488–493
50. Otton S, Schadel M, Cheung SW, Kaplan HL, Busto UE, Sellers EM (1993) CYP2D6 phenotype determines the metabolic conversion of hydrocodone to hydromorphone. Clin Pharmacol Ther 54(5):463–472
51. Ritschel W, Parab PV, Denson DD, Coyle DE, Gregg RV (1987) Absolute bioavailability of hydromorphone after peroral and rectal administration in humans: saliva/plasma ratio and clinical effects. J Clin Pharmacol 27(9):647–653
52. Murray A, Hagen NA (2005) Hydromorphone. J Pain Symptom Manage 29(5):57–66
53. Parab PV, Ritschel WA, Coyle DE, Gregg RV, Denson DD (1988) Pharmacokinetics of hydromorphone after intravenous, peroral and rectal administration to human subjects. Biopharm Drug Dispos 9(2):187–199
54. Dilaudid and Dilaudid-HP Injection (hydromorphone hydrochloride). Prescribing information. Manufactured by Hospira, Inc., Lake Forest, IL 60045, USA for Purdue Pharma L.P. Stamford, CT 06901–3431. Revised June 2008
55. Umans JG, Inturrisi CE (1982) Antinociceptive activity and toxicity of meperidine and normeperidine in mice. J Pharmacol Exp Ther 223(1):203–206
56. Kirkwood CF, Edwards DJ, Lalka D, Lasezkay G, Hassett JM, Slaughter RL (1986) The pharmacokinetics of meperidine in acute trauma patients. J Trauma 26(12):1090–1093
57. Inturrisi CE, Colburn WA, Kaiko RF, Houde RW, Foley KM (1987) Pharmacokinetics and pharmacodynamics of methadone in patients with chronic pain. Clin Pharmacol Ther 41(4):392–401

58. Oda Y, Kharasch ED (2001) Metabolism of methadone and levo-α-acetylmethadol (LAAM) by human intestinal cytochrome P450 3A4 (CYP3A4): potential contribution of intestinal metabolism to presytemic clearance and bioactivation. J Pharmacol Exp Ther 298(3):1021–1032
59. Wolff K, Rostami-Hodjegan A, Shires S, Hay AWM, Feely M, Calvert R, Raistrick D, Tucher GT (1997) The pharmacokinetics of methadone in healthy subjects and opiate users. Br J Clin Pharmacol 44:325–334
60. Nilsson M-I, Widerlöv E, Meresaar U, Änggåard E (1982) Effect of urinary pH on the disposition of methadone in man. Eur J Clin Pharmacol 22(4):337–342
61. Olsen GD, Bennett WM, Porter GA (1975) Morphine and phenytoin binding to plasma proteins in renal and hepatic failure. Clin Pharmacol Ther 17(6):677–684
62. Yeh SY, Gorodetzky CW, Krebs HA (1977) Isolation and identification of morphine 3- and 6-glucuronides, morphine 3,6-diglucuronide, morphine 3-ethereal sulfate, normorphine, and normorphine 6-glucuronide as morphine metabolites in humans. J Pharm Sci 66(9):1288–1293
63. Cone EJ, Huestis MA (2007) Interpretation of oral fluid tests for drugs of abuse. Ann N Y Acad Sci 1098(1):51–103
64. Pöyhiä R, Vainio A, Kalso E (1993) A review of oxycodone's clinical pharmacokinetics and pharmacodynamics. J Pain Symptom Manage 8(2):63–67
65. Lalovic B, Kharasch E, Hoffer C, Risler L, Liu-Chen L-Y, Shen DD (2006) Pharmacokinetics and pharmacodynamics of oral oxycodone in healthy human subjects: role of circulating active metabolites. Clin Pharmacol Ther 79(5):461–479
66. Adams MP, Ahdieh H (2005) Single- and multiple-dose pharmacokinetic and dose-proportionality study of oxymorphone immediate-release tablets. Drugs R D 6:91–99
67. Adams MP, Ahdieh H (2004) Pharmacokinetics and dose-proportionality of oxymorphone extended release and its metabolites: results of a randomized crossover study. Pharmacother J Human Pharmacol Drug Ther 24(4):468–476
68. Cone EJ, Darwin WD, Buchwald WF, Gorodetzky CW (1983) Oxymorphone metabolism and urinary excretion in human, rat, guinea pig, rabbit and dog. Drug Metab Dispos 11(5):446–450
69. Lee CR, McTavish D, Sorkin EM (1993) Tramadol: a preliminary review of its pharmacodynamics and pharmacokinetic properties, and therapeutic potential in acute and chronic pain states. Drugs 46(2):313–340
70. Lintz W, Erlacin S, Frankus E et al (1981) Biotransformation of tramadol in man and animal (in German). Arzneimittel Forschung 31(11):1932–1943
71. Paar WD, Poche S, Gerloff J, Dengler HJ (1997) Polymorphic CYP2D6 mediates O-demethylation of the opioid analgesic tramadol. Eur J Clin Pharmacol 53(3–4): 235–239
72. Meuldermens W, Woestenborghs R, Noorduin H, Cmu F, van Steenberge A, Heykants J (1986) Protein binding of the analgesics alfentanil and sufentanil in maternal and neonatal plasma. Eur J Clin Pharmacol 30(2):217–219
73. Meuldermans W, Van Peer A, Hendrickx J et al (1988) Alfentanil pharmacokinetics and metabolism in humans. Anesthesiology 69(4):527–534
74. Labroo RB, Thummel KE, Lunze KL, Podoll T, Trager WF, Kharasch ED (1995) Catalytic role of cytochrome P4503A4 in multiple pathways of alfentanil metabolism. Drug Metab Dispos 23(4):490–496
75. Scholz J, Steinfath M, Schulz M (1996) Clinical pharmacokinetics of alfentanil, fentanyl and sufentanil, an update. Clin Pharmacokinet 31(4):275–292
76. Meuldermans WEB, Hurkmans RMA, Heykants JJP (1982) Plasma protein binding and distribution of fentanyl, sufentanil, alfentanil and lofentanil in blood. Arch Int Pharmacodyn Ther 257(1):4–19
77. McClain DA, Hug CC (1980) Intravenous fentanyl kinetics. Clin Pharmacol Ther 28(1):106–114

78. Labroo RB, Paine MF, Thummel KE, Kharasch ED (1997) Fentanyl metabolism by human hepatic and intestinal cytochrome P450 3A4: implications for interindividual variability in disposition, efficacy, and drug interactions. Drug Metab Dispos 25(9):1072–1080
79. Bovill JG, Sebel PS (1980) Pharmacokinetics of high-dose fentanyl. Br J Anaesth 52(8):795–801
80. Glass PSA, Gan TJ, Scott H (1999) A review of the pharmacokinetics and pharmacodynamics of remifentanil. Anesth Analg 89(4 Suppl):7
81. Egan TD, Lemmens HJM, Fiset P et al (1993) The pharmacokinetics of the new short-acting opioid remifentanil (GI87084B) in healthy adult male volunteers. Anesthesiology 79(5):881–892
82. Glass PSA, Hardman D, Kamiyama Y et al (1993) Preliminary pharmacokinetics and pharmacodynamics of an ultra-short-acting opioid: remifentanil (GI87084B). Anesth Analg 77(5):1031–1040
83. Westmoreland CL, Hoke JF, Sebe PS, Hug CC, Muir KT (1993) Pharmacokinetics of remifentanil (GI87084B) and its major metabolite (GI90291) in patients undergoing elective inpatient surgery. Anesthesiology 79(5):893–903
84. Bovill JG, Seel PS, Blackburn CL, Oei-Lim V, Heykants JJ (1984) The pharmacokinetics of sufentanil in surgical patients. Anesthesiology 61(5):502–506
85. Tateishi T, Krivoruk Y, Ueng Y-F, Wood AJJ, Guengerich FP, Wood M (1996) Identification of human liver cytochrome P-450 3A4 as the enzyme responsible for fentanyl and sufentanil N-dealkylation. Anesth Analg 82(1):167–172
86. Scholz J, Bause H, Schulz M et al (1994) Pharmacokinetics and effects on intracranial pressure of sufentanil in head trauma patients. Br J Clin Pharmacol 38(4):369–372
87. Garrett ER, Chandran VR (1985) Pharmacokinetics of morphine and its surrogates VI: bioanalysis, solvolysis kinetics, solubility, pK_a values, and protein binding of buprenorphine. J Pharm Sci 74(5):515–524
88. Kuhlman JJ, Lalani S, Magluilo J et al (1996) Human pharmacokinetics of intravenous, sublingual, and buccal buprenorphine. J Anal Toxicol 20(6):369–378
89. Cone EJ, Gorodetzky CW, Yousefnejad D, Buchwald W, Johnson RE (1984) The metabolism and excretion of buprenorphine in humans. Drug Metab Dispos 12(5):577–581
90. Gaver RC, Vasijev M, Wong H et al (1980) Disposition of parenteral butorphanol in man. Drug Metab Dispos 8(4):230–235
91. Shyu WC, Pittman KA, Robinson DS, Barbhaiya RH (1993a) The absolute bioavailability of transnasal butorphanol in patients experiencing rhinitis. Eur J Pharmacol 45(6): 559–562
92. van Dorp EL, Romberg R, Sarton E, Bovill JG, Dahan A (2006) Morphine-6-glucuronide: morphine's successor for postoperative pain relief? Anesth Analg 102(6):1789–1797
93. Wasan AD, Michna E, Janfaza D, Greenfield S, Teter CJ, Jamison RN (2008) Interpreting urine drug tests: prevalence of morphine metabolism to hydromorphone in chronic pain patients treated with morphine. Pain Med 9(7):918–923
94. Somogyi AA, Barratt DT, Coller JK (2007) Pharmacogenetics of opioids. Clin Pharmacol Ther 81(3):429–444
95. Sadhasivam S, Chidambaran V (2012) Pharmacogenomics of opioids and perioperative pain management. Pharmacogenomics 13(15):1719–1740
96. Gasche Y, Daali Y, Fathi M et al (2004) Codeine intoxication associated with ultrarapid CYP2D6 metabolism. N Engl J Med 351(27):2827–2831
97. Kaplan HL, Busto UE, Baylon GJ et al (1997) Inhibition of cytochrome P450 2D6 metabolism of hydrocodone to hydromorphone does not importantly affect abuse liability. J Pharmacol Exp Ther 281(1):103–108
98. Murtagh FE, Chai MO, Donohoe P, Edmonds PM, Higginson IJ (2007) The use of opioid analgesia in end-stage renal disease patients managed without dialysis: recommendations for practice. J Pain Palliat Care Pharmacother 21(2):5–16
99. Mercadante S, Arcuri E (2004) Opioids and renal function. J Pain 5(1):2–19

100. Filitz J, Griessinger N, Sittl R, Likar R, Schüttler J, Koppert W (2006) Effects of intermittent hemodialysis on buprenorphine and norbuprenorphine plasma concentrations in chronic pain patients treated with transdermal buprenorphine. Eur J Pain 10(8):743–748
101. Hand CW, Sear JW, Uppington J, Ball MJ, McQuay HJ, Moore RA (1990) Buprenorphine disposition in patients with renal impairment: single and continuous dosing, with special reference to metabolites. Br J Anaesth 64(3):276–282
102. Kestenbaum MG, Vilches AO, Messersmith S et al (2014) Alternative routes to oral opioid administration in palliative care: a review and clinical summary. Pain Med 15(7):1129–1153
103. Nestorov I (2003) Whole body pharmacokinetic models. Clin Pharmacokinet 42(10): 883–908
104. Mathias NR, Hussain MA (2010) Non-invasive systemic drug delivery: developability considerations for alternate routes of administration. J Pharm Sci 99(1):1–20
105. Plosker GL (2011) Buprenorphine 5, 10 and 20 μg/h transdermal patch. A review of its use in the management of chronic nonmalignant pain. Drugs 71(18):2491–2509
106. Shyu WC, Mayol RF, Pfeffer M, Pittman KA, Gammans RE, Barbhaiya RH (1993b) Biopharmaceutical evaluation of transnasal, sublingual, and buccal disk dosage forms of butorphanol. Biopharm Drug Dispos 14(5):371–379
107. Lötsch J, Walter C, Parnham MJ, Oertel BG, Geisslinger G (2013) Pharmacokinetics of non-intravenous formulations of fentanyl. Clin Pharmacokinet 52(1):23–36
108. Exalgo (hydromorphone HCl) Extended-Release Tablets. Prescribing Information. Mallinckrodt Brand Pharmaceutical, Inc. Hazelwood, MO 63042. Revised: April 2014
109. Babul N, Darke AC (1993) Disposition of morphine and its glucuronide metabolites after oral and rectal administration: evidence of route specificity. Clin Pharmacol Ther 54(3):286–292
110. Lintz W, Barth H, Osterloh G, Smith-Böthelt E (1998) Bioavailability of enteral tramadol formulations. 3rd communication: suppositories. Arzneimittel Forschung 48(9):889–899
111. Panagiotou I, Mystakidou K (2010) Intranasal fentanyl: from pharmacokinetics and bioavailability to current treatment applications. Expert Rev Anticancer Ther 10(7):1009–1021
112. Lane ME (2013) The transdermal delivery of fentanyl. Eur J Pharm Biopharm 84(3): 449–455
113. Grond S, Radbruch L, Lehmann KA (2000) Clinical pharmacokinetics of transdermal opioids: focus on transdermal fentanyl. Clin Pharmacokinet 38(1):59–89
114. Beaver WT, Feise GA (1977) A comparison of the analgesic effect of oxymorphone by rectal suppository and intramuscular injection in patients with postoperative pain. J Clin Pharmacol 17(5–6):276–291
115. IUPHAR/BPS Guide to Pharmacology. Available at: www.guidetopharmacology.org. Last accessed on 23 Mar 2015
116. Volpe DA, McMahon Tobin GA, Mellon RD et al (2011) Uniform assessment and ranking of opioid μ receptor binding constants for selected opioid drugs. Regul Toxicol Pharmacol 59(3):385–390
117. Yaksh T, Wallace M (2014) Chapter 18: Opioids, analgesia, and pain management. In: Goodman & Gilman's the pharmacological basis of therapeutics, 12th ed. The Mc Graw Hill Company, Inc. (e-version). McGraw-Hill publishing, Boston, MA.
118. Olkkola KT, Kontinen VK, Saari TI, Kalso EA (2013) Does the pharmacology of oxycodone justify its increasing use as an analgesic? Trends Pharmacol Sci 34(4):206–214
119. Washington State Agency Medical Directors' Group. Opioid dose calculator. Available at: http://agencymeddirectors.wa.gov/mobile.html. Last accessed 23 Mar 2015
120. VA/DoD Clinical Practice Guidelines (2010) Management of opioid therapy (OT) for chronic pain. Available at: www.healthquality.va.gov/guidelines/Pain/cot/. Last accessed 23 Mar 2015
121. Vieweg WV, Lipps WF, Fernandez A (2005) Opioids and methadone equivalents for clinicians. Prim Care Companion J Clin Psychiatry 7(3):86–88
122. Center to Advance Palliative Care. Methadone for the treatment of pain. Fast Fact #75. Available at: https://www.capc.org/fast-facts/75-methadone-treatment-pain/. Last accessed 23 Mar 2015

123. Waxman SA (2013) Clinical neuroanatomy, 27th edn. McGraw-Hill Education, New York
124. Lexi-Comp Online [Internet] (2015) Hudson, OH: Lexi-Comp. Last accessed and cited 23 Mar 2015 from institutional university access database
125. Hewitt DJ (2000) The use of NMDA-receptor antagonists in the treatment of chronic pain. Clin J Pain 16(2 Suppl):S73–S79
126. Drolet G, Dumont EC, Gosselin I, Kinkead R, Laforest S, Trottier JF (2001) Role of endogenous opioid system in the regulation of the stress response. Prog Neuropsychopharmacol Biol Psychiatry 25(4):729–741
127. Xi ZX, Stein EA (2002) GABAergic mechanisms of opiate reinforcement. Alcohol Alcohol 37(5):485–494
128. Bailey CP, Connor M (2005) Opioids: cellular mechanisms of tolerance and physical dependence. Curr Opin Pharmacol 5(1):60–68
129. Christie MJ (2008) Cellular neuroadaptations to chronic opioids: tolerance, withdrawal and addiction. Br J Pharmacol 154(2):384–396
130. Dang VC, Christie MJ (2012) Mechanisms of rapid opioid receptor desensitization, resensitization and tolerance in brain neurons. Br J Pharmacol 165(6):1704–1716
131. Morgan MM, Christie MJ (2011) Analysis of opioid efficacy, tolerance, addiction and dependence from cell culture to human. Br J Pharmacol 164(4):1322–1334
132. Pattinson KT (2008) Opioids and the control of respiration. Br J Anaesth 100(6):747–758
133. O'Connor RE, Brady W, Brooks SC et al (2010) Part 10: acute coronary syndromes: 2010 American Heart Association Guidelines for Cardiopulmonary Resuscitation and Emergency Cardiovascular Care. Circulation 122(18 Suppl 3):S787–S817
134. Krantz MJ, Martin J, Stimmel B, Mehta D, Haigney MC (2009) QTc interval screening in methadone treatment. Ann Intern Med 150(6):387–395
135. Hemstapat K, Monteith GR, Smith D, Smith MT (2003) Morphine-3-glucuronide's neuro-excitatory effects are mediated via indirect activation of N-methyl-D-aspartic acid receptors: mechanistic studies in embryonic cultured hippocampal neurones. Anesth Analg 97(2):494–505, table of contents
136. Seifert CF, Kennedy S (2004) Meperidine is alive and well in the new millennium: evaluation of meperidine usage patterns and frequency of adverse drug reactions. Pharmacotherapy 24(6):776–783
137. Wood JD, Galligan JJ (2004) Function of opioids in the enteric nervous system. Neurogastroenterol Motil 16(Suppl 2):17–28
138. Rosow CE, Gomery P, Chen TY, Stefanovich P, Stambler N, Israel R (2007) Reversal of opioid-induced bladder dysfunction by intravenous naloxone and methylnaltrexone. Clin Pharmacol Ther 82(1):48–53
139. Suri A, Estes KS, Geisslinger G, Derendorf H (1997) Pharmacokinetic-pharmacodynamic relationships for analgesics. Int J Clin Pharmacol Ther 35(8):307–323
140. Lötsch J (2005) Pharmacokinetic-pharmacodynamic modeling of opioids. J Pain Symptom Manage 29(5 Suppl):S90–S103
141. Inturrisi CE, Colburn WA, Kaiko RF, Houde RW, Foley KM (1987) Pharmacokinetics and pharmacodynamics of methadone in patients with chronic pain. Clin Pharmacol Ther 41(4):392–401
142. Inturrisi CE, Portenoy RK, Max MB, Colburn WA, Foley KM (1990) Pharmacokinetic-pharmacodynamic relationships of methadone infusions in patients with cancer pain. Clin Pharmacol Ther 47(5):565–577
143. Lötsch J, Skarke C, Schmidt H, Grösch S, Geisslinger G (2001) The transfer half-life of morphine-6-glucuronide from plasma to effect site assessed by pupil size measurement in healthy volunteers. Anesthesiology 95(6):1329–1338
144. Martini C, Olofsen E, Yassen A, Aarts L, Dahan A (2011) Pharmacokinetic–pharmacodynamic modeling in acute and chronic pain: an overview of the recent literature. Expert Rev Clin Pharmacol 4(6):719–728

145. Mazoit JX, Butscher K, Samii K (2007) Morphine in postoperative patients: pharmacokinetics and pharmacodynamics of metabolites. Anesth Analg 105(1):70–78
146. Olofsen E, van Dorp E, Teppema L et al (2010) Naloxone reversal of morphine- and morphine-6-glucuronide-induced respiratory depression in healthy volunteers: a mechanism-based pharmacokinetic-pharmacodynamic modeling study. Anesthesiology 112(6): 1417–1427
147. Scott JC, Cooke JE, Stanski DR (1991) Electroencephalographic quantitation of opioid effect: comparative pharmacodynamics of fentanyl and sufentanil. Anesthesiology 74(1): 34–42
148. Scott JC, Stanski DR (1987) Decreased fentanyl and alfentanil dose requirements with age. A simultaneous pharmacokinetic and pharmacodynamic evaluation. J Pharmacol Exp Ther 240(1):159–166
149. Scott JC, Ponganis KV, Stanski DR (1985) EEG quantitation of narcotic effect: the comparative pharmacodynamics of fentanyl and alfentanil. Anesthesiology 62(3):234–241
150. Skarke C, Darimont J, Schmidt H, Geisslinger G, Lötsch J (2003) Analgesic effects of morphine and morphine-6-glucuronide in a transcutaneous electrical pain model in healthy volunteers. Clin Pharmacol Ther 73(1):107–121
151. Staahl C, Upton R, Foster DJ et al (2008) Pharmacokinetic-pharmacodynamic modeling of morphine and oxycodone concentrations and analgesic effect in a multimodal experimental pain model. J Clin Pharmacol 48(5):619–631
152. Yassen A, Kan J, Olofsen E, Suidgeest E, Dahan A, Danhof M (2006) Mechanism-based pharmacokinetic-pharmacodynamic modeling of the respiratory-depressant effect of buprenorphine and fentanyl in rats. J Pharmacol Exp Ther 319(2):682–692
153. Yassen A, Olofsen E, Romberg R et al (2007) Mechanism-based PK/PD modeling of the respiratory depressant effect of buprenorphine and fentanyl in healthy volunteers. Clin Pharmacol Ther 81(1):50–58
154. Shiran MR, Lennard MS, Iqbal MZ et al (2012) Pharmacokinetic-pharmacodynamic modeling of mood and withdrawal symptoms in relation to plasma concentrations of methadone in patients undergoing methadone maintenance treatment. J Clin Psychopharmacol 32(5):666–671
155. Boulton DW, Arnaud P, DeVane CL (2001) Pharmacokinetics and pharmacodynamics of methadone enantiomers after a single oral dose of racemate. Clin Pharmacol Ther 70(1):48–57
156. Murthy BR, Pollack GM, Brouwer KL (2002) Contribution of morphine-6-glucuronide to antinociception following intravenous administration of morphine to healthy volunteers. J Clin Pharmacol 42(5):569–576
157. Romberg R, Olofsen E, Sarton E, den Hartigh J, Taschner PE, Dahan A (2004) Pharmacokinetic-pharmacodynamic modeling of morphine-6-glucuronide-induced analgesia in healthy volunteers: absence of sex differences. Anesthesiology 100(1):120–133
158. Nakamura A, Hasegawa M, Ito H et al (2011) Distinct relations among plasma concentrations required for different pharmacological effects in oxycodone, morphine, and fentanyl. J Pain Palliat Care Pharmacother 25(4):318–334
159. Dyer KR, White JM, Foster DJ, Bochner F, Menelaou A, Somogyi AA (2001) The relationship between mood state and plasma methadone concentration in maintenance patients. J Clin Psychopharmacol 21(1):78–84
160. Florian J, Garnett CE, Nallani SC, Rappaport BA, Throckmorton DC (2012) A modeling and simulation approach to characterize methadone QT prolongation using pooled data from five clinical trials in MMT patients. Clin Pharmacol Ther 91(4):666–672

Chapter 12
Stimulants and Other Non-stimulants for Attention-Deficit/Hyperactivity Disorder (ADHD)

John S. Markowitz and Guo Yu

Abstract Methylphenidate, amphetamines, and atomoxetine are established agents used to treat children, adolescents, and adults with attention-deficit/hyperactivity disorder (ADHD). Methylphenidate remains the commonly prescribed drug for ADHD throughout the world. The dosage formulations for the majority of methylphenidate preparations contain a racemic mixture (50:50) of *d*- and *l*-isomers. The *d*-isomer is the therapeutically active compound. Amphetamine formulations are marketed as mixtures of *d*- and *l*-isomers, or the *d*-isomer only, where in the *d*-isomer is about three to five times more potent than the *l*-isomer. A variety of sustained or extended-release products have been developed to provide patients with either once or twice-daily dosing regimens for methylphenidate and amphetamine. Methylphenidate is almost exclusively metabolized by the hepatic enzyme carboxylesterase 1 (CES1) in a stereoselective manner. A single nucleotide polymorphism (SNP) encoding for *CES1* variant p.Gly143Glu was found in various populations resulting in impairment of methylphenidate metabolism and clearance. Amphetamine is mainly metabolized by oxidative deamination and a minor route via CYP2D6. Atomoxetine was the first non-stimulant agent developed for ADHD pharmacotherapy. The CYP2D6 system primarily metabolizes atomoxetine, and it was found that poor metabolizers have about a ten-fold decrease in oral drug clearance. The pharmacodynamic benefits and adverse effects of methylphenidate, amphetamines, and atomoxetine may be linked to their pharmacokinetic profiles. Guanfacine and clonidine are more recent additions to the ADHD armamentarium but are not considered first-line treatments.

J.S. Markowitz, PharmD (✉)
Department of Pharmacotherapy and Translational Research, Center for Pharmacogenomics, University of Florida, Gainesville, FL, USA
e-mail: jmarkowitz@cop.ufl.edu

G. Yu, PhD
Laboratory of Pharmacogenomics and Pharmacokinetic Research, Medical Research Center, Subei People's Hospital, Yangzhou University, Yangzhou, Jiangsu Province, China
e-mail: appleyuguo@gmail.com

M. Jann et al. (eds.), *Applied Clinical Pharmacokinetics and Pharmacodynamics of Psychopharmacological Agents*,
DOI 10.1007/978-3-319-27883-4_12

Keywords Methylphenidate • Amphetamine • Atomoxetine • Attention-deficit/hyperactivity disorder (ADHD) • Carboxylesterase 1 (CES1) • Guanfacine • Clonidine

12.1 Introduction

Attention-deficit/hyperactivity disorder (ADHD) is a neurodevelopmental disorder characterized by developmentally inappropriate and impairing levels of hyperactive, impulsive, and inattentive behaviors [1]. Symptoms of ADHD typically begin during early childhood or adolescence, persist over time, and are pervasive across settings. Three subtypes of ADHD are recognized: predominantly hyperactive-impulsive, predominantly inattentive, and the combined type which is the most frequently diagnosed. ADHD is the most common neurobehavioral disorder of childhood with prevalence in school-age children estimated to be between 8 and 10 % [2, 3] and often persists into adulthood.

A variety of guidelines and suggested algorithms are available regarding treatment approaches to ADHD, but multimodal approaches are universally advocated. Nonpharmacological treatments include behavioral interventions, school-based interventions, social skills training, and psychotherapeutic interventions and should be considered initially and in combination with pharmacotherapy when it is utilized [4–6]. Although the underlying causes and pathophysiology of ADHD remains incompletely understood, converging evidence suggests abnormalities of monoamines dopamine (DA) and norepinephrine (NE) as well as their metabolism and transport, particularly within the frontal cortex and subcortical neural networks [3, 7, 8]. Furthermore, at the neuronal level, medications with the greatest efficacy in ADHD largely target central DA and NE transporters. Taken together, these observations suggest that irregularities in DA and NE metabolism and turnover, as well as alterations in associated transporters and receptors, are the major determinants of the pathophysiology of ADHD.

The psychostimulants methylphenidate (MPH) and amphetamine (AMP) are the first-line pharmacological treatments of ADHD in children and adult patients. These two agents, in continuous clinical use for over 60 years, are arguably the most effective agents in all of clinical psychopharmacology with impressive response rates consistently reported [9]. Furthermore, when one class of stimulant fails, the alternative can then be initiated to increase the overall treatment effectiveness to as high as 85 %. The net primary pharmacologic action of both AMP and MPH is an enhancement of synaptic concentrations of monoamine neurotransmitters through their interaction with both the DA transporter (DAT) and the NE transporter (NET), albeit through significantly different modes of action [10–14]. Overall, based on meta-analyses of effect sizes, it appears that AMP formulations may be moderately more efficacious than MPH preparations among children and adolescents, and both tend to be more effective than available non-stimulant medications FDA-approved for use in ADHD [9]. The non-stimulant medications FDA approved for ADHD include the selective NE reuptake inhibitor atomoxetine (Strattera®) as well as the α_2-agonists clonidine and guanfacine more recently approved under the proprietary names Kapvay® and Intuniv®, respectively. In the present chapter, the ADME (absorption, distribution, metabolism, and excretion) of each of these agents will be discussed followed by a section on formulation and dosing parameters.

12.2 The Stimulants

12.2.1 Methylphenidate

Methylphenidate, in clinical use since 1955, remains the most commonly utilized medication in treating ADHD throughout the world [15]. The majority of MPH dosage forms are orally administered tablets or capsules containing racemic (50:50) mixtures of *d*- and *l*-MPH isomers with formulations differing only in their general release and dispersal pattern dictated by various modified-release (MR) technologies [15, 16]. The *d*-isomer of MPH is the therapeutically active isomer, and a limited number of enantiopure formulations are also available. All available long-acting MPH formulations are presented in Table 12.1 [17–19]. For purposes of the present chapter, the abbreviation "MPH" will refer to racemic methylphenidate unless otherwise indicated. Large interindividual differences in MPH pharmacokinetics pharmacodynamics, and, accordingly, dose requirements are recognized [18], and the metabolism of MPH can be at least partially influenced by genetic factors [20]. In spite of the relatively low bioavailability and large intersubject variability in the extent of systemic exposure to MPH, these are not factors which limit therapeutic effectiveness of the drug once dosing has been individualized for a given patient.

12.2.2 Absorption

Following oral dosing with standard immediate-release (IR) tablets, the hydrochloride salt of MPH is readily soluble in the fluids of the GI tract and is rapidly absorbed from the intestine to the colon [15]. MPH does not appear to be a major substrate of the P-glycoprotein (P-gp) transporter [21]. The intestinal absorption of [^{14}C]-MPH was found to be nearly complete as indicated by a near complete recovery of radioactivity in the urine [22]. Due to extensive and stereoselective first-pass metabolism, the absolute bioavailability (F) is limited to approximately 23 % for *d*-MPH and 5 % for the *l*-isomer [23]. Peak plasma concentrations following a 0.30 mg/kg dose are approximately 10 ng/ml on average, with a T_{max} of 1–2 h. The maximum plasma concentration (C_{max}) values however show considerable

Table 12.1 Long-acting methylphenidate dosage forms available in the USA

Product	Formulation	Pharmacokinetic release profile	Available dosage strengths (mg)	Can dosage form be opened and sprinkled?
Concerta® (*d,l*-MPH)	OROS™, osmotically active trilayer CR system; 22 % IR, 78 % SR	Compares with tid dosing of IR MPH	Tablets: 18, 27, 36, 54	No
Metadate® CD (*d,l*-MPH)	Diffucaps®, beaded CR system; 30:70 ratio of IR:ER beads	Biphasic: mimics twice dosing	Capsules: 10, 20, 30, 40, 50	Yes
Ritalin® LA (*d,l*-MPH)	SODAS®, beaded CR system; 50:50 ratio of IR:ER beads	Biphasic: mimics twice dosing	Capsules: 10, 20, 30, 40	Yes
Focalin® XR (*d*-MPH)	SODAS®, beaded CR system; 50:50 ratio of IR:ER beads	Biphasic: mimics twice dosing	Capsules: 5,10, 15, 20, 25, 30, 35, 40	Yes
Quillivant XR® (*d,l*-MPH)	ER oral suspension	Compares with bid dosing of IR MPH	25 mg per 5 mL	N/A
Daytrana® (*d,l*-MPH)	DOT Matrix™ transdermal patch	Compares with tid dosing of IR MPH but dependent on duration of wear time	10 mg/9 h, 15 mg/9 h, 20 mg/9 h, 30 mg/9 h	N/A

MPH methylphenidate, *IR* immediate-release, *SR* sustained-release, *ER* extended -release, *OROS* osmotic release oral system, *CR* controlled-release, *LA* long-acting, *SODAS, N/A* not applicable

intersubject variability. The area under the plasma concentration-time curve (AUC) and the C_{max} are generally proportional to the dose. Therapeutic drug monitoring of MPH has not proven useful in managing ADHD treatment. In five children dosed with IR MPH, F was found to range between 11 and 53 %, with a mean of 28 % in the fasted state, and 31 % when dosing was with breakfast. [24] The extent of absorption of essentially all MPH dosage forms is unaffected by food intake, although consumption of a high-fat meal may result in a 1–2 h delay in the T_{max} which most likely reflects a delay in gastric emptying [15].

For IR dosing, the elimination half-life ($t_{1/2}$) is typically reporting in the range of 2–3 h. However, in a number of more recent studies utilizing the newer MR dosage forms, significantly longer half-lives have been reported. However, this is thought to be an artifact of the prolonged absorption of MPH from these dosage forms which are programmed to continue to release MPH into the elimination phase masking the true elimination $t_{1/2}$ [15, 16]. The pharmacokinetics of MPH have not been found to

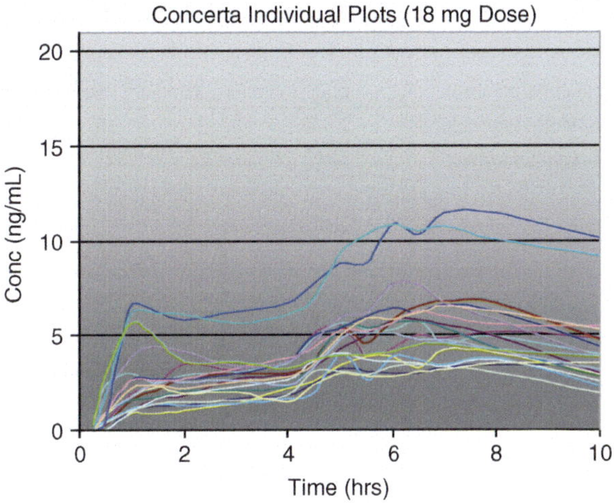

Fig. 12.1 Intersubject variability can be appreciated from the individual AUCs of 19 healthy adult subjects participating in a normal volunteer PK study of the methylphenidate modified-release formulation Concerta®

differ significantly between children, adolescents, or adults, although it appears that the relative bioavailability of MPH may be greater in adult men relative to women receiving similar dosages [15, 25]. There is little evidence that intra-subject variability in MPH pharmacokinetics is of the same magnitude generally observed between subjects (i.e., interindividual variability). On the other hand, intra-subject variability of MPH has undergone relatively little formal study with the newer MR formulations. This intersubject variability can be illustrated in Fig. 12.1 in which a PK "spaghetti" plot depicts individual AUCs from 19 healthy adult subjects participating in a normal volunteer pharmacokinetic study of the MR Concerta® dosage form [26]. Such variation in individual AUCs is typical of all MR formulations of MPH [27].

12.2.3 Distribution

Upon reaching the systemic circulation, MPH is rapidly distributed to the various tissues including the CNS. The steady-state volume of distribution (V_d) is estimated at 2 L/kg. With regard to the specific isomers, the V_d has been reported as 2.65 ± 1.11 L/kg for *d*-MPH and 1.80 ± 0.91 L/kg for *l*-MPH. Clearance of MPH is also rapid, with little or no accumulation of the drug from day to day, even with the longer-acting MR formulations [16]. Thus, true steady-state conditions are essentially never attained with MPH pharmacotherapy due to its short half-life. In the blood, MPH becomes distributed in the plasma (57 %) and the erythrocytes (43 %). MPH exhibits low plasma protein binding at ~15 % [15]. Some basic pharmacokinetic parameters of IR MPH are presented in Table 12.2.

Table 12.2 General comparison of immediate-release psychostimulant formulations

Psychostimulant	T_{max} (h)	$t_{1/2}$ (h)	Typical dose range (mg/day)	Usual dosing frequency
dl-Methylphenidate	2.5–3.5	2–3.5	10–60	2–3 times daily
d-Amphetamine	3–4	~7	5–40	2 times daily

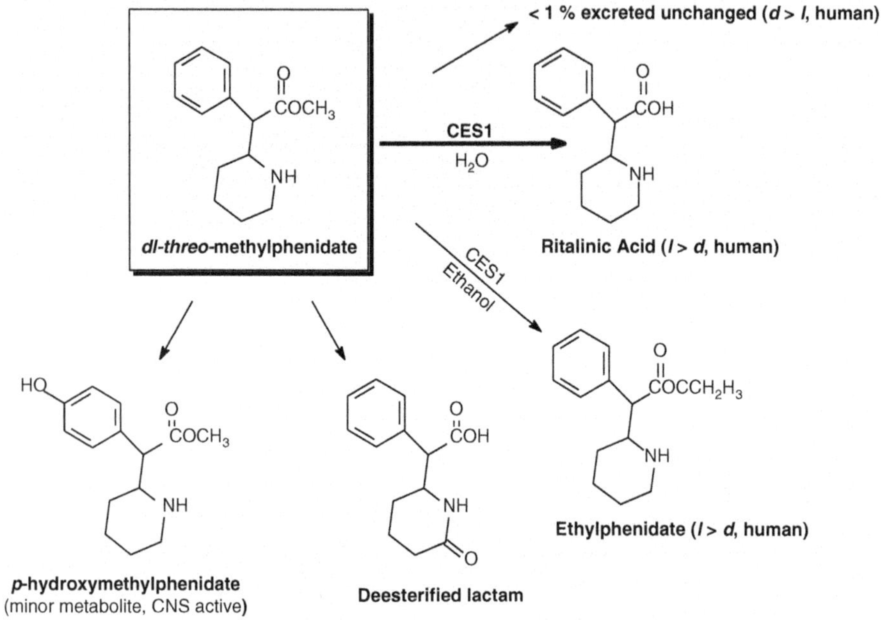

Fig. 12.2 The metabolism of methylphenidate in man

12.2.4 Metabolism

Biotransformation of MPH is rapid, stereoselective, and extensive and occurs almost exclusively via de-esterification (hydrolysis) of the parent compound to the primary and inactive metabolite, ritalinic acid (RA) (Fig. 12.2). MPH undergoes only a limited amount of metabolism by other phase I enzymes including aromatic hydroxylation to form small amounts of *p*-hydroxymethylphenidate (~1 %) which has CNS activity, as well as a de-esterified lactam, and their respective glucuronides [22]. With regard to the major metabolite RA, concentrations may attain systemic levels that are 50–60 times that of circulating MPH [15]. The half-life of RA is approximately twice that of MPH, and the mean systemic clearance is 0.17 L/h/kg. This metabolic pathway is exclusively catalyzed by the major hepatic enzyme carboxylesterase 1 (CES1) [28]. Furthermore, MPH hydrolysis is highly stereoselective, with the catalytic efficiency of CES1 estimated to be six- to sevenfold higher for the largely inactive *l*-isomer relative to *d*-MPH [28]. Indeed, enantioselective PK studies of racemic MPH formulations consistently demonstrate that the plasma concentrations of the *l*- isomer are only ~1 % that of *d*-MPH. Further to the point, in an enantiospecific study of MPH in which the drug was administered intravenously, both isomers exhibited similar initial distribution characteristics, though the terminal elimination phase of the *l*-isomer was far more rapid [19]. Interestingly, the transdermal patch formulation of racemic MPH results in a near 1:1 ratio of *d*- and *l*-MPH in the systemic circulation since its continuous delivery through the skin avoids the substantial first-pass effect and stereoselective metabolism affecting MPH oral dosage forms. CES1 is also known to mediate an unusual transesterification reaction when MPH is co-ingested with ethanol. The enzymatic reaction entails the conversion of the methyl ester in MPH into the corresponding ethyl ester to form *ethyl*phenidate, a metabolite with CNS activity [29]. A single nucleotide polymorphism (SNP) in the human *CES1* gene encoding for CES1 was recently found to confer dysfunctional enzymatic activity [20]. This *CES1* variant p.Gly143Glu (rs71647871), discovered in the course of a healthy volunteer PK study of MPH, has a minor allele frequency (MAF) estimated to be 3.7, 4.3, and 2.0 % in Caucasian, Blacks, and Hispanic populations, respectively, and is believed to result in a significant impairment in MPH metabolism and clearance [20].

12.2.5 Excretion

Following the oral administration of IR MPH, the drug is rapidly eliminated from the plasma with a mean $t_{1/2}$ of approximately 2 h. The systemic clearance is 0.40 ± 0.12 L/h/kg for *d*-MPH and 0.73 ± 0.28 L/h/kg for *l*-MPH. Within 48–96 h, 78–97 % of an administered dose is excreted in the urine and 1–3 % in the feces in the form of metabolites described above. Very little (<1 %) unchanged MPH appears in the urine with the bulk of the dose (60–86 %) excreted in the urine as RA [15, 22].

Since 2000, there have been at least 12 new FDA approvals of psychostimulants indicated for the treatment of ADHD. However, essentially all of these approvals merely represented a different pharmaceutical dosage form that provided an alternative delivery pattern of one of the two molecules (i.e., MPH and AMP). The majority of these newer formulations include various modified-release (MR) oral dosage forms of MPH (e.g., Concerta®) or mixed AMP salts (*d*-AMP: *l*-AMP, 3:1; Adderall®) enantiopure MPH formulations (e.g. Focalin®), a transdermal formulation of MPH, an oral solution of MPH, and an oral suspension of MPH (see Table 12.1). Regarding newer developments with AMP formulations, the orally administered prodrug lisdexamfetamine (Vyvanse®) is comprised of *d*-AMP covalently bound to the amino acid L-lysine via an amide linkage, which is subsequently hydrolyzed in vivo by hydrolases thereby liberating the active *d*-AMP molecule.

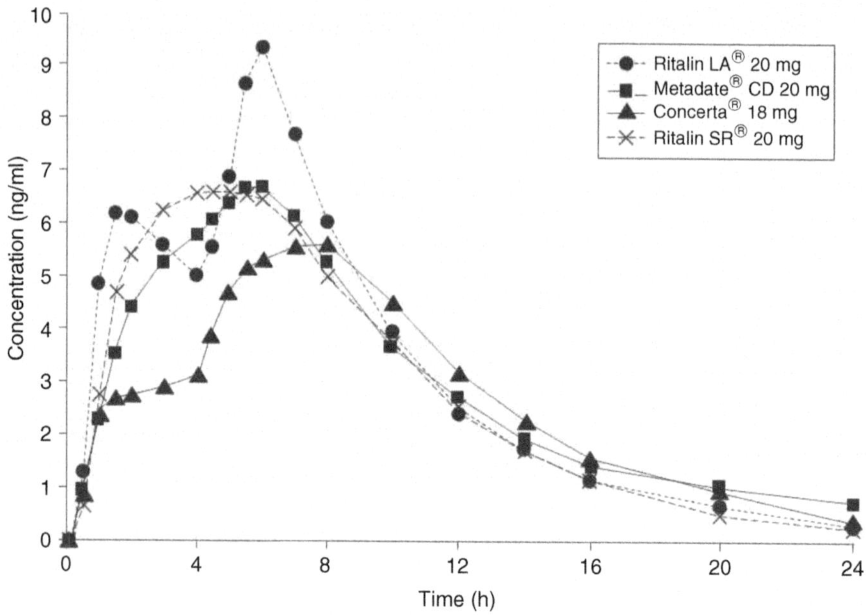

Fig. 12.3 Superimposed pharmacokinetic profiles of sustained-release methylphenidate and newer modified-release (MR) methylphenidate formulations (*LA* long acting, *CD* controlled delivery, *SR* sustained release Reproduced with permission: Wiley publishing from: Markowitz et al. [15])

12.2.6 Newer Methylphenidate Oral Dosage Forms

The rapid metabolism of MPH limits its half-life to just 2–3 h. In order to provide drug coverage throughout the school or work day, this brief half-life necessitates multiple daily dosing when IR MPH is employed in treatment. This situation resulted in inconvenience, potentially decreased compliance, security concerns at schools relevant to controlled substance storage and administration, and the potential stigmatization by peers during school day administration to children. As a result, a number of long-acting MPH formulations suitable for once-daily dosing were developed in an effort to offset these limitations. A number of modified-release (MR) formulations were developed which included combinations of IR and extended-release (ER) technologies that provided extended, yet distinctive drug release profiles. These newer, once-daily MPH MR formulations have now been widely accepted by patients, parents, and clinicians such that they now dominate the marketplace [15, 16]. Since the nomenclature used to describe long-acting dosage forms can be confusing, for the purposes of this chapter, the term modified-release (MR) will be used throughout since the object products are formulated with a combination of IR and ER components. The first attempt to provide a clinically acceptable long-acting MPH dosage form was a sustained-release (SR) formulation with a wax-matrix vehicle designed to provide slow release of MPH over the school day and was introduced in 1983 as Ritalin SR®. Clinician experiences and some anecdotal reports suggested the formulation were somewhat unfavorable compared to the IR formulations which had been used up until its introduction. In Fig. 12.3, a comparison of the MPH-SR formulation's AUC "shape" is presented for purposes of comparison with other newer formulations which were subsequently introduced into the clinical arena [15].

12.2.7 Newer Modified-Release Formulations of MPH

MR oral dosage forms are designed to release drug in a controlled manner to achieve desired exposure, efficacy, and safety profiles. A number of MPH product terms have been used to describe these products such as controlled delivery (CD) and long acting (LA). The initial once-daily MPH product to follow the MPH-SR dosage form was marketed some 17 years later under the proprietary name Concerta® that was introduced in 2000. With this formulation, an existing osmotic release oral system (OROS™) technology was utilized whereby osmotic pressure delivered MPH at a programmed rate through a trilayer core (Table 12.1). The tablet overcoat contains 22 % of the MPH dose and dissolves rapidly to provide an initial MPH absorption "pulse" or peak, that is generally followed by a brief plateau as water permeates the osmotically active polymer portion, releasing MPH through a laser-drilled orifice that results in a second steep rise in concentration (Fig. 12.3). The remainder of the dosage form remains intact and is passed in the stool as an insoluble core. The formulation was designed to provide the same drug coverage as *thrice*-daily IR MPH, approximating a 12-h duration of action.

The Concerta® formulation has been extremely successful both commercially and in the clinic and has remained the market leader among once-daily formulations [16]. The next entrant to the MPH MR market was called Metadate® CD (Table 12.1). This dosage form utilized the Diffucaps™ technology and provided the coverage expected of a *twice*-daily schedule of IR MPH. The disparate nature of the MPH-containing beads within the capsule allow for rapid dissolution of 30 % of the MPH dose, while the remaining 70 % is released in an extended fashion (Fig. 12.3). Initial formulation development studies suggested that an IR:ER dose ratio of 30:70 provided more consistent treatment effects than either a 20:80 or 40:60 ratio. A formulation marketed as Ritalin® LA was the next MPH MR formulation approved by the FDA and incorporated a spheroidal oral drug absorption system (SODAS™) bead technology as well. This was a biphasic dosage form in a capsule containing a 50:50 ratio of IR:ER beads. The ER beads are polymer coated to offer an approximate 4-h latency before the dissolving of this coat in the GI tract to release the second pulse of MPH, resulting in a biphasic profile mimicking *twice*-daily IR MPH [16].

Lastly, an enantiopure formulation of *d*-MPH (dexmethylphenidate; Focalin® XR) was later introduced that also employed the SODAS™ bead technology and is analogous to racemic Ritalin® LA in terms of release mechanism and general AUC shape. As can be appreciated from Fig. 12.3, each formulation produces a distinctly different plasma profile, often with similar overall exposures to MPH relative to the equivalent IR dose. It should also be appreciated that substantial interindividual variability exists with all of the newer MPH MR formulations. Food, diurnal rhythms, and GI function and transit times may all influence the performance of MR dosage forms (Fig. 12.1)

12.2.8 Amphetamine

Amphetamine is usually viewed as being as effective as MPH and is often used as the initial pharmacologic treatment by many clinicians. Racemic amphetamine sulfate (Benzedrine, *d*-AMP and *l*-AMP, 1:1) was the first psychostimulant documented in the treatment of children with behavioral disorders by Bradley in 1937 [30]. However, in the USA, for several decades, the only AMP formulations available for clinical use were either enantiopure *d*-AMP formulations (e.g., Dexedrine®) or, later, mixtures of *d*- and *l*-AMP isomer salts in a 3:1 ratio referred to as "mixed amphetamine salts" that were neither enantiopure nor racemic, but *scalemic* formulations. *d*-AMP has been reported to be three to five times more potent than the *l*-AMP isomer in blocking the uptake of DA while exhibiting approximately the same potency in blocking the uptake of NE. However, the rationale for the exclusion/inclusion of the *l*-isomer in various marketed formulations has not always been obvious. In September, 2014, racemic AMP (i.e., *d*- and *l*-AMP isomers in a 1:1 ratio) re-entered the clinical pharmacopoeia in the USA following the FDA approval of *dl*-AMP sulfate marketed under the proprietary name of Evekeo™ with an indication for the treatment of ADHD in children >3 years of age [31]. Table 12.3 provides a listing of available FDA-approved AMP formulations for ADHD.

12.2.9 Absorption

Following oral administration, both isomers of AMP are well absorbed, and there appears to be little effect of food on the extent or rate of absorption. AMP does not appear to be a substrate of the P-gp transporter [23]. The bioavailability of AMP is approximately 25 %. The T_{max} of IR AMP generally occurs within 2–3 h, though substantial intersubject variability has been reported. For the ER formulations of mixed amphetamine salts and *d*-AMP formulations, a T_{max} of 7–8 h is typical. The mean C_{max} after 0.25 or 0.5 mg/kg doses of IR AMP are approximately 40 and 70 ng/mL, respectively. Therapeutic drug monitoring of AMP formulations has not proven useful in the management of ADHD. A half-life of ~7 h is typical [32]. After the administration of a single dose 10 or 30 mg of IR mixed AMP salts to healthy volunteers under fasted conditions, peak plasma concentrations occurred approximately 3 h post-dose for both *d*-AMP and *l*-AMP [33]. The mean elimination half-life ($t_{1/2}$) for *d*-AMP was shorter than the $t_{1/2}$ of the *l*-isomer (9.77–11 h vs.

Table 12.3 Amphetamine containing dosage forms approved for treating ADHD

Brand name (generic name)	Formulations and strengths available
Adderall® (mixed salts of *d*- and *l*-amphetamine in ratio of 3:1)	Formulation: immediate-release tablet Available strengths: 5, 7.5, 10, 12.5, 15, 20, and 30 mg
Adderall XR® (mixed salts of *d*- and *l*-amphetamine in the ratio of 3:1)	Formulation: extended-release capsule Available strengths: 5, 10, 15, 20, 30 mg
Vyvanse® (lisdexamfetamine) lysine-conjugate prodrug	Formulation: immediate-release capsule Available strengths: 20, 30, 40, 50, 70 mg
Zenzedi® (*d*-amphetamine) Others	Formulations: immediate-release tablets Available strengths: 2.5, 5, 7.5, 10, 15, 20, 30 mg
Dexedrine Spansule® (*d*-amphetamine)	Extended-release capsules: 5, 10, 15 mg
Evekeo™ (racemic i.e. *dl*-amphetamine)	Formulation: immediate-release tablets Available strengths: 5, 10 mg
Desoxyn® (methamphetamine)	Formulation: immediate-release tablets Available strengths: 5 mg

11.5–13.8 h) [33]. It has been postulated that stereoselective differences in metabolic deamination might account for this difference. Although both enantiomers accumulate in the brain, *d*-AMP may attain higher concentrations [18].

12.2.10 *Metabolism*

The metabolism of AMP proceeds primarily through oxidative deamination forming an intermediate phenylacetone which is then oxidized to benzoic acid and then conjugated with glycine to form hippuric acid (Fig. 12.4), part of which is eliminated as a sulfate conjugate [32, 34, 35]. Aromatic hydroxylation is a more minor pathway believed to be mediated by the cytochrome P450 (CYP) 2D6 pathway and leads to the formation of 4-hydroxyamphetamine. Additionally, β-hydroxylation is stereoselective for the *d*-isomer of AMP to form norephedrine (phenylpropanolamine). Norephedrine and 4-hydroxyamphetamine are both active, and each is subsequently *N*-oxidized to form 4-hydroxynorephedrine. These metabolites may then be subject to conjugation with sulfate or glucuronic acid. Approximately one third of a dose is excreted unchanged in the urine at physiologically normal pH (i.e., ~6.5–7.5) [18, 32, 34, 35].

12.2.11 *Distribution*

Amphetamines are highly lipid soluble and are concentrated in the kidney, lungs, cerebrospinal fluid, and brain. Plasma protein binding is approximately 15–40 %, and the volume of distribution is similar for both isomers at approximately 3–4 L/kg. The plasma clearance of *d*-AMP is 5.39 mL/min/kg [18, 34].

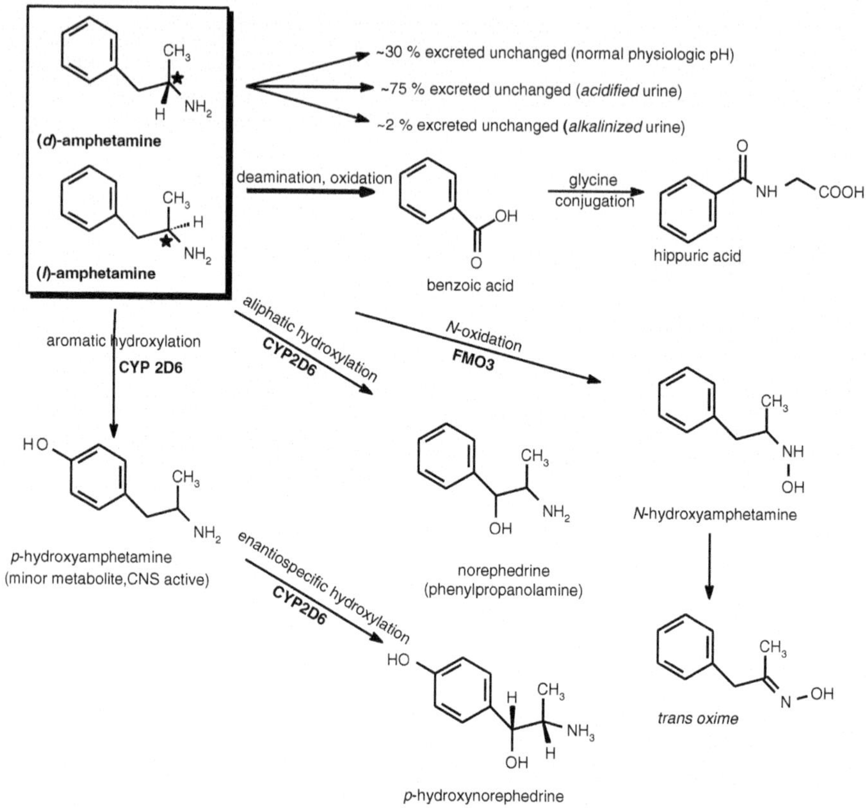

Fig. 12.4 The metabolism of amphetamine in man

12.2.12 Excretion

Approximately 5–30 % of amphetamine is excreted unchanged, while the balance of an administered dose is eliminated as benzoic acid and its corresponding glycine conjugate, hippuric acid. Excretion of AMP is highly dependent on urinary pH under normal pH conditions with acidic urine greatly enhancing excretion of the parent compound and alkaline conditions having the opposite effect [18]. Under acidic conditions, amphetamines are largely ionized, and there is little reabsorption in the kidneys, while under alkaline conditions, unionized amphetamines are readily reabsorbed in the kidneys and excretion in urine decreases. Other minor metabolites include benzoyl glucuronide as well as 4-hydroxyamphetamine, norephedrine, and their respective conjugates (Fig. 12.4). The elimination half-life of *d*-AMP is 10–12 h for adults and 6–8 h for children [32, 34].

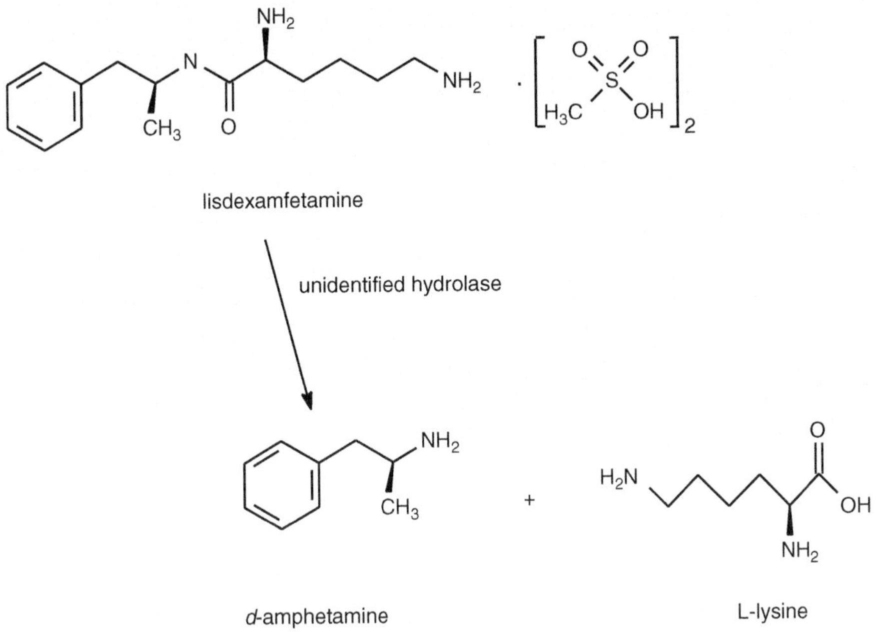

Fig. 12.5 The metabolism of lisdexamfetamine in man

12.2.13 Lisdexamfetamine

Lisdexamfetamine dimesylate is an orally administered, pharmacologically inactive prodrug consisting of *d*-AMP covalently bound to the amino acid L-lysine via an amide linkage. This bond is subsequently hydrolyzed in vivo releasing the active *d*-AMP molecule (Fig. 12.5) [36]. The resulting release profile supports once-daily administration without the necessity to employ sustained-release dosage technologies. There had been some hopes by the innovators of this formulation that there might be some relaxation of the C-II controlled substance scheduling since recreational users of stimulants may prefer i.v. or intranasal routes of administration because the rate of entry into the brain is much more rapid and reinforcing of drug-seeking/rewarding behavior than might be observed following oral administration of conventional, non-prodrug amphetamine formulations. Although it may offer some advantages in this area, it is classified as a C-II drug as are all of the available psychostimulants.

12.2.14 Absorption

After oral administration, lisdexamfetamine is rapidly absorbed from the GI tract. The administration of lisdexamfetamine with a high-fat meal produces no changes in the observed AUC and C_{max} of *d*-AMP. However, administration with food is observed to prolong the T_{max} by approximately 1 h (from 3.8 h at fasted state to 4.7 h after a high-fat meal). The plasma elimination half-life of the parent prodrug, lisdexamfetamine, typically averages less than 1 h [36, 37].

12.2.15 Metabolism

Following the oral administration of a 70 mg dose of radiolabeled lisdexamfetamine dimesylate, >90 % of oral dose radioactivity was recovered in the urine of normal volunteers and only 0.3 % recovered in the feces over a period of 120 h. Lisdexamfetamine appears to be extensively converted to *d*-AMP and L-lysine primarily in blood due to hydrolytic activity occurring within red blood cell by an as yet unidentified hydrolase. The lisdexamfetamine parent molecule itself is not metabolized by CYP450 enzymes, and only 2 % of the dose is excreted in the urine as the intact molecule [36, 37]. Once released, *d*-AMP is then subject to the metabolic processes described previously for *d*-AMP and illustrated in Fig. 12.5. *d*-AMP PK appear to be linear after single dose administration over the dose range of 30–70 mg. There is no accumulation of *d*-AMP at steady state in healthy adults and no accumulation of lisdexamfetamine after once-daily dosing for 7 consecutive days [36].

12.2.16 Distribution

Plasma concentrations of intact lisdexamfetamine are low and transient, generally becoming non-quantifiable by hour 8 post-administration. Plasma concentrations of unconverted lisdexamfetamine are low and transient and essentially absent 8 h after administration. There is no accumulation of *d*-AMP at steady state in healthy adults and no accumulation of lisdexamfetamine after once-daily dosing for 7 consecutive days [36].

12.2.17 Excretion

Only 2 % of the dose is excreted as the intact prodrug in the urine. Of the metabolites recovered in the urine, the situation is nearly identical to that observed with *d*-AMP oral administration (Fig. 12.4) [36].

12.3 The Non-stimulants

In spite of the lengthy clinical track record and extensive documentation of efficacy and response rates, >30 % of individuals treated with psychostimulants may experience an inadequate response to both MPH and AMP, making the availability of

Table 12.4 Non-stimulant medications approved for the treatment of ADHD

Brand name (generic name)	Formulations and strengths available
Strattera® (atomoxetine)	Formulation: immediate-release capsule Available strengths: 10, 18, 25, 40, 60, 80, 100 mg
Intuniv® (guanfacine)	Formulation: extended-release tablet Available strengths: 1, 2, 3, 4 mg
Kapvay® (clonidine)	Formulation: extended-release tablet Available strengths: 0.1, 0.2 mg

non-stimulant options desirable [38]. Beyond patients who simply do not respond adequately to an appropriate trial of a psychostimulant, other individuals may be appropriate candidates for non-stimulant medications as well. These include those intolerant of psychostimulant-associated side effects, those who have medical issues which may be a relative contraindication to their use, and those patient populations presenting with comorbid disorders such as Tourette syndrome or tic disorders or symptoms such as anxiety or insomnia [39, 40]. Furthermore, both AMP and MPH have high abuse potential and are classified as C-II narcotics under federal law in the USA. Accordingly, in certain patients with caregivers who wish to avoid controlled substances or if legitimate concerns over potential misuse or drug diversion by the patient or other members of the household exists, non-stimulant agents should be considered [38]. Available non-stimulant medications, presented in Table 12.4, may also be judiciously used in combination with stimulant medications in cases where neither agent alone is adequately controlling target symptoms.

12.3.1 Atomoxetine

The first truly novel non-stimulant medication to be developed and FDA approved for ADHD which was not already marketed for another indication was the selective NE reuptake inhibitor atomoxetine (Strattera®). Atomoxetine, approved by the FDA in 2002, is marketed as the *R* (−) isomer of the racemic compound, which is ~9-fold more potent as an inhibitor of NET than the *S* (+) isomer. Currently, atomoxetine is the only approved NE reuptake inhibitor for the treatment of ADHD and the only non-stimulant medication approved for adult ADHD. Atomoxetine selectively blocks the NET and increases the availability of intra-synaptic NE. This action is believed to lead to improvements in higher cognitive functions that are typically impaired in patients with ADHD [39–42].

Notably, the cytochrome P450 CYP2D6 pathway is heavily involved in the metabolism and disposition of atomoxetine (Fig. 12.6). It is recognized that *CYP2D6* genes are highly polymorphic with numerous allelic variants resulting in varying degrees of loss of metabolic function (i.e., extensive, intermediate, and poor metabolizer [PM] phenotypes). Additionally, gene duplication may result in the "ultra-rapid" metabolizer (UM) phenotype. Further, there are significant differences in the

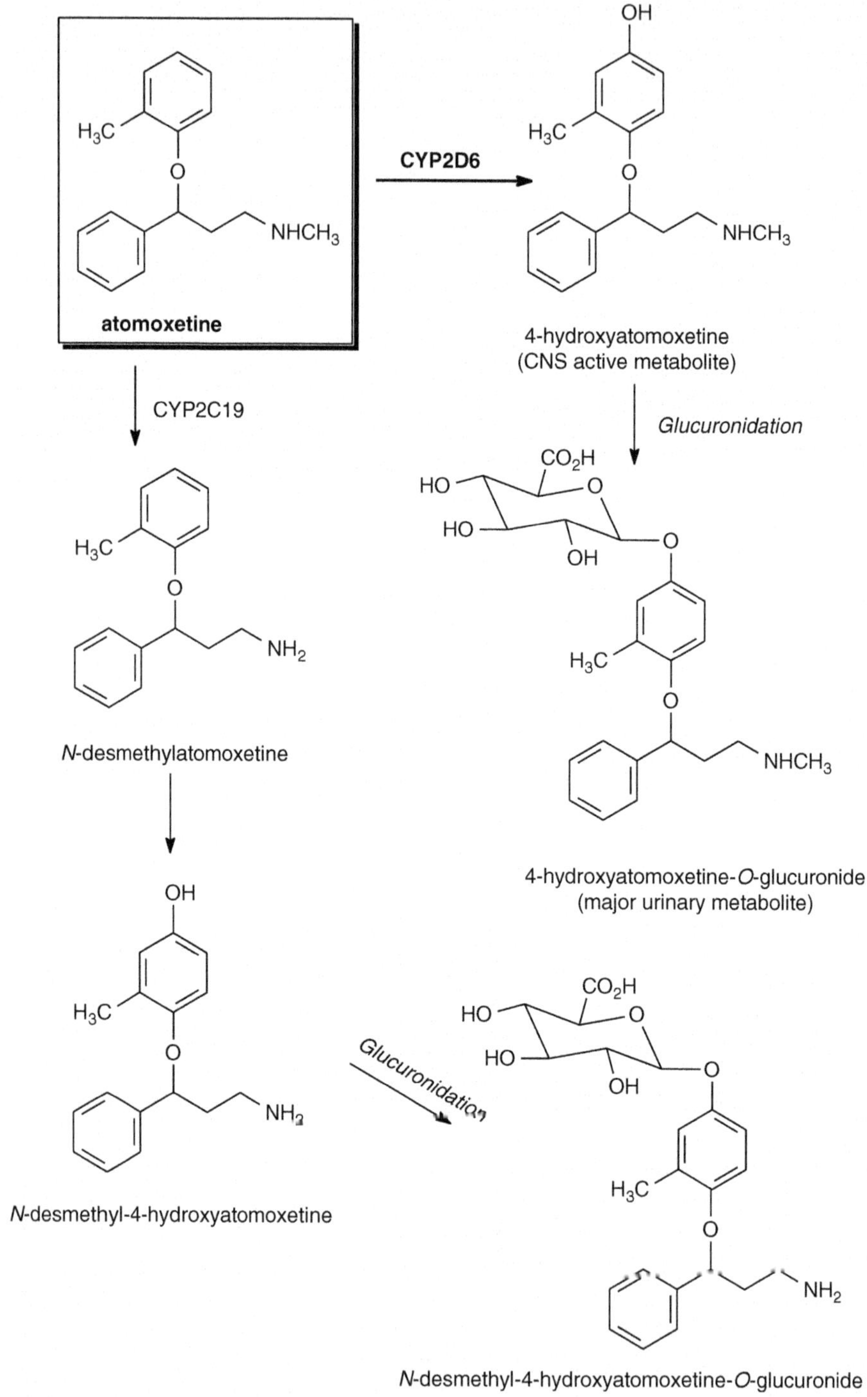

Fig. 12.6 The metabolism of atomoxetine in man

frequencies of the variant alleles between different racial and ethnic populations. Atomoxetine has undergone more extensive study with regard to pharmacogenomics (i.e., *CYP2D6*) than all of the other compounds discussed in this chapter combined. However, although the fundamental influences of CYP2D6 metabolizer status with regard to atomoxetine metabolism and disposition will be discussed in the following section, an in-depth review of CYP2D6 pharmacogenomics and atomoxetine is beyond the scope of the present chapter.

12.3.2 Absorption

Atomoxetine is rapidly absorbed after oral administration, and crossover (pilot) bioavailability studies in healthy subjects revealed that the F of atomoxetine (40 mg oral capsule) in CYP2D6 EMs and PMs were 63 % and 94 %, respectively [44], indicating high intestinal permeability and oral absorption of atomoxetine in both groups. After oral administration of atomoxetine, the median T_{max} of the parent drug in CYP2D6 EMs and PMs were approximately 1.0 h and 4.0–6.0 h, respectively, suggesting a rapid rate of balance between absorption and disposition in CYP2D6 EMs. A relative bioavailability study found identical oral bioavailability between atomoxetine capsule and solution; thus, oral absorption and bioavailability would not be influenced by the capsule formulation [44]. Atomoxetine can be administered without regard to food. Administration with a standard high-fat meal in adult subjects did not affect the extent of absorption (AUC), but did decrease the rate of absorption, resulting in a 37 % lower C_{max} and delayed T_{max} by 3 h. The average time to reach C_{max} at steady state was approximately 1–2 h. At steady state, the C_{max} for atomoxetine was almost six-fold higher in PMs than in EMs, and the mean plasma AUC was approximately eight-fold higher [43, 44]. The bioavailability of atomoxetine was unchanged during coadministration with Maalox (aluminum/magnesium hydroxides) or omeprazole; thus, concurrent administration of drugs that alter gastric acid secretion (such as omeprazole) or neutralize gastric acid (such as aluminum/magnesium hydroxides) do not appear to affect the absorption and bioavailability of atomoxetine [44].

12.3.3 Distribution

The steady-state volume of distribution of atomoxetine after intravenous administration is 0.85 L/kg, which is similar with the total volume of body water, suggesting that the distribution of atomoxetine is mainly into total body water [45]. The concentrations of atomoxetine in postmortem liver and fluids in two persons whose death was unrelated to the drug, and notwithstanding the potential influence of potential postmortem redistribution, were as follows: liver, <0.44–3.9 mg/kg; aortic blood, <0.1–0.65 mg/L; femoral blood, <0.1–0.33 mg/L; and vitreous humor, 0.1 mg/L

[46]. At therapeutic doses, atomoxetine and its metabolite 4-hydroxyatomoxetine presented in human oral fluid, with significant lower levels relative to those in plasma [47]. The oral fluid-to-plasma concentration ratio of atomoxetine ranged from 0.01 to 0.12 and that of 4-hydroxyatomoxetine from 0.16 to 1.96, with the minimum at 1 and 2 h post-administration, respectively [47].

Binding of atomoxetine to human plasma protein *in vitro* was ~98 % and was almost entirely to albumin [48]. Plasma protein binding of the two metabolites, N-desmethyl atomoxetine and 4-hydroxyatomoxetine, were 99.1 % and 66.6 %, respectively [48]. The plasma protein binding of atomoxetine was lower in subjects with end-stage renal disease (94.8 % ± 6.9 %, mean ± SEM, $N=6$) and subjects with moderate and severe liver disease (96.4 % ± 1.56 %, mean ± SEM, $N=10$) relative to healthy subjects (98.0–98.7 %) [44, 48]. This is presumably the result of the decrease in albumin associated with severe renal or hepatic impairment.

12.3.4 Metabolism

Atomoxetine is extensively metabolized (Fig. 12.6) with more than 80 % of a radiolabeled dose being detected in the urine as metabolites and less than 3 % unchanged parent compound [49]. The primary phase I metabolic pathways that govern the biotransformation of atomoxetine in humans are aromatic ring hydroxylation, benzylic oxidation, and N-demethylation [49]. The O-glucuronidation of the hydroxylated metabolites is the only phase II metabolic pathway involved in the biotransformation of atomoxetine [49]. The major phase I metabolite is 4-hydroxyatomoxetine produced via aromatic ring hydroxylation, which is subsequently glucuronidated forming 4-hydroxyatomoxetine-O-glucuronide [49]. CYP2D6 is the primary enzyme responsible for the formation of 4-hydroxyatomoxetine, whereas a variety of other CYP enzymes have shown capability in metabolizing atomoxetine to 4-hydroxyatomoxetine in the absence of CYP2D6, albeit at a considerably slower rate. N-desmethyl atomoxetine, a minor metabolite, is predominantly formed via CYP2C19 and undergoes further hydroxylation mediated via CYP2D6 and subsequent O-glucuronidation [48–50]. While 4-hydroxyatomoxetine has similar pharmacologic activity to atomoxetine in terms of NET inhibition, the inhibitory *potency* of N-desmethyl atomoxetine is nearly 20-fold less [44]. In addition, on the basis of the metabolic profiles of CYP2D6 EMs and PMs, the same metabolites were identified regardless of phenotypes, and no CYP2D6 phenotype-specific metabolites were observed [44, 50]. A summary of major differences in these parameters observed by metabolizer type is presented in Table 12.5.

A within study comparison showed that the average steady-state oral clearance (CLss/F) of atomoxetine in CYP2D6 EMs (0.373 L/h/kg) is approximately ten-fold greater than that of PMs (0.0357 L/h/kg), demonstrating the predominant role of CYP2D6 in the metabolic clearance of atomoxetine. Atomoxetine circulates principally in the plasma of CYP2D6 EMs as the parent and the major metabolite

Table 12.5 Pharmacokinetic parameters of atomoxetine and selected metabolites in extensive versus poor metabolizers of CYP2D6 [40, 43]

Parameter	Extensive metabolizers CYP2D6	Poor metabolizers CYP2D6
Bioavailability (%)	63	94
T_{max} (h)	1–2	3–4
$C_{max,ss}$ (ng/mL) ± SD	159.70 ± 51.9	914.72 ± 30.5
Half-life (h)	5.2	21.6
Primary metabolites		
4-Hydroxyatomoxetine	2.03 ± 17.5	–
4-Hydroxyatomoxetine-*O*-glucuronide		
Half-life (h)	6–8	–
$C_{max,ss}$ (ng/mL) ± SD	413.88 ± 35.5	88.00 ± 16.9
N-Desmethylatomoxetine		
Half-life (h)	–	34–40
$C_{max,ss}$ (ng/mL) ± SD	7.02 ± 71.5	259.22 ± 39.6

Sauer et al. [59]

4-hydroxyatomoxetine-O-glucuronide, but in PMs, atomoxetine circulates principally as the parent compound and the metabolite N-desmethyl atomoxetine [44]. In adult CYP2D6 EM subjects, after dosing with 20 mg twice daily for 5 days, the exposure to 4-hydroxyatomoxetine is only around 1 % (based on $C_{ss,max}$) of that of atomoxetine, while the exposure of N-desmethyl atomoxetine is approximately 5 % (based on $C_{ss,max}$ and AUC during a dosage interval [AUCτ]) of that of atomoxetine [48]. In adult CYP2D6 PMs, after 75 mg twice daily over 5 days, the exposure of 4-hydroxyatomoxetine is just 0.1 % of that of atomoxetine, while the exposure of N-desmethyl atomoxetine is about 45 % of that of atomoxetine [44]. Taken together, exposure to 4-hydroxyatomoxetine ranges from 0.1 % of the parent compound in CYP2D6 PMs and 1 % in EMs, but exposure to N-desmethyl atomoxetine ranged from 5 % of the parent compound in CYP2D6 EMs and 45 % of the parent compound in PMs. 4-Hydroxyatomoxetine-O-glucuronide plasma concentrations in CYP2D6 EMs are 2.6-fold that of atomoxetine and over 40-fold greater than N-desmethylatomoxetine, but the levels in PMs are numerically less than either the parent or N-desmethyl atomoxetine [48].

12.3.5 Excretion

Because of extensive metabolism, the largest fraction of an atomoxetine dose is excreted into the urine as the 4-hydroxyatomoxetine-O-glucuronide [48]. Less than 3 % of the administered dose is excreted into the urine as unchanged the parent compound, suggesting a minimal role for renal excretion in overall clearance of the drug. The cumulative fraction of a radioactive dose excreted into the urine is about 96 % in EMs and 80 % in PMs. The cumulative fraction of a radioactive dose excreted via the feces is approximately 2 % in CYP 2D6 EMs and 17 % in PMs. In CYP2D6 EMs, almost all of a radiolabeled dose was cleared from the body within 48 h, but in PMs, all of the dose was not eliminated until beyond the 144 h time point. [48] When about 90 % of the radiolabeled amount had been cleared in CYP2D6 EMs within 24 h post-dose, only 30 % of the dose was excreted in PMs. [48]

12.3.6 α_2-Agonists: Guanfacine and Clonidine

With regard to other non-stimulant medications, the α_2-agonists and imidazoline derivatives clonidine and guanfacine, initially marketed as centrally acting antihypertensive medications, had found extensive use as "off-label" medications to treat ADHD symptoms as adjunctive therapy to existing stimulant regimens or as monotherapy. These agents gained FDA approval for the treatment of ADHD relatively recently and have been reformulated as ER tablets that provide a significantly reduced C_{max} compared to the same dosage of their respective IR formulations presently marked as antihypertensive agents. Basic pharmacokinetic parameters of these two related agents are presented in Table 12.6. Both clonidine and guanfacine act on the presynaptic and postsynaptic α_2 neuronal receptors. This action is believed to improve working memory by stimulating and strengthening the functional connectivity of prefrontal networks [38, 41]. These agents may be employed as adjunctive treatments or as monotherapies for ADHD. The amelioration of ADHD symptoms is believed to rely on the specific stimulation of the postsynaptic α_{2A} subtype of receptor. Of note, relative to clonidine, guanfacine is a much more selective α_{2A} adrenergic receptor agonist, while clonidine binds at all α_2 receptor subtypes (i.e., A, B, and C) [51, 52]. Relative to clonidine ER, there is much more available published pharmacokinetic data with guanfacine ER at present.

Table 12.6 Comparison of pharmacokinetic parameters of clonidine and guanfacine following the single dose of the respective agents in healthy adults

Mean pharmacokinetic parameters (± SD)	Extended-release clonidine (Kapvay®) 0.1 mg	Extended release guanfacine (Intuniv®) 1 mg
C_{max} (ng/mL)	1.0 ± 0.3	0.26 ± 0.033
$AUC_{0-\infty}$ (ng.h/mL)	32 ± 9	6.73 ± 1.65
T_{max} (h)	6	6.5
$t_{1/2}$ (h)	18 ± 4	12.7 ± 3.6
Influence of high-fat meal	No effect	↑ mean C_{max} ~75 % ↑ mean AUC ~40 %

Data do not represent a comparative crossover study but are derived from the separate studies described in the Full Prescribing Information for Kapvay® and Intuniv® [51, 52]

12.3.7 Guanfacine

12.3.7.1 Absorption

Guanfacine is readily absorbed and from the GI tract and is not a substrate or a potent inhibitor of the of the P-gp transporter [53]. The F of guanfacine is ~80 %. Following oral administration, the T_{max} is approximately 6 h. When a single dose of guanfacine 4 mg was administered with a high-fat breakfast, the mean exposure increased significantly (i.e., C_{max} ~75 % and AUC ~40 %) compared to dosing in a fasted state [51].

12.3.7.2 Distribution

The plasma protein binding of guanfacine as determined by equilibrium dialysis ranges from 64 to 72 %, and it is widely distributed throughout the body. The V_d is 6.3 L/kg (276–347 L) suggesting intracellular distribution, and approximately 60 % of guanfacine in the blood is bound to red blood cells. Exposure to guanfacine was higher in children (ages 6–12 years) compared to adolescents (ages 13–17 years) and adults, and following the oral administration of multiple 4 mg doses of guanfacine the C_{max} was 10 ng/mL compared to 7 ng/mL, and the AUC was 162 ng h/mL compared to 116 ng h/mL in children (ages 6–12) and adolescents (ages 13–17), respectively [51]. These differences are believed to be attributable to the lower body weight of children compared to adolescents and adults. The pharmacokinetics of guanfacine generally appear to be linear and dose proportional [51, 54–56].

12.3.7.3 Metabolism

Approximately 50 % of an administered dose is metabolized in the liver with the 3-hydroxy-derivative of guanfacine; its respective O-glucuronide and sulfate conjugates represent the major metabolites. Other oxidized mercapturic acid derivatives are also present as minor metabolites. About 30 % of an administered dose of guanfacine is excreted unchanged in the urine [51, 54, 55]. *In vitro* studies have demonstrated that guanfacine is primarily metabolized by CYP3A4. Accordingly, as a substrate of CYP3A4/5, exposure is affected by coadministration with CYP3A4/5 inducers/inhibitors [51].

12.3.7.4 Elimination

Guanfacine is excreted by the kidney by filtration and active secretion, although reabsorption by the tubule cannot be ruled out. Renal excretion is ~50 %, and the elimination $t_{1/2}$ is 17 h (range, 10–30 h) [51].

12.3.8 *Clonidine*

12.3.8.1 Absorption

Following a single dose of clonidine ER (0.1 mg) in fasted adult subjects, clonidine was absorbed more slowly relative to the IR formulation achieving a C_{max} at 6.5 h (T_{max}). The bioavailability is approximated at 70 %. Neither food nor coadministration with a high-fat meal had any significant effect on plasma concentrations, bioavailability, or elimination half-life of clonidine [52, 57].

12.3.8.2 Distribution

Clonidine is ~20–40 % protein bound, primarily to albumin. Clearance rates of clonidine were independent of the dosage of clonidine ER across a range of 0.2–0.4 mg/day, in children and adolescents with ADHD. However, clearance rates of clonidine decreased with increasing age over the range of 6–17 years and females had a 23 % lower clearance rate than males. The V_d is estimated at 3–6 L/kg [52, 57]. Clonidine pharmacokinetics appear to be linear and dose proportional. Basic pharmacokinetic parameters are presented in Table 12.6.

12.3.8.3 Metabolism

Approximately 40–60 % of orally administered clonidine is excreted unchanged in the urine with the remainder undergoing hepatic metabolism to produce inactive metabolites, mainly 4-hydroxyclonidine. *In vitro* studies indicate that CYP2D6 is the primary isoform catalyzing the formation of 4-hydroxyclonidine with much smaller roles contributed by CYP1A2, 3A4, 1A1, and 3A5 [52, 57, 58].

12.3.8.4 Excretion

Clonidine is predominantly renally eliminated with 40–60 % excreted into the urine unchanged, 20 % is excreted in feces. Less than 10 % of an administered dose is excreted as 4-hydroxyclonidine.

12.4 Conclusions

Stimulants and nonstimulants are indicated for the treatment of child, adolescent, and adult ADHD. The pharmacodynamic benefits of these agents appear to be related to their pharmacokinetic profiles. From a pharmacokinetic perspective, the stimulants are rapidly absorbed agents with relatively short half lives. This situation necessitates multiple daily dosing regimens in order to maintain effectiveness across the treatment day. Modified-release methylphenidate formulations permit once daily dosing and a number of variable formulations are now available. The metabolism of MPH is almost entirely dependent on the CES1 enzyme, and investigations continue into the potential impact of *CES1* genetic variants upon MPH disposition and response. Similarly, once daily formulations of amphetamines were developed to enhance patient adherence to treatment. Atomoxetine was the first non-stimulant agent used for ADHD treatment and is primarily metabolized by CYP2D6. Patients who are CYP2D6 PMs may require dosage adjustments with atomoxetine. Guanfacine and clonidine are not considered first-line treatments for ADHD. Nevertheless, these agents continue to be used in those patients intolerant of, or otherwise suboptimally responsive to the stimulants or atomoxetine.

References

1. National Institute of Mental Health (2015) Attention deficit hyperactivity disorder (ADHD). http://www.nimh.nih.gov/health/topics/attention-deficit-hyperactivity-disorder-adhd/index.shtml. Accessed 2 Apr 2015
2. Polanczyk G, de Lima MS, Horta BL, Biederman J, Rohde LA (2007) The worldwide prevalence of ADHD: a systematic review and metaregression analysis. Am J Psychiatry 164:942–948
3. Warikoo N, Faraone SV (2013) Background, clinical features and treatment of attention deficit hyperactivity disorder in children. Expert Opin Pharmacother 14:1885–1906
4. Pliszka SR, Crismon ML, Hughes CW, Corners CK, Emslie GJ, Jensen PS et al (2006) The Texas Children's Medication Algorithm Project: revision of the algorithm for pharmacotherapy of attention-deficit/hyperactivity disorder. J Am Acad Child Adolesc Psychiatry 45(6):642–657
5. Greenhill LL, Pliszka S, Dulcan MK (2002) Practice parameters for the use of stimulant medications in the treatment of children, adolescents, and adults. J Am Acad Child Adolesc Psychiatry 41(Suppl):26S–49S
6. Pliszka S (2007) Practice parameter for the assessment and treatment of children and adolescents with attention-deficit/hyperactivity disorder. J Am Acad Child Adolesc Psychiatry 46(7):94–921
7. Pliszka SR (2005) The neuropsychopharmacology of attention-deficit/hyperactivity disorder. Biol Psychiatry 57(11):1385–1390
8. Cortese S, Faraone SV, Sergeant J (2011) Misunderstandings of the genetics and neurobiology of ADHD: moving beyond anachronisms. Am J Med Genet B Neuropsychiatr Genet 156:513–516
9. Faraone SV, Buitelaar J (2010) Comparing the efficacy of stimulants for ADHD in children and adolescents using meta-analysis. Eur Child Adolesc Psychiatry 19:353–364
10. Wilens TE (2008) Effects of methylphenidate on the catecholaminergic system in attention-deficit/hyperactivity disorder. J Clin Psychopharmacol 28:S46–S53
11. Volkow ND, Wang GJ, Fowler JS, Ding YS (2005) Imaging the effects of methylphenidate on brain dopamine: new model on its therapeutic actions for attention-deficit/hyperactivity disorder. Biol Psychiatry 57:1410–1415
12. Robertson SD, Matthies HJ, Galli A (2009) A closer look at amphetamine- induced reverse transport and trafficking of the dopamine and norepinephrine transporters. Mol Neurobiol 39:73–80
13. Seeman P, Madras BK (1998) Anti-hyperactivity medication: methylphenidate and amphetamine. Mol Psychiatry 3:386–396
14. Wood S, Sage JR, Shuman T, Anagnostaras SG (2013) Psychostimulants and cognition: a continuum of behavioral and cognitive activation. Pharmacol Rev 66(1):193–221

15. Markowitz JS, Straughn AB, Patrick KS (2003) Advances in the pharmacotherapy of attention-deficit hyperactivity disorder: focus on methylphenidate formulations. Pharmacotherapy 23(10):1281–1299
16. Patrick KS, Gonzalez MA, Straughn AB, Markowitz JS (2005) New methylphenidate formulations for the treatment of attention-deficit/hyperactivity disorder. Expert Opin Drug Deliv 2(1):121–143
17. Patrick KS, Caldwell RW, Ferris RM, Breese GR (1987) Pharmacology of the enantiomers of threo- methylphenidate. J Pharmacol Exp Ther 241(1):152–158
18. Patrick KS, Markowitz JS (1997) Pharmacology of methylphenidate, amphetamine enantiomers and pemoline in attention-deficit hyperactivity disorder. Hum Psychopharmacol 12:527–546
19. Markowitz JS, Patrick KS (2008) Differential pharmacokinetics and pharmacodynamics of methylphenidate enantiomers: does chirality matter? J Clin Psychopharmacol 28:S54–S61
20. Zhu HJ, Patrick KS, Yuan HJ, Wang JS, Donovan JL, DeVane CL et al (2008) Two CES1 gene mutations lead to dysfunctional carboxylesterase 1 activity in man: clinical significance and molecular basis. Am J Hum Genet 82(6):1241–1248
21. Zhu H-J, Wang J-S, DeVane CL et al (2006) The role of the polymorphic efflux transporter p-glycoprotein on the brain accumulation of d-methylphenidate and d-amphetamine. Drug Metab Dispos 34:1116–1121
22. Faraj BA, Israili ZH, Perel JM et al (1974) Metabolism and disposition of methylphenidate-14C: studies in man and animals. J Pharmacol Exp Ther 191:535–547
23. Srinivas NR, Hubbard JW, Korchinski ED et al (1993) Enantioselective pharmaokinetics of dl-threo-methylphenidate in humans. Pharm Res 10:14–21
24. Chan Y-P, Swanson JM, Soldin SS et al (1983) Methylphenidate hydrochloride given with or before breakfast: II. Effects on plasma concentration of methylphenidate and ritalinic acid. Pediatrics 72:56–59
25. Sonuga-Barke EJS, Coghill D, Markowitz JS, Swanson JM, Vandenberghe M, Hatch SJ (2007) Sex differences in the response of children with ADHD to once daily formulations of methylphenidate. J Am Acad Child Adolesc Psychiatry 46:701–710
26. Markowitz JS, Straughn AB, Patrick KS, DeVane CL, Pestreich L, Lee J, Wang Y, Muniz R (2003) Pharmacokinetics of methylphenidate after oral administration of two modified-release formulations in healthy adults. Clin Pharmacokinet 42:393–401
27. Rochdi M et al (2004) Dose-proportional pharmacokinetics of a methylphenidate extended-release capsule. Int J Clin Pharmacol Ther 42(5):285–292
28. Sun Z, Murry DJ, Sanghani SP, Davis WI, Kedishvili NY, Zou Q et al (2004) Methylphenidate is stereoselectively hydrolyzed by human carboxylesterase CES1A1. J Pharmacol Exp Ther 310(2):469–476
29. Patrick KS, Straughn AB, Yeatts S et al (2007) Influence of ethanol and gender on methylphenidate pharmacokinetics and pharmacodynamics. Clin Pharmacol Ther 81:346–353
30. Bradley C (1937) The behavior of children receiving benzedrine. Am J Psychiatry 94:577–588
31. Evekeo™ (amphetamine sulfate), Full Prescribing Information, Arbor Pharmaceuticals, LLC. Revised Apr 2014
32. Heal DJ, Smith SL, Gosden J, Nutt DJ (2013) Amphetamine, past and present-a pharmacological and clinical perspective. J Psychopharmacol 27:479–496
33. Adderall XR® (mixed salts of a single-entity amphetamine product), Full Prescribing Information, Shire US Inc. Revised Apr 2015
34. Dexedrine Spansule® (dextroamphetamine sulfate), Full Prescribing Information, Amedra Pharmaceuticals LLC. Revised Feb 2015
35. Zenzedi™ (dextroamphetamine sulfate), Full Prescribing Information, Arbor Pharmaceuticals, LLC. Revised Jan 2014
36. Vyvanse® (lisdexamfetamine dimesylate) Full Prescribing Information, Shire US Inc. Revised Apr 2015
37. Hutson PH, Pennick M, Secker R (2014) Preclinical pharmacokinetics, pharmacology and toxicology of lisdexamfetamine: a novel d-amphetamine pro-drug. Neuropharmacology 87:41–50

38. Childress AC, Sallee FR (2014) Attention-deficit/hyperactivity disorder with inadequate response to stimulants: approaches to management. CNS Drugs 28:121–129
39. Rizzo R, Gulisano M, Calì PV, Curatolo P (2013) Tourette Syndrome and comorbid ADHD: current pharmacological treatment options. Eur J Paediatr Neurol 17:421–428
40. Christman AK, Fermo JD, Markowitz JS (2004) Atomoxetine: a novel treatment for attention-deficit/hyperactivity disorder. Pharmacotherapy 24:1020–1036
41. Robbins TW, Arnsten AF (2009) The neuropsychopharmacology of fronto-executive function: monoaminergic modulation. Annu Rev Neurosci 32:267–287
42. Swanson CJ, Perry KW, Koch-Krueger S, Katner J, Svensson KA, Bymaster FP (2006) Effect of the attention deficit/hyperactivity disorder drug atomoxetine on extracellular concentrations of norepinephrine and dopamine in several brain regions of the rat. Neuropharmacology 50:755–760
43. Strattera® (atomoxetine), Full Prescribing Information, Lilly USA, Inc. Revised Jan 2015
44. US Food and Drug Administration. Atomoxetine approval package. http://www.accessdata.fda.gov/drugsatfda_docs/nda/2002/21-411_Strattera.cfm. Accessed 24 Apr 2014
45. US Food and Drug Administration (2014) Atomoxetine label. http://www.accessdata.fda.gov/drugsatfda_docs/label/2014/021411s044lbl.pdf. Accessed 24 Apr 2015
46. Garside D, Ropero-Miller JD, Riemer EC (2006) Postmortem tissue distribution of atomoxetine following fatal and nonfatal doses – three case reports. J Forensic Sci 51(1):179–182
47. Papaseit E, Marchei E, Farré M, Garcia-Algar O, Pacifici R, Pichini S (2013) Concentrations of atomoxetine and its metabolites in plasma and oral fluid from paediatric patients with attention deficit/hyperactivity disorder. Drug Test Anal 5(6):446–452
48. Sauer JM, Ponsler GD, Mattiuz EL, Long AJ, Witcher JW, Thomasson HR et al (2003) Disposition and metabolic fate of atomoxetine hydrochloride: the role of CYP2D6 in human disposition and metabolism. Drug Metab Dispos 31(1):98–107
49. Chalon SA, Desager JP, Desante KA, Frye RF, Witcher J, Long AJ et al (2003) Effect of hepatic impairment on the pharmacokinetics of atomoxetine and its metabolites. Clin Pharmacol Ther 73(3):178–191
50. Ring BJ, Gillespie JS, Eckstein JA, Wrighton SA (2002) Identification of the human cytochromes P450 responsible for atomoxetine metabolism. Drug Metab Dispos 30(3):319–323
51. Intuniv® (guanfacine extended-release tablets), Full Prescribing Information, Shire US Inc. Revised Mar 2015
52. Kapvay® (clonidine extended-release tablets), Full Prescribing Information, Concordia Pharmaceuticals Inc. Revised Jan 2014
53. Gillis NK, Zhu H-J, Markowitz JS (2011) An in vitro evaluation of guanfacine as a substrate for P-glycoprotein. Neuropsychiatr Dis Treat 7:501–505
54. Swearingen D, Pennick M, Shojaei A, Lyne A, Fiske K (2007) A phase I, randomized, open-label, crossover study of the single-dose pharmacokinetic properties of guanfacine extended-release 1-, 2-, and 4-mg tablets in healthy adults. Clin Ther 29:617–625
55. Boellner SW, Pennick M, Fiske K, Lyne A, Shojaei A (2007) Pharmacokinetics of a guanfacine extended-release formulation in children and adolescents with attention-deficit–hyperactivity disorder. Pharmacotherapy 27:1253–1262
56. Martin P, Satin L, Vince BD, Padilla AF, White C, Corcoran M, Stevenson A, Erme J (2014) Pharmacokinetics and pharmacodynamics of guanfacine extended release in adolescents aged 13–17 years with attention-deficit/hyperactivity disorder. Clin Pharmacol Drug Develop 3:252–261
57. Croxtall JD (2011) Clonidine extended-release In attention-deficit hyperactivity disorder. Pediatr Drugs 13(5):329–336
58. Claessens AJ, Risler LJ, Eyal S, Shen DD, Easterling TR, Hebert MF (2010) CYP2D6 mediates 4-Hydroxylation of clonidine In vitro: implication for pregnancy-induced changes in clonidine clearance. Drug Metab Dispos 38:1393–1396
59. Sauer JM, Ring BJ, Witcher JW (2005) Clinical pharmacokinetics of atomoxetine. Clin Pharmacokinet 44(6):571–590

Chapter 13
Antidementia Drugs

Chad M. VanDenBerg and Michael W. Jann

Abstract Alzheimer's disease (AD) is the most commonly occurring dementia and consists of both cognitive impairment and behavioral disturbances. Two types of medication classes are approved by the regulatory agencies for AD treatment. The cholinesterase inhibitors (ChEIs) are used for patients with mild, moderate, and severe AD. Memantine (MEM) is indicated for moderate to severe AD patients. ChEIs and MEM are often combined together for treatment. The pharmacokinetics (PK) of the ChEIs is well known. Donepezil and galantamine display linear PK, whereas rivastigmine has nonlinear PK. Donepezil and galantamine are metabolized by the CYP2D6 and CYP3A4 enzymes. Rivastigmine is metabolized by the hepatic esterases. MEM is not significantly metabolized by the hepatic enzymes and is primarily excreted by the kidneys. Dosage adjustments are recommended for patients with severe hepatic and renal impairment. The clinical pharmacodynamic (PD) properties for the ChEIs and MEM can be assessed by various biomarkers that include cholinesterase enzyme inhibition, clinical rating scales for cognitive impairment and behavioral symptoms, and PET scan evaluations. Pharmacogenetic status is in its early utilization phase of clinical utility in AD patients. PET scans may provide useful information on patient response to ChEIs and MEM. The gastrointestinal adverse side effects limit ChEIs, but these effects are transient and associated with dose titration. Population PK analysis can integrate the PK, PD, and pharmacogenetic data to optimize treatment in patients with AD.

Keywords Alzheimer's disease • Rivastigmine • Donepezil • Galantamine • Memantine • Acetylcholinesterase • Butyrylcholinesterase • Transdermal patch • Extended release • Positron emission tomography (PET) • Pharmacogenetics

C.M. VanDenBerg, PharmD
Institute of Healthcare Innovation, Midwestern University,
Glendale, AZ, USA

M.W. Jann, PharmD (✉)
Department of Pharmacotherapy, University of North Texas System College of Pharmacy (UNTSCP) and University of North Texas Health Science Center (UNTHSC),
Fort Worth, TX, USA
e-mail: Michael.jann@unthsc.edu

M. Jann et al. (eds.), *Applied Clinical Pharmacokinetics and Pharmacodynamics of Psychopharmacological Agents*,
DOI 10.1007/978-3-319-27883-4_13

13.1 Introduction

Dementia can result from a variety of diseases; however, Alzheimer's disease (AD) is by far the most common and accounts for 50–60 % of cases associated with cognitive impairments and behavioral disturbances [1]. Other types of medical conditions where dementia can take place are Lewy body, vascular, mixed, frontotemporal, Huntington's disease, Creutzfeldt-Jakob disease, and Parkinson's disease. For a further description of the various underlying dementia pathophysiology, the reader is referred to other references where early recognition and treatment are key aspects to maintain the patient's quality of life [1, 2]. Mild cognitive impairment (MCI) is a recently recognized syndrome where a patient displays cognitive complaints without sufficient severity to warrant a diagnosis of dementia. About 10–15 % of MCI patients progress to AD [1]. Despite the recognition of the different dementia types and MCI, there are relatively few pharmacotherapeutic interventions available.

Alzheimer's disease is generally accepted to be related to a cholinergic deficit in the cerebral cortex and other areas of the brain. The cholinesterase inhibitors (ChEIs) which prevent the action of cholinesterase enzymes in the synaptic cleft (tacrine, donepezil, rivastigmine, and galantamine) were the first category of drugs approved for the treatment of Alzheimer's disease [3]. However, the efficacy of ChEIs is modest; therefore, the focus of research has shifted toward disease-modifying (and possibly disease prevention) strategies, revolving especially around amyloid and tau proteins. Still, consistently positive results with multiple ChEIs have clearly confirmed the relevance of the cholinergic hypothesis and their use in AD therapy. Since present oral doses of ChEIs do not approach the limit of potential cholinesterase inhibition in the brain [4] due to dose-limiting adverse events, if it were possible to boost central cholinergic transmission further, without significant gastrointestinal and peripheral side effects, then ChEIs might have a continuing role in AD pharmacotherapy.

Two categories of pharmacotherapy agents have been used for dementia with an initial focus on patients with AD. Use of these agents for the other dementia diseases continues to be explored and in some cases demonstrate efficacy and regulatory agency approval. These two groups of drugs are the cholinesterase inhibitors (ChEI) and the NMDA receptor antagonist memantine (MEM) [5, 6]. Tacrine was the first ChEI approved by the US FDA in 1993 for patients with mild to moderate AD, but its use has been starkly limited to due hepatotoxicity and this agent has not been included in treatment guidelines due to presence of the other, less problematic ChEIs [1, 7, 8]. However, tacrine will be included only in comparison to the other ChEIs' pharmacokinetic (PK) and pharmacodynamic (PD) properties for completeness. Memantine blocks the NMDA receptor by blocking the binding of glutamate and is thought to provide therapeutic benefit to patients with moderate to severe AD [5].

13.2 Clinical Pharmacokinetics of the Cholinesterase Inhibitors (ChEIs)

A summary of the clinical pharmacokinetic properties of the antidementia drugs is displayed in Table 13.1.

13.2.1 Donepezil

Donepezil immediate-release (IR) formulations of 5 and 10 mg have been approved in the United States to treat mild to moderate AD, while the 10 mg and sustained-release formulation of 23 mg have been approved for mild to moderate and severe AD.

Absorption Donepezil bioavailability after oral dosing regardless of formulation is near 100 %. The mean observed T_{max} of donepezil 5–10 mg tablets is longer than other ChEIs and occurs 3–5 h after dosing [9, 10]. The T_{max} for donepezil 23 mg sustained-release tablets is achieved approximately 6–8 h after dosing [11, 12]. Despite the longer rate of absorption, mean peak plasma concentrations are almost

Table 13.1 Summary of the clinical pharmacokinetic properties of the antidementia drugs

Property	Tacrine	Donepezil	Rivastigmine	Galantamine	Memantine
FDA approval	1993	1996	2000	2001	2003
Daily dose	40–160 mg	5–10 mg, 23 mg[a]	3–12 mg (c, s), 9.5 (p)	16–24 mg, 28 mg[b]	20 mg
Pharmacokinetics	Nonlinear	Linear	Nonlinear	Linear	Linear
Bioavailability (%)	37	100	35 (3 mg), 70 (6 mg)	100	100
T_{max} (h)	1–2	4 (IR, odt), 6 (SR)	1 (c), 8 (p)	1 (IR), 4–5 (ER)	3–8
Protein binding (%)	75	93	40	17	45
$t_{½}$ (h)	1.3–7	70	1.5–2 (c), 3.4 (p)	6–8	60–70
Metabolism	CYP1A2, 2D6	CYP3A4, 2D6	Esterases	CYP3A4, 2D6	Minor extent Major renal excretion

Adapted from Refs. [6, 21, 32]

IR immediate-release, T_{max} time to reach peak plasma concentration, $t_{½}$ elimination half-life, *c* capsule, *p* patch, *s* solution, *odt* oral disintegrating tablet, *CYP* cytochrome P450

[a] *SR* sustained-release

[b] *ER* extended-release

twofold higher for donepezil 23 mg tablets compared to the 10 mg tablets, suggesting relative linearity [11]. Similarly mean AUC for the 5, 10, and 23 mg displays relative dose proportionality [11, 13]. The rate and extent of absorption of donepezil tablets are not influenced by food [9, 11], but administration with food may decrease gastrointestinal adverse events common with all ChEIs.

Distribution The steady-state volume of distribution is 12–16 L/kg. Donepezil is approximately 96 % bound to human plasma proteins, mainly to albumins (about 75 %) and alpha1-acid glycoprotein (about 21 %) over the concentration range of 2–1000 ng/mL. Although protein binding is high, its relative affinity for binding is low, meaning that donepezil does not displace other drugs that are tightly bound to plasma proteins [3].

Metabolism Donepezil is metabolized by CYP2D6 and 3A4 and undergoes glucuronidation. After oral administration donepezil undergoes extensive first-pass metabolism. Following administration of 14C-labeled donepezil, plasma radioactivity, expressed as a percent of the administered dose, was present primarily as intact donepezil (53 %) and as 6-O-desmethyl donepezil (11 %), which has been reported to inhibit AChE to the same extent as donepezil *in vitro* and was found in plasma at concentrations equal to about 20 % of donepezil [14]. Examination of the effect of CYP2D6 genotype in Alzheimer's patients showed differences in clearance values among CYP2D6 genotype subgroups. When compared to the extensive metabolizers, poor metabolizers had a 31.5 % slower clearance and ultrarapid metabolizers had a 24 % faster clearance. These results suggest CYP2D6 has a minor role in the metabolism of donepezil [3].

No significant differences exist between elderly subjects with dementia and healthy young volunteers with regard to the pharmacokinetics of donepezil; [15] nor do gender differences seem to play a significant role in drug metabolism [16]. No significant racial differences (Japanese and Caucasian) have ever been reported, and a recent study in African-Americans demonstrated efficacy comparable to that found in other groups [17]. Pharmacokinetics of donepezil (C_{max}, AUC, Css, and degree of accumulation) did not differ between healthy and moderately impaired renal patients at a dose of 5 mg, suggesting that donepezil can be administered safely to patients with moderate renal impairment [18].

Excretion Following multiple-dose administration, the mean terminal half-life of donepezil is about 70 h, and steady state is reached within 15 days [9]. The mean apparent plasma clearance (Cl/F) is 0.13–0.19 L/h/kg [11]. The total plasma clearance and renal clearance of donepezil are dose independent [9]. Donepezil is both excreted in the urine intact and extensively metabolized to four major metabolites, two of which are known to be active, and a number of minor metabolites, not all of which have been identified. Approximately 57 and 15 % of the total radioactivity were recovered in urine and feces, respectively, over a period of 10 days, while 28 % remained unrecovered, with about 17 % of the donepezil dose recovered in the urine as unchanged drug [14]. The lower, but clinically effective, dose of donepezil

5 mg/day can be safely given to individuals with mild to moderate hepatic disease [19] and renal impairment [18].

Formulation Impact Donepezil is available for oral administration in film-coated tablets containing 5, 10, or 23 mg of donepezil hydrochloride. In addition, donepezil is available in orally disintegrating tablets (ODTs) containing 5 or 10 mg of donepezil hydrochloride. While the original tablet is meant to be swallowed whole, the ODT formulation is a rapidly disintegrating tablet meant to be dissolved on the tongue and followed with water. The 5 and 10 mg donepezil ODTs are bioequivalent to donepezil 5 mg and 10 mg tablets, respectively [11]. The ODT formulation may be preferred in patients with difficulty swallowing or other conditions where rapid disintegration of the tablet may be beneficial such as willful noncompliance.

Pharmacokinetic Dosing Regimen The recommended starting dose of donepezil is 5 mg once daily. Evidence from the controlled trials in mild to moderate Alzheimer's disease indicates that the 10 mg dose, with a 1 week titration, is likely to be associated with a higher incidence of cholinergic adverse events compared to the 5 mg dose. In open-label trials using a 6-week titration, the type and frequency of these same adverse events were similar between the 5 and 10 mg dose groups. Therefore, because donepezil steady state is achieved about 15 days after it is started and because the incidence of untoward effects may be influenced by the rate of dose escalation, a dose of 10 mg should not be administered until patients have been on a daily dose of 5 mg for 4–6 weeks. A dose of 23 mg once daily can be administered once patients have been on a dose of 10 mg once daily for at least 3 months.

13.2.2 Rivastigmine

Absorption Rivastigmine is administered orally and is absorbed rapidly and completely (96 %), reaching peak plasma concentrations within 0.5–1.7 h [20, 21]. The absolute bioavailability of rivastigmine is 36 % due to a significant first-pass effect [22]. Rivastigmine displays a nonlinear relationship with capacity-limited elimination and dose to AUC such that when doses of 2, 8, and 12 mg were administered, the corresponding mean AUCs were 6.2 ± 3.2, 41.7 ± 13.0, and 55.9 ± 16.5 μg · h/L, respectively [6, 21]. When administered with food, the time to maximum concentration is increased, resulting in a decrease in C_{max} of about 30 % [23]. Despite the decrease in C_{max}, the AUC is increased by approximately 30 % [21]. Considering the increased extent of absorption and improved tolerability to GI adverse events, it is recommended that rivastigmine should be administered with food.

Distribution Rivastigmine is weakly bound to plasma proteins (~40 %) [21, 24]. The volume of distribution of rivastigmine and its metabolite (NAP 226-90) are 1.8–2.7 and 4.3–5.9 L/kg, respectively [21, 25]. It readily crosses the blood–brain barrier, reaching CSF peak concentrations in 1.4–2.6 h [24]. Peak CSF concentrations were about 40 % of those detected in plasma, with rapid clearance characterized by a $t_{1/2}\beta$ that ranged from 0.3 to 3.0 h. A significant correlation was found between dose and AUC for rivastigmine and its NAP-226-90 metabolite ($r=0.84$, $p<0.0001$; $r=0.92$, $p<0.0001$, respectively). Similar results were found comparing rivastigmine plasma and CSF AUCs ($r=0.93$, $p<0.0001$).

Metabolism Rivastigmine is rapidly metabolized and one metabolite, NAP 226-90, has been found in the CSF, plasma, and urine [26]. The metabolite may undergo N-demethylation as well as conjugation [27]. The mean T_{max} for NAP-226-90 was 2.93 h and mean C_{max} was 3.14 ± 0.57 μg/L; however this metabolite shows minimal inhibition of acetylcholinesterase (<10 %) [24]. NAP-226-90 appears to be reduced in patients with renal and mild to moderate hepatic impairment; therefore dosage recommendations to titrate according to individual tolerability should be closely followed in these patients [26].

Excretion The pharmacokinetic half-life of rivastigmine in patients with AD is about 1.5 h, whereas the pharmacodynamic (see Sect. 13.4) half-life is about 10.0 h [28]. Rivastigmine binds to the esteratic site of the AChE enzyme causing a "pseudo-irreversible" state, resulting in a much longer pharmacodynamic effect than the short plasma half-life of the drug would predict [22, 27]. Rivastigmine is inactivated by cleavage to a phenolic product during the process of inhibiting acetylcholinesterase and is excreted as the metabolite NAP 226-90 via the kidneys [23]. As in patients with hepatic impairment, dose adjustment in patients with renal dysfunction does not appear to be warranted because the starting dose is low and followed by titration to tolerance or the maximum dose [27].

Formulation Impact In addition to the oral capsules and oral solution, rivastigmine is also available as a transdermal patch. For patients switching from an oral dosage to the transdermal formulation, those who are on a total daily dose of <6 mg of oral rivastigmine can be switched to the 4.6 mg/24 h transdermal patch and patients on a total daily dose of 6–12 mg of oral rivastigmine can be switched to the 9.5 mg/24 h patch [24]. Patients initiating therapy on the transdermal formulation or patients who are re-initiating therapy after a dosing hiatus (>3 days) should start titration at the 4.6 mg/24 h dose for a minimum of 4 weeks before considering dose escalation based on tolerability. After the initial application of the transdermal formulation, there is a lag time of 0.5–1 h in the absorption of rivastigmine. Concentrations then rise slowly typically reaching a maximum after 8 h, although maximum values (C_{max}) can also occur later (at 10–16 h). A transdermal dose of 9.5 mg/24 h results in exposure approximately equal to an oral dose of 6 mg twice daily (i.e., 12 mg/day) [24]. Less metabolite is formed following transdermal dosing versus oral dosing due to the bypass of first-pass metabolism.

Pharmacokinetic Dosing Regimen Due to the incidence of nausea and vomiting, rivastigmine requires a titration period of 4–12 weeks to reach effective doses versus donepezil (0–6 weeks) [29]. Tolerance of effective doses varies greatly among patients, resulting in significant variation in titration time to an effective dose of rivastigmine (6–12 mg/day) from patient to patient. Initiation of oral therapy should occur at the lowest dose (3 mg/day divided oral dose) for a minimum of 2 weeks before dose escalation with a target dose of 6–12 mg/day. Initiation of transdermal should occur at 4.6 mg/24 h for a minimum of 4 weeks with a target dose of 9.5–13.3 mg/24 h [17]. Once the maximally tolerated dose is achieved, the compound is well tolerated and has shown no evidence of liver or hematopoietic toxicity [29].

13.2.3 Galantamine

Absorption Galantamine is well absorbed with absolute oral bioavailability of about 90 %. Galantamine is rapidly and completely absorbed with time to peak concentration about 1 h. Bioavailability of the tablet was the same as the bioavailability of an oral solution. Food did not affect the AUC of galantamine but C_{max} decreased by 25 % and T_{max} was delayed by 1.5 h [31].

Distribution The mean volume of distribution of galantamine is 175 L. The plasma protein binding of galantamine is 18 % at therapeutically relevant concentrations. In whole blood, galantamine is mainly distributed to blood cells (52.7 %). The blood to plasma concentration ratio of galantamine is 1.2 [21, 31].

Metabolism Galantamine is metabolized by hepatic cytochrome P450 enzymes, glucuronidated, and excreted unchanged in the urine. *In vitro* studies indicate that cytochrome CYP2D6 and CYP3A4 were the major cytochrome P450 isoenzymes involved in the metabolism of galantamine, and inhibitors of both pathways increase oral bioavailability of galantamine modestly. O-demethylation, mediated by CYP2D6, was greater in extensive metabolizers of CYP2D6 than in poor metabolizers. In plasma from both poor and extensive metabolizers, however, unchanged galantamine and its glucuronide accounted for most of the sample radioactivity. In studies of oral 3H-galantamine, unchanged galantamine and its glucuronide accounted for most plasma radioactivity in poor and extensive CYP2D6 metabolizers. Up to 8 h post-dose, unchanged galantamine accounted for 39–77 % of the total radioactivity in the plasma and galantamine glucuronide for 14–24 %. After i.v. or oral administration, about 20 % of the dose was excreted as unchanged galantamine in the urine in 24 h, representing a renal clearance of about 65 mL/min, about 20–25 % of the total plasma clearance of about 300 mL/min [30].

Excretion By 7 days, 93–99 % of the radioactivity had been recovered, with about 95 % in urine and about 5 % in the feces. Total urinary recovery of unchanged galantamine accounted for, on average, 32 % of the dose and that of galantamine glucuronide for another 12 % on average. In patients with moderately impaired hepatic or renal function, dose titration should proceed cautiously. The use of galantamine in patients with severe hepatic or renal impairment is not recommended [30, 31, 33].

Formulation Impact Galantamine 24 mg extended-release (ER) capsules administered once daily under fasting conditions are bioequivalent to galantamine tablets 12 mg administered twice daily with respect to AUC and C_{min}. The C_{max} and T_{max} of the ER capsules were lower and occurred later, respectively, compared with the immediate-release tablets, with C_{max} about 25 % lower and median T_{max} occurring about 4.5–5.0 h after dosing. Dose proportionality is observed for galantamine ER capsules over the dose range of 8–24 mg daily, and steady state is achieved within a week. There was no effect of age on the pharmacokinetics of galantamine ER capsules. CYP2D6 poor metabolizers had drug exposures that were approximately 50 % higher than for extensive metabolizers. There are no appreciable differences in pharmacokinetic parameters when galantamine ER capsules are given with food compared to when they are given in the fasted state.

Pharmacokinetic Dosing Regimen Galantamine tablets and oral solution should be administered twice per day, preferably with the morning and evening meals. Dose escalation should follow a minimum of 4 weeks at prior dose. If therapy has been interrupted for more than 3 days, the patient should be restarted with the lowest dose and then re-titrated to an appropriate dosage. Recommended starting dosage for galantamine tablets and oral solution is 4 mg twice daily; increase dose to initial maintenance dosage of 8 mg twice daily after a minimum of 4 weeks. Based upon assessment of clinical benefit and tolerability, dosage may be increased to 12 mg twice daily after a minimum of 4 weeks at 8 mg twice daily. Galantamine extended-release (ER) capsules should be administered once daily in the morning, preferably with food. Recommended starting dosage for galantamine ER is 8 mg/day in the morning; increase dose to an initial maintenance dose of 16 mg/day after a minimum of 4 weeks. Based upon assessment of clinical benefit and tolerability, dosage may be increased to 24 mg/day after a minimum of 4 weeks at 16 mg/day. Conversion from galantamine tablets or oral solution to galantamine ER should occur at the same daily dosage with the last dose of galantamine tablets/oral solution taken in the evening and starting galantamine ER once daily treatment the next morning [34].

13.3 Population Pharmacokinetics of the ChEIs

An extensive population PK study with donepezil was conducted in AD patients ($N = 129$) that included plasma drug concentrations and pharmacogenetic data [35]. The pharmacogenetic data included CYP2D6 status, CYP3A, ABCB1, POR, and NR1/2. The CYP POR is a protein that transfers electrons from NADPH to microsomal CYP enzymes and might be a "general" limiting factor in drug metabolism. The pregnane X receptor (PXR) is a nuclear receptor encoded by the NR1/2 gene that regulates detoxifying enzymes and transporters. A one-compartment model with first-order absorption and elimination best described the donepezil data and a two-compartment model also tested did not enhance the final model. The model found that CYP2D6 PMs had a reduced donepezil clearance by 32 % and ultrarapid metabolizers (UMs) had an increased drug clearance by 24 % compared to the EMs. A donepezil therapeutic plasma concentration range of 30–75 ng/mL was suggested for AD patients. The other pharmacogenetic variables were found not to be significant factors. A population pharmacokinetic analysis indicates ($n = 539$ males and 550 females) that galantamine clearance is about 20 % lower in females than in males (explained by lower body weight in females), while race ($n = 1029$ White; 24 Black; 13 Asian; and 23 other) did not affect the clearance of galantamine. Galantamine clearance was influenced by age and hepatic and renal impairment where CYP2D6 PMs demonstrated lower clearance rates but dosage adjustments were not necessary in the population [6, 31, 36]. A small rivastigmine population PK study was conducted in AD patients ($N = 18$) that used a one-compartment model with first-order absorption and elimination [37]. Plasma and CSF concentrations for rivastigmine and its metabolite were analyzed. The population PK clearance for rivastigmine and its metabolite was found to be 120 L/h and 100 L/h, respectively. The plasma/CSF ratio for rivastigmine and its metabolite was 0.398 and 0.895, respectively. Rivastigmine bioavailability for the 6 mg dose was reported to be 40 % greater than the lower drug doses and similar to the previous bioavailability study [38].

13.4 Clinical Pharmacodynamics of the ChEIs

Assessment of the ChEIs pharmacodynamic (PD) activities can involve various biomarkers and, like other CNS disorders, clinical rating scales designed to detect differences between a placebo control group and the treatment group. Clinical drug trials typically employ at least two different drug doses versus the placebo control group. Rarely, a dementia clinical drug trial will examine greater than three drug doses due to the large number of patients required to detect a statistical difference based upon power analysis, the study's cost, and time. Dementia clinical trials are the longest in duration and require a placebo control usually for at least six months but can be as long as for 1–2 years. Various biomarkers include cholinesterase enzyme inhibition, plasma drug concentrations, PET scan data, and clinical rating scales. The key feature is how to integrate the data into a cohesive manner to differentiate a true drug effect from the placebo group.

Cholinesterase Enzyme Inhibition A summary of PD actions for the antidementia drugs is shown in Table 13.2. Two enzymes are responsible for the breakdown of acetylcholine in the synapse and are known as acetylcholinesterase (AChE) and butyrylcholinesterase (BChE). The ChEIs prevent the breakdown of acetylcholine by inhibiting the actions of these enzymes, thereby prolonging neurotransmission

Table 13.2 Summary of the pharmacodynamic properties of the antidementia drugs

Property	Tacrine	Donepezil	Rivastigmine	Galantamine	Memantine
Inhibition	Rapid reversible	Rapid reversible	Pseudo-irreversible	Rapid reversible	NMDA antagonist
AChE/BChE	BChE>AChE	AChE>>BChE	AChE=BChE	AChE>BChE	N/A
CNS vs peripheral	Yes	Yes	Yes	No	N/A
ACh isoform	No	No	G1>G4	No	N/A
Nicotinic effect	No	No	No	Yes	N/A

Adapted from Refs. [6, 21]
ACh acetylcholine, *AChE* acetylcholinesterase, *BChE* butyrylcholinesterase, *CNS* central nervous system

Fig. 13.1 Relationship between ChEI dose/concentration and enzyme inhibition

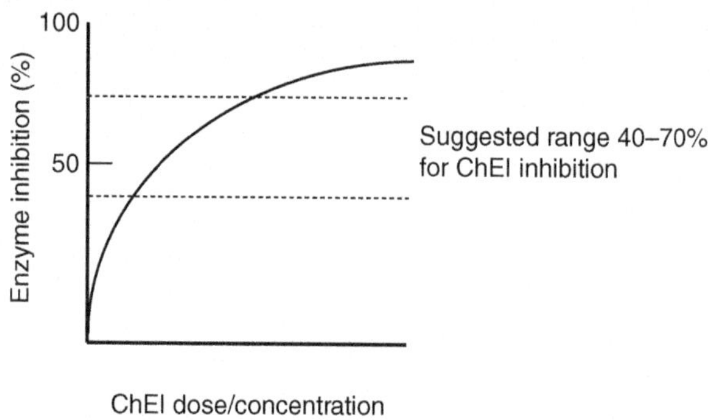

[5, 6, 21]. The PD model for cholinesterase enzyme inhibition follows the hyperbolic curve (shown in Fig. 13.1) that is based upon the sigmoidal E_{max} Model: $E=E_{max} \bullet C/EC_{50}+C$ [39]. As drug dosages increase with subsequent elevations in plasma drug concentrations, enzyme inhibition will reach a plateau at about 70–80 % and will not exceed 100 %. Cholinesterase inhibition can be measured from plasma, red blood cells (RBCs), and CSF [6, 21, 28, 40].

Tacrine is a rapidly reversible ChEI with affinity to both acetyl cholinesterase (AChE) and butyrylcholinesterase (BChE) but is no longer on the market in developed countries and therefore will not be addressed here. At present, three ChEIs are available for treatment of AD; donepezil, rivastigmine, and galantamine. Donepezil is the most selective, rapidly reversible, mixed competitive and noncompetitive AChE inhibitor. Galantamine is a selective, rapidly reversible, competitive ChEI and may act as an allosteric potentiating ligand of nicotinic acetylcholine receptors. Rivastigmine is a dual inhibitor of AChE and BChE, with a pseudo-irreversible mode of inhibition. It is the only ChEI that produces sustained inhibition without any significant increase in the expression of the target enzymes. A PK-PD model for rivastigmine in AD patients ($N=18$) showed that a one-compartment PK model analyzed with the sigmoidal E_{max} PD model described drug dose, plasma, and CSF concentrations to AChE inhibition [37]. A conceptual model proposed that a range of 40–70 % for total cholinesterase inhibition produced the optimal therapeutic benefit and inhibition greater than 80 % leads to adverse side effects limiting their use in patients [21].

Rivastigmine was found to have a dose-dependent effect for CSF AChE inhibition reaching 62 % at the maximum 6 mg twice-daily oral dose. This dose-dependent effect was not found for BChE inhibition but still produced inhibition of 62 % at the maximum 6 mg twice daily oral dose [28]. ChEIs prescribed at their regulatory agency "approved" doses achieve an enzyme inhibition of about 40–70 % [21]. Rivastigmine and galantamine have additional PD features that differ from donepezil. Rivastigmine was reported to preferentially inhibit the AChE G1 form as the G4 form becomes reduced as the disease progresses, which may aid in its therapeutic benefits and reduction in adverse side effects such as muscle cramps and weakness [41]. Galantamine was shown to bind to the presynaptic nicotinic receptors leading to an allosteric modulation that stimulates acetylcholine release [31]. Due to these actions on the cholinergic system by the ChEIs, common GI adverse side effects occur as indicated by nausea, vomiting, and diarrhea. A longitudinal AD patient study (N = 171) evaluated CYP2D6 status and BChE inhibition with various ChEIs. A lack of correlation was found between these two variables and clinical response to the ChEIs [42].

Plasma ChEI Concentrations A population PK study using model-based simulations reported that donepezil 10 mg in AD patients (N = 129) had a therapeutic plasma concentration range of 30–75 ng/mL and an average of 51 ng/mL [35]. Donepezil 5 mg was evaluated in Taiwanese AD patients (N = 37) and plasma concentrations obtained after 6 months of treatment [43]. Cognition was assessed using the Cognitive Abilities Screening Instrument (CASI) that contains nine different measures for memory. A significant correlation between the total CASI score and donepezil plasma concentration was not found (mean ± S.D.) 68.7 ng/mL ± 33.3. A subscale analysis found that only long-term memory was noted to improve with a mean plasma concentration of 75.1 ng/mL ± 32.2. Plasma concentrations and clinical response studies have not been reported with the other ChEIs.

Clinical Trials with ChEIs It is beyond the scope of this chapter to review all the clinical registration trials with the ChEIs and the reader is referred to other sources [21, 31, 32, 44]. ChEI clinical trials are initially focused on patients with mild to moderate AD. The primary clinical efficacy rating scales used were the Alzheimer's Disease Assessment Scale cognition subscale (ADAS Cog) and the Clinician's Interview-Based Impression of Change Plus Caregiver Input (CIBIC-Plus). The clinical trials were at least 6 months with usually about four assessments obtained during the study. The PD goal was to achieve minimal cognitive decline over time that statistically differentiates drug from the placebo group.

The clinical drug trials outside of evaluating PK studies have involved different formulations in mild to moderate AD patients such as with the transdermal rivastigmine patch (see Section 13.2.2, Formulation Impact) and ChEI SR and ER products.

However, donepezil 23 mg will be briefly presented as this product represented a formulation change (higher dose) and expanded disease indication (moderate to severe AD). A large multicenter clinical trial ($N=1371$) compared donepezil 23 mg SR to donepezil 10 mg daily in moderate to severely ill AD patients [45]. The primary indicators for efficacy were the clinical rating scale Severe Impairment Battery (SIB), which is a 40-item tool that assesses cognitive function in patients with advanced dementia and the Clinician's Interview-Based Impression of Change Plus Caregiver Input (CIBIC-Plus) obtained at baseline and at week 24 of the study. A statistically significant difference in the mean (±SEM) SIB scores were found comparing donepezil 23 mg SR and donepezil 10 mg groups (+2.6 [0.58] versus +0.4 [0.66], $p<0.001$). A significant difference in the CIBIC-Plus scores was not found between the groups. Donepezil 23 mg was well tolerated but had a greater incidence of nausea (11.8 % versus 3.4 %) and vomiting (9.2 % versus 2.5 %) than the donepezil 10 mg dose. However, these GI adverse effects occurred typically during the first month and substantially lessened afterwards [46].

Positron Emission Tomography (PET) Studies PET studies in AD patients have revealed reductions in the metabolic activity of cholinergic neurons. An *in vivo* PET study was conducted using ^{11}C-donepezil 5 mg that was intravenously administered to mild and moderate AD patients and was compared to an elderly group of normal subjects [47]. Patients with mild and moderate AD had about a 20 and 30 % reduction of donepezil binding to the neocortex and hippocampus, respectively. A significant correlation between the volume of hippocampal density and Mini-Mental Status Exam score was found ($r=0.659$, $p<0.038$). PET utilization may be a tool for assessing therapeutic response to ChEIs as noted in these preliminary studies [48, 49].

Using ^{18}F-fluorodeoxyglucose to measure brain metabolism, rivastigmine was compared to placebo in AD patients ($N=27$) when PET scans were obtained at baseline and at week 26 [50]. Rivastigmine produced a significant increase in overall brain metabolism ($p<0.01$) with specific areas like the prefrontal cortex 41 % ($p<0.05$) and hippocampus 32 % ($p<0.03$) in AD patients with CIBIC-Plus scores that remain stable or improved. Patients who had declining CIBIC-Plus scores did not display metabolic improvements noted in the PET scans. A longitudinal PET study was conducted in AD patients ($N=11$) treated with rivastigmine and compared to untreated AD patients ($N=10$) over a 1 year time period [51]. Rivastigmine doses of 10–12 mg/day had a positive correlation between cognitive tests and cerebral glucose metabolism especially noted in the frontal cortical and temporo-parietal regions. These results suggest that rivastigmine may provide a "stabilization" effect for long-term treatment. A longitudinal PET study in mild AD patients ($N=11$) was conducted with rivastigmine that combined PET scan data, CSF AChE and BChE inhibition, and cognitive assessments [52]. Data was collected at baseline, 3 months and 12 months after starting rivastigmine with 9–12 mg used throughout the study. The PET scan assessed ^{11}C-nicotine binding sites as cortical nicotinic receptors were noted to decline over time in patients with AD. After 3 months, cortical nicotine binding sites were significantly increased ($p<0.05$) and significantly correlated with AChE inhibition ($r=0.68$, $p<0.03$) and with BChE inhibition ($r=0.70$, $p<0.03$). A positive association with attention and nicotinic binding was reported but details were not provided on other cognitive assessments. This study emphasized that the complex nature of evaluating patients with dementia requires the use of various PK and PD assessments in attempting to integrate a pharmacotherapeutic approach to therapy.

An open-label PET study with galantamine 16–24 mg in mild to moderate AD patients ($N=19$) was conducted to assess brain metabolism with ^{18}F-deoxyglucose and treatment response [53]. The PET scan results indicate that an increased left caudate metabolism and significant activation of the thalamofrontal network with galantamine treatment. This occurrence was not present in patients who worsened. A significant correlation was found between the ADAS Cog and the left anterior cingulate metabolism ($r=0.70$, $p=0.02$). This initial PET study with galantamine showed improvements in the prefrontal network and thalamic activation. A subsequent set of PET studies with galantamine was conducted by the same investigators using PET, CSF AChE inhibition, and nicotine binding [54, 55]. Galantamine 16–24 mg/day was used in AD patients ($N=12$) and compared with AD patients taking placebo ($N=6$) and data collected at baseline and 9 months later [54]. The AChE inhibition ranged between 30 and 36 % throughout the study and significantly correlated with the nicotinic binding ($r=0.99$, $p<0.0001$). A significant correlation was reported between RBC AChE inhibition and plasma galantamine concentrations ($r=0.81$, $p<0.0001$). A positive correlation was found with plasma AChE inhibition and cognitive assessments with attention and visuospatial ability ($r=0.68$, $p<0.005$; $r=0.51$, $p<0.05$, respectively). A significant correlation between plasma and CSF galantamine concentration was reported ($r=0.96$, $p<0.0001$) and plasma galantamine with nicotinic binding at 3 months ($r=0.65$, $p<0.04$) but not at 12 months ($r=0.46$, $p<0.10$) [55]. Significant correlations were found between cognitive assessments and the left anterior cingulate cortex at 12 months ($r=0.68$, $p<0.05$) and left frontal cortex ($r=0.61$, $p<0.04$). These studies indicate that galantamine produced long-term AChE inhibition associated with significant correlations between nicotinic binding, cognition, enzyme inhibition, and drug concentrations.

13.5 Clinical Pharmacokinetics of the NMDA Receptor Antagonist

Memantine (MEM) is presently the only NMDA receptor antagonist agent that was FDA approved in 2003 for antidementia pharmacotherapy. MEM is specifically indicated for patients with moderate to severe AD [56]. MEM can be used as monotherapy but is more commonly prescribed with a ChEI [56, 57]. MEM pharmacokinetic (PK) properties are shown in Table 13.1. Following oral administration, MEM is highly absorbed with peak concentrations reached in about 3–7 h. MEM has linear pharmacokinetics over the therapeutic dose range. Food has no effect on the absorption of MEM. Mean $AUC_{0-\infty}$ increased by 4 %, 60 %, and 115 % in subjects with mild, moderate, and severe renal impairment, respectively, compared to healthy subjects. The mean volume of distribution of MEM is 9–11 L/kg and the plasma protein binding is low (45 %). MEM undergoes partial hepatic metabolism. The hepatic microsomal CYP450 enzyme system does not play a significant role in the metabolism of MEM. MEM is excreted predominantly (about 48 %) unchanged in urine and has a terminal elimination half-life of about 60–80 h [56, 58]. The remainder is converted primarily to three polar metabolites which possess minimal NMDA receptor antagonistic activity: the N-glucuronide conjugate, 6-hydroxy MEM, and 1-nitroso-deaminated MEM. A total of 74 % of the administered dose is excreted as the sum of the parent drug and the N-glucuronide conjugate [58]. Renal clearance involves active tubular secretion moderated by pH-dependent tubular reabsorption. No dosage adjustment is recommended for patients with mild and moderate renal impairment. The terminal elimination half-life increased by 18 %, 41 %, and 95 % in subjects with mild, moderate, and severe renal impairment, respectively, compared to healthy subjects. Dosage should be reduced in patients with severe renal impairment [59, 60].

Formulation Impact MEM is available as both an extended release capsule and an oral solution. No pharmacokinetic differences are expected between the different formulations.

Pharmacokinetic Dosing Regimen The recommended starting dose of the extended release capsule is 7 mg once daily. Dose increases should occur at a minimum of one week to the recommended maintenance dose of 28 mg once daily. The recommended starting dose of MEM oral solution is 5 mg (2.5 mL) once daily. The dose should be increased in 5 mg increments to 10 mg/day (2.5 mL twice daily), 15 mg/day (2.5 and 5 mL as separate doses), and 20 mg/day (5 mL twice daily). The minimum recommended interval between dose increases is 1 week. The dosage shown to be effective in controlled clinical trials is 20 mg/day (5 mL twice daily).

Population Pharmacokinetics MEM pharmacokinetics was evaluated following the administration of single oral doses of 20 mg in eight subjects with moderate hepatic impairment (Child-Pugh Class B, score 7–9) and eight subjects who were age-, gender-, and weight-matched to the hepatic-impaired subjects. There was no change in memantine exposure (based on C_{max} and AUC) in subjects with moderate hepatic impairment as compared with healthy subjects. However, terminal elimination half-life increased by about 16 % in subjects with moderate hepatic impairment as compared with healthy subjects. No dose adjustment is recommended for patients with mild and moderate hepatic impairment. MEM should be administered with caution to patients with severe hepatic impairment as the pharmacokinetics of MEM has not been evaluated in that population. Following multiple-dose administration of MEM 20 mg daily, females had about 45 % higher exposure than males, but there was no difference in exposure when body weight was taken into account. A population PK MEM model was reported that a two-compartment open model with first-order absorption described MEM disposition [61]. The population MEM CL was 4.95 L/h and the volume of distribution 294 L. The final regression model indicated that body weight, presence of concomitant medications, and formulation (tablets versus solution) were significant factors that influenced MEM CL and explained for 61 % of the interpatient variability. A later MEM population PK study ($N=108$) also included genotyping for the renal cation transporters (SLC22A1/2/5, SLC47A1, and ABCB1) and nuclear receptors (NR1/2, NR1/3, PXR, and PPAR) involved with transporter expression [61]. This study found that a one-compartment open model with first-order absorption provided the best fit for the data with a population MEM CL of 5.2 L/h and the volume of distribution of 194 L. Renal function, sex, and the NR1/2 genotype influenced MEM CL and explained for 27 % of the interpatient variability. Patients with the NR1/2 CT/TT genotypes had a 16 % reduced MEM CL compared to the CC genotypes.

A MEM PK study compared 10 mg twice daily to 20 mg once daily with simulated data using a one-compartment model dosed for 21 days using population PK parameters for a 70 kg person [62]. These results showed that MEM plasma concentration time curves were similar for both doses and that MEM can be conveniently given on a once-daily basis. Recently, a once-daily MEM 7 mg, 14 mg, 21 mg, and 28 mg extended-release (ER) formulations were FDA approved in 2013. The sponsor discontinued manufacturing original MEM tablets on August 15, 2014, and only recommends the use of the ER formulation. Patients were suggested to be transitioned from MEM 10 mg twice daily to the ER 28 mg once daily. A PK simulation study reported that the 28 mg ER dose yielded a 37 % higher MEM steady-state trough concentration, whereas the 21 mg ER had similar profile of the 10 mg twice-daily product [63]. Therefore, careful patient monitoring is needed, and the suggestion was to initially transition the patient to the 21 mg ER product instead of the 28 mg ER formulation.

13.6 Clinical Pharmacodynamics of the NMDA Receptor Antagonist

MEM is an NMDA receptor antagonist with possible neuroprotective effects that prevents abnormal glutamate neurotransmission. It has been suggested that excess glutamate levels and chronic neuronal depolarization results in NMDA receptor dysfunction with excessive calcium neuronal influx leading to cell death [56]. MEM serum and CSF concentrations were examined in patients ($N=6$) and an average CSF/serum concentration ratio of 0.52 was found [64]. MEM CSF levels were significantly correlated to the serum MEM concentrations ($r=0.99$, $p<0.002$). One patient was treated with MEM 20 mg/day and had a MEM serum and CSF concentration of 0.374 μM and 0.207 μM, respectively. The K_i value for the NMDA receptor was determined to be at 0.5 μM using preclinical human frontal cortex tissue. Therefore, it was suggested that the MEM 20 mg/day dose could provide adequate drug concentrations for NMDA receptor antagonism.

Clinical MEM Trials It is beyond the scope of this chapter to discuss the number of MEM clinical trials and the reader is referred elsewhere [56]. This section will only focus on the once-daily dosing regimen and the recent MEM 28 mg ER formulation. A once-daily MEM dosing study was conducted patients with moderate to severe AD ($N=78$) where patients were assigned three different regimens: 10 mg twice daily (control) and 20 mg once daily with two different starting dosing strategies (10 mg/day increased weekly versus 5 mg/day increased weekly) [65]. The results showed that all three regimens were adequately tolerated and that patients can be given 20 mg once daily irrespective of the starting dosing schedule.

A multinational clinical trial with MEM 28 mg ER was conducted in patients with moderate to severe AD ($N=677$) where patients were randomized to placebo or MEM for 24 weeks [66]. The mean SIB score for the MEM group significantly differed from the placebo group (MEM 2.7 versus placebo 0.3, $p<0.001$). A similar finding for the MEM group was reported with the mean CIBIC-Plus score ($p<0.008$), which lead to the FDA approval for the 28 mg ER product. MEM was well tolerated with most adverse events occurring less than 6 %. Diarrhea was noted at 5 % but the placebo rate reported an incidence of 3.9 %. The incidence of nausea was lower for the MEM group than the placebo group (1.5 % versus 2.1 %).

Positron Emission Tomography (PET) MEM Studies An early PET study with ^{18}F-MEM in healthy volunteers ($N=5$) was conducted to determine the feasibility of using this ligand for AD patients [67]. It was found that ^{18}F-MEM was distributed to various gray matter in the cortex and basal ganglia and described by a one-compartment tissue model. The compound was distributed into the white matter similar to the gray matter and thereby did not reflect regional NMDA receptor specificity. As such, this ligand was reported to be unsuitable for further research in AD patients.

Patients ($N=16$) with frontotemporal dementia (FTD) were treated with MEM 20 mg/day for 2 months and were assessed by PET scan with fluorodeoxyglucose for cerebral metabolic activity prior to and after MEM treatment [68]. The primary endpoint was enhancement of cortical metabolic activity and secondary endpoints were mood and behavioral disturbance, executive function, and motor disturbance. MEM produced an enhanced cortical metabolic activity by 4–13 % in the left frontal cortex ($p<0.01$) among 8 of the 16 patients. Correlations between metabolic activity and behavioral inventories were not found. A subsequent study followed six patients (among the 8 patients with enhanced metabolic activity) that continued with MEM 20 mg/day treatment and were assessed at the 6 month time period [69]. The results showed a sustained cortical metabolic activity ($p<0.013$) from the baseline. Additional studies were suggested and to include a longer time period for at least 1 year.

An early PET study evaluated the addition of MEM 10 mg twice daily to patients with mild to moderate AD ($N=17$) taking stabilized doses of any ChEIs [70]. MEM treatment was for 10 weeks and PET scans were taken prior to MEM and at the study endpoint. Preliminary results indicated that increased metabolic activity was observed in the inferior temporal gyrus and angular/supramarginal gyrus, but significant improvements in dementia rating scores were not found. However, significant improvements were reported with the behavioral ratings ($p<0.009$) associated with increased metabolism in the right parietal and temporal cortex. A PET study in patients with moderate to severe AD ($N=22$) with MEM 20 mg/day was conducted where scans were obtained at baseline and 24 weeks later [71]. PET cerebral metabolic rate for glucose (CMRg) was determined with fluorodeoxyglucose. CSF beta-amyloid and tau protein concentrations were also obtained with cognitive assessments. A small but statistically significant improvement ($p<0.03$) in CMRg was reported at the 24-week time period. However, significant treatment effects were not found in the CSF beta-amyloid or tau proteins. PET scans will continue to be used in various studies with patients with different dementia types in an effort to identify biomarkers for therapeutic response.

13.7 Conclusion

Presently, pharmacotherapeutic interventions for patients with dementia provide treatments for only the symptoms without addressing the disease's underlying pathophysiology. AD represents the most common type of dementia. MCI is a new challenge for pharmacotherapeutic intervention and currently no medications have been approved by the regulatory agencies. Treatment for the other types of dementia (e.g., FTD) remains to be fully developed. Two pharmacologic categories of medications are approved by the regulatory agencies for dementia, which are the ChEIs and the NMDA receptor antagonist MEM. Donepezil remains the most frequently prescribed ChEI [72]. MEM is often combined with any of the ChEIs. This drug combination represents the only "approved" therapeutic approach to dementia. Therefore, a major goal for the ChEIs is to maximize their utility by early disease recognition, diagnosis, and drug dosage titration to the maximal tolerated dose [73]. Many patients may not reach the maximal ChEI dose due to the GI adverse effects, but these problems usually occur during the dose titration phase and tend to be transient. Therefore, patient and caregiver education regarding adherence is an important attribute for long-term treatment.

The PK properties of the ChEIs and MEM are well known and linked to their PD actions. Utilization of pharmacogenetic markers is relatively early in this population and will continue to be collected and analyzed [6, 35, 61, 74, 75]. As dementia is associated with the presence of beta-amyloid and tau proteins, measure of these proteins as potential biomarkers and cholinesterase inhibition in the CSF and plasma will continue to be explored [48, 49, 76]. The challenge for future molecule development (e.g., beta-site amyloid cleaving enzyme, BACE) as a treatment approach will be to determine if these molecules can significantly alter the disposition of these proteins as measured by the PET scans or other imaging methods. Imaging data can then be correlated with symptom improvement or disease stabilization. PET studies are limited due to their small patient numbers, extensive procedures, and expense. However, PET assessments have been included as a standard tool for clinical dementia drug trials. Clinical rating scales have been developed to assess the cognitive and behavioral aspects of dementia at the various stages of mild, moderate, and severe impairment. The ADAS Cog and SIB are the cognitive assessment instruments. The Neuropsychiatric Inventory (NPI) is employed to evaluate the behavioral symptoms in patients with AD. Population PK analysis may provide additional information integrating the PK, PD, pharmacogenetics, and clinical rating assessments. New pharmacological agents for dementia have not emerged for over a decade despite the advances in understanding the biological processes. Advances in drug and biological development continue with the hope of identifying a disease-state-modifying agent for the treatment of patients with dementia.

References

1. Slattum PW, Peron EP, Hill AM (2014) Alzheimer's disease. In: DiPiro JT, Talbert RL, Yee GC et al (eds) Pharmacotherapy: a pathophysiologic approach, 9th edn. McGraw-Hill, New York, pp 817–833
2. Steele CD, Steinberg M, Milles G, Jann MW (1999) Recognition and management of early Alzheimer's disease. JCOM 6:52–67
3. Seltzer B (2007) Donepezil: an update. Expert Opin Pharmacother 8:1011–1023
4. Kuhl DE, Minoshima S, Frey KA, Foster NL, Kilbourn MR, Koeppe RA (2000) Limited donepezil inhibition of acetylcholinesterase measured with positron emission tomography in living Alzheimer cerebral cortex. Ann Neurol 48:391–395
5. Jann MW, Small GW (2009) Cholinesterase inhibitors and similarly acting compounds. Chapter 31.15. In: Sadock BJ, Sadock VA, Ruiz R (eds) Comprehensive textbook of psychiatry, 9th edn. Lippincott, Williams, and Wilkens, Philadelphia, PA, pp. 3089–3099
6. Noetzli M, Eap CB (2013) Pharmacodynamic, pharmacokinetic, and pharmacogenetic aspects of drugs used in the treatment of Alzheimer's disease. Clin Pharmacokinet 52:225–251
7. Jann MW (1998) Pharmacology and clinical efficacy of cholinesterase inhibitors. Am J Health Syst Pharm 55(Suppl 2):S22–S25
8. Jann MW, Grossberg G (2000) Cholinesterase inhibitors in the treatment of Alzheimer's disease. Consult Pharm 15(Suppl B):7–15
9. Mihara M, Ohnishi A, Tomono Y et al (1993) Pharmacokinetics of E2020, a new compound for Alzheimer's disease, in healthy male volunteers. Int J Clin Pharmacol Ther Toxicol 31(5):223–229
10. Rogers SL, Friedhoff LT (1998) Pharmacokinetic and pharmacodynamic profile of donepezil HCl following single oral doses. Br J Clin Pharmacol 46(Suppl 1):1–6
11. Eisai (2014) ARICEPT® (donepezil hydrochloride) tablets: prescribing information. Eisai Inc., Woodcliff Lake, NJ
12. FDA (2010) Application number: 022568. Center for Drug Evaluation and Research; Clinical Pharmacology and Biopharmaceutics Review(s)
13. Rogers C, Sukovaty P, Lee F (1998) Pharmacokinetic and pharmacodynamic profile of donepezil HCl following multiple oral doses. Br J Clin Pharmacol 46(S1):7–12
14. Tiseo PJ, Perdomo CA, Friedhoff LT (1998) Metabolism and elimination of 14C-donepezil in healthy volunteers: a single-dose study. Br J Clin Pharmacol 46(Suppl 1):19–24
15. Ohnishi A, Mihara M, Kamakura H et al (1993) Comparison of the pharmacokinetics of E2020, a new compound for Alzheimer's disease, in healthy young and elderly subjects. J Clin Pharmacol 33:1086–1091
16. Haywood WM, Mukaetova-Ladinska EB (2006) Sex influences on cholinesterase inhibitor treatment in elderly individuals with Alzheimer's disease. Am J Geriatr Pharmacother 4:273–286

17. Griffith P, Lichtenberg P, Goldman R, Payne-Parrish J (2006) Safety and efficacy of donepezil in African Americans with mild-to-moderate Alzheimer's disease. J Natl Med Assoc 98:1590–1597
18. Nagy CF, Kumar D, Cullen EI et al (2004) Steady-state pharmacokinetics and safety of donepezil HCl in subjects with moderately impaired renal function. Br J Clini Pharmacol 58(Suppl 1):18–24
19. Reyes JF, Vargas R, Kumar D, Cullen EI, Perdomo CA, Pratt RD (2004) Steady-state pharmacokinetics, pharmacodynamics and tolerability of donepezil hydrochloride in hepatically impaired patients. Br J Clin Pharmacol 58(Suppl 1):9–17
20. Nordberg A, Svensson A-L (1998) Cholinesterase inhibitors in the treatment of Alzheimer's disease. Drug Saf 19:465–480
21. Jann MW, Shirley KL, Small GW (2002) Clinical pharmacokinetics and pharmacodynamics of cholinesterase inhibitors. Clin Pharmacokinet 41:719–739
22. Polinsky RJ (1998) Clinical pharmacology of rivastigmine: a new-generation acetylcholinesterase inhibitor for the treatment of Alzheimer's disease. Clin Ther 20:634–647
23. Anand R, Gharabawi G, Enz A (1996) Efficacy and safety results of the early phase studies with Exelon (TM)(ENA-713) in Alzheimer's disease: an overview. J Drug Dev Clin Pract 8:109–116
24. Novartis (2015) Exelon® Patch (rivastigmine transdermal system), full prescribing information. Novartis Pharmaceuticals Corporation, East Hanover, NJ
25. Kennedy JS, Polinsky RJ, Johnson B et al (1999) Preferential cerebrospinal fluid acetylcholinesterase inhibition by rivastigmine in humans. J Clin Psychopharmacol 19:513–521
26. Spencer CM, Noble S (1998) Rivastigmine. A review of its use in Alzheimer's disease. Drugs Aging 13:391–411
27. Williams BR, Nazarians A, Gill MA (2003) A review of rivastigmine: a reversible cholinesterase inhibitor. Clin Ther 25:1634–1653
28. Cutler NR, Polinsky RJ, Sramek JJ et al (1998) Dose-dependent CSF acetylcholinesterase inhibition by SDZ ENA 713 in Alzheimer's disease. Acta Neurol Scand 97:244–250
29. Krall WJ, Sramek JJ, Cutler NR (1999) Cholinesterase inhibitors: a therapeutic strategy for Alzheimer disease. Ann Pharmacother 33:441–450
30. Janssen (2013) RAZADYNE® ER (galantamine hydrobromide) full prescribing information. Janssen Pharmaceuticals, Inc., Titusville, NJ
31. Farlow MR (2003) Clinical pharmacokinetics of galantamine. Clin Pharmacokinet 42:1383–1392
32. VanDenBerg CM, Kazmi Y, Jann MW (2000) Cholinesterase inhibitors for the treatment of Alzheimer's disease in the elderly. Drugs Aging 16:123–138
33. Zhao Q, Iyer GR, Verhaeghe T et al (2002) Pharmacokinetics and safety of galantamine in subjects with hepatic impairment and healthy volunteers. J Clin Pharmacol 42:428–436
34. Gomolin JH, Smith C, Jeitner TM (2011) Cholinesterase inhibitors: applying pharmacokinetics to clinical decision making. Am J Geriatr Pharmacother 9:259–263
35. Noetzli M, Guidi M, Ebbing K et al (2014) Population pharmacokinetic approach to evaluate the effect of CYP2D6, CYP3A, ABCB1, POR, NR1/2 genotypes on donepezil clearance. Br J Clin Pharamacol 78:135–144
36. Piotrovsky V, Van Peer A, Van Osselaer N et al (2003) Galantamine population pharmacokinetics in patients with Alzheimer's disease: modeling and simulation. J Clin Pharmacol 43:514–523
37. Gobburu JV, Tammara V, Lesko L et al (2001) Pharmacokinetic-pharmacodynamic modeling of rivastigmine, a cholinesterase inhibitor, in patients with Alzheimer's disease. J Clin Pharmacol 41:1082–1090
38. Hossain M, Jhee SS, Shiovitz T et al (2002) Estimation of the absolute bioavailability of rivastigmine in patients with mild-moderate dementia of the Alzheimer's type. Clin Pharmacokinet 41:225–234
39. Holford NH, Sheiner LB (1982) Kinetics of pharmacologic response. Pharmacol Ther 16:143–166

40. Sramek JJ, Cutler NR (2000) RBC cholinesterase inhibition: a useful surrogate marker for cholinesterase inhibitor activity in Alzheimer's disease therapy? Alzheimer's Dis Assoc Disord 14:216–227
41. Weinstock M (1999) Selectivity of cholinesterase inhibition: clinical implications for the treatment of Alzheimer's disease. CNS Drugs 12:307–323
42. Chianella C, Gragnaniello D, Maisanio Delser P et al (2011) BCHE and CYP2D6 genetic variation in Alzheimer's disease patients treated with cholinesterase inhibitors. Eur J Clin Pharmacol 67:1147–1157
43. Yang YH, Chen CH, Chou MC et al (2013) Concentration of donepezil to the cognitive response in Alzheimer's disease. J Clin Psychopharmacol 33:351–355
44. Jann MW (2000) Rivastigmine, a new generation cholinesterase inhibitor for the treatment of Alzheimer's disease. Pharmacotherapy 20:1–12
45. Farlow MR, Salloway S, Tariot PN et al (2010) Effectiveness and tolerability of high-dose (23 mg/d) versus standard-dose (10 mg/d) in moderate to severe Alzheimer's disease: a 24-week, randomized, double-blind study. Clin Ther 32:1234–1251
46. Christensen DD (2012) Higher dose (23 mg/day) donepezil formulation for the treatment of patients with moderate-severe Alzheimer's disease. Postgrad Med 124:110–116
47. Okamura N, Funaki Y, Tashiro M et al (2008) In vivo visualization of donepezil binding in the brain of patients with Alzheimer's disease. Br J Clin Pharmacol 65:472–479
48. Shimada A, Hashimoto H, Kawabe J et al (2011) Evaluation of therapeutic response to donepezil by positron emission tomography. Osaka City Med J 57:11–19
49. Kasuya M, Meguro K, Okamura N et al (2012) Greater responsiveness to donepezil in Alzheimer's patients with higher levels of acetylcholinesterase based on attention task scores and a donepezil PET study. Alzheimer's Dis Assoc Disord 26:113–118
50. Potkin S, Anand R, Fleming K et al (2001) Brain metabolic and clinical effects of rivastigmine in Alzheimer's disease. Int J Neuropsychopharmacol 4:223–230
51. Stefanova E, Wall A, Almkvist O et al (2006) Longitudinal PET evaluation of cerebral glucose metabolism in rivastigmine treated patients with mild Alzheimer's disease. J Neural Transm 113:205–218
52. Kadir A, Darreh-Shori T, Almkvist O et al (2007) Changes in brain 11C-nicotine binding sites in patients with mild Alzheimer's disease following rivastigmine treatment as assessed by PET. Psychopharmacology 191:1005–1014
53. Mega MS, Dinov ID, Porter V et al (2005) Metabolic patterns associated with the clinical response to galantamine therapy. Arch Neurol 62:721–728
54. Darreh-Shori T, Kadir A, Almkvist O et al (2008) Inhibition of acetylcholinesterase in CS versus brain assessed by 11C-PMP PET in AD patients treated with galantamine. Neurobiol Aging 29:168–184
55. Kadir A, Darreh-Shori T, Almkvist O et al (2008) PET imaging of the in vivo brain acetylcholinesterase activity and nicotine binding in galantamine-treated patients with AD. Neurobiol Aging 29:1204–1217
56. McKeage K (2009) Memantine: a review of its use in moderate to severe Alzheimer's disease. CNS Drugs 23:881–897
57. Atri A, Hendrix SB, Pejovic V et al (2015) Cumulative, additive benefits of memantine-donepezil combination component monotherapies in moderate-to-severe Alzheimer's dementia: a pooled area under the curve analysis. Alzheimers Res Ther 7(1):28. doi:10.1186/s13195-015-0109-2
58. Kornhuber J, Kennepohl EM, Bleich S et al (2001) Memantine pharmacotherapy. Clin Pharmacokinet 46:599–612
59. Periclou A, Ventura D, Rao N, Abramowitz W (2006) Pharmacokinetic study of memantine in healthy and renally impaired subjects. Clin Pharmacol Ther 79:134–143
60. Moritoyo T, Hasunuma T, Harada K et al (2012) Effect of renal impairment on the pharmacokinetics of memantine. J Pharmacol Sci 119:324–329
61. Noetzli M, Guidi M, Ebbing K et al (2013) Population pharmacokinetic study of memantine: effects of clinical and genetic factors. Clin Pharmacokinet 52:211–223

62. Gomolin IH, Smith C, Jietner TM (2010) Once-daily memantine pharmacokinetic and clinical considerations. JAGS 58:1812–1813
63. Lam S, Smith C, Gomolin IH (2015) Memantine standard tablet and extended-release dosing considerations: a pharmacokinetic analysis. JAGS 63:183–184
64. Kornhuber J, Quack G (1995) Cerebrospinal fluid and serum concentrations of the N-methyl-D-aspartate (NMDA) receptor antagonist memantine in man. Neurosci Lett 195:137–139
65. Jones RW, Bayer A, Inglis F, Barkers A, Phul R (2007) Safety and tolerability on once-daily versus twice-daily memantine: a randomized, double-blind study in moderate to severe Alzheimer's disease. Int J Geriatr Psychiatry 22:258–262
66. Grossberg GT, Manes F, Allegri RF et al (2013) The safety, tolerability, and efficacy of once-daily memantine (28 mg): a multinational, randomized, double-blind, placebo-controlled trial in patients with moderate-to-severe Alzheimer's disease taking cholinesterase inhibitors. CNS Drugs 27:469–478
67. Ametamey SM, Bruehlmeier M, Kneifel S et al (2002) PET studies of 18F-memantine in healthy volunteers. Nucl Med Biol 29:227–231
68. Chow TW, Graff-Guerrero A, Verhoeff NP et al (2011) Open-label study of the short-term effects of memantine on FDG-PET in frontotemporal dementia. Neuropsychiatr Dis Treat 7:415–424
69. Chow TW, Farm D, Graff-Guerrero A et al (2013) FDG-PET in semantic dementia after 6 months of memantine: an open-label study. Int J Geriatr Psychiatry 28:319–325
70. Sultzer DL, Melrose RJ, Harwood DG, Campa O, Mandelkern MA (2010) Effects of memantine treatment on regional cortical metabolism in Alzheimer's disease. Am J Geriatr Psychiatry 18:606–614
71. Wang T, Huang Q, Reiman EM et al (2013) Effects of memantine on clinical ratings, fluorodeoxyglucose positron emission tomography measurements, and cerebrospinal fluid assays in patients with moderate to severe Alzheimer's dementia. J Clin Psychopharmacol 33:636–642
72. Prvulovic D, Schneider B (2014) Pharmacokinetic and pharmacodynamics evaluation of donepezil for the treatment of Alzheimer's disease. Expert Opin Drug Metab Toxicol 10:1039–1050
73. Small GW, Bullock R (2011) Defining optimal treatment with cholinesterase inhibitors in Alzheimer's disease. Alzheimer's Demen 7:177–184
74. Zhong Y, Zheng X, Miao Y et al (2013) Effect of CYP2D6*10 and APOE polymorphisms on the efficacy of donepezil in patients with Alzheimer's disease. Am J Med Sci 34:222–226
75. Noetzli M, Guidi M, Ebbing K et al (2013) Relationship of CYP2D6, CYP3A, POR, ABCB1, genotypes with galantamine steady-state plasma concentrations. Ther Drug Monit 35:270–275
76. Giacobini E, Spiegel R, Enz A, Veroff AE, Cutler NR (2002) Inhibition of acetyl – and butyrylcholinesterase in the cerebrospinal fluid of patients with Alzheimer's disease by rivastigmine: correlation with cognitive benefit. J Neural Transm 109:1053–1065

Chapter 14
Anti-addiction Agents

Michael W. Jann

Abstract Pharmacotherapeutic interventions for addiction focus on treatment and prevention of dependence. Addiction is a complex biological process and its complete underlying pathophysiology remains elusive. Successful treatment involves both short-term and long-term maintenance pharmacologic approaches linked with various psychosocial support avenues. However, specific agents have been developed for alcohol, nicotine, and opiate dependence. Disulfiram has been used since the 1950s as an aversive therapeutic technique where its metabolites when exposed to alcohol lead to the patient experiencing symptoms of nausea and vomiting, encouraging the patient to abstain from alcohol. Acamprosate is indicated for alcohol abstinence maintenance with the chemical component acetyl-homotaurine measured in pharmacokinetic studies. Acamprosate is primarily renally excreted. Varenicline is a partial agonist of the central nicotinic acetylcholine receptor and approved for the treatment of nicotine dependence. Varenicline is mainly renally excreted where a combined pharmacokinetic-pharmacodynamic model described this compound with an open two-compartment pharmacokinetic model with a linear pharmacodynamic model. Naloxone and naltrexone are opiate antagonists used in a variety of clinical settings. Naloxone is a "rescue" agent for opiate overdose. Naltrexone is used for alcohol dependence and available in an oral and a monthly long-acting depot injection. Naloxone has been combined with pentazocine, buprenorphine, and oxycodone to prevent abuse. Levo-alpha acetyl methadol (LAAM) is a potent derivative of methadone but QTc prolongation occurrences have limited its clinical use.

Keywords Alcohol • Nicotine • Opiate antagonist • Acamprosate • Disulfiram • Varenicline • Naloxone • Naltrexone • Pentazocine • Buprenorphine • Oxycodone • Levo-alpha acetyl methadol (LAAM) • Long-acting depot

---

M.W. Jann, PharmD
Department of Pharmacotherapy, University of North Texas System College of Pharmacy (UNTSCP) and University of North Texas Health Science Center (UNTHSC), Fort Worth, TX, USA
e-mail: Michael.jann@unthsc.edu

M. Jann et al. (eds.), *Applied Clinical Pharmacokinetics and Pharmacodynamics of Psychopharmacological Agents*,
DOI 10.1007/978-3-319-27883-4_14

14.1 Introduction

The treatment of patients with substance abuse and addiction is a complex phenomenon and continues to challenge clinicians, patients, families, and healthcare systems. Pharmacologic interventions for anti-addictive pharmacotherapy remain in an early development phase where many specific treatment regimens are lacking. For example, addition of an opiate antagonist with an opiate agonist or partial agonist as a combination product does not solve the basic underlying pathophysiology of addiction as our knowledge of this medical condition remains limited. Simply providing a pharmacologic intervention is only one component needed to address the multifaceted problem of addiction. Proper support avenues must be also included such as treatment centers, psychosocial therapy, family, and employment opportunities that prepare the patient for the short- and long-term successes needed to cease the addiction.

This chapter will focus on the agents where clinical pharmacokinetic (PK) and pharmacodynamic (PD) studies have been conducted with an emphasis on treatment and prevention of dependence. The agents included in this chapter are for the treatment of alcohol and nicotine dependence, opiate antagonists, their combination products with opiate agonists, partial agonists, and levo-acetyl-alpha-methadol (LAAM). Methadone was originally developed to treat opiate addiction; however, this agent was soon discovered to be as addictive as the opiates and covered in Chap. 11. Agents such as clonidine were not included as PK studies were not initially designed for opiate withdrawal treatment and the reader is referred to other sources for a general review of these medications [1]. Bupropion pharmacokinetics and use for nicotine dependence are presented in Chap. 9. Representative PK and PD studies were selected to be presented in this chapter, as in some areas, a large number of studies with these agents were available.

14.2 Alcohol Dependence

Acamprosate This agent is a psychotropic agent approved by regulatory agencies for the treatment of alcohol dependence after detoxification with a focus on abstinence maintenance [2, 3]. It was approved in Europe prior to the USA [4]. Acetyl-homotaurine (ACH) is the chemical component of acamprosate and is measured in all pharmacokinetic studies [5]. ACH is not bound to plasma proteins and is not a P-gp substrate. From the various studies, the mean absolute oral bioavailability was 11 ± 1 % with a t_{max} range of 3.5–18.6 h with the oral tablets. The elimination half-life ($t_{½}$) range was 13–20 h under multiple dosing conditions with the oral tablets. From the infusion studies, the mean volume of distribution at steady state was 24 ± 1 L. ACH is not metabolized by hepatic CYP enzymes and primarily excreted by renal mechanisms. About 90 % of the dose is found unchanged in the urine. The mean (±S.D.) total body clearance (CL) was reported to be 15.78 ± 0.72 L/h with a mean renal CL of 7.92 ± 1.08 L/h from infusion studies. Renal CL from oral tablet administration was reported to be higher at 15 L/h. The mechanism for renal CL was suggested to occur via tubular secretion and possible non-renal elimination thought to take place by biliary excretion.

Acamprosate exhibits a linear PK relationship with dose for AUC and C_{max} ($r^2 = 0.99$). Gender differences and hepatic impairment classified by the Child-Pugh groups A and B reported no significant differences in ACH disposition compared to the normal volunteers. Two patient groups were assessed regarding renal impairment and acamprosate disposition as the groups were divided by creatinine CL. Moderate and severe renal impairment were defined as 1.8–3.6 L/h/1.73 m^2 and 0.3–1.74 L/h/m^2, respectively. As expected, acamprosate disposition is significantly impacted by renal impairment with mean elimination half-lives of 33.4 ± 6.6 h and 46.6 ± 12.9 h, respectively. The mean renal CLs for the moderate and severe impairment groups were 3.29 ± 0.85 L/h and 1.10 ± 0.21 L/h, respectively. Based upon these studies, it was recommended that acamprosate be very carefully dosed or avoided in patients with moderate or severe renal impairment.

Exact cellular mechanisms for acamprosate's action to reduce alcohol consumption and abstinence maintenance remain unknown. Several PD approaches have been proposed with the main focus on inhibition of neuronal hyperexcitability by antagonizing the excitatory amino acid activity particularly the glutamate actions associated with NMDA receptors [2, 3]. Other actions proposed have included antagonism of opiate and noradrenergic activity, stimulation of serotonergic activity, stimulation of inhibitory GABA neurotransmission, and possible antiacetylaldehyde activity [3]. Clinical trials have demonstrated the efficacy and safety of acamprosate in the management of alcohol dependence after detoxification with doses of 1.3 g for patients with body weight <60 kg and 2 g for patients with body weight >60 kg. The most common adverse side effects were gastrointestinal, mainly diarrhea which is dose related (7 % with 1.3 g and 12 % with 2 g). Other side effects reported were nausea, vomiting, pruritis, dizziness, confusion, drowsiness, and headache [2, 3]. The length of treatment is recommended to be at least 1 year.

Disulfiram (DSF) The pharmacologic approach to alcohol dependence with DSF was and continues to be based upon an aversive therapeutic intervention. DSF has been used since the 1950s [6, 7], yet data regarding its PK properties are relatively sparse due to the small number of studies. However, the PD actions are well known as the DSF metabolites are exposed to alcohol leading to adverse reactions such as nausea and vomiting; thereby, patients are encouraged not to consume any alcoholic products [6, 7]. A brief review of the DSF PK and PD aspects will be presented and the reader is referred to the reference for a complete review [8]. After oral ingestion, more than 80 % of the dose is absorbed as DSF is converted to form diethyldithiocarbamic acid (DDC), which is unstable and undergoes phase II glucuronidation metabolism to form diethylthiomethylcarbamate (Me-DDC). The Me-DDC is further metabolized by CYP450 enzymes (specific enzymes were not reported in the article) to form sulfoxide and sulfone metabolites and all three compounds can inhibit aldehyde dehydrogenase (ALDH). DSF and Me-DDC are highly protein bound to albumin at 96 % and 79.5 %, respectively. Approximately 65 % of the dose is renally eliminated, 20 % by the feces, and the remainder via pulmonary mechanisms. The eliminated half-life for DSF and Me-DDC in alcoholic patients with single and multiple doses was reported to be 9.2 h and 10 h, respectively. Acetylaldehyde is the first metabolite formed by alcohol oxidative metabolism and then further metabolized to acetic acid by the hepatic ALDH. DSF and Me-DDC preferentially inhibit ALDH activity, leading to the dramatic increase in acetylaldehyde blood concentrations. The increased acetylaldehyde levels result in the PD actions of facial flushing, headache, nausea, vomiting, hypotension, tachycardia, and dizziness [1]. DSF ALDH inhibition is irreversible and enzyme activity depends upon de novo enzyme synthesis that takes places several days following DSF discontinuation, and the patient can still experience the unwanted PD effects after drug cessation. The intensity and duration of the PD effects are dependent upon the DSF dose and amount of alcohol consumed [6].

14.3 Nicotine Dependence

Treatment to initiate smoking cessation and continued abstinence maintenance involves a variety of nonprescription and prescription products. The nonprescription products typically involve nicotine replacement therapies in various dosage formulations (e.g., gum, lozenge, patch) and the reader is referred elsewhere [9]. The PK and PD of nicotine have been well studied and will not be discussed in this chapter and the reader is again referred to other resources [10, 11]. Bupropion is approved for the treatment of smoking cessation and maintenance therapy and its PK and PD properties are reviewed in Chap. 9. The only other agent used for smoking cessation is varenicline.

Varenicline (VCL) From oral administration, VCL is almost completely absorbed from the GI tract with systemic bioavailability >90 % with an overall drug recovery rate from the urine that ranges from 81 to 95 %. VCL was reported not to be a P-gp substrate and a volume of distribution at a steady state of 5.9 L/kg. Protein binding for the unbound VCL ranged from 88 to 94 % [12]. VCL does not undergo hepatic phase I oxidation metabolism with the metabolite N-carbamoylglucuronide representing <10 % of the dose formed by the uridine diphosphate glucuronosyltransferase (UGT) 2B7 [12]. The elimination half-life ($t_{1/2}$) ranges from 23.8 to 33.0 h with multiple dosing. VCL is primarily excreted renally with a mean CL of 94.4 ± 34.5 mL/min, and doses must be adjusted in patients with moderate (CLcr ≥30 to ≤50 mL/min) and severe (CLcr <30 mL/min) impairment. Active tubular secretion via the human organic cation transports (hOCTs) type 2 was reported to have moderate affinity for VCL with an apparent Michaelis-Menten Km of 370 μmol/L [13]. Single, multiple-dose, and population pharmacokinetic analysis have not reported any significant effects from age, ethnicity, and gender that affect VCL disposition [14–16]. The recommended dosage is 1 mg twice daily and a dosage reduction to 1 mg daily for patients with severe renal impairment [12, 14].

VCL is a partial agonist of the central nicotinic acetylcholine receptor α4β2 nAChR, and when subjects are smoking, the significantly higher receptor affinity of VCL over nicotine prevents access of nicotine to the receptor [12]. Various clinical trials have demonstrated the efficacy and safety of VCL in adults who initiate a smoking cessation program. A PK-PD analysis described a model for VCL that included using a two-compartment PK model with a linear PD model with first-order onset/offset rate constants [17]. Craving reduction scores were associated with VCL plasma concentrations with a rapid onset under 1 h peaking at 3 h and were maintained for the next 4 h (the maximum time period studied). A pharmacogenetic analysis ($N=2699$) was conducted from three placebo-controlled, double-blind, clinical trials comparing bupropion and VCL [18]. A number of genes were assessed – nicotine and bupropion metabolism, nicotinic receptors, VCL transporter and genes for Chr15q25, and serotonin receptors 5HT3A and 5HT3B. VCL abstinence was reported to be associated with nAChr subunit genes CHRNB2, CHRNA5, and CHRNA4 ($p<0.005$). Bupropion abstinence was associated with CYP2B6 ($p<0.001$). The nausea incidence was found to be associated with several nAChR subunit genes and time to relapse with 5HT3B gene ($p<0.001$). Several loci contributed to successful smoking cessation and response. Perhaps a combined PK-PD model that incorporates pharmacogenetic data would be the next step to data analysis to predict optimal response while minimizing the adverse side effects for patients treated with VCL.

14.4 Opioid Antagonists and Dependence

Naloxone (NLX) NLX was the first opiate antagonist discovered to be used clinically to reverse the clinical signs and symptoms of a narcotic overdose [19]. Its safety and lack of intrinsic agonist properties were favored over the use of earlier agents nalorphine and levallorphan [20]. NLX has been incorporated into many first-responder's emergency medical kits. Along with oxygen and dextrose 50 %, NLX should be given to any unconscious patient regardless of age when a drug overdose is suspected [21]. NLX is a potent opiate antagonist for the three opiate receptors – μ, κ, and σ receptors [22].

Naloxone (NLX) After intravenous (IV) 0.4 mg administration, clinical response can be observed within 1–2 min with a duration of effect between 45 and 90 min [21]. Although NLX has been used extensively in the clinical arena, its PK parameters were not widely assessed in preclinical or human studies. NLX disposition was reported in two male subjects where one subject had a history of opiate dependence [23]. NLX-78-^{3}H isotope was given with plasma samples obtained for the next 6 h and urine samples collected for 72 h. The NLX PK parameters reported were an elimination half-life of 90 min, a volume of distribution (Vd) 2500 L/day, and a clearance 2.83 L/kg/day. A later study with nine healthy volunteers age 25–54 years (five men, four females) reported a mean (±S.D.) elimination half-life of 64 ± 12 min. After 2 min post IV administration of 0.4 mg, the mean amount of NLX measured was 0.01 ± 0.001 μg/mL and 5 min later noted at 0.0043 ± 0.0003 μg/mL [24]. NLX distribution half-life was reported to be 4.7 min. The preclinical data with rat brain concentrations showed that brain to serum concentration ratios ranged from 2.7 to 4.6 indicating higher brain concentrations and that amounts decline paralleling serum concentration elimination. NLX concentrations rapidly exit from the rat brain and when compared to morphine given earlier that outlasted NLX actions, and the morphine effect was sustained for over 1 h [25]. These results explain the rationale for continued NLX administration when treating patients for an acute opiate overdose.

NLX is rapidly metabolized by phase II glucuronidation to NLX-3-glucuronide with 65 % of the dose excreted into the urine [26]. The other minor metabolites formed are reduced-NLX and N-dealkylation [27]. NLX has low protein binding with 46 % primarily to albumin with alpha-one acid glycoprotein and β-lipoprotein [28]. NLX was shown not to be a P-glycoprotein (P-gp) substrate or inhibitor [29]. The onset of activity when NLX is given from the intramuscular (IM), subcutaneous (SC), or oral route is about 15 min [30]. However, the absolute NLX bioavailability was very low from 1 to 2 % [29]. Iontophoretic transdermal delivery for NLX has been investigated as an alternative administration route to provide prolonged NLX therapy and continues to be researched [31, 32]. A population PK study with NLX was reported from six male volunteers given NLX IV, IM, and IN (intranasal) [30]. The population PK parameter estimates from 128 plasma samples obtained at various times reported were an absolute bioavailability for NLX IM and IN of 36 % and 4 %, respectively. Other parameters reported were clearance 91 L/h (2184 L/day) with a median time to peak plasma concentrations of 12 min for the IM and 6–9 min for the IN. A review of NLX IN device has been developed for opiate overdose situations [33]. Other NLX administration routes have been examined and included subcutaneous, intraosseous, and endotracheal routes assessed in preclinical and clinical studies [33, 34].

As NLX PK and PD parameters became well known, IV continuous infusion methods were developed to provide sustained treatment for opiate overdose patients [35]. The basic maintenance dose (M.D.) equation was used – M.D. (mg) = loading dose (mg) × $1 - e^{-k\tau}$ (τ = minutes). Following a 2 or 4 mg loading dose, patients were treated with a 1.5 or 3 mg/h continuous NLX infusion that resulted in plasma NLX concentrations preventing recurrent respiratory depression. Higher NLX doses may be needed to treat patients with septic shock as plasma levels of 3.78 mcg/mL were noted without significant side effects [36]. Prolonged opioid antagonism was reported with a patient in chronic renal failure with respiratory depression secondary to morphine intoxication [37]. Serum NLX concentrations obtained 2.3 and 4.5 h after NLX infusion were 33.33 and 21.33 ng/mL, respectively. The extended NLX actions were attributed to the potential reduction in renal glucuronidation but only extensive renal PK studies would confirm that hypothesis.

Population PK-PD models for NLX reversal of opiate agonist (morphine) and partial opiate agonist-induced (buprenorphine) respiratory depression in healthy volunteers provide clinicians with precise information on NLM's duration and magnitude of clinical effect [38, 39]. Both studies used the NLX PK parameters and incorporated a biphasic equilibrium (or slow phase) PD model incorporating the opiate receptor association-dissociation kinetics. These studies indicated that reversal of respiratory depression can be modeled by NLX and that a biphasic NLX equilibrium model predicted clinical activity with opiate overdose situations.

NLX is well known to reverse the respiratory depression from opiates; however, a pilot study in three patients when given oral NLX showed that opiate-induced constipation can be ameliorated [40]. NLX 12 mg given at least 6 h apart was recommended as withdrawal symptoms with constipation occurred with NLX AUC >550 ng/mL with dosing intervals <3 h. Since this report, oral or enteral NLX up to 16 mg/day has been used in a variety of situations where opiate-induced constipation can be effectively treated including in the intensive care unit environment [41].

Naltrexone (NTX) NTX was developed in the 1960s as an opiate antagonist and is 17 times more potent than NLX [42]. Later in the 1990s, NTX was discovered to be effective in the treatment of patients with alcohol dependence with FDA approval in 1994 [43]. NTX was shown to reduce alcohol consumption, reduce alcohol use, and promote abstinence. Preclinical studies reported that NTX is metabolized to an active metabolite β-naltrexol (β-NTL) with an antagonist property of 1:53 compared to NTX in rats [44]. NTX was 12 times more potent than the metabolite in the dog model [45]. NTX disposition was described in four male post-addict volunteers given oral daily NTX 100 mg doses for 7 days [46]. Following oral NTX administration, T_{max} occurred for NTX and β-NTL at 1 and 2 h, respectively. PD objective responses (e.g., pupillography) and subjective responses (e.g., Addiction Research Center Inventory Scale) were also collected during the PK analysis. Under the chronic dosing conditions, the mean elimination half-life of NTX and β-NTL were 9.7 ± 1.1 h and 11.4 ± 2.0 h, respectively. A 25 mg heroin challenge was co-administered with NTX and NTX provided antagonism for following 48 h. Peak plasma levels of β-NTL were about twice the amounts of NTX. A significant correlation was found between NTX plasma levels and opiate antagonism ($r = 0.91$) and the individual NTX elimination half-life ($r = 0.99$). The duration of mu-opiate receptor occupancy by NTX 50 mg was evaluated using positron emission tomography (PET) in nine healthy volunteers (seven males and two females) using ^{11}C-carfentanil [47]. The elimination half-life range for the mu receptor blockade from NTX was from 72 to 108 h which is longer than the PK elimination half-life. These findings can explain for the prolonged PD benefits of opiate antagonism from NTX.

A long-acting (LA) NTX injection formulation given once monthly was developed to provide patients with alcoholic dependence a reliable method of treatment without the interruption of daily oral administration [48]. The PK of LA NTX was reported in 16 alcohol-dependent subjects given 300 mg in a 6-week open-label study [49]. The median t_{max} values for NTX and β-NTL were 540 h and 336 h, respectively. The mean β-NTL to NTX $AUC_{0-42\ (days)}$ ratio was 3.4 as plasma metabolite levels remained about three times greater than NTX at all times. Injection site reactions were the most common adverse event; otherwise, the NTX was well tolerated. A single- and multiple-dose PK study with LA NTX microsphere formulation was conducted in healthy subjects given 190 or 380 mg or placebo [50]. After a single 380 mg dose, NTX plasma concentrations were detectable in all subjects 31 days post dose and the plasma concentrations were proportional to the dose. The mean apparent elimination half-life for both NTX and β-NTL ranged from 5 to 7 days and serious adverse events were not reported.

Patients with alcoholic dependence are likely to have comorbid liver compromise, and the LA NTX disposition in patients with mild ($N=6$) and moderate ($N=6$) hepatic impairment was assessed and compared to age-matched healthy volunteer controls ($N=5$, one subject withdrew consent after 14 days and was not replaced) [51]. Hepatic impairment was defined by the Child-Pugh scale grade A = mild and grade B = moderate. NTX and β-NTL PK parameters (C_{max}, t_{max}, AUC, $t_{1/2}$) did not significantly differ between the control group and the mild and moderate hepatic impairment groups. The elimination half-life for both NTX and β-NTL in all the subjects ranged from 5 to 9 days. Studies with patients with severe hepatic impairment have not been conducted, but if LA NTX were to be used, a significant dose reduction would likely be prescribed for general safety reasons.

A population PK study with the NTX clinical trial studies ($N=453$) was conducted, and the patients ranged in age from 18 to 76 years with 28 subjects that were >65 years [49]. Data from the patients included 3821 NTX and 3766 β-NTL plasma samples. Subjects (59 %) were alcohol dependent and some subjects (27 %) were both alcohol and opiate dependent. Population NTX clearance was 140 L/h and volume of distribution 38,300 L, which were weight dependent (changes of 0.548 L/h/kg) and were higher by 23–35 % in subjects with alcohol and/or opioid dependence. NTX clearance was dependent on age while β-NTL clearance was associated with creatinine clearance and alkaline phosphatase. NTX CL was increased by 18 % in subjects who smoked. Although these covariates were identified, these parameters were not considered to be clinically significant to reflect any dosing adjustments necessary for LA NTX based upon weight, age, gender, smoking, creatinine clearance, and hepatic function.

14.5 Opioid Agonist and Antagonist Combination Products

The dependence on opioids alone and in combination with other CNS drugs such as benzodiazepines has resulted in a significant impact in the USA where over 19,000 fatalities occurred per year in the last decade [52]. However, prior to the 2000s, opiate dependence was recognized to be a major healthcare negative influence in society. In response to the growing opiate dependence problem in society, the pharmaceutical industry initiated various combination products adding NLX or NTX to reduce the potential for abuse and dependence. This section will examine the different opiate agonist or partial agonist combination products with NLX or NTX.

Pentazocine (PTZ)/Naloxone PTZ dependence is similar to other opiates, but overdoses are relatively uncommon. A review of PTZ use in over 10-year time period reported 57 cases of overdose combined with other products. Only 23 patients (40 %) ingested PTZ alone [53]. Most patients remained awake with respiratory rates >12/min. Overdose symptoms reported included grand mal seizures, hypertension, hypotonia, dysphoria, hallucinations, delusions, and agitation. NLX IV 0.4–2.4 mg was given to 11 of the 23 patients that ingested only PTZ and only two patients improved. When PTZ was taken with other agents such as alcohol or sedative-hypnotics, three of five patients that were in a coma were given IV NLX 0.4–1.2 mg and had a positive response. Besides the symptoms previously described, a case report of PTZ overdose of 1.5 g reported additional laboratory findings of ventricular arrhythmias and metabolic acidosis [54]. While in the ICU, the patient was given 0.4 mg IV NLX and continued to receive NLX until respiratory depression and other opiate overdose symptoms were reversed. This case reported use of up to 5–20 mg of IV NLX, and the suggestion is that higher NLX doses may be necessary for PTZ overdose situations.

The premise of NLX addition to the PTZ formulation was to reduce opiate dependence and to manufacture a nonabusable form of PTZ as a potential niche for this combination product [55–57]. Pharmacokinetic studies could not be found with this combination product. PTZ dependence was reported since the 1960s, and the company proposed in 1981 to manufacture this combination product. The product Talwin Nx® was FDA approved in 1982 and PTZ as a single entity ceased in 1983. Data from the Drug Abuse Warning Network (DAWN) reported in 1981 to the first quarter of 1983 4678 PTZ overdoses from emergency rooms. [58] From Talwin Nx®'s introduction to 1985, only 1706 emergency room visits were noted with a tenfold drop in medical examiners' notes from autopsies. Abuse from PTZ/tripelennamine use was also noted to decline [58]. However, reports surfaced noting abuse of the PTZ/NLX combination [59]. An explanation for possible abuse by the combination product was shown by a study where the PTZ analgesia was potentiated by low-dose NLX in postoperative patients ($N = 105$) with moderately severe pain [60]. Nevertheless, this product led to the development of other opioid agonist or partial agonist products combined with NLX.

Buprenorphine (BUP)/Naloxone (NLX) The combination product of BUP/NLX consists of the partial mu-opioid receptor agonist BUP and the opiate antagonist NLX. Due to the very low oral bioavailability of NLX, the sublingual (SL) combination preparation was developed [61]. This combination product was devised for the treatment of opiate dependence, and when the product is crushed for parental administration, the NLX addition would lead to withdrawal symptoms, discouraging the person to abuse the BUP [62].

The PK parameters of BUP were previously described in Chap. 11. Various PK studies have reported that BUP and NLX do not interact with each other. BUP is primarily metabolized by CYP3A4 to nor-BUP, which possesses weak (about 25 % of BUP) mu-opioid receptor agonist activity. NLX is primarily metabolized by phase II glucuronidation (see above NLX section). While BUP is highly bound to plasma proteins α and β globulin (96 %), NLX has low protein binding (46 %) mainly to albumin. The likelihood of a drug-drug interaction by protein-binding displacement is minimal [61]. The bioavailability of the SL tablet was compared to the oral solution with different dose combinations of BUP 2–8 mg and NLX 4–8 mg [63]. The BUP and NLX bioavailability ranged from 30 to 51 % and 7 to 9 %, respectively. The oral liquid and SL tablets were found to be equally bioavailable [61]. A PK study with non-dependent opiate volunteers was given ascending BUP/NLX doses of 4/1, 8/2, and 16/4 mg [64]. BUP serum concentrations increased with dose, but not proportionally with the mean BUP AUC_{48} as the 4/1 mg dose was 12.52 ng•h/mL, 8/2 mg dose was 20.22 ng•h/mL, and 16/4 mg was 34.89 ng•h/mL. Therefore, although linear PK disposition for the BUP/NLX product was determined, clinicians should be aware of the increasing doses and its relationship to serum drug concentrations.

The BUP/NLX product Suboxone® was reported to have a bitter taste or aftertaste from the polyethylene oxide in the drug formulation [65]. A different formulation used a dry mixing manufacturing method producing a small and fast-dissolving tablet (OX219) that used menthol and sucralose as a sweetener to mask the bitter taste [66]. This formulation was reported to be bioavailable as the Suboxone® oral tablet and SL products. BUP/NLX tablets were crushed and given by the IV and intranasal route to healthy non-opioid-dependent volunteers ($N = 10$). Intranasal drug administration in another route was used by patients with substance abuse problems [62]. Significant NLX concentrations were found with intranasal BUP/NLX administration, which may potentially attenuate BUP effects. Although NLX concentrations were measured, these findings have not yet been assessed in opiate-dependent patients.

The BUP/NLX combination in a 4:1 dose ratio was discovered to be the most reasonable product that balances the PD therapeutic benefits and minimizes unwanted adverse effects [67]. The 4:1 ratio was evaluated against the other ratios of 2:1 and 8:1 [68]. When IV BUP/NLX was given, it produced a dose-dependent precipitated withdrawal with the 2:1 ratio having the highest withdrawal score (Clinical Institute Narcotic Assessment, CINA). The 8:1 ratio had the least severe symptoms. Withdrawal symptom duration was 30 min for the 2:1 ratio and 15 min for the 4:1 and 8:1 ratios. BUP-induced pupil constriction was significantly attenuated by the 2:1 and 4:1 ratio combinations, but not the 8:1 ratio. Both the 2:1 and 4:1 ratio precipitated substantial withdrawal; however, the 2:1 ratio could be separated from the 4:1 ratio on some withdrawal ratings [69]. The BUP/NLX 4:1 ratio in doses of 8/2, 16/4, and 32/8 mg was assessed in eight healthy volunteers for neurocognitive effects [70]. Various cognitive tests were included such as the digit symbol substitution test (DSST), trial-making A and B, recognition memory, and several other tools. Only the 32/8 mg dose produced a significant impairment effect with the recognition memory test ($p < 0.05$) while the other assessments did not show significant impairment. These findings support that BUP/NLX does not significantly impair cognition while treating opiate-dependent patients. BUP/NLX was evaluated in opiate-dependent patients ($N = 9$) when given BUP 8 mg SL and different doses of NLX 0, 4, and 8 mg [71]. It was found that combined BUP and NLX displayed opiate withdrawal symptoms after introduction of the SL BUP/NLX treatment. BUP oral and NLX IV produced similar effects of BUP SL without precipitating opiate withdrawal symptoms.

BUP monotherapy has established efficacy in the treatment of opioid dependence and in a medically supervised withdrawal treatment [61]. When BUP/NLX has been evaluated versus BUP alone, the results are largely indistinguishable between the two agents. BUP/NLX has been compared to methadone, different counseling and/or medication dispensing regimens, clonidine, and "real-world" settings. In each set of studies, BUP/NLX was reported either greater than or comparable efficacy rates to the other treatments [61]. BUP/NLX pharmacotherapy involves short-term use as in the medically supervised withdrawal therapy. In contrast, opioid dependence as maintenance therapy can be viewed as long-term management. BUP like methadone was susceptible to illegal diversion and incorporation of NLX was designed to address this problem. BUP/NLX usage continues to be closely monitored by professional and regulatory agencies.

Methadone (MTH)/Naloxone In the early 1970s, a methadone/naloxone (MTH/NLX) product was proposed for patients with opiate dependence treated with MTH. MTH alone can also lead to dependence and this combination product was developed to curb abuse and dependence. A pilot study with ten patients stabilized on MTH agreed to participate and was given IV MTH/NLX 20 mg/0.4 mg (50:1 ratio) [72]. Serum drug concentrations were not measured and PD effects were assessed by pupillary measurements obtained 3 min prior to administration with subsequent measurements taken 3, 6, 15, and 30 min post administration. The IV MTH/NLX caused a significant withdrawal syndrome that peaked at 6 min ($p<0.01$) and declined after 15 min, returning to baseline at 30 min. Pupillary response was significantly elevated at 3 min with the MTH/NLX formulations 10:1 and 20:1 ratios and similar findings were reported [73]. A large multicenter trial ($N=1413$) with the 20:1 ratio tablet was completed; however, the study results were not published but reported at a conference. The investigators noted that the MTH/NLX was well tolerated and not associated with significant adverse effects. The product was expensive and the perception at that time was the little need for this combination in the market [74]. Finally, a small pilot study ($N=10$) with oral MTH/NLX 50:1 ratio reported no significant drug-drug interactions between MTH and NLX [75]. Similar to previous findings, withdrawal symptoms were noted to occur with the oral formulation that peaked later at 15–30 min, returning to baseline at 60 min. It is unlikely that the MTH/NLX combination product will see a commercial market.

Oxycodone (OXY)/Naloxone (NLX) The oxycodone/naloxone product like the previous combination products (e.g., BUP/NLX) was developed for reducing the potential for abuse and then expanded to the treatment of opioid-induced constipation [76]. The available OXY/NLX doses are in a ratio of 2:1 with 5/2.5 mg, 10/5 mg, 20/10 mg, and 40/20 mg [77]. The optimal 2:1 ratio was reported in a four-arm clinical trial ($N=202$) where subjects were treated with OXY dosed 40 and

80 mg daily and NLX with varying doses of 0, 10, 20, and 40 mg [78]. Bowel function and pain intensity were assessed by a simple numerical analog scale. The Bowel Function Index (BFI) is a validated instrument that was also used and consists of three items: defection ease, feeling of incomplete bowel emptying, and personal judgment of constipation. Significant difference between analgesia was not found and the dose ratio improved constipation while avoiding diarrhea. Subsequent studies have similar results with the OXY/NLX 2:1 ratio [79]. Nausea and diarrhea were the most often reported adverse event and detected when the dose ratio was shifted toward a higher NLX dose.

An extensive single- ($N=23$) and multiple-dose ($N=28$) PK study with the OXY/NLX prolonged-release (PR) formulation in healthy male and female volunteers was conducted [80]. The OXY/NLX PR doses evaluated were $4\times10/5$ mg, $2\times20/10$ mg, and $1\times40/20$ mg, which was compared to OXY PR alone 40 mg formulation and the NLX PR alone 20 mg formulation. The products were considered bioequivalent when the confidence interval (CI) for relative bioavailability came within a range of 80–125 % for the single products. Both the single- and multiple-dose studies reported that the combined OXY/NLX PR doses were bioequivalent to the OXY PR and NLX PR products. Further, OXY/NLX combined formulation did not significantly affect each other's bioavailability. The adverse event profile did not differ between each product. A small PD study was conducted to assess the effects of a single NLX dose to reverse the OXY-induced effect on colon transit time [81]. Fifteen healthy male volunteers participated and each received placebo, OXY 10 and 20 mg, and OXY/NLX 10/5 mg and 20/10 mg as a capsule with a radiolabeled resin (surrogate biomarker for GI contents). Colon arrival time did not statistically significantly differ between the OXY and the OXY/NLX products (mean 7.19 h versus 5.16 h, $p=0.065$). The mean colon arrival time for the placebo was 5.15 h and similar to the OXY/NLX. The OXY/NLX 20/10 mg significantly reduced the mean colonic transit time by 2.1 h ($p=0.037$), indicating clinical efficacy for opioid-induced constipation. Subsequent clinical trials with OXY/NLX in patients with various pain conditions (e.g., cancer, chronic pain) have demonstrated the efficacy of OXY/NLX in alleviating pain symptoms while improving the opioid-induced bowel dysfunction [82]. Clinicians should constantly monitor patients using this product for both chronic pain management and constipation pharmacotherapy [77].

Morphine (MS)/Naltrexone (NTX) The morphine extended release (ER) that contains sequestered naltrexone (NTX) has been developed [83]. MS ER is a polymer-coated pellet where each pellet has an NTX sequestered core and is released only when the capsules are tampered. The formulation is intended to reduce or eliminate diversion and abuse [84]. When MS/NTX is taken orally, NTX was inconsistently absorbed with very minimal or nondetectable plasma concentrations of NTX or its 6 β naltrexol metabolite [83]. NTX and its metabolite after repeated MS/NTX administration do not accumulate, and plasma concentrations were not associated with dose, age, or sex [83]. NTX was shown to have a higher volume of distribution with single-dose compared to multiple-dose administration (16.1 L/kg versus 14.2 L/kg, $p<0.05$). Oral NTX had a reported elimination half-life of 8.9 h

[83]. MS and NTX PK did not significantly differ between the MS/NTX combination product and either MS or NTX alone. Therefore, MS and NTX did not interfere with each other's PK profile [84]. Food was shown not to have a significant impact upon MS/NTX disposition in healthy volunteers ($N = 36$), and MS PK parameters were within the 80–125 % confidence intervals and the C_{max} was delayed by 2.5 h [85]. NTX remained sequestered with only trace amounts detected.

When the MS/NTX is crushed, a rapid release of NTX occurs equal to the bioequivalence of oral NTX solution [86]. A healthy volunteer ($N = 24$) study reported that the t_{max} for both the MS/NTX and oral NTX solution was about 1 h. The C_{max} NTX concentrations and NTX AUC for both the crushed MS/NTX and oral NTX solution were between the 80 and 125 % bioavailability with the 95 % confidence interval. A similar finding in PK properties occurred when non-dependent opioid users ($N = 32$) were given crushed MS/NTX and oral NTX solution (e.g., t_{max} 1.1 h) [84]. Co-administration with quinidine, a P-gp inhibitor, was reported to increase the MS exposure by twofold when given with the MS/NTX product, and caution was advised if these two agents were prescribed together [83].

MS/NTX was compared to ER MS treated in patients ($N = 72$) in a double-blind randomized clinical trial for the treatment of chronic pain associated with knee or hip osteoarthritis [87]. Pharmacokinetic profiles of both agents were determined over a 12 h time period and pharmacodynamic assessments were conducted with a validated pain scale (Western Ontario and McMaster Universities, WOMAC) and a visual analog scale (VAS) 0–100 mm as 0 = no pain with 100 = extreme pain. The study results reported that the ER MS and MS/NTX products were PK bioequivalent (95 % CI $AUC_{0-12\,h}$). Both WOMAC and VAS scores did not significantly differ between both products. These results showed that MS/NTX was equal to ER MS in both PK parameters and PD effects. The results of three different studies were reported in one publication where the PK and PD of MS/NTX were evaluated in healthy volunteers, non-opioid and recreational opioid users, and chronic pain patients >3 months [88, 89]. The different formulations used were the oral, crushed MS/NTX, and immediate-release (IR) MS products. The PD measurements included VAS scores, drug-liking effects, and the Cole/Addiction Research Center Inventory (Cole/ARCI) Stimulation-Euphoria scale. When MS/NTX product was crushed, the NTX bioavailability was equal to NTX oral solution. The MS/NTX was also equally bioavailable compared to the IR MS. When the VAS and Cole/ACRI scores were assessed with the product, these three studies indicate that when taken as directed by the prescriber, MS/NTX can be an effective agent for pain treatment with bioequivalence to MS with effective PD actions in pain management.

The overall adverse event profile for MS/NTX was comparable to MS monotherapy [83]. The most commonly reported adverse effects were constipation, nausea, and somnolence. The highest dose approved by the regulatory agencies for MS/NTX is 100 mg/4 mg. It is used only for patients who are tolerant to opiates and may lead to respiratory depression if used in other patients. The combination MS/NTX is FDA approved for the treatment of moderate to severe pain when continuous therapy is required for long-term use [83].

14.6 Levo-Alpha Acetyl Methadol (LAAM)

LAAM was FDA approved in 1993 for use in medication therapy for opiate addiction [90]. LAAM is a derivative of methadone (see Fig. 14.1a and Chap. 11) developed in 1948 for analgesia. Interest in LAAM occurred in the early 1960s as a substitute for methadone with numerous clinical studies conducted from 1969 to 1981. Lack of research funding during the 1980s limited further research. However, the National Institute on Drug Abuse (NIDA) initiated the process of obtaining FDA approval in 1990 and conducted the additional required clinical trials. In summary, LAAM was demonstrated to be either equally as or more effective than methadone in maintaining opiate abstinence [91]. Unfortunately, LAAM has been linked to prolonged QT intervals and possible torsades de pointes and is no longer commonly used [92, 93]. In Europe, LAAM was suspended for use in 2001 and US FDA issued a "black box" warning on the product's label [93].

LAAM Pharmacokinetics and Pharmacodynamics LAAM may be considered a "prodrug" as it is metabolized by N-demethylation to two primary metabolites, nor-LAAM and dinor-LAAM by the cytochrome P450 (CYP) 3A4 shown in Fig. 14.1b [94]. Other CYP enzymes that are reported to be involved with LAAM metabolism to a lesser extent are 2B6, 2C8, and 2C18 [95]. LAAM and its two metabolites were reported with in vitro models to be P-gp substrates [96]. Ketoconazole was reported to markedly increase LAAM disposition in opioid-naïve subjects ($N=13$) when given oral LAAM 5 mg/70 kg and a single 400 mg ketoconazole dose [9, 97]. Co-administration with ketoconazole resulted in a mean 3.22-fold ($p<0.001$) increase in LAAM C_{max} and mean 5.29-fold ($p<0.001$) increase in AUC. The nor-LAAM and dinor-LAAM mean C_{max} significantly increased by 0.77-fold and 0.55-fold ($p<0.001$), respectively. Subsequent nor-LAAM and dinor-LAAM mean AUC significantly increased by 2.25-fold ($p<0.001$) and 1.21-fold ($p<0.005$), respectively. Mean pupil diameter was significantly decreased with a t_{max} for miosis by 2.92-fold ($p<0.001$) From a single ketoconazole dose, clinically relevant increases in LAAM and metabolite concentrations were found and that may affect physiologic function such as QT intervals which suggests that CYP3A4 inhibitors and LAAM should be contraindicated.

Nor-LAAM was shown to be five to ten times more potent than LAAM and dinor-LAAM leading to the longer duration of action for LAAM reflected in its dosing schedule [98]. The disposition of LAAM and its two metabolites were described in six healthy male adult volunteers [99]. Each subject was given oral and IV LAAM 20 and 40 mg with physiologic, subjective, and pharmacokinetic samplings. The bioavailability for LAAM was found to be about 50 % with a mean (±S.D.) elimination half-life of 7.9 (±1.2) hours for the oral 20 mg dose and 18.5 (±4.9) hours for the 40 mg dose. The LAAM t_{max} was 2.5 and 2.6 h for the oral 20 and 40 mg doses, respectively. The nor-LAAM t_{max} occurred slightly later than LAAM at 3–4 h and had a greater AUC than LAAM (20 mg dose; mean 994 ± 192 ng/mL•h versus 393 ± 85 ng/mL•h). The nor-LAAM mean elimination half-life was 33.6 ± 4.2 h. The dinor-LAAM mean t_{max} and elimination half-life was later and longer than LAAM

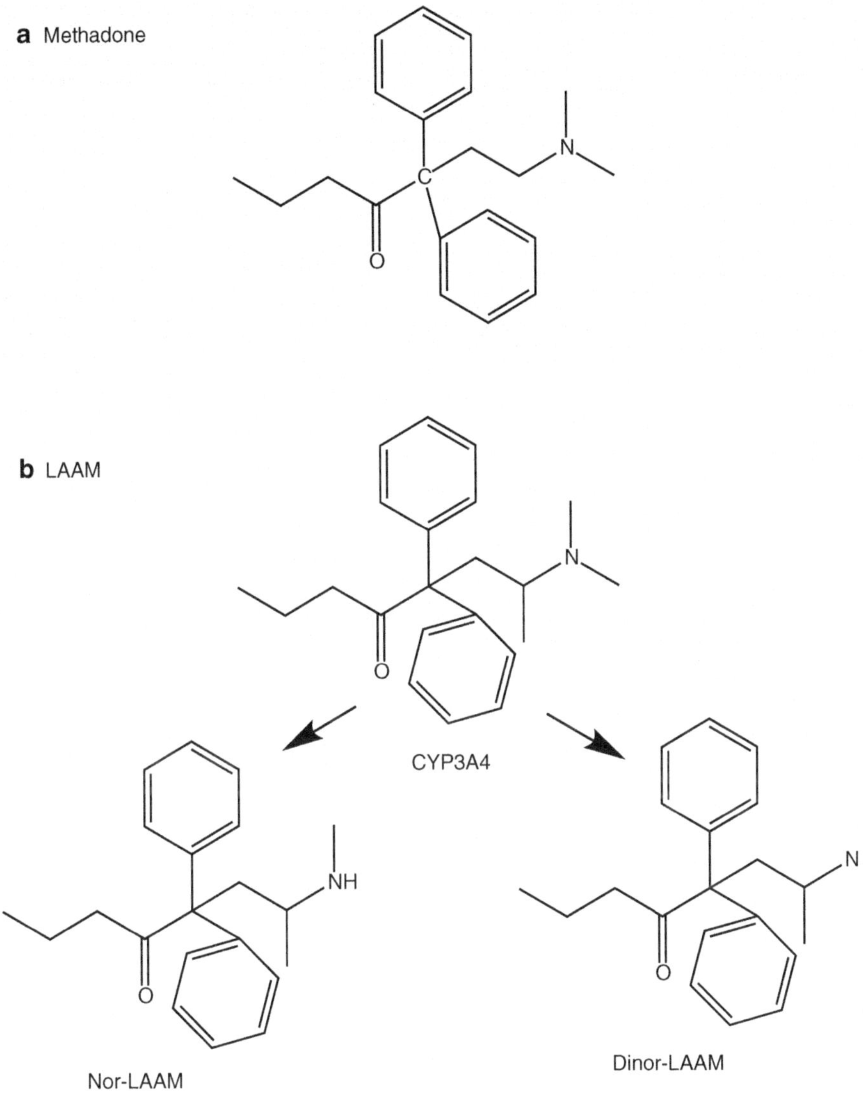

Fig. 14.1 Structure of methadone (**a**) and LAAM metabolism (**b**)

and nor-LAAM at 17.9±7.3 h and 75.6±15.4 h, respectively. Pupil diameter decreased with all doses and routes with the IV route reported to have greater subjective feelings of any drug effect and liking the drug from baseline to 3 h. LAAM disposition was reported in two groups of male subjects where one group received methadone 50 mg/day for 3 months ($N=5$) and the other group were heroin addicts without prior exposure to methadone or LAAM ($N=5$) [100]. The methadone group received LAAM 60 mg and then under chronic conditions 85 mg/dose three times a week for 3 months with plasma samples obtained to determine LAAM disposition.

The second group started with LAAM 25 mg which was increased to the 85 mg/dose three times a week. Under the acute conditions, LAAM plasma concentrations had a biexponential decline with a mean t_α=4.6 h (range 3.1–9.9 h) and a t_β=53.3 h (range 31.5–115.5 h). The mean t_{max} was 3.3±1.2 h. With chronic dosing administration, nor-LAAM and dinor-LAAM plasma concentrations increased by five- to tenfold with an elimination half-life of 31 h and >100 h, respectively.

The PD effects of LAAM and methadone were compared in nine occasional opioid users with oral doses of 15, 30, and 60 mg/70 kg given to each subject. The NLX challenge dose of 1 mg/70 kg was given to determine if NLX can reverse PD effects of LAAM or methadone [101]. In a variety of PD measurements (e.g., VAS scores), LAAM was reported to produce a more PD significant effect than methadone. For example, pupil diameter changes were significantly of a greater magnitude than methadone by a factor of 1.63 ($p<0.05$). Three subjects were withdrawn from the study due to respiratory depression induced by the LAAM 60 mg dose. Unlike methadone findings, NLX failed to reverse LAAM 60 mg induced pupil constriction. These results can assist clinicians determining appropriate LAAM doses when converting patients from methadone to LAAM. Also, LAAM may possess more potent PD effects than methadone and lower doses may be indicated.

Methadone and LAMM PK and PD were compared in 16 stable patients on methadone maintenance [102]. Half of the subjects were known as "non-holders" where inadequate methadone doses led to unpleasant withdrawal symptoms. Methadone and LAAM mean daily doses were identical in the methadone holder mean 73±32 and 73±34, respectively. For the non-holders, the LAAM mean dose was a 1.1 factor higher (mean 93±52 mg versus 83±49 mg). The methadone PK profile did not differ between the two groups. However, withdrawal symptoms were initially reduced up to 9 h after methadone dosing in the non-holders and significantly elevated afterwards ($p<0.001$), while holders did not experience any withdrawal symptoms. Interestingly, LAAM PD effects in the non-holders showed that withdrawal symptoms and scores remained reduced 2 h after dosing and remained consistently reduced up to 24 h (also significantly lower when given methadone noted at 24 h, $p<0.001$). The withdrawal symptoms scores for LAAM non-holders only slightly increased at 36 and 48 h later. Therefore, methadone non-holder patients can be effectively treated with LAAM.

A randomized 24-week clinical trial compared the QT interval changes between methadone and LAAM [92]. LAAM-treated patients ($N=31$) showed a significant increase in QTc interval prolongation (0.409±0.022 s versus 0.418±0.28 s, $p<0.046$), whereas methadone-treated patients ($N=22$) did not. More LAAM patients with borderline prolonged and prolonged QTc intervals were observed than methadone-treated patients (LAAM seven patients versus methadone one patient, $p=0.1$). This study showed that LAAM produced a higher incidence of prolonged QTc intervals than methadone with careful ECG monitoring recommended [92]. As previously mentioned, regulatory agencies have place severe restrictions with LAAM.

Based upon the information with LAAM, if prescribed in the USA and outside of Europe, it is given in juice like methadone but every other day or three times a week. Patients switched from methadone to LAAM can be dosed 1.2–1.3 times higher therapeutic concentrations achieved within 2 weeks. If LAAM is given more than every other day, the drug accumulates and a fatal overdose may result. Drug interactions particularly with CYP3A4 inhibitors should not be prescribed in LAAM-treated patients. Since LAAM elimination half-life is longer, the drug remains detectable for up to 72 h post dose but provides a stable plateau of plasma concentrations, preventing withdrawal symptoms. As previously mentioned, the QTc interval prolongation severely limits LAAM usage today.

14.7 Conclusion

The pharmacologic treatment for addiction remains elusive. Few products are available that directly treat alcohol, nicotine, and drug dependence such as acamprosate and varenicline. The promise of methadone to treat opiate dependence soon became a separate dependence problem. LAAM was initially shown to be beneficial for opioid dependence, but due to QTc interval prolongation, its use has become discouraged due to safety and regulatory issues. NLX is widely accepted as the antagonist for opiate overdose and is included in many first-responder's medical emergency kits. NTX is approved for opiate and alcohol dependence. The combination products that contain an opiate agonist or partial agonist and an opiate antagonist have found several roles in therapy for short-term use in the medically supervised withdrawal therapy, long-term use as for opioid dependence as maintenance therapy, and the prevention or treatment of opiate-induced constipation. However, addition of an opiate antagonist agent in a combination product has not averted the substance abuse challenges with the opiate agonists or partial agonists but may effectively address the opiate-induced constipation problems. Opiate, alcohol, and other types of drug dependence continue to be a worldwide medical problem facing our society.

References

1. Doering PL, Li RM (2014) Chapter 49. Substance-related disorders II. In: DiPiro JT, Talbert RL, Yee GC et al. (eds) Pharmacotherapy, 9th edn. McGraw Hill, New York. pp. 1003–1018
2. Wilde MI, Wagstaff AJ (1997) Acamprosate. Drugs 53:1038–1053
3. Scott LJ, Figgitt DP, Keam SJ, Waugh J (2005) Acamprosate. CNS Drugs 19:445–464
4. Mason BJ (2001) Treatment of alcohol-dependent outpatients with acamprosate: a clinical review. J Clin Psychiatry 62(Suppl 20):42–48
5. Saivin S, Hulot T, Chabac S et al (1998) Clinical pharmacokinetics of acamprosate. Clin Pharmacokinet 35:331–345
6. Peachy JE, Brien JF, Roach CA, Loomis CW (1981) A comparative review of the pharmacological and toxicological properties of disulfiram and calcium carbimide. J Clin Psychopharmacol 1:21–26
7. Peachy JE, Sellers EM (1981) The disulfiram and calcium carbimide acetaldehyde-mediated ethanol reactions. Pharmacol Ther 15:89–97

8. Johnansson B (1992) A review of the pharmacokinetics and pharmacodynamics of disulfiram and its metabolites. Acta Psychiatr Scand Suppl 369:15–26
9. Hudmon KS, Kroon LA, Corelli RL (2012) Chapter 47. Smoking cessation. In: Krinsky DL, Berardi RR, Ferreri SP (eds) Handbook of nonprescription drugs, 17th edn. American Pharmacists Association, Washington DC, pp 885–910
10. Svensson CK (1987) Clinical pharmacokinetics of nicotine. Clin Pharmacokinet 12:30–40
11. Benowitz NL, Hukkanen J, Jacob P III (2009) Nicotine chemistry, metabolism, kinetics, and biomarkers. Handb Exp Pharmacol 192:29–60
12. Faessel HM, Obach RS, Rollema H et al (2010) A review of the clinical pharmacokinetics and pharmacodynamics of varenicline for smoking cessation. Clin Pharmacokinet 49:799–816
13. Feng B, Obach RS, Burstein AH et al (2008) Effect of human renal cationic transporter inhibition on the pharmacokinetics of varenicline, a new therapy for smoking cessation: an in vitro – in vivo study. Clin Pharmacol Ther 83:567–576
14. Ravva P, Gastonguay MR, Tensfeldt TG, Faessel HM (2009) Population pharmacokinetic analysis of varenicline in adult smokers. Br J Clin Pharmacol 68:669–681
15. Faessel HM, Gibbs MA, Clark DJ et al (2006) Multiple-dose pharmacokinetics of the selective nicotinic receptor partial agonist, varenicline, in healthy smokers. J Clin Pharmacol 46:1439–1448
16. Kikkawa H, Maruyama N, Fujimoto Y, Hasunuma T (2011) Single and multiple-dose pharmacokinetics of the selective nicotinic receptor partial agonist, varenicline, in healthy Japanese adult smokers. J Clin Pharmacol 51:527–537
17. Ravva P, Gastonguay MR, Faessel HM, Lee TC, Niaura R (2014) Pharmacokinetic-pharmacodynamic modeling of the effect of varenicline on nicotine craving in adult smokers. Nicotine Tob Res 17(1):106–113. doi:10.1093/intr/ntu154
18. King DP, Paciga S, Pickering E et al (2012) Smoking cessation pharmacogenetics: analysis of varenicline and bupropion in placebo-controlled clinical trials. Neuropsychopharmacol 37:641–650
19. Blumberg H, Dayton HB, Wolf PS (1966) Counteraction of narcotic antagonist by the narcotic antagonist Naloxone. Proc Soc Exp Biol Med 123:755–758
20. Evans LE, Swainson CP, Roscoe P, Prescott LF (1973) Treatment of drug overdose with naloxone, a specific narcotic antagonist. Lancet 1(7601):452–455
21. Handal KA, Schauben JL, Salamone FR (1983) Naloxone. Ann Emerg Med 12:438–445
22. Berkowitz BA (1976) The relationship of pharmacokinetics to pharmacologic activity: morphine, methadone, and naloxone. Clin Pharmacokinet 1:219–230
23. Fishman J, Roffwarg H, Hellman L (1973) Disposition of naloxone in normal narcotic dependent men. J Pharmacol Exp Ther 187:575–580
24. Weinstein SH, Pfeffer M, Schor JM et al (1971) Metabolites of naloxone in human urine. J Pharm Sci 60:1567–1568
25. Ngal SH, Berkowitz BA, Yang JC, Hempstead J, Spector S (1976) Pharmacokinetics of naloxone in rats and man. Anesthesiology 44:398–401
26. Berkowitz BA, Ngal SH, Hempstead J, Spector S (1975) Disposition of naloxone: use of a new radioimmunoassay. J Pharmacol Exp Ther 195:499–504
27. Cone EF (1976) General procedure for the isolation and identification of a 6-α and 6-β hydroxyl metabolites of narcotic agonists and antagonists with a hydroxymorphine structure. J Chromatogr 129:355–361
28. Asali LA, Brown KF (1984) Naloxone protein binding in adult and foetal plasma. Eur J Clin Pharmacol 27:459–463
29. Kanaan M, Daali Y, Dayer P, Desmeules J (2009) P-glycoprotein is not involved in the differential oral potency of naloxone and naltrexone. Fundam Clin Pharmacol 23:543–548
30. Dowling J, Isbister GK, Kirkpatrick CM, Naidoo D, Graudins A (2008) Population pharmacokinetics of intravenous, intramuscular, and intranasal naloxone in human volunteers. Ther Drug Monit 30:490–496

31. Yamamoto R, Takasuga S, Yoshida Y et al (2012) In vitro and in vivo transdermal iontophoretic delivery of naloxone, an opioid antagonist. Int J Pharm 422:132–138
32. Sanaei-Zadeh H (2012) Is transdermal iontophoretic delivery of naloxone sufficient for the management of intoxication in opioid-overdosed patients? Int J Pharm 428:187
33. Robinson A, Wermeling DP (2014) Intranasal naloxone administration for treatment of opioid overdose. Am J Health Syst Pharm 71:2129–2135
34. Greenberg MI, Roberts JR, Baskin SI (1980) Endotracheal naloxone reversal of morphine-induced respiratory depression in rabbits. Ann Emerg Med 9:289–292
35. Goldfrank L, Weisman RS, Errick JK, Lo MW (1986) A dosing nomogram for continuous infusion intravenous naloxone. Ann Emerg Med 15:566–570
36. Groeger JS, Inturrisi CE (1987) High-dose naloxone: pharmacokinetics in patients in septic shock. Crti Care Med 15:751–756
37. Hanes SD, Franklin M, Kuhl DA, Headley AS (1999) Prolonged opioid antagonist with naloxone in chronic renal failure. Pharmacother 19:897–901
38. Olofsen E, van Dorp E, Teppema L et al (2010) Naloxone reversal of morphine and morphine-6-glucuronide-induced respiratory depression in healthy volunteers. Anesthesiology 112:1417–1427
39. Yassan A, Oolofsen E, van Dorp E et al (2007) Mechanism-based pharmacokinetic-pharmacodynamic modeling of the reversal of buprenorphine-induced respiratory depression by naloxone: a study in healthy volunteers. Clin Pharmacokinet 46:965–980
40. Culpepper-Morgan JA, Inturrisi CE, Portenoy RK et al (1992) Treatment of opioid-induced constipation with oral naloxone: a pilot study. Clin Pharmacol Ther 52:90–95
41. Gibson CM, Pass SE (2014) Enteral naloxone for the treatment of opioid-induced constipation in the medical intensive care unit. J Crit Care 29:803–807
42. Martin WR, Jasinski DR, Mansky PA (1973) Naltrexone, an antagonist for the treatment of heroin dependence in man. Arch Gen Psychiatry 28:784–791
43. Gonzalez JP, Brogden RN (1988) Naltrexone: a review of its pharmacodynamics and pharmacokinetic properties and therapeutic efficacy in the management of opioid-dependence. Drugs 35:192–313
44. Fujimoto JM, Roerig S, Wang RI, Cahtterjie N, Inturrisi CE (1975) Narcotic antagonistic activity of several metabolites of naloxone and naltrexone tested in morphine dependent mice (38558). Proc Soc Exp Biol Med 148:443–448
45. Cone EJ, Gorodedtzky CW, Yeh S (1974) The urinary excretion profile of naltrexone and metabolites in man. Drug Metab Dispos 2:506–512
46. Verebey K, Volavka J, Mule SJ, Resnick RB (1976) Naltrexone: disposition, metabolism, and effects after acute and chronic dosing. Clin Pharmacol Ther 20:315–328
47. Lee MC, Wagner HN, Tanada S et al (1988) Duration of occupancy of opiate receptors by naltrexone. J Nucl Med 29:1207–1211
48. Galloway GP, Koch M, Cello R, Smith DE (2005) Pharmacokinetics, safety, and tolerability of a depot formulation naltrexone in alcoholics: an open-label trial. BMC Psychiatry 5:18. doi:10.1186/1471-244X-5-18
49. Dunbar JL, Truncliff RZ, Hayes SC, Farrell CB (2007) Population pharmacokinetics of extended-release injectable naltrexone (XR-NTX) in patients with alcohol dependence. J Stud Alcohol Drugs 68:862–870
50. Dunbar JL, Turncliff RZ, Dong Q et al (2006) Single and multiple-dose pharmacokinetics of long-acting injectable naltrexone. Alcohol Clin Exp Res 30:480–490
51. Turncliff RZ, Dunbar JL, Dong Q et al (2005) Pharmacokinetics of long-acting naltrexone in subjects with mild to moderate hepatic impairment. J Clin Pharmacol 45:1259–1267
52. Bart G (2012) Maintenance medication for opiate addiction: the foundation of recovery. J Addcit Dis 31:207–225
53. Challoner KR, McCarron MM, Newton EJ (1990) Pentazocine (Talwin) intoxication: report of 57 cases. J Emerg Med 8:67–74
54. Stahl SM, Kasser IS (1983) Pentazocine overdose. Ann Emerg Med 12:63–65

55. Legros J, Khalili-Varasteh H, Margetts G (1984) Pharmacologic study of pentazocine-naloxone combination: interest as a potentially nonabusable oral form of pentazocine. Arch Int Pharmacodyn Ther 271:11–21
56. Swift JQ, Hargreaves KM (1993) Pentazocine analgesia: is there a niche for Talwin Nx? Compendium 14:1048
57. Lahmeyer HW, Craig RJ (1987) Pentazocine-naloxone: another "addiction-proof" drug of abuse. Int J Addict 22:1163–1166
58. Baum C, Hsu JP, Nelson RC (1987) The impact of the addition of naloxone on the use and abuse of pentazocine. Public Health Rep 102:426–429
59. Reed DA, Schnoll SH (1986) Abuse of pentazocine-naloxone combination. JAMA 256:2562–2564
60. Levine JD, Gordon CG, Taiwo YO, Coderra TJ (1988) Potentiation of pentazocine analgesia by low-dose naloxone. J Clin Invest 82:1574–1577
61. Orman JS, Keating GM (2009) Buprenorphine/naloxone. Drugs 69:577–607
62. Middleton LS, Nuzzo PA, Lofwall MR, Moody DE, Walsh SL (2011) The pharmacodynamics and pharmacokinetic profile of intranasal crushed buprenorphine/naloxone tablets in opioid-abusers. Addiction 106:1460–1473
63. Nath RP, Upton RA, Everhart ET et al (1999) Buprenorphine pharmacokinetics: relative bioavailability of sublingual tablet and liquid formulations. J Clin Pharmacol 39:619–623
64. Center for Drug Evaluation and Research. Clinical pharmacology and biopharmaceutics review: application number: 20–732, 20–733 (Suboxone®) [online]. Available from URL: http://fda.gov/cder. Accessed 22 Nov 2014
65. Suboxone commercial web page (2014) Reckitt-Benckiser Inc. Available from: http://www.suboxone.com/. Accessed 22 Nov 2014
66. Fischer A, Jonsson M, Hjelmstrom P (2015) Pharmaceutical and pharmacokinetic characterization of a novel sublingual buprenorphine/naloxone tablet formulation in healthy volunteers. Drug Dev Ind Pharm 41(1):79–84; early on-line 1–6
67. Mendelson J, Jones RT (2003) Clinical and pharmacologic evaluation of buprenorphine and naloxone combinations: why the 4:1 ratio for treatment. Drug Alcohol Depend 70:S29–S37
68. Chaing CN, Hawks RL (2003) Pharmacokinetics of the combination tablet of buprenorphine and naloxone. Drug Alcohol Depend 70:S39–S47
69. Mintzer MZ, Correia CJ, Strain EC (2004) A dose-effect study of repeated administration of buprenorphine/naloxone on performance in opioid-dependent volunteers. Drug Alcohol Depend 74:205–209
70. Harris DS, Mendelson JE, Lin ET, Upton RA, Jones RT (2004) Pharmacokinetics and subjective effects of sublingual buprenorphine, alone or in combination with naloxone. Clin Pharmacokinet 43:329–340
71. Harris DS, Jones RT, Wlem S et al (2000) Buprenorphine and naloxone co-administration in opiate-dependent patients stabilized on sublingual buprenorphine. Drug Alcohol Depend 61:85–94
72. Parwatikar SD, Knowles RR (1973) Methadone-naloxone in combination for the treatment of heroin addicts. Clin Pharmacol Ther 14:941–948
73. Nutt JG, Jasinski DR (1974) Methadone-naloxone mixtures for use in methadone maintenance programs. Clin Pharmacol Ther 15:156–166
74. Loimer N, Presslich O, Grunberger J, Linzmayer L (1991) Combined naloxone-methadone preparations for opiate substitution therapy. J Subst Abuse Treat 8:157–160
75. Bell J, Shearer J, Ryan A et al (2009) The acceptability, safety, and tolerability of methadone-naloxone in a 50:1 ratio. Exp Clin Psychopharmacol 17:146–153
76. Mueller-Lissner S (2010) Fixed combination of oxycodone with naloxone: a new way to prevent and treat opioid-induced constipation. Adv Ther 27:581–590
77. Leppert W (2014) Oxycodone/naloxone in the management of patients with pain and opioid-induced bowel dysfunction. Curr Drug Targets 15:124–135
78. Meissner W, Leyendecker P, Mueller-Lissner S et al (2009) A randomized controlled trial with prolonged-release oral oxycodone and naloxone to prevent and reverse opioid-induced constipation. Eur J Pain 13:56–64

79. Vondrackova D, Leyendecker P, Meissner W et al (2008) Analgesic effect and safety of oxycodone in combination with naloxone as prolonged release tablets in patients with moderate to severe chronic pain. J Pain 9:1144–1154
80. Smith K, Hopp M, Mundin G et al (2008) Single- and multiple dose pharmacokinetic evaluation of oxycodone and naloxone in an opioid agonist/antagonist prolonged-release combination in healthy adult volunteers. Clin Ther 30:2051–2068
81. Smith K, Hopp M, Mundin G et al (2011) Naloxone as part of a prolonged release oxycodone/naloxone combination reduces oxycodone-induced slowing of gastrointestinal transit in healthy volunteers. Expert Opin Investig Drugs 20:427–439
82. Mercadante S, Ferrera P, Adile C (2011) High doses of oxycodone-naloxone combination may provide poor analgesia. Support Care Cancer 19:1471–1472
83. Duggan ST, Scott LJ (2010) Morphine/Naltrexone. CNS Drugs 24:527–538
84. Johnson F, Setnik B (2011) Morphine sulfate and naltrexone hydrochloride extended release capsules: naltrexone release, pharmacodynamics and tolerability. Pain Physician 14: 391–406
85. Johnson F, Ciric S, Boudriau S, Swearingen D, Stauffer J (2010) Food effects on the pharmacokinetics of morphine sulfate and naltrexone hydrochloride extended release capsules. Adv Ther 27:846–858
86. Johnson FK, Stark JG, Bieberdorf FA, Stauffer J (2010) Relative oral bioavailability of morphine and naltrexone derived from crushed morphine sulfate and naltrexone hydrochloride extended-release capsules versus intact product and versus naltrexone solution: a single-dose, randomized-sequence, open-label, three-way crossover trial in healthy volunteers. Clin Ther 32:1149–1164
87. Katz N, Sun S, Jonhson F, Stauffer J (2010) ALO-01 (morphine sulfate and naltrexone hydrochloride) extended release capsules in the treatment of chronic pain of osteoarthritis of the hip or knee: pharmacokinetics, efficacy, and safety. J Pain 11:303–311
88. King Pharmaceuticals Inc. Embeda® (morphine sulfate and naltrexone hydrochloride) extended release capsules for oral use [online]. Available from URL: http://www.accessdata.fda.gov/drugsatfda_docs/label/2009/
89. Stauffer J, Setnik B, Sokolowski M (2009) Subjective effects and safety of whole and tampered morphine sulfate and naltrexone hydrochloride (ALO-01) extended-release capsules versus morphine solution and placebo in experienced non-dependent opioid users: a randomized, double-blind, placebo-controlled, crossover study. Clin Drug Investig 29:777–790
90. Finn P, Wolcock K (1997) Levo-alpha acetyl methadol (LAAM). J Subst Abuse Treat 14:559–564
91. Center for Substance Abuse Treatment (1995). Treatment Improvement Protocol (TIP) Series, No 22. LAAM in the treatment of opiate addiction. Rockville, MD: Department of Health and Human Services
92. Weineke H, Conrads H, Wolstein J et al (2009) Levo-α-acetylmethadol (LAAM) induced QTc prolongation – results from a controlled clinical trial. Eur J Med Res 14:7–12
93. US Food and Drug Administration: Product Discontinuation Notice (2003) ORLAAM® (Levomethadyl hydrochloride) Oral Solution, 10 mg/mL, CII. Available at http://www.fda.gov
94. Kharasch ED, Whittington D, Hoffer C et al (2005) Paradoxical role of cytochrome P450 3A in the bioactivation and clinical effects of levo-α-acetylmethadol. Clin Pharmacokinet 44:731–751
95. Henderson GL, Wilson BK, Lau DH (1977) Plasma l-alpha-acetylmethadol (LAAM) after acute and chronic administration. Clin Pharmacol Ther 21:16–25
96. Crettol S, Digon P, Golay KP, Brawand M, Eap CB (2007) In vitro P-glycoprotein-mediated transport of (R), (S), (R, S)-methadone, LAAM and their main metabolites. Pharmacology 80:304–311
97. Moody DE, Walsh SL, Rollins DE, Neff JA, Huang W (2004) Ketoconazole, a cytochrome P450 3A4 inhibitor, markedly increases concentrations of levo-acetyl-alpha-methadol in opioid-naïve individuals. Clin Pharmacol Ther 76:154–166
98. Huang W, Bemis PA, Slawson MH, Moody DE (2003) Determination of l-α-acetylmethadol (LAAM), norLAAL, and dinorLAAM in clinical and in vitro samples using liquid chromatography with electrospray ionization and tandem mass spectrometry. J Pharm Sci 92:10–20

99. Eissenberg T, Stitzer ML, Bigelow GE, Buchhalter AR, Walsh SL (1999) Relative potency of levo-α-acetylmethadol and methadone in humans under acute dosing conditions. J Pharmacol Exp Ther 289:936–945
100. Henderson GL, North-Root H, Kuttab SH (1977) Metabolism and disposition of l-α-acetylmethadol in the rat. Drug Metab Dispos 5:321–328
101. Walsh SL, Johnson RE, Cone EJ, Begelow GE (1998) Intravenous and oral l-α-acetylmethadol: pharmacodynamics and pharmacokinetics in humans. J Pharmacol Exp Ther 285:71–82
102. Newcombe DA, Bochner F, White JM, Somogyi AA (2004) Evaluation of levo-alpha-acetylmethadol (LAAM) as an alternative treatment for methadone maintenance patients who regularly experience withdrawal: a pharmacokinetic and pharmacodynamic analysis. Drug Alcohol Depend 76:63–72

Chapter 15
Anesthetic Drugs Pharmacokinetics and Pharmacodynamics

Michael W. Jann

Abstract Patients undergoing surgery require anesthesia that involves using a variety of medications that promote sedation, pain mitigation, and abate any response to stimulation. Early agents used for sedation induction were thiopental and etomidate. Although ketamine is commonly used in veterinary medicine, this agent is often employed in combination with a benzodiazepine to induce analgesia and sedation. Ketamine is a racemic mixture where the S(+) isomer is two to four times more potent. Midazolam is a water-soluble benzodiazepine where at pH>4, the molecule's ring structure closes, and it becomes a highly lipophilic agent. Both ketamine and midazolam pharmacokinetics fit into a two-compartment open model and primarily metabolized by CYP3A4. The muscle relaxant agents succinyolcholine, d-tubocurarine, roncuronium, and vencuronium induce muscle paralysis used for anesthesia. Succinylcholine pharamacokinetics has been described as a one-compartment open model whereas the other agents a two- or three-compartment open model. Their pharmacodynamics effects are closely linked with their pharmacokinetic profiles. The short-acting opioids fentanyl, sufentanil, and alfentanil are used in anesthesia for pain management and maintain cardiovascular stability. The pharmacokinetics of these agents are expressed as either a two- or three-compartment open model and mainly metabolized by CYP3A4. Propofol and thiopental display a three-compartment open model. Various factors can alter anesthetic drug disposition and their pharmacodynamic actions.

Keywords Etomidate • Ketamine • Midazolam • Succinylcholine • d-Tubocurarine • Roncuronium • Vecuronium • Muscle relaxants • Opioids • Fentanyl • Sufenantil • Alfentanil • Propofol • Thiopental

---

M.W. Jann, PharmD
Department of Pharmacotherapy, University of North Texas System College of Pharmacy (UNTSCP) and University of North Texas Health Science Center (UNTHSC), Fort Worth, TX, USA
e-mail: Michael.jann@unthsc.edu

M. Jann et al. (eds.), *Applied Clinical Pharmacokinetics and Pharmacodynamics of Psychopharmacological Agents*,
DOI 10.1007/978-3-319-27883-4_15

15.1 Introduction

Anesthesia induction of patients undergoing surgery requires various combinations of medications to promote sleep or loss of consciousness, alleviate pain, and diminish response to any stimulation. Anesthesia is commonly achieved with a minimum of two different types of pharmacologic agents such as a hypnotic and an opioid analgesic [1]. In addition to the pharmacologic agents for hypnosis and analgesia, inhalation anesthetics and muscle relaxants are often employed prior to their usage. Physical signs have served as distinct pharmacodynamic (PD) biomarkers for the anesthesia that include respiratory patterns, somatic muscle tone, ocular signs, hemodynamic parameters, and the minimum alveolar concentration (MAC) [2]. This chapter will focus only on the pharmacologic agents used in anesthesia. For a review of the inhalational anesthetic agents, these agents display a three-compartment model as shown in Fig. 15.1 and the reader is referred to these references [3, 4].

A summary of the anesthetic agents covered in this chapter is presented in Table 15.1. Pharmacologic anesthetic agents given intravenously (IV) or orally were used since the 1930s with thiopental, but integrating their pharmacokinetic properties with the PD effects occurred 45 years later. Since then, sophisticated PK/PD modeling methods have been developed and continually to be revised that enhances the clinical utility of these agents and development of newer agents. Anesthetic agents PK and PD have increased the comprehension of other central nervous system (CNS) drugs that have been employed to treat neurological and psychiatric medical conditions. This chapter will include the muscle relaxants used in anesthesia as distinct PK/PD models that are used in clinical practice. Some of the anesthetic agents have an extensive array of PK and PD studies (e.g., midazolam, propofol) and

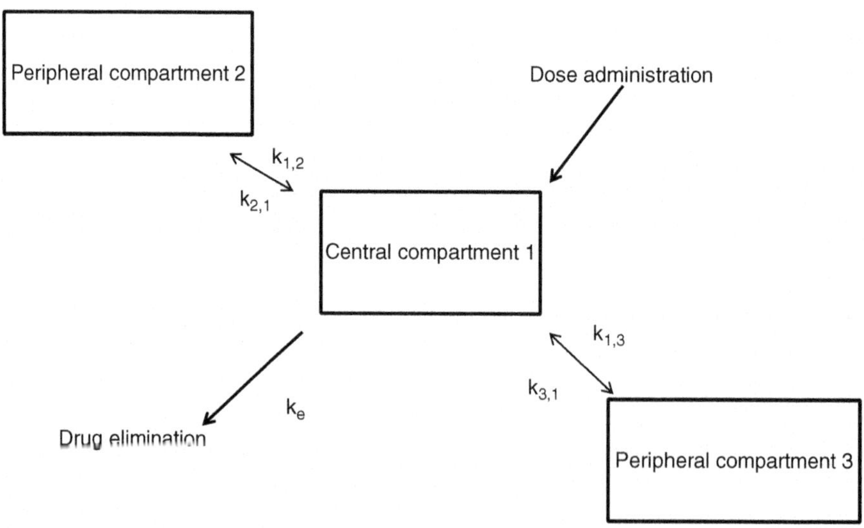

Fig. 15.1 Three-compartment open pharmacokinetic model

Table 15.1 Summary of the pharmacokinetic parameters of selected anesthetic agents

Drug	Vd (L/kg)	CL (mL/kg/min)	Protein binding (%)	Metabolism	$T_{1/2\beta}$ (h)	Action duration (min)
Alfentanil[a]	0.3–1.0	3–7.6	92	CYP3A4[b]	0.6–1.5	5–10
Etomidate	2.5–4.5	18–25	77	Hydrolysis[c]	2.9–5.3	3–5
Ketamine	3.1	12–17	12	CYP3A4[d]	2–4	5–10
Midazolam	1.1–1.7	6.4–11	94	CYP3A4[e]	1.7–2.6	15–20
Propofol	2–10	20–30	97	CYP2B6[f]	4–23	3–5
Thiopental	2.5	3.4	83	N.R.	11	5–10

[a]Adapted from Eilers and Niemann [1]
[b]Davis and Cook [59]
[c]Kharasch et al. [120]
[d]Geise and Staney [7]
[e]Santamaria et al. [121]
[f]Kronbach et al. [26]
[g]Turpeinen and Zanger [94]

only selected key articles were selected for inclusion in this chapter. Although at least two different anesthetic drugs are used in clinical practice, the PK/PD of these agents is reviewed individually and the reader is referred to the drug-drug interactions with the anesthetic drugs in Chap. 24.

15.2 Etomidate

Etomidate (ETD) is a carboxylated imidazole with hypnotic properties and the FDA approved the drug as an IV anesthetic induction agent [5]. Preclinical studies reported that ETD may possess a wider margin of safety compared to thiopental [6]. CNS depressant actions were related to the stimulation of the gamma-aminobutyric acid (GABA) receptors. However, pain upon injection and myoclonia were reported to be ETD's most undesirable adverse side effects. Nausea and vomiting occurring more frequently (as high as 50 %) have been reported in various studies with multiple ETD dosing [7].

ETD Pharmacokinetics and Pharmacodynamics ETD has been described similar to thiopental with an open three-compartment pharmacokinetic (PK) model shown in Fig. 15.1. Table 15.1 describes the general ETD PK parameters. ETD 0.3 mg/kg was administered IV to eight patients who underwent eye or ear surgery with 14 blood samples obtained over the following 10 h [8]. The following PK properties (mean ± s.d.) were found with ETD that included volume of distribution (Vd) of 4.5 ± 2.2 L/kg, CL of 860 ± 230 mL/min, and elimination half-life of 4.6 ± 2.6 h. The free fraction of ETD was about 7 % and the hepatic extraction ratio of 0.5 was determined. A later study reported that ETD with a rapid distribution half-life of 2.81 ± 1.64 min and a protein binding of 77 % almost totally to albumin was metabolized by hydrolyzation in the plasma and in the liver at the ETD ester forming carboxylic acid [7].

A PD dose-response relationship was found with ETD in patients undergoing electroconvulsive therapy (ECT) that received no other premedication treatment [9]. ETD was given at doses of 0.1, 0.2, and 0.4 mg/kg. The higher ETD doses had significantly greater effects on waking time and the late recovery time ($p<0.01$). The ETD 0.1 mg/kg dose had a reported mean (± s.d.) waking time of 7.52 ± 1.07 min and a mean recovery time of 20.41 ± 1.17 min. The ETD doses of 0.2 mg/kg and 0.4 mg/kg reported mean waking times of 10.02 ± 0.78 min and 14.05 ± 1.46 min, respectively. The ETD 0.2 mg/kg and 0.4 mg/kg reported mean late recovery times of 27.60 ± 1.74 min and 38.05 ± 2.70 min, respectively. ETD ($N=10$) 0.3 mg/kg was compared to thiopental ($N=5$) 3.5 mg/kg in patients with various elective surgeries and PD actions assessed by the EEG [10]. The main differences between the two agents were the lack of beta activity and a longer duration of "deep stage" sleep with ETD. ETD had higher incidences of pain and myoclonic and tonic movements than thiopental but these effects were not associated with epileptiform discharges.

15.3 Ketamine

Ketamine (KTM) is an N-methyl-D-aspartate (NMDA) receptor antagonist that blocks glutamatergic functions with opioid receptor activity [11, 12]. KTM has been used in veterinary medicine and when combined with benzodiazepine anesthetics employed for analgesia and sedation in adult and pediatric populations [13]. KTM has efficacy in neuropathic and nociceptive pain. A variety of administration routes for KTM have been utilized including parenteral, oral, rectal, subcutaneous, transdermal, and intranasal [11]. Only the routes of administration when KTM is used for anesthesia will be presented in this chapter.

KTM Pharmacokinetics and Pharmacodynamics KTM PK was investigated in five adult healthy male volunteers given a single dose of 0.125 and 0.250 μg/kg separated by 1 week [14]. Blood samples were obtained prior to drug administration and for 7 h afterward. Pain assessment was conducted by using sphygmomanometers known as "tourniquet time." KTM plasma concentration time data were fitted by a two-compartment open model. The KTM metabolite nor-KTM was also characterized. The mean KTM PK parameters for both doses reported were clearance (CL) of 17 mL/min/kg, elimination half-life of 186 ± 8 min, and volume of distribution (Vd) of 3.1 L/kg. Nor-KTM peak plasma concentrations (mean ± S.E.M.) were reached at 75 min (40 ± 14 ng/mL) and 45 min (21 ± 3 ng/mL) for the 0.250 μg/kg and 0.125 μg/kg doses, respectively. Both KTM doses extended the period of pain-free time at KTM plasma concentrations greater than 100 ng/mL. KTM 0.5 mg/kg single dose was given intramuscularly (IM) and an oral solution to six healthy volunteers and the pain evaluation was conducted by the tourniquet test by ischemic exercise [15]. KTM bioavailability was found to be 93 % and 16 % for the IM and oral solution, respectively. The mean (± s.d.) peak plasma concentration occurred at 22 ± 4 min and 30 ± 5 min for the IM and oral solution, respectively. The mean elimination half-life for the IM and oral routes were 115 ± 12 min and 174 ± 50 min, respectively, with plasma concentrations associated with analgesia at 150–160 ng/mL [15, 16]. Nor-KTM plasma concentrations were 2- to 5-fold higher than KTM plasma concentrations noted from oral administration. Nor-KTM plasma concentrations were generally lower than the KTM plasma levels when given by the IM route [15].

KTM is also a racemic mixture of two enantiomers S(+) KTM and R(−) KTM where the S isomer has been suggested to be two to four times more potent in pain alleviation and causes fewer adverse side effects than the racemic KTM [17]. The S(+) isomer was also reported to be twice as potent as the R(−) isomer on the NMDA receptors [18]. KTM is extensively metabolized by hepatic CYP3A4 (to nor-KTM) and to a lesser extent CYP2B6 and CYP2C9 [19]. Potential drug-drug interactions can occur with KTM via CYP enzymes (see Drug-Drug Interactions Anesthetic Agents Chapter).

The PK properties for racemic and S(+) KTM were evaluated in 50 adult patients undergoing minor surgery [20]. The patients were divided into two groups of 25 patients that received racemic KTM 2 mg/kg and S(+) KTM 1 mg/kg. Using the change of systolic arterial pressure, the sample size of 22 patients per group was calculated that achieved at 90 % power (alpha) at a 5 % level (beta). The PK parameters of S(+) KTM did not significantly differ from the racemic KTM. For example, the S(+) KTM mean (± s.d.) elimination half-life was 2.39 ± 1.26 h, CL 16.4 ± 5.7 mL/min/kg, and Vd 2.84 ± 1.59 L/kg. Systolic and diastolic arterial pressure significantly increased with both agents ($p < 0.005$). S(+) KTM had significantly ($p < 0.005$) higher systolic and diastolic arterial pressure than racemic KTM noted at 1, 3, and 15 min after drug administration. S(+) and R(−) KTM PK were examined in ten healthy male volunteers given two infusion cycles of S(+) KTM 0.1 and 0.2 μg/mL/min of R(−) KTM (11). KTM PK was estimated using a 2- and 3-compartment model. S(+) KTM showed a significantly ($p < 0.05$) higher mean (± s.d.) CL of 26.3 ± 3.5 mL/min/kg than R(−) KTM 13.8 ± 1.3 mL/min/kg. The authors suggested that R(−) KTM may inhibit S(+) KTM elimination although a mechanism was not proposed. Further studies would be needed to confirm the actions of R(−) KTM on S(+) KTM PK.

15.4 Midazolam

Midazolam (MDZ) is the first water-soluble benzodiazepine and used for sedation and sleep induction for anesthesia [21, 22]. Under the environmental pH = 4, the ring diazepine structure opens reversibly that produces a highly water-soluble molecule. At pH > 4, the ring closes resulting in a highly lipophilic molecule that under physiological pH rapidly enters the CNS after drug administration [21]. MDZ can be given IV, IM, and orally to induce sedation and anesthesia. Due to wealth of information with MDZ, the pharmacokinetic and pharmacodynamic sections were separated with selected information presented.

MDZ Pharmacokinetics A summary of MDZ PK is presented in Table 15.1 and its elimination half-life was shown not to be significantly different when given either IV, IM, or oral administration [21]. MDZ PK will be briefly presented in this section as an open two-compartment model was described after IV administration [23]. MDZ PK was examined in six healthy volunteers given 5 mg IV, 10 mg oral solution, and 10 mg oral tablet [23]. The mean (± s.d.) MDZ bioavailability was reported to be low at 0.36 (±0.09) indicating a significant first-pass effect. The mean Vd and total MDZ CL after the IV dose were 1.14±0.57 L/kg and 0.383±0.094 L/kg/h, respectively. The mean terminal elimination half-life was 1.77±0.83 h from the three different administration routes. After IV administration, sleep induction occurred within 1–2 min with continued sedation for an average of 1.33 h. Sleep induction took place later with the oral solution and tablet with an average of 0.38 h (range 0.25–0.55 h) and sedation was maintained for an average of 1.17 h (range 0.5±to 2.33 h). MDZ bioavailability was investigated with the oral doses 10 mg, 20 mg, and 40 mg versus an IV dose of 0.15 mg/kg in six healthy volunteers [24]. The mean MDZ bioavailability range for the 10 and 20 mg dose was identical (0.46±0.11 and 0.48±0.12, respectively). The MDZ bioavailability was greater with the 40 mg dose (range 0.63–0.72), but only three subjects were able to tolerate the high dose. The MDZ distribution of blood/plasma concentration coefficient (λ) was reported to be 0.53 indicating only a small extent of binding to red blood cell erythrocytes. MDZ is primarily metabolized by the CYP3A4 to its 1-OH and 4-OH MDZ metabolite. The 1-OH metabolite is converted to another metabolite 1,4 OH compound. All three metabolites are glucuronidated and then renally eliminated [21, 25].

Factors That Influence MDZ Pharmacokinetics The factors reported to affect MDZ PK disposition were age and obesity [26]. It was found that in elderly males versus adult males, a decrease in drug CL took place. Differences in MDZ PK between elderly females and adult females were not found. Vd was slightly increased in the elderly females and males, but it was not significant. Based upon these findings, MDZ doses should be reduced by about 50 % in elderly men. MDZ disposition was significantly altered in morbidly obese persons reflected by the Vd with enhanced drug distribution into peripheral adipose tissues. This action produces a significant ($p<0.05$) prolongation in MDZ elimination half-life. Therefore, MDZ doses should be increased proportionally to the patient's total body weight. Significant differences in MDZ PK were not found between patients with chronic renal failure and normal controls and dosage adjustments are not recommended.

MDZ Pharmacodynamics MDZ can induce and maintain anesthesia, used as a premedication agent prior to surgery and as an adjunct to local or regional anesthesia for sedation [26]. During anesthesia, MDZ affects respiration via CNS depression, but lacks significant cardiovascular effects, and produces only a slight decrease in cerebral perfusion and oxygenation [27]. IV MDZ 0.15 mg/kg was given to healthy unpremedicated volunteers ($N=20$) where CNS and cardiovascular effects were monitored [28]. Significant adverse effects were not found and blood pressure only slightly decreased after 3 min postdrug administration. Anterograde amnesia and drowsiness were observed in all subjects,

The PD effects of oral MDZ 10 mg, 20 mg, and 40 mg or IV MDZ 0.15 mg/kg were investigated in six healthy volunteers [29]. The PD tests included the tracing test, reaction time, subject's self-assessment (sedation, muscle relaxation, and concentration capacity), and investigator subjective assessment. After drug administration, MDZ PK parameters were determined and the plasma concentrations were linked with the PD effects using the sigmoid Hill Equation E_{max} model: $E = E_{max} \times Cp/EC_{50} \times Cp$ where E = the intensity of action, E_{max} = maximal effect, Cp = concentration linked to the effect, and EC_{50} = plasma concentration at 50 % of E_{max}. Peak effects from the oral route occurred at 30 min in reducing the PD effects. The duration of the PD effects were 2 h for the IV route and the 10 mg oral dose. The 20 and 40 mg doses had a significantly longer effect of 4 h ($p < 0.05$). The minimum effective MDZ plasma concentration to affect the subject's reduced PD actions ranged from 30 to 100 ng/ml. The PD effects were correlated with the E_{max} model. The respiratory and cardiovascular effects of MDZ and diazepam (DZ) were compared in eight healthy volunteers [30]. MDZ 0.05 mg/kg and DZ 0.15 mg/kg were given via the IV route using a randomized double-blind crossover method. Blood pressure, blood gases, and Pa_{CO2} with plasma drug concentrations were obtained. The PD effects of blood pressure and Pa_{CO2} followed a sigmoidal E_{max} model where the MDZ EC_{50} was from 50 to 60 ng/ml. Correlation between respiratory effects and plasma drug concentrations was not found. In another study with IV MDZ 0.15 mg/kg and DZ 0.3 mg/kg given to eight healthy volunteers, both agents produced an equal effect in respiratory depression measured by ventilatory and mouth occlusion pressure response to CO_2 [31]. Therefore, MDZ like DZ can cause significant respiratory depression. Physostigmine 2.0 mg given IV was reported in three case reports to reverse the MDZ-induced sedation [32]. Flumazenil, a benzodiazepine receptor antagonist, was reported to reverse the respiratory depression effects of MDZ alone and MDZ plus alfentanil in healthy volunteers ($N = 20$) using a starting dose of 1 mg IV followed by an infusion of 20 μg/min [33]. Flumazenil has become the standard "rescue" medication for reversing the actions of MDZ and other benzodiazepines. MDZ has been compared to other anesthetics and benzodiazepines for anesthesia induction with comparable effects [21].

15.5 Muscle Relaxants

Muscle relaxants are commonly used as adjunctive medications for anesthesia for endotracheal intubation and to reduce muscle tone during surgery [34]. These agents are given to patients undergoing general anesthesia and usually not to normal healthy volunteers. Patients with normal hepatic and renal function are considered as "normal" patients. Muscle relaxant PK and PD actions contributed toward the understanding of integrating PK to PD effects. A large number of muscle relaxants are available and beyond the scope of this chapter to cover. Muscle relaxants are neuromuscular-blocking agents with their main pharmacologic action to inhibit transmission of nerve impulses by acetylcholine at the skeletal neuromuscular junction [34]. Inactivation of neuromuscular blockers occurs via plasma cholinesterase by hydrolysis dependent on three factors: (1) intrinsic speed of reaction, (2) drug concentration, and (3) esterase concentration [35]. Based upon these pharmacologic mechanism, neuromuscular agents either depolarizing (non-competitive) or non-depolarizing (competitive) agents are deactivated [34]. Extensive review articles on the clinical pharmacokinetics of these agents have been published with various factors including pregnancy that can influence their disposition [34, 36–39]. This section will present only selected agents with succinylcholine as the depolarizing agent. Tubocurarine (d-isomer) is considered the prototypical non-depolarizing agent and the "newer" agents rocuronium and vecuronium are discussed in this section.

Succinylcholine (SCL) Pharmacokinetics and Pharmacodynamics The typical adult dose of SCL is about 1.0 mg/kg that results in complete neuromuscular blockade with a 50 % recovery time in approximately 10 min [37]. SCL PK can be estimated by a one-compartment model and elimination: $C_0 = C \times e^{-k\tau}$. The PD model can be determined as $E = E_0 - k_m \times t_d/2.30$, where E_0 = the effect at time zero and t_d = the time to whatever blockade percentage is selected at minute in a typical 70 kg patient with 3.5 l of plasma. It was reported that the in vivo rate of SCL hydrolysis was between 3 and 7 mg/L/min and that an infusion rate of 4 mg/min was needed to maintain a 90 % reduction in the human twitch movement [36]. About 1/2800 persons possess an atypically low amount of plasma cholinesterase which results in a slower rate of hydrolysis and in those persons, the SCL dose was suggested to be significantly reduced by tenfold or greater [40]. However, presently, patient identification is not yet possible and clinicians must carefully monitor every patient.

Tubocurarine (dTC) Pharmacokinetics and Pharmacodynamics Early dTC PK reported studies have been limited to blood sampling collection times of up to 60 min postdrug administration. The use of dTC has been reported since the 1960s [41]. dTC PK studies with longer sample collection times up to 24 h reported a terminal half-life as long as 3.5 h, but a rapid recovery from muscle relaxant effects occurred after 15 min of drug cessation. The volume of distribution from the central compartment (V_c) for dTC was estimated to be 72–97.7 mL/kg [37]. From the central compartment shown in Fig. 15.1, the k_e leads to the sigmoidal E_{max} PD model [37]. A significant linear correlation between serum dTC concentration and muscle twitch tension was found and recovery from the twitch tension was estimated to be 0.7 μg/mL [42].

dTC infusion was given to patients ($N = 12$) to maintain a "steady-state" concentration of 1.09 μg/mL and after the infusion cessation, twitch response returned in half of patients with a full recovery for all patients in 30 min [43]. Based upon these results, a dTC bolus dose of 540 μg/kg and infusion rate of 2.0 μg/kg should produce continuous paralysis in the average patient. PK of dTC was reported not to significantly differ between infants, children, and adults and patients with hypothermia [44, 45]. dTC was simultaneously modeled using the open three-compartment model and the sigmoidal E_{max} model [46]. The results reported that the mean rate constant for dTC equilibrium for a paralysis effect from infusion was a serum concentration of 0.13±0.04 μg/min and the mean steady-state serum concentration of 0.37±0.05 μg/mL to achieve 50 % paralysis. These studies suggest that dTC has been well characterized for its PK and PD effects in a variety of patient populations [34, 46].

Rocuronium (RCM) Pharmacokinetics and Pharmacodynamics RCM is a neuromuscular-blocking drug that has a similar PK profile as vecuronium (see vecuronium section) and time course of action except that it has a more rapid onset of action with an ED_{95} of 0.3 mg/kg [38]. RCM had an average CL and terminal elimination half-life was 0.27 L/h/kg and 83 min, respectively. Age, renal failure, smoking, and hypothermia were reported not be significant factors in RCM CL and Vd when comparing these parameters to the adult population [38, 47]. RCM protein binding was found to be at 25 % and the only metabolite detected was 17-desacetyl-RCM present in very low concentrations. The metabolite is only 1/20 as potent as RCM and likely clinically insignificant [38]. RCM PK and PD was evaluated in patients ($N=10$) who were stabilized under either propofol or isoflurane anesthesia [48]. Differences in RCM PK were not found between the two groups. After a second RCM bolus dose of 0.5 mg/kg, the duration of neuromuscular blockade was significantly longer in the isoflurane group versus the propofol group (20±6 min versus 39±8 min, $p<0.05$). Using the sigmoidal E_{max} model, the EC_{50} was significantly higher under propofol anesthesia (1008 μg/L versus 592 μg/L, $p<0.05$).

The effects of RCM PK in patients with mild to moderate cirrhosis ($N=17$) was compared to healthy patients ($N=21$) given an RCM bolus dose of 0.6 mg/kg [49]. Blood samples were obtained for the next 8 h after RCM administration with the twitch response assessed. Using a three-compartment open model, RCL CL was significantly reduced in the cirrhotic group (2.66 mL/kg/min versus 3.70 mL/kg/min, $p<0.005$) and elimination half-life was also significantly prolonged in the cirrhotic group (28.3±12.1 min versus 16.8±4.6 min, $p<0.005$; 143±80 min versus 92±40 min, $p<0.05$, respectively). The time for clinical effect did not differ between the groups, but the mean time to recovery was significantly longer in the patients with cirrhosis (T50 % recovery 73.9±33.9 min versus 52.6±19.8 min, $p<0.05$). The increased PD recovery time reflects the prolonged PK effects of RCM in patients with cirrhosis. A similar finding in RCM PK and PD (recovery time) was reported in patients with obstructive jaundice (OJ, $N=27$) and control patients ($N=26$) given RCM of 0.9 mg/kg [50]. RCM plasma concentrations were significantly higher ($p<0.05$) from 30 to 120 min post RCM bolus injection with a corresponding longer recovery time (T25 % OJ 80.8±16.9 min versus 62.8±13.2 min, $p<0.01$). From these studies, hepatic impairment but not renal impairment can significantly alter RCM disposition and prolong PD effects.

Vecuronium (VCM) Pharmacokinetics and Pharmacodynamics VCM and its active 3-desacetyl VCM metabolite PK and PD were reported in 12 healthy volunteers [51]. Animal models reported that 3-desacetyl VCM had about 50–70 % neuromuscular-blocking activity as VCM [52]. The VCM and metabolite PK data were fit into a two- and three-compartment open model with the PD twitch model analysis using the sigmoidal E_{max} model. The VCM CL was significantly greater than the metabolite (5.39 [range 5.04–7.19] mL/kg/min versus 3.51 [range 2.11–6.57] mL/kg/min, $p<0.05$). The metabolite had significantly greater Vd and longer elimination half-life than VCM (254 [range 215–411] L/kg versus 152 [range 111–170] L/kg; 116 [44–672] minutes versus 34 [range 25–61] minutes, $p<0.05$). The EC_{50} for the VCM and its metabolite was 123 [range 109–154] ng/mL versus 102 [range 71–123] ng/mL ($p<0.05$), respectively. These findings show that the 3-desacetyl VCM is a potent active metabolite and can prolong VCM PD actions in patients [51].

The PK and PD of VCM were compared to pancuronium (PCM) in nine patients undergoing surgery [53]. VCM was shown to have a 50% shorter mean elimination half-life than PCM (71 ± 20 min versus 140 ± 25 min, $p<0.05$) and corresponding increase in CL. The EC_{50} was similar for both agents. The PK and PD of VCM were compared to PCM in twelve children aged 3–6 years [54]. The elimination half-life of VCM did not significantly differ from PCM. However, the VCM Vd and CL were significantly greater than PCM with shorter VCM duration of action and recovery index ($p<0.05$). The shorter action duration for VCM was suggested to be probably due to the larger Vd and higher CL. Elderly patients (age 70–84 years) were found not to have any significant differences in PK and PD actions compared to young adults (age 30–57 years) when given VCM and PCM [55].

VCM PK and PD effects were compared in normal patients ($N=7$) and patients with renal failure ($N=12$) given 0.1 mg/kg [56]. Mean VCM CL was significantly reduced in patients with renal failure (3.08 ± 0.83 mL/kg/min versus 5.29 ± 2.17 mL/kg/min, $p<0.05$) and duration of action significantly longer (98.6 ± 37.7 min versus 54.1 ± 25.2 min, $p<0.05$). A significant correlation between VCM CL and duration of action was found to be $r^2=0.869$. VCM PK was significantly altered in burn patients ($N=20$) compared to normal patients ($N=20$) given a single bolus of 0.12 mg/kg [57]. A three-compartment open model best described the VCM profile with an enhanced VCM CL in burn patients (0.12 L/min versus 0.095 L/min, $p<0.001$) and shorter elimination half-life (5.5 h versus 6.6 h, $p<0.001$). This shorter time period of VCM exposure in burn patients may explain the resistance to VCM in these patients.

15.6 Opioids

The role of opioids in anesthesia has evolved from use as a premedicant or adjunctive agent to the inhalants and postoperative pain management to a primary anesthetic drug due to their PD actions to maintain cardiovascular stability during surgery [58].

Table 15.2 Summary of the opioid pharmacokinetic parameters [13]

Drug	Vd (L/kg)	CL (L/kg/h)	Protein binding (%)	Metabolism	$T_{1/2\beta}$ (min)	Onset (min)
Alfentanil	0.75	0.48	92	CYP3A4	94	0.75
Sufentanil	3.2	0.76	92.5	CYP3A4	164	1
Fentanyl	4.5	0.78	84.4	CYP3A4	219	1.5
Morphine	3.2	0.9	30	Glucuronidation	177	7.5

Vd volume of distribution at steady state, *CL* clearance, $T_{1/2\beta}$ elimination half-life, *min* minutes

Only the short-acting opioid agents fentanyl (Fen), sufentanil (Suf), and alfentanil (Alf) will be presented in this section as these agents are the most commonly used opioids in anesthesia. Fen was introduced in the 1960s with Suf and Alf being the "newer" opioids. The main advantages of these opioids over morphine are a faster onset of analgesia and shorter elimination half-life shown in Table 15.2 and that allows for enhanced dosing flexibility in anesthesia management [58]. Additionally, these three drugs also have a lack of hyperglycemic response to surgery, decreased catecholamine levels, and increased lipid solubility [59].

Opioid Pharmacokinetics and Pharmacodynamics Fen and Suf PK have been described as a three-compartment open model [58]. Suf and Alf PK were described as both a two- and three-compartment model [58, 60]. The Gepts Model has been utilized as a foundational PK approach for Suf studies [61]. Peak brain concentrations in patients ($N = 19$) were reached for Alf at 45 s, Suf at 5 min, and Fen at 6 min during the postacute stage of head injury with normal intracranial pressure [62]. These opioid PK parameters and their comparison to morphine are presented in Table 15.2 [58, 62]. Suf Vd and elimination half-life were found to be between Fen and Alf. All three opioids are highly protein bound [63]. Fen and Alf are metabolized by hepatic CYP3A4 [64, 65]. Suf is also metabolized by N-dealkylation and O-demethylation, but a specific CYP enzyme was not reported [66]. Later, it was reported that CYP3A4 was responsible for Suf metabolism to the N-dealkylation metabolite [67]. Erythromycin is a known CYP3A4 inhibitor and was shown not to significantly affect Suf disposition [68]. An explanation for the lack of erythromycin effect on Suf PK may be due to its extraction ratio. Fen and Suf are agents with high hepatic extraction ratios of 0.8 and 1.0, respectively [69]. Compounds with a high extraction ratio could be less prone to metabolic inhibitors and more dependent on hepatic blood flow. Alf was found to have a low to moderate hepatic extraction ratio from 0.14 to 0.4 [58, 69, 70]. The three opioids were also reported not to be P-glycoprotein substrates but were shown to be inhibitors using the Caco-2 cell model [70]. The PD effects of Alf using the ED_{95} serum concentration-response curves to maintain hemodynamic stability in surgical patients ($N = 64$) were reported be 300 ng/ml and 400 ng/ml for superficial and intra-abdominal operations, respectively [71]. Concentration-response relationships for hemodynamic control under target-controlled infusion (TCI) with Suf and Fen were achiever with concentrations of 0.71 ± 0.13 ng/mL and 7.3 ± 1.3 ng/mL, respectively [72]. Higher Suf and Fen mean concentrations of ≥ 1.25 ng/mL and 13.5 ng/mL, respectively, did not improve hemodynamic control. Slightly lower Suf Fen mean concentrations were reported also to be effective for patients undergoing CABS with 0.59 ± 0.13 ng/mL and 5.8 ± 1.9 ng/mL, respectively [73]. Using the Gepts Model for Suf TCI, anesthesia was managed for patients (N = 34) with CABS with Suf concentrations as low as 0.4 ng/mL and equally effective as 0.8 ng/mL [74].

Factors That Can Alter Opioid Pharmacokinetics and Pharmacodynamics Opioids are typically administered as a bolus injection and/or by continuous infusion. Other administration routes that can be used include epidural, intrathecal, transdermal, and intranasal in which each of these routes alters the PK of these three opioids [75]. Factors have been shown to influence opioid PK that include age, obesity, plasma protein content, acid-base status, hepatic, and surgical procedures such as cardiopulmonary bypass [75]. Renal impairment was reported not to significantly alter opioid disposition due to their PK profiles and hepatic extraction ratios. Age-related effects for opioid disposition result from changes in increased body fat, decreases in protein binding, hepatic blood flow, and enzyme capacity [75]. Children ages 9 months to 10 years had reported significantly higher Alf CL than adults ($p < 0.05$) and a much shorter elimination half-life (41.6 min versus 55 min, $p < 0.05$). These PK changes were likely due to the increased CYP3A4 hepatic enzyme activity found in the children [76]. A similar finding with Suf was reported with children ages 2–8 years with an average CL of 1.83 L/kg/h [77]. Using EEG assessments, it was found that a 50 % reduction in Alf or Fen dose in the elderly was needed to produce similar effects in EEG suppression compared to the adults although significant PK differences were not found between the elderly and the adults [78].

Obesity was found to be a significant factor in opioid PK as these agents are highly lipophilic due to the peripheral compartment (either two or three) that contains a high adipose content. This factor increases opioid Vd which prolongs the drug's elimination half-life. All three agents are highly protein bound (see Table 15.2); however, only 50 % of Fen and Suf are bound to albumin. Alf binding to albumin is lower at 33 % [63, 75]. These agents are also bound to α_1-acid glycoprotein (AAG) and changes in AAG levels can either increase or decrease free drug concentrations. Acid-base changes in pH influence protein binding as alkalosis leads to increased protein binding and acidosis results in decreased protein binding. The pH changes has greater effects for Fen > Suf > Alf [63]. As previously mentioned, hepatic blood flow is a major factor in opioid PK due to their extraction ratio. Hepatic impairment could affect opioid disposition but varying results have been reported and therefore, dosage adjustments may not be necessary except for patients with moderate to severe impairment [75]. Different surgical procedures including cardiovascular bypass have been reported to alter opioid PK properties [79–83]. Surgery such as in CABS produces factors such as hemodilution, relative hypotension, and hypothermia [75]. Hemodilution results in lower plasma protein binding and increases drug Vd. Hypotension reduces hepatic blood flow and hypothermia reduces enzyme metabolic capacity. Each factor alters opioid serum or plasma concentrations and those changes can lead to an enhanced or reduced PD effects by prolonging or diminishing the opioid pharmacologic actions.

15.7 Propofol

Propofol (Ppf) is an anesthetic agent introduced in the 1980s to induce anesthesia. Unfortunately, a high incidence of pain upon IV injection and anaphylactoid reactions resulted in the development of an emulsion formation [84]. Ppf can be given as a bolus injection and by controlled infusion to induce and maintain anesthesia. Selected articles are presented to describe Ppf disposition and its PD effects.

Ppf Pharmacokinetics and Pharmacodynamics Ppf disposition was reported in 12 adult patients (six males and six females) given a single bolus IV injection of 2.5 mg/kg with blood samples collected for 8 h post-administration [85]. Ppf displayed a three-compartment open model as shown in Fig. 15.1; however, a subsequent second peak drug concentration occurred indicating a redistribution effect at 60 min. Ppf PK did not significantly differ between males and females and the mean (±SEM) CL was 1.80 L/kg for both groups. The elimination half-life for males was slightly greater than females (56.0 ± 4.0 min versus 44.9 ± 4.0 min, p = n.s.). Ppf PK was compared between the elderly (N = 12) aged 65–80 years and the adults (N = 12) aged 18–35 years [86]. Ppf doses were a single bolus of 2.0 mg/kg and 2.5 mg/kg for the elderly and adult groups, respectively. Ppf CL was significantly lower in the elderly group than the adult group (1.43 ± 0.09 L/min versus 1.78 ± 0.12 L/min, $p = 0.03$) and a smaller Vd (19.6 ± 5.2 L versus 26.3 ± 2.9 L, $p = 0.046$). Plasma protein binding did not differ between the groups.

Ppf PK covariates given by bolus injection and a 60 min infusion were evaluated in 24 patients with the PK data fitted to a three-compartment model [87]. Using a population PK approach, age was reported to be a significant covariate for volume of distribution and CL. Ppf CL was influenced by weight, lean body weight, and height. When taken together, these three variables significantly improved the model ($p < 0.01$). PK of Ppf in children ($N = 20$) aged 2–10 years was compared to adults under infusion to maintain a target Ppf plasma concentration of 15 μg/mL for anesthesia (10 μg/mL is used for the adults) [88]. The volume of distribution in the central compartment (Vc) was about 50 % greater than adults (343 mL/kg versus 228 mL/kg) and a higher CL (34.30 mL/kg/min versus 27.36 mL/kg/min). A larger Ppf bolus dose of 50 % and a higher maintenance infusion dose of 25 % were recommended for children. Lower Ppf Vd and CL were reported with the Asian population (Indian and Chinese) and dosage adjustments may be needed [89, 90].

Ppf was reported with in vitro models to be metabolized mainly by CYP2B6 (although this enzyme is about 3–6 % of the total hepatic enzyme content) and to a lesser extend CYP2C9 [91–93]. The CYP2B6 and UGT1A9 genotypes were reported to be significantly affected by Ppf plasma concentrations in patients ($N=51$) aged 42–81 years [92]. The group had a mean age of 65 years with 29 subjects >65 years and statistical analysis indicated patients with advanced age of 65 years had a higher Ppf risk score when factored with the two genotypes that influence Ppf PK and PD.

A number of studies have indicated that Ppf PK can be scaled allometrically and directly proportionally to lean body mass (LBM) [94, 95]. Ppf PK and PD effects were reported in adult patients ($N=42$) and the sigmoidal Emax model was used to determine effective concentration (EC) to achieve a Bispectral Index Score (BIS) between 40 and 60 [96]. The Ppf maintenance EC_{50} was found to be 2.23 mg/L (95 % C.I. 1.95–2.51). Ppf LBM was sued in dosing and sex was found not to influence the PK model. Using body weight as the key indicator for Ppf dosing, this concept was evaluated in adult morbidly obese patients ($N=66$, BMI ≥ 40 kg/m^2) that used a preset Ppf concentration of 2.5 µg/mL during infusion to maintain anesthesia [97]. The Bispectral Index <60 score (BIS) was used as the biomarker for anesthesia that determined the effective concentration (ECe). A probit regression model was used to calculate the ECe_{50} and ECe_{95} for Ppf. Total body weight (TBW) was found to be the best factor in Ppf dosing and the ECe_{50} was 3.4 µg/mL and ECe_{95} was 4.2 µg/mL. A higher Ppf target concentration was needed in morbidly obese patients most likely due to the much larger Ppf Vd. Similar findings using TBW for Ppf dosing and BIS in morbidly obese children and adolescents were found [98, 99].

Although initial Ppf studies did not report sex as a significant factor, later studies that measured Ppf metabolites reported that females had significantly higher Ppf glucuronide (1.25 fold, $p<0.03$), 4-OH Ppf-1-glucuronide (2.1 fold, $p=0.0009$), and 4-OH Ppf-4-glucuronide (1.7 fold, $p=0.02$) concentrations than males [100, 101]. Significant effects of CYP2B6 and UGT1A9 genotypes were not found to be factors. However, females tended to recover faster than males from Ppf anesthesia and that PD effect can be due to the increased Ppf metabolism.

Surgery can influence Ppf disposition. CABS effects on Ppf disposition was reported in patients ($N=19$) given 4 mg/kg/h infusion [102]. Total Ppf concentrations remained unchanged, but unbound Ppf amounts increased by twofold during surgery and decreased back to baseline levels at surgery completion. Careful patient monitoring is recommended during surgery. Ppf CL appears to change during liver transplantation as described in ten patients [103]. The following mean (± s.d.) Ppf CL were reported in the dissection, anhepatic, and reperfusion phases as 1.89 ± 0.48 L/min, 1.08 ± 0.25 L/min, and 1.53 ± 0.51 L/min, respectively. The Ppf mean extraction ratio was found to be 0.24 ± 0.12 without changes in Ppf concentrations between radial and pulmonary arteries. Ppf CL decreased about 42 % during the anhepatic phase and after reperfusion, Ppf metabolism resumes to prior capacity. A population PK and PD model for Ppf in patients ($N=23$) undergoing lung cancer surgery reported a lower EC_{50} of 1.4 mg/L during Ppf infusion 8 mg/kg/h [104]. However, the Population PK variables for CL was 2.38 L/min and volume of distribution was 189 L, which did not differ from previous Ppf studies. It was suggested that the use of Fen 3 µg/kg IV bolus dose may have influence the Ppf EC_{50} or cancer patients could be more sensitive due to chemotherapy and other therapeutic approaches to cancer. Other factors may influence Ppf PK and PD that remains to be elucidated. However, when making these assessments, Ppf modeling has generally utilized two specific approaches examining Ppf effect-site concentrations [105]. Computer simulation models have observed Ppf concentrations to range between 1.3 and 4.4 μg/mL with a desired effect noted at 2 min after the bolus dose. Continuous infusion dosing may require an EC_{50} from 1.5 to 4.0 μg/mL depending upon the patient's body weight and other factors that influence Ppf PK and PD.

15.8 Thiopental

Thiopental (TPL) is a barbiturate agent which was introduced into clinical anesthetic practice in 1934 and a popular anesthetic agent for many years. Unfortunately, thiopental produces respiratory and myocardial depression; causes spontaneous tremor, muscle movements, and hiccoughs in some patients; and is contraindicated in patients with porphyria and demyelinating diseases [106].

TPL Pharmacokinetics and Pharmacodynamics Thiopental's very short PD actions were originally thought to be related to drug metabolism. It was not until the 1950s and 1960s that TPL PK was modeled to describe its redistribution from the brain and plasma to less perfused fat tissues in the body that accounted for its actions [106]. A low extraction ratio for thiopental of 0.1 was reported that suggests that hepatic metabolism may not account for the PD actions [107]. The basic PK parameters of thiopental are shown in Table 15.1. After a bolus intravenous (IV) injection of TPL, a basic PK model with a distribution and elimination phase was described [108]. However, early studies initially suggested that thiopental protein binding markedly decreases at plasma concentrations of 100 μg/mL or greater indicating increased availability of additional free thiopental concentrations [109]. Based upon these findings, studies reported the lack of fit in describing TPL using a one- or two-compartment model [108].

It was not until the 1980s that a three-compartment model was shown to accurately describe thiopental PK with one central compartment feeding into two separate peripheral compartments with rate constants (e.g., $k_{1,2}$ and $k_{2,1}$, $k_{1,3}$ and $k_{3,1}$) to and from each compartment [109]. Drug dosing proceeds directly into the central compartment with metabolism and elimination (k_e) from the central compartment. Using the following equations, the total cumulative thiopental lost from the central compartment from metabolism was metabolic loss = CL × ∫ Cpssdt from zero to time t and total drug loss = V × [Cpss (0) – Cpss (t)] where V = volume of distribution, CL = total body clearance, Cpss thiopental plasma concentration, 0 = time zero, and t = thiopental plasma concentration at time t. Using this mathematical approach, the following thiopental PK parameters were reported in 11 surgical patients (mean ± s.d.): CL = 3.4 ± 0.4 mL/min/kg; V (central compartment) = 0.53 ± 0.18 L/kg; Vd (steady state) = 2.34 ± 0.75 L/kg; and terminal elimination half-life = 719 ± 329 min. Further, protein binding was examined and found to be not different with TPL plasma concentrations >100 μg/mL and remained consistent at about 83 % [110]. The hepatic extraction ratio from the central compartment was reported to be 0.14. A TPL isomer (1-ethylpropyl) was identified but was present in only about 6–7 % in the TPL preparation. The isomer displayed similar PK properties as thiopental and anesthetic potency in mice [111]. TPL metabolism including its CYP profile has not yet been reported due to early development of the drug.

Factors Influencing Thiopental Pharmacokinetics and Pharmacodynamics Various factors were evaluated that could affect TPL disposition. TPL PK was reported to not significantly differ between young women ($N=8$) and young men ($N=8$) with an age range from 20 to 40 years that used a three-compartment model as previously described [112]. TPL protein binding and PK were determined in a pediatric population ($N=24$) age range from 5 months to 13 years and compared to adult patients ($N=11$) where each patient received a single thiopental bolus IV injection [113]. Protein binding (87 %) and Vd at steady state of TPL were similar between the pediatric and adult groups. Total TPL drug CL was significantly greater in the pediatric patients than the adult patients (6.6±2.2 mL/min/kg versus 3.1±0.5 mL/min/kg, $p<0.001$). Elimination half-life was also significantly longer in the pediatric group compared to the adult group (6.1±3.3 h versus 12±6 h, $p<0.005$). The shorter elimination half-life in infants and children was solely due to the greater hepatic CL.

TPL was given to elderly women ($N=8$) and elderly men ($N=8$) age range from 60 to 79 years and was described by a three-compartment model [114]. The TPL PK parameters volume of distribution, elimination half-life, and CL did not significantly differ between the elderly women and men. When the elderly data was compared to previous studies of young men and young women [112], both elderly populations had significantly higher Vd than the young adult group ($p<0.05$) and longer elimination half-lives (elderly women mean 990 min, range 616–2223; elderly men mean 791 min, range 440–1580). However, only CL was found to be significantly greater in the elderly women (mean 0.19 L/min, range 0.137–0.269; $p<0.05$) when compared to young adult women (mean 0.131 L/min, range 0.047–0.209). Induction of sleep onset had lower TPL plasma concentrations in both elderly women and 3.9 % elderly men compared to young adult women and men but this finding was not statistically significant. The average induction dose for TPL dose was significantly lower for the elderly groups versus the young adult groups ($p<0.05$). Therefore, the elderly can have a longer TPL elimination half-life due to the volume of distribution but need lower drug doses which induce sleep at an earlier time frame [115].

TPL PK parameters were reported to be similar between patients with chronic renal failure ($N=7$) and with age-matched normal patients undergoing surgery [116]. Intrinsic TPL CL was reported to be significantly lower in patients undergoing renal transplantation ($p<0.05$) and higher protein binding (83 % versus 89 %, $p<0.05$); however, the PD cardiovascular effects and cardiac output were unchanged for both groups [116]. Thiopental PK in patients with cirrhosis ($N=8$)

was compared to patients with normal hepatic and renal function undergoing elective or orthopedic surgery [117]. The TPL Vd was significantly lower in patients with cirrhosis than normal patients (2.3 ± 0.5 L/kg versus 3.5 ± 1.9 L/kg, $p < 0.05$) although CL did not significantly differ. Mean TPL protein binding in patients with cirrhosis was almost twice that of the normal patients (25.2 ± 3.9 % versus 14.5 ± 3.4 %, $p < 0.05$) which can be explained by the lower serum albumin concentrations [117]. However, due to TPL's low extraction ratio, dosing adjustments and PD effects are not clinically needed. Significant differences were not found between patients with chronic alcoholism ($N = 10$) and normal control patients ($N = 9$) when given TPL [118, 119].

15.9 Conclusions

Anesthetic agents have specific PD functions to induce sleep, reduce pain, and maintain anesthesia. A single anesthetic drug does not fulfill all these requirements. Yet, the understanding of their PK and PD individually contributes to the overall anesthesia management of patients undergoing surgery. Without anesthetic drugs, medical treatments are significantly impacted. Anesthetic agents have formed the basis of the two- and three-compartment PK models and integration with their PD effects has shaped the foundations for modeling central nervous system drugs.

References

1. Eilers H Niemann (2003) Clinically important drug interactions with intravenous anesthetic agents in older patients. Drug Aging 20:969–980
2. Stanski DR, Shafer SL (1995) Quantifying anesthetic drug interactions. Anesthesiology 83:1–5
3. Feingold A, Holaday DA (1997) The pharmacokinetics of metabolism of inhalation anaesthetics. Br J Anaesth 49:155–162
4. Tanner G (1982) Pharmacokinetics of inhalation anesthetics: a three-compartment linear model. Anesth Analg 61:587–594
5. Doenicke A (1975) Etomidate: a new intravenous hypnotic. Acta Anaesthesia Belg 25:5–8
6. Morgan N, Lumley J, Whitwam JA (1975) Etomidate, a new water insoluble nonbarbiturate intravenous induction agent. Lancet 1:955–956
7. Geise JL, Stanley TH (1983) Etomidate: a new intravenous anesthetic induction agent. Pharmacotherapy 3:251–258
8. Van Hamme MJ, Ghoneim MM, Ambre JJ (1978) Pharmacokinetics of etomidate, a new intravenous anesthetic. Anesthesiology 49:274–277
9. Kay B (1976) A dose-response relationship for etomidate, with some observations on cumulation. Br J Anaesth 48:213–216
10. Ghoneim MM, Yamada T (1977) Etomidate: a clinical and electroencephalographic comparison to thiopental. Anesthesia Analg 56:479–485
11. Austin KR (1976) Ketamine hydrochloride: a potent analgesic. Br Med J 2:943–945

12. Kronenberg RH (2002) Ketamine as an analgesic: parenteral, oral, rectal, subcutaneous, transdermal, and intranasal administration. J Pain Palliat Care Pharmacother 16:27–35
13. Hatch RC (1973) Ketamine – excellent anesthetic. J Am Vet Assoc 162:835
14. Clements JA, Nimmo WS (1981) Pharmacokinetics and analgesic effect of ketamine in man. Br J Anaesth 53:27–30
15. Grant IS, Nimmo WS, Clements JA (1981) Pharmacokinetics and analgesic effects of IM and oral ketamine. Br J Anaesth 53:805–810
16. Clements JA, Nimmo WS, Grant IS (1982) Bioavailability, pharmacokinetics, and analgesic activity of ketamine in humans. J Pharm Sci 71:539–541
17. Oye I, Paulsen O, Maurset A (1992) Effects of ketamine on sensory perception: evidence for a role of NMDA receptors. J Pharmacol Exp Ther 260:1209–1213
18. Zeilhofer HU, Swandulala D, Geisslinger G, Brune K (1992) Differential effects of ketamine enantiomers on NMDA receptor currents in cultured neurons. Eur J Pharmacol 213:155–158
19. Hijazi Y, Boulieu R (2002) Contribution of CYP3A4, CYP2B6, and CYP2C9 isoforms to N-demethylation of ketamine in human liver microsomes. Drug Metab Dispos 30:853–858
20. Geisslinger G, Hering W, Thomann P et al (1993) Pharmacokinetics and pharmacodynamics of ketamine enantiomers in surgical patients using a stereoselective analytical method. Br J Anaesth 70:666–671
21. Ihmsen H, Geisslinger G, Schuttler J (2001) Stereoselective pharmacokinetics of ketamine: R(−) ketamine inhibits the elimination of S(+) ketamine. Clin Pharmacol Ther 70:431–438
22. Kanto JH (1985) Midazolam: the first water-soluble benzodiazepine. Pharmacotherapy 5:138–155
23. Kanto JH, Allonen H (1983) Pharmacokinetics and the sedative effect of midazolam. Int J Clin Pharmacol Ther Toxic 21:460–463
24. Smith MH, Eadie MJ, Brophy TO (1981) The pharmacokinetic of midazolam in man. Eur J Clin Pharmacol 19:271–278
25. Heizmann P, Eckert M, Ziegler WH (1983) Pharmacokinetics and bioavailability in man. Br J Clin Pharmacol 16:43S–49S
26. Kronbach T, Mathys D, Umeno M et al (1989) Oxidation of midazolam and triazolam by human liver cytochrome P450IIIA4. Mol Pharmacol 30:89–96
27. Reves JG, Fragen RJ, Vinik R, Greenblatt DJ (1985) Midazolam: pharmacology and uses. Anesthesiology 62:310–324
28. Crevoisier C, Ziegler WH, Eckert M, Heizmann P (1983) Relationship between plasma concentration and effect of midazolam after oral and intravenous administration. Br J Clin Pharmacol 16:51S–61S
29. Gemperle M, Kapp WK (1983) Midazolam and anaesthesia. Br J Clin Pharmacol 16:187S–190S
30. Forster A, Gardaz JP, Suter PM, Gemperle M (1980) IV midazolam as an induction agent for anaesthesia: a study in volunteers. Br J Anaesth 52:907–911
31. Sunzel M, Paalzow L, Berggren L, Eriksson I (1988) Respiratory and cardiovascular effects in relation to plasma levels of midazolam and diazepam. Br J Clin Pharmacol 25:561–569
32. Forster A, Gardaz JP, Suter PM, Gemperle M (1980) Respirator depression by midazolam and diazepam. Anesthesiology 53:494–497
33. Caldwell CB, Gross JB (1982) Physostigmine reversal of midazolam-induced sedation. Anesthesiology 57:125–127
34. Gross JB, Blouin RT, Zandsberg S et al (1996) Effect of flumazenil on ventilatory drive during sedation with midazolam and alfentanil. Anesthesiology 85:713–720
35. Ramzan MI, Somogyi AA, Walker JS et al (1981) Clinical pharmacokinetics of the non-depolarising muscle relaxants. Clin Pharamcokinet 6:25–60
36. Kalow W (1956) The relation of plasma cholinesterases to response to clinical doses of succinylcholine. J Arch Can Anaesth 3:22–30
37. Wingard LB, Cook DR (1977) Clinical pharmacokinetics of muscle relaxants. Clin Pharmacokinet 2:330–343

38. Agoston S, Vandenbrom RH, Wierda JM (1992) Clinical pharmacokinetics of neuromuscular blocking drugs. Clin Pharmacokinet 22:94–115
39. Paul D, Atherton L, Huter JM (1999) Clinical pharmacokinetics of the newer neuromuscular blocking drugs. Clin Pharmacokinet 36:169–189
40. Guay J, Grenier Y, Varin F (1998) Clinical pharmacokinetics of neuromuscular relaxants in pregnancy. Clin Pharmacokinet 34:483–497
41. Kalow W, Gunn DR (1959) Some statistical data on atypical cholinesterase of human serum. Am J Hum Genet 23:239–250
42. Ryan AR (1964) Tubocurarine administration based upon its disappearance and accumulation curves in anaesthesized man. Br J Anaesth 38:287
43. Matteo RS, Spector S, Horowitz PE (1974) Relation of serum d-tubocurarine concentration to neuromuscular block in man. Anesthesiology 41:440–448
44. Ramzan MI, Shanks CA, Triggs EJ (1980) Pharmacokinetics of tubocurarine administered by combined IV bolus and infusion. Br J Anaesth 52:893–899
45. Fisher DM, O'Keefe C, Stanski DR et al (1982) Pharmacokinetics and pharmacodynamics of d-tubocurarine in infants, children, and adults. Anesthesiology 57:203–208
46. Ham J, Stanski DR, Newfield P, Miller RD (1981) Pharmacokinetics and dynamics of d-tubocurarine during hypothermia in humans. Anesthesiology 55:631–633
47. Sheiner LB, Stanski DR, Vozeh S et al (1979) Simultaneous modeling of pharmacokinetics and pharmacodynamics: application to d-tubocurarine. Clin Pharmacol Ther 25:358–371
48. Ltorre F, deAlemeida MC, Stanek A, Kleeman PP (1997) The effect of smoking on neuromuscular transmission after rocuronium. Anaesthesist 46L:493–495
49. Drage A, Varin F, Plaud B, Donati F (2002) Rocuronium pharmacokinetics-pharmacodynamic relationship under stable propofol or isoflurane anesthesia. Can J Anesth 49:353–360
50. Van Miert MM, Estwood NB, Boyd AH et al (1997) The pharmacokinetic and pharmacodynamics of rocuronium in patients with hepatic cirrhosis. Br J Clin Pharmacol 44:139–144
51. Wang ZM, Zhang P, Lin MJ et al (2013) Influence of obstructive jaundice on pharmacodynamics of rocuronium. PLoS One 8:e78052
52. Caldwell JE, Szenohradszky J, Segredo V et al (1994) The pharmacodynamics and pharmacokinetics of the metabolite 3-desacetylvencuronium (ORG 7268) and its parent compound, vecuronium, in human volunteers. J Pharm Exp Ther 270:1216–1222
53. Marshall IG, Gibb AJ, Durant NN (1983) Neuromuscular and vagal blocking actions of pancuronium bromide, its metabolites, and vecuronium bromide (Org NC45) and its potential metabolites in the anesthetized cat. Br J Anaesth 55:703–714
54. Cronnelly R, Fisher DM, Miller RD et al (1983) Pharmacokinetics and pharmacodynamics of vecuronium (ORG NC 45) and pancuronium in anaesthesized patients. Anesthesiology 58:405–408
55. Meistelman C, Agoston S, Kersten UW et al (1996) Pharmacokinetics and pharmacodynamics of vencuronium and pancuronium in anesthetized children. Anesth Analg 65:1319–1322
56. Rupp SM, Castagnoili KP, Fisher DM, Miller RD (1987) Pancuronium and vencuronium pharmacokinetics and pharmacodynamics in younger and elderly adults. Anesthesiology 67:45–49
57. Lyman DP, Cronnelly R, Castagnoli KP et al (1988) The pharmacodynamics and pharmacokinetics of vecuronium in patients anesthetized with isoflurane with normal renal function or with renal failure. Anesthesiology 69:227–231
58. Vego-villa KR, Kaneda K, Yamashita S et al (2014) Vecuronium pharmacokinetics in patients with major burns. Br J Anaesthesia 112:304–310
59. Davis PJ, Cook DR (1986) Clinical pharmacokinetics of the newer intravenous anaesthetic agents. Clin Pharmacokinet 11:18–35
60. Willens JS, Myslinski NR (1993) Pharmacodynamics, pharmacokinetics, and clinical uses of fentanyl, sufentanil, and alfentanil. Heart Lung 22:239–251
61. Fung DL, Eisele JH (1980) Fentanyl pharmacokinetics in awake volunteers. J Clin Pharmacol 20:652–658

62. Gepts E, Shafer SL, Camu F et al (1998) Linearity of pharmacokinetics and model estimation of sufentanil. Anesthesiology 83:1194–1204
63. Metz C, Gobel L, Gruber M et al (2000) Pharmacokinetics of human cerebral opioid extraction: a comparative study on sufentanil, fentanyl, and alfentanil in a patient after severe head injury. Anesthesiology 92:1559–1567
64. Meuldermans WE, Hurkmans RM, Heykants JJ (1982) Plasma protein binding and distribution of fentanyl, sufentanil, alfentanil and lofentanil in blood. Arch Int Pharmacodyn Ther 257:4–19
65. Labroo RB, Paine FP, Thummel KE, Khararsch ED (1997) Fentanyl metabolism by human hepatic and intestinal cytochrome P450 3A4: implications for interindividual variability in disposition, efficacy, and drug interactions. Drug Metab Dispos 25:1072–1080
66. Yun CH, Wood M, Wood AJ (1992) Identification of the pharmacogenetic determination of alfentanil metabolism cytochrome P450 3A4. An explanation of the variable elimination clearance. Anesthesiology 77:467–474
67. Roscow CE (1984) Sufentanil citrate: a new opioid analgesic for use in anesthesia. Pharmacotherapy 4:11–19
68. Lundberg S, Roelofse JA (2011) Aspects of pharmacokinetics and pharmacodynamics of sufentanil in pediatric practice. Paediatr Anaesth 21:274–279
69. Bartkowski RR, Goldberg ME, Huffnagle S, Epstein RH (1993) Sufentanil disposition. Is it affected by erythromycin administration? Anesthesiology 78:260–265
70. Ibrahim AE, Feldman J, Karim A, Kharasch ED (2003) Simultaneous assessment of drug interactions with low and high extraction opioids. Anesthesiology 98:853–861
71. Wandel C, Kim R, Wood M, Wood A (2002) Interaction of morphine, fentanyl, sufentanil, alfentanil, and loperamide with the efflux drug transporter P-glycoprotein. Anesthesiology 96:913–920
72. Shafer A, Sung ML, White PF (1986) Pharmacokinetic and pharmacodynamics of alfentanil infusions during general anesthesia. Anesth Analg 65:1021–1028
73. Thomson IR, Henderson BT, Singh K, Hudson RJ (1998) Concentration-response relationship for fentanyl and sufentanil in patients undergoing coronary artery bypass grafting. Anesthesiology 89:852–861
74. Thompson IR, Harding G, Hudson RJ (2000) A comparison of fentanyl and sufentanil in patients undergoing coronary artery bypass graft surgery. J Cardiothoracic Vas Anesth 14:652–656
75. Jeleazcov C, Saari TI, Ihmsen H et al (2012) Changes in total and unbound concentrations of sufentanil during target controlled infusion for cardiac surgery with cardiopulmonary bypass. Br J Anaesth 109:698–706
76. Scholz J, Steinfath M, Schulz M (1996) Clinical pharmacokinetics of alfentanil, fentanyl, and sufentanil. An update. Clin Pharmacokinet 31:275–292
77. Davis PJ, Killian A, Stiller RL et al (1988) Alfentanil pharmacokinetics in premature infants and older children. Anesthesiology 69:A758
78. Guay J, Gaudreault P, Tang A et al (1992) Pharmacokinetics of sufentanil in normal children. Can J Anaesth 39:14–20
79. Scott JC, Stanski DR (1987) Decreased fentanyl and alfentanil dose requirements with age: a simultaneous pharmacokinetic and pharmacodynamics evaluation. J Pharmacol Exp Ther 240:159–163
80. Bovill JG, Sebel PS, Blackburn CL, Oei-Lim V, Heykants JJ (1984) The pharmacokinetics of sufentanil in surgical patients. Anesthesiology 61:502–506
81. Hudson RJ, Bergstrom RG, Thomson IR et al (1989) Pharmacokinetics of sufentanil in patients undergoing abdominal aortic surgery. Anesthesiology 70:426–431
82. Hudson RJ, Thomson IR, Burgess PM, Rosenbloom M (1991) Alfentanil pharmacokinetics in patients undergoing abdominal aortic surgery. Can J Anaesth 38:61–67
83. Baylaen WA, Herregods LL, Mortier EP et al (1989) Cardiopulmonary bypass and the pharmacokinetics of drugs. An update. Clin Pharmacokinet 17:10–22

84. Hall R (1991) The pharmacokinetic behavior of opioids administered during cardiac surgery. Can J Anaesth 38:747–756
85. Cummings GC, Dixon J, Kay NH et al (1984) Dose requirements of ICI 35868 (propofol, Diprivan) in a new formulation for induction of anaesthesia. Anaesthesia 39:1168–1173
86. Kay NH, Sear JW, Uppington J et al (1986) Disposition of propofol in patients undergoing surgery. Br J Anaesth 58:1075–1079
87. Kirkpatirck T, Cockshott ID, Douglas EJ, Nimmo WS (1988) Pharmacokinetics of propofol (Diprivan) in elderly patients. Br J Anaesth 60:146–150
88. Schnider TW, Minto CF, Gambus PL et al (1998) The influence of method of administration and covariates on the pharmacokinetics of propofol in adult volunteers. Anesthesiology 88:1170–1182
89. Marsh B, White M, Morton N, Kenny GNC (1991) Pharmacokinetic model driven infusion of propofol in children. Br J Anaesth 67:41–48
90. Puri A, Medhi B, Panda NB et al (2012) Propofol pharmacokinetics in young healthy Indian subjects. Indian J Pharmacol 44:402–406
91. Ye HB, Li JH, Rui JZ et al (2012) Propofol pharmacokinetics in China: a multicentric study. Indian J Pharmacol 44:393–397
92. Court MH, Duan SX, Hesse LM et al (2001) Cytochrome P450 2B6 is responsible for interindividual variability of propofol hydroxylation by human liver microsomes. Anesthesiology 94:110–119
93. Guitton J, Buronfosse T, Desage M et al (1998) Possible involvement of multiple human cytochrome P450 isoforms in the liver metabolism of propofol. Br J Anaesth 80:788–795
94. Turpeinen M, Zanger UM (2012) Cytochrome P450 2B6: function, genetics, and clinical relevance. Drug Metab Drug Interact 27:185–197
95. Kansaku F, Kuma T, Sasaki K et al (2011) Individual differences in pharmacokinetics and pharmacodynamics of anesthetic agent propofol with regard to CYP2B6 and UGR1A9 genotype and patient age. Drug Metab Pharmacokinet 26:532–537
96. Coetzee JF (2012) Allometric or lean body mass scaling of propofol pharmacokinetics. Clin Pharmacokinet 51:137–145
97. Martin-Mateos I, Perez JAM, Reboso JA, Leon A (2013) Modeling propofol pharmacodynamics using BIS-guided anaesthesia. Anaesthesia 68:1132–1140
98. Echevarria CG, Elgueta MF, Donoso MT et al (2012) The effective effect-site propofol concentration for induction and intubation with two pharmacokinetic models in morbidly obese patients using total body weight. Anesth Analg 115:823–829
99. Diepstraten J, Chidambaran V, Sadhasivan S et al (2012) Propofol clearance in morbidly obese children and adolescents. Clin Pharmacokinet 51:543–551
100. Chidambaran V, Sadhasivan S, Diepstraten J et al (2013) Evaluation of propofol anesthesia in morbidly obese children and adolescents. BMC Anesthesiol 13:1–9
101. Loryan I, Lindqvist M, Johansson I et al (2012) Influence of sex on propofol metabolism, a pilot study: implications for propofol anesthesia. Eur J Clin Pharmacol 68:397–406
102. Choong E, Loryan I, Lindqvist M et al (2013) Sex difference in formation of propofol metabolites: a replication study. Basic Clin Pharmacol Toxic 113:126–131
103. Hiraoka H, Yamamoto K, Okana N et al (2004) Changes in drug plasma concentrations of an extensively bound and highly extracted drug propofol, in response to altered plasma binding. Clin Pharmacol Ther 75:324–330
104. Takizawa D, Sato E, Hiraoka H et al (2005) Changes in apparent systemic clearance of propofol during transplantation of living related donor liver. Br J Anaesth 95:643–647
105. Przybylowski K, Tyczka J, Szczesny D et al (2015) Pharmacokinetic and pharmacodynamics of propofol in cancer patients undergoing major kung surgery. J Pharmacokinet Pharmacodyn 42:111–122
106. Glen JB (2013) Propofol effect-site concentration: hunt the Keo. Anesth Anal 117:535–536
107. Guerra F (1980) Thiopental forever after. In: Aldrete JA, Stanley TH (eds) Trends in intravenous anesthesia. Yearbook, Chicago, pp 143–151

108. Bischoff KB, Dedrick RL (1968) Thiopental pharmacokinetics. J Pharm Sci 57:1346–1351
109. Morgan DJ, Blackman GL, Paull JD et al (1981) Pharmacokinetics and plasma binding of thiopental. I. Studies in surgical patients. Anesthesiology 54:468–473
110. Stanski DR (1981) Pharmacokinetic modelling of thiopental. Anesthesiology 54:446–448
111. Burch PG, Stanski DR (1983) The role of metabolism and protein binding in thiopental anesthesia. Anesthesiology 58:146–152
112. Stanski DR, Burch PG, Harapat S, Richards RK (1983) Pharmacokinetics and anesthetic potency of a thiopental isomer. J Pharm Sci 72:937–940
113. Christensen JH, Andreasen F, Jansen JA (1980) Pharmacokinetics of thiopentone in a group of young women and a group of young men. Br J Anesth 52:913–918
114. Sorbo S, Hudson RJ, Loomis JC (1984) The pharmacokinetics of thiopental in pediatric surgical patients. Anesthesiology 61:666–670
115. Christensen JH, Andreasen F, Jansen JA (1981) Influence of age and sex on the pharmacokinetics of thiopentone. Br J Anesth 53:1189–1195
116. Christensen JH, Andreasen F, Jansen JA (1982) Pharmacokinetics and pharmacodynamics of thiopentone, a comparison between young and elderly patients. Anaesthesia 37:398–404
117. Christensen JH, Andreasen F, Jansen JA (1983) Pharmacokinetics and pharmacodynamics of thiopentone in patients undergoing renal transplantation. Acta Anaesthesiol Scand 27:513–518
118. Pandele G, Chaux F, Salvadori C et al (1985) Thiopental pharmacokinetics in patients with cirrhosis. Anesthesiology 59:123–125
119. Couderc E, Ferrier C, Haberer JP et al (1984) Thiopentone pharmacokinetics in patients with chronic alcoholism. Br J Anaesth 56:1393–1397
120. Kharasch KD, Russell M, Mautz D et al (1997) The role of cytochrome P450 3A4 in alfentanil clearance. Implications for interindividual variability in disposition and perioperative drug interactions. Anesthesiology 87:36–50
121. Santamaria R, Pailleux F, Beaudry F (2013) *In vitro* ketamine CYP3A-mediated metabolism study using mammalian liver S9 fractions, cDNA expressed enzymes and liquid chromatography tandem mass spectrometry. Biomed Chromatogr. doi:10.1002/bmc3199

Part III
Clinically Significant Drug Interactions with Psychopharmacological Agents

Lawrence J. Cohen, PharmD
Department of Pharmacotherapy
University of North Texas
System College of Pharmacy
Fort Worth, TX
USA
e-mail: Lawrence.Cohen@unthsc.edu

Chapter 16
Clinically Significant Interactions with Antipsychotics

Mong-Liang Lu and Hsien-Yuan Lane

Abstract Second-generation antipsychotics (SGAs) have become the mainstay of treatment for patients with schizophrenia and bipolar disorder. The antipsychotic drugs are often prescribed with other medications to improve clinical efficacy or treat comorbid diseases. Drug combinations can cause pharmacokinetic and/or pharmacodynamic drug-drug interactions. Pharmacokinetic interactions can occur during any pharmacokinetic phases, absorption, distribution, metabolism, or excretion. Smoking, caffeine, and food might have influences on the pharmacokinetic profiles of SGAs. Pharmacodynamic drug-drug interactions occur when drugs act at the same or interrelated sites of action, resulting in additive, synergistic, or antagonistic effects of each drug.

Among the genes involved in pharmacokinetics, the members of cytochrome P450 family display large interindividual and interethnic variations in activity. Other enzyme systems such as UDP-glucuronosyltransferases also exhibit genetic polymorphism with potential clinical relevance in psychopharmacology. The demographic characteristics might also have impact on pharmacokinetic and/or pharmacodynamic profiles of SGAs. The potential pharmacokinetic interactions would guide antipsychotic dosage adjustments. For antipsychotics, optimal dose titration should be guided by measuring plasma concentrations. Therapeutic drug monitoring (TDM) is a valid tool for tailoring the dosage of antipsychotic drugs. Clinicians must have the knowledge of potential interactions of SGAs and carefully monitor patients to minimize potentially adverse events and maximize therapeutic efficacy.

M.-L. Lu, MD, MS (✉)
Department of Psychiatry, Wan Fang Hospital and School of Medicine, College of Medicine, Taipei Medical University, Taipei, Taiwan
e-mail: mongliang@hotmail.com

H.-Y. Lane, MD, PhD
Department of Psychiatry, China Medical University and Hospital, Taichung, Taiwan
e-mail: hylane@gmail.com

M. Jann et al. (eds.), *Applied Clinical Pharmacokinetics and Pharmacodynamics of Psychopharmacological Agents*,
DOI 10.1007/978-3-319-27883-4_16

Keywords Absorption • Caffeine • Children and adolescent • Cytochrome P450 (CYP) enzymes • Distribution • Dosage adjustments • Elderly patients • Elimination • Metabolic disturbance • Metabolism pharmacodynamic • Pharmacokinetic • Pregnancy & breast-feeding • Smoking • Therapeutic drug monitoring (TDM)

Patients with schizophrenia, bipolar disorder, or any other psychiatric diseases that require the use of antipsychotics will encounter the following situation. These psychiatric diseases are chronic and require long-term medication to control psychopathology. Sometimes, even lack of evidence-based data, the combination of antipsychotics and other psychotropic agents to treat psychiatric illness is common in clinical practice. Besides, these psychiatric patients who also suffer from medical diseases require the use of medication other than psychotropic agents. If these medications are combined, the potential of drug-drug interactions would increase and might lead to increased adverse reactions and/or efficacy. It is estimated that one-fourth of patients with schizophrenia are exposed to potentially harmful drug-drug interactions [1]. Knowledge of drug-drug interactions, careful medication titration and patient monitoring, and individualized medication regimen are important to clinical outcomes.

16.1 Pharmacokinetics and Pharmacodynamics of Drug-Drug Interactions

A drug interaction is a situation in which one drug affects the activity of another drug when both are administered together. Drug interactions can be classified into two categories: pharmacokinetic interactions and pharmacodynamic interactions.

Pharmacokinetic interactions have consequences for the amount of the drug reaching the sites of action. They can occur during any pharmacokinetic phases, absorption, distribution, metabolism, or excretion. Pharmacodynamic interactions occur at the drug's action sites and produce a change in the drug's activity. This action can be synergistic (when the drug's effect is increased) or antagonistic (when the drug's effect is decreased) or a new effect can be produced that neither produces on its own.

16.2 Pharmacokinetic Interactions

Modifications in the effect of a drug are caused by differences in the absorption, distribution, metabolism, or excretion of one or both of the drugs compared with the expected behavior of each drug when taken individually. These changes are basically modifications in the concentration of the drugs.

16.2.1 Absorption

Most antipsychotics are taken orally. Interactions during the absorption phase affect the influx of drugs from the gut into the bloodstream. Examples are changes in gastrointestinal pH or motility. Other examples are interactions at the levels of drug transporters. The availability of some antipsychotic drugs is limited by the action of drug efflux transporters in the endothelial cells [2].

The most important efflux transporter is P-glycoprotein (P-gp). P-gp is an adenosine triphosphate (ATP)-dependent efflux transporter located mainly in the gastrointestinal tract and the blood-brain barrier [3]. P-gp is also known as ATP-binding cassette subfamily member B1 (ABCB1) and multidrug resistance protein 1 (MDR1) [4]. Several SGAs, including amisulpride, aripiprazole, olanzapine, risperidone, and paliperidone, are substrates for P-gp in therapeutic concentrations [5].

16.2.2 Distribution

Antipsychotic drugs are highly lipophilic, resulting in high volume of distribution. Another factor affecting drug interactions is protein binding. When two or more drugs are coadministered, competition for the protein binding sites occurs. Coadministration of drugs can result in a highly bound drug displacing a weakly bound drug from its binding sites. Drugs bound to plasma proteins are not membrane permeable and pharmacologically inactive. As free drug is a major determinant of pharmacologic effects, these drug interactions could result in toxicity and/or enhanced efficacy [6]. Since most SGAs are highly protein bound, coadministration with another medication could theoretically produce protein binding displacement interaction. However, changes in plasma protein binding have little clinical relevance [7].

16.2.3 Metabolism

16.2.3.1 Phase I Metabolism: Modification

In phase I metabolism, a variety of enzymes act to introduce reactive and polar groups into their substrates. Phase I metabolism involves oxidative, reductive, and hydrolytic processes. One of the most common modifications is hydroxylation catalyzed by cytochrome P450 (CYP) enzymes. Hepatic phase I metabolism, catalyzed primarily by CYP enzymes, represents the major pathway of metabolism of SGAs. Most of the antipsychotic drugs are metabolized primarily by CYP enzymes. However, exceptions exist; for example, ziprasidone is metabolized primarily by the aldehyde oxidase pathway [8], and olanzapine is metabolized primarily by the

Table 16.1 Summary of the pharmacokinetic parameters of second-generation antipsychotics [11–16]

Drugs	Bioavailability (%)	T_{max} (h)	Half-life (h)	Protein binding (%)	Primary metabolic pathways	Active metabolites
Aripiprazole	90	3–5	75	99	CYP3A4, CYP2D6	Dehydroaripiprazole
Asenapine	35	0.5–1.5	24	95	CYP1A2, UGT1A4	–
Clozapine	50–60	2.5	6–30	95	CYP3A4, CYP1A2, CYP2C19	Norclozapine
Lurasidone	9–19	1–3	29–37	99	CYP3A4	ID-14283
Olanzapine	93	6	33	93	CYP1A2, UGT1A4, FMO, CYP2D6	N-Desmethylolanzapine
Paliperidone	28	24	24	74	UGT	–
Risperidone	68	1	22	89	CYP2D6, CYP3A4	9-Hydroxyrisperidone
Quetiapine	83	1.5	6	83	CYP3A4, CYP2D6	Norquetiapine
Ziprasidone	99	4	4–10	99	Aldehyde oxidase, CYP3A4, CYP2D6	–

uridine diphosphate glucuronosyltransferase (UGT) pathway [9]. These two drugs are still metabolized by the CYP enzymes, but to a much lesser extent. Paliperidone is not metabolized extensively in the liver, and renal excretion is the major route of elimination. Biotransformation of paliperidone occurs through oxidative N-dealkylation, monohydroxylation, alcohol dehydrogenation, and benzisoxazole scission, the latter in combination with glucuronidation or alicyclic hydroxylation [10]. Each of these pathways accounts for up to a maximum of 6.5 % of the biotransformation of paliperidone dose. Because of this, paliperidone has demonstrated minimal clinically significant drug-drug interactions. Table 16.1 summaries the pharmacokinetic parameters of second-generation antipsychotics.

Most significant drug interactions with SGAs occur within the CYP system [16, 17]. When two drugs that are metabolized by the same CYP enzyme system are given together, metabolic inhibition or metabolic induction can develop. These effects can be either reversible or irreversible, depending on the medication and the CYP enzyme involved. Knowledge of the properties of common CYP pathways can provide the cues to clinicians as to the likelihood of clinically significant drug interactions.

Moreover, individual genetic variations in CYP enzymes also occur and must be considered when evaluating the potential drug-drug interactions. However, there may be alternate CYP pathways that operate in antipsychotic drug elimination in certain individuals, particularly those with diminished metabolic capacity along the major CYP pathways [18].

16.2.3.2 Phase II Metabolism: Conjugation

In phase II metabolism, xenobiotic metabolites are conjugated with charged species. Products of conjugation reactions have increased molecular weight and tend to be less active than their substrates. Glucuronidation is the most common phase II metabolic pathway. UGT enzymes predominantly catalyze glucuronidation reactions. UGT exists as a superfamily of 22 proteins, which are divided into 5 families and 6 subfamilies on the basis of sequence identity [19]. The genetic variation and environmental factors have influences on the UGT activity [19].

16.2.4 Elimination

The major routes of excretion of antipsychotic agents are through urine and feces. Most of the antipsychotic agents undergo substantial metabolism prior to excretion, with one exception: paliperidone. Most of the agents undergo excretion primarily in the urine, with two exceptions: aripiprazole and ziprasidone. We divided the agents into one of three groups: (1) primarily excreted unchanged and primarily excreted in the urine (paliperidone), (2) primarily excreted changed and primarily excreted in the urine (clozapine, olanzapine, quetiapine, risperidone), and (3) primarily excreted changed and primarily excreted in the feces (aripiprazole, ziprasidone) [15]. Lower doses of antipsychotic agents are generally recommended in elderly patients due to decreased renal clearance.

16.3 Protein Binding Interactions

Binding to plasma proteins plays a major role in drug therapy as this binding provides a depot for many compounds, affects the pharmacokinetics and pharmacodynamics of drugs, and may influence the metabolic modification of ligands. In general, antipsychotics are highly protein bound, with affinity for α-1-acid glycoprotein (AGP) and albumin. Decreased levels of these proteins will lead to decreased protein binding ability and a resultant increase in the percentage of free drug, which provide the potential of toxicity. When two drugs exist simultaneously in the plasma, competition for protein binding sites may occur. This may result in displacement of a previously bound drug which, in the free state, becomes pharmacologically active.

16.4 Smoking, Caffeine, Food, and Other Types of Interactions

Tobacco smoking is associated with induction of drug-metabolizing enzymes. Polycyclic aromatic hydrocarbons (PAHs) present in cigarette smoke induce hepatic aryl hydrocarbon hydroxylases, thereby increasing metabolic clearance of drugs that are substrates for these enzymes. PAHs have been shown to induce three hepatic CYP enzymes, primarily CYP1A1, CYP1A2, and CYP2E1 [20]. The most common effect of smoking on drug disposition in humans is an increase in biotransformation rate, consistent with induction of drug-metabolizing enzymes [21]. Smokers taking clozapine have up to 50 % lower plasma concentrations than nonsmokers. Smoking as few as 7–12 cigarettes daily may be sufficient to cause the maximum enzyme induction [22]. Tobacco cessation can cause an increase in clozapine level, which might lead to adverse effects such as seizure and postural hypotension. Therefore, dosage reductions of 30–40 % are required to achieve pre-cessation concentrations [23]. Other antipsychotics affected include olanzapine (plasma levels may reduce up to 50 %) [24] and haloperidol (about 20 % reduction in plasma levels) [25].

Case Study
A 30-year-old schizophrenic male patient, a heavy smoker, was successfully treated with olanzapine 15 mg/d during hospitalization. His cigarette consumption increased rapidly from 0 to 12 cigarettes per day following his discharge. Two weeks later, his delusion of persecution, levels of hostility, and aggressive behavior worsened. The plasma levels of olanzapine during hospitalization and after hospitalization were 52.1 ng/mL and 21.2 ng/mL, respectively. Based on our observations of this case, we suggest that the reduced levels of plasma olanzapine and exacerbated clinical symptoms are closely related to the increased consumption of cigarettes. A possible explanation would be that heavy smoking induced cytochrome P4501A2, the major enzyme involved in olanzapine metabolism.

Caffeine is metabolized by CYP1A2 and exhibits dose-dependent kinetics. Moreover, caffeine also acts as a competitive inhibitor of CYP1A2 and might contribute to interindividual variability [26]. Caffeine in 400–1000 mg/day may significantly inhibit the metabolism of clozapine, which is due to completion of the same enzymes [27]. Theoretically, olanzapine metabolism may also be affected by caffeine in the same way [28].

Grapefruit juice can inhibit the activity of CYP3A4 in the intestine and in the liver and may elevate plasma levels of substrates for CYP3A4 [29]. Grapefruit juice increases the bioavailability of some orally administered drugs that are metabolized by CYP3A and normally undergo extensive presystemic extraction. With regard to this, plasma levels of clozapine and haloperidol were not affected by ingestion of grapefruit juice [30–32].

Food intake exerts a complex influence on the bioavailability of drugs. The majority of clinically relevant food-drug interactions are caused by food-induced changes in the bioavailability of the drug. It may interfere not only with tablet disintegration, drug dissolution, and drug transit through the gastrointestinal tract but may also affect the metabolic transformation of drugs in the gastrointestinal wall and in the liver [33]. Coadministration of food decreased the rate of clozapine absorption but had no effect on the extent of clozapine absorption [34]. The product labels of ziprasidone and lurasidone note that bioavailability is increased in the presence of food. Ziprasidone is recommended to be taken with a meal >500 kcal, irrespective of fat content [35, 36]. Low-calorie meals (250 kcal) resulted in 60–90 % decrease in bioavailability and approached exposures seen under fasting conditions [35]. Lurasidone is recommended to be administered with at least 350 cal of food in order to optimize bioavailability [37].

16.5 Pharmacodynamic Drug Interactions

Pharmacodynamic drug-drug interactions occur when drugs act at the same or interrelated sites of action, resulting in additive, synergistic, or antagonistic effects of each drug. Pharmacodynamic interactions, which result in a potentiation of the pharmacologic effects at the receptor, can be clinically important. Some examples of psychiatric pharmacodynamic drug interactions are discussed below.

16.5.1 Anticholinergic Intoxication

Dry mouth, blurred vision, constipation, urinary retention, disturbed accommodation, impaired cognition, delirium, and seizure are clinical consequences of blockade of acetylcholine M1 receptors. There are a number of psychotropic drugs exhibiting anticholinergic activity [38]. Among antipsychotics, marked anticholinergic activity was found for clozapine and thioridazine, followed by chlorpromazine, olanzapine, and quetiapine [38]. With regard to anticholinergic drug interactions, one should avoid combination of an antipsychotic and another drug when both exhibit anticholinergic activity.

16.5.2 QTc Prolongation and Torsades de Pointes (TdP)

A pharmacodynamic drug interaction may be the result of combining two or more drugs with established risk of prolongation of QTc interval, e.g., thioridazine, haloperidol, or ziprasidone, placing the patient at a greater risk for adverse effects. QT interval prolongation of at least 500 milliseconds (ms) generally has been shown to correlate with an increased risk of TdP. QTc interval prolongation indicates prolonged ventricular repolarization, mostly under high levels of the drug. The prolonged repolarization results from the decrease in repolarizing current by increased inward current or decreased outward current [39]. This current is generated by potassium flow through the hERG ion channel which is susceptible to be blocked by various drugs [40]. Since drug-induced QTc prolongation seems to be concentration dependent [41], pharmacokinetic interactions may also play an important role in the pathogenesis of QTc prolongation.

16.5.3 *Blood Dyscrasias*

Almost all classes of psychotropic agents have been reported to cause blood dyscrasias. Leukopenia, neutropenia, thrombocytopenia, eosinophilia, anemia, agranulocytosis, and altered platelet function are some of the hematologic side effects that may be encountered with psychiatric medication therapy. Clozapine is well known as a drug that causes dyscrasias; however, many other agents, including olanzapine, antidepressants, anticonvulsants (e.g., divalproex, carbamazepine), and other atypical antipsychotics, can cause similar problems [42].

16.5.4 *Metabolic Disturbance*

Weight gain and metabolic dysfunction is a severe health burden of antipsychotic drugs [43]. The low-potency FGAs, such as chlorpromazine and thioridazine, are associated with a higher potential for weight gain than are the high-potency FGAs, such as haloperidol and fluphenazine [44]. SGAs carry different risks of causing weight gain and metabolic dysregulation: clozapine and olanzapine have the highest risk; quetiapine and risperidone a moderate risk; and aripiprazole, amisulpride, and ziprasidone the lowest risks [44, 45]. The affinities of antipsychotic drugs for H1, 5-HT2C, M3, 5-HT1A, D2, and adrenergic receptors might be implicated in causing metabolic abnormalities [43]. Several cross-sectional studies revealed that antipsychotic polypharmacy increases the risk of metabolic abnormalities [46, 47]. However, adjunctive aripiprazole may counteract antipsychotic-induced weight gain and metabolic adverse effects in schizophrenia [48, 49].

16.6 Clinical Significance of PK and PD Interactions (Case Study)

16.6.1 *Incorporate Genetic Polymorphisms*

Among the genes involved in pharmacokinetics, the members of CYP family display large interindividual and interethnic variation in activity [50]. The US Food and Drug Administration issues the Table of Pharmacogenomic Markers in Drug

Labeling that contains around 150 drugs (27 of which are agents with a primary indication in psychiatry), half of them CYP-dependent drugs (http://www.fda.gov/drugs/scienceresearch/researchareas/pharmacogenetics/ucm083378.htm). Of the 32 neuropsychiatric drugs listed, 27 (84 %) have CYP2D6 metabolizer status listed as an important biomarker, 3 (9 %) identify CYP2C19 metabolizer status as an important biomarker, and 3 (9 %) pertain to other genetic markers (e.g., major histocompatibility complex human leukocyte antigen [HLA] allele HLA-B*1502 and HLA-A*3101 for carbamazepine and HLA-B*1502 for phenytoin). The presence of polymorphic alleles for CYP may result in lack of expression, altered levels of expression, or altered function of CYP450 isoenzymes [51]. Such genetic variations affecting metabolism may lead to alterations in the bioavailability of certain antipsychotics, resulting in loss of efficacy (decreased plasma levels) or increased toxicity (elevated plasma levels).

Other enzyme systems such as UDP-glucuronosyltransferases also exhibit genetic polymorphism, and their effects of potential clinical relevance in psychopharmacology are also recognized [52]. Lower plasma olanzapine concentrations in heterozygous carriers of UGT1A4*3 were reported in a study in Caucasians [53]. In contrast with these data originating from studies in Caucasians, a study performed in a Japanese population failed to detect any influence of the UGT1A4*3 allele on plasma olanzapine levels in patients with schizophrenia [54]. The UGT1A1*28 and UGT1A4*3 alleles contribute significantly to the variability in clozapine metabolism [55].

Pharmacogenetic testing of drug metabolism consists of two approaches [56]. Biochemical tests are used to evaluate the rate of metabolism by a patient after he or she takes a probe drug, which is a well-characterized target of a recognized metabolic pathway. The excretion of the parent drug and its metabolite is measured at regular intervals and a rate of metabolism calculated. The result is often referred to as an individual's phenotype, although the use of the term to describe functional aspects of drug metabolism differs from its meaning in genetics. For example, caffeine has been shown to provide an accurate phenotypic probe for measuring CYP1A2 activity [57, 58]. The other approach is the use of molecular genetic testing to characterize the alleles of a patient's gene related to metabolic enzymes, the drug target, or receptors. The genes of interest often have a number of alleles, and polymorphisms present in these alleles may result in lack of expression, altered levels of expression, or altered function [51]. The multiallelic nature of CYP450 enzyme genetics can result in various phenotypes. These polymorphisms reflect gene insertions and deletions, gene duplications, copy number variations, and single nucleotide polymorphisms (SNPs). The resulting phenotypes associated with these genetic variants are usually classified as one of four groups: poor metabolizers (PMs), intermediate metabolizers (IMs), extensive metabolizers (EMs), and ultrarapid metabolizers (UMs).

Association of an enzyme with metabolism of a drug is necessary but not sufficient justification for pharmacogenetic testing, as many drugs may be metabolized by alternative pathways. Further, pharmacogenetic results should be interpreted with caution. Other factors will also influence efficacy and toxicity of antipsychotic agents, such as comorbidities, adherence, body weight, and smoking [59]. In addition to pharmacogenetic considerations, CYP isoenzymes can be induced and inhibited by certain drugs, which can substantially alter metabolism of other drugs through drug-drug interactions.

There are wide interindividual variations (40- to 130-fold) in CYP1A2 expression and activity [60]. There is also marked racial difference in CYP1A2 activity. A higher CYP1A2 activity has been found in Caucasians, compared to Asian and African populations [61]. It is estimated that about 72.5 % of interindividual difference in CYP1A2 activity is due to genetic factors [62]. To date, more than 40 variant alleles of CYP1A2 gene (http://www.cypalleles.ki.se/cyp1a2.htm) and 493 SNPs in CYP1A2 upstream sequence, introns, and exons (http://www.ncbi.nlm.nih.gov/snp) have been found. *CYP1A2*1A* is referred to as the wild type. The CYP1A2*1C allele is associated with decreased inducibility and occurs in 21–27 % of Asians, 7 % of Africans, and 1–4 % of Caucasians [63]. In addition, CYP1A2*1F polymorphism may contribute to the risk of developing prolonged QT interval in patients who are treated with chlorpromazine equivalent doses of above 300 mg/day [64].

The CYP2C9 gene is mapped to the long arm of chromosome 10, located in a densely packed region also containing genes encoding CYP2C8, CYP2C18, and CYP2C19 [65]. CYP2C9 is one of the most abundant CYP enzymes in the human liver (about 20 % of hepatic total CYP content), where it metabolizes approximately 15 % of clinical drugs [66]. To date, more than 67 variant alleles of CYP2C9 gene (http://www.cypalleles.ki.se/cyp2c9.htm) and 2672 SNPs in CYP2C9 upstream sequence, introns, and exons (http://www.ncbi.nlm.nih.gov/snp) have been identified. CYP2C9*1A is referred to the wild type. There are significant ethnic differences in the frequency of CYP2C9 variants.

The CYP2C19 gene is mapped to the long arm of chromosome 10, located in a densely packed region also containing genes encoding CYP2C8, CYP2C9, and CYP2C18 [65]. CYP2C19 is primarily present in hepatic tissue, but a significant amount is also found in the gut wall, particularly the duodenum [67]. CYP2C19 is responsible for the metabolism of approximately 10 % of commonly used drugs [68]. To date, more than 46 variant alleles of CYP2C19 gene (http://www.cypalleles.ki.se/cyp2c19.htm) and 4854 SNPs in CYP2C19 upstream sequence, introns, and exons (http://www.ncbi.nlm.nih.gov/snp) have been identified. CYP2C19*1A is referred to the wild type. The distribution of common variant alleles of CYP2C19 has been found to vary among different ethnic groups. The allelic frequency of CYP2C19*2 has been shown to be 7 % in African-Americans, 30 % in Chinese, and 15 % in Caucasians [69]. CYP2C19*3 has been shown to be more frequent in the Chinese (5 %) and less frequent in African-Americans (0.4 %) and Caucasians (0.04 %) [70]. These two alleles account for almost all PMs in Asian and Black African populations.

The CYP2D6 gene is mapped to chromosome 22q13.1. CYP2D6 accounts for only a small percentage of all hepatic CYPs (<2 %); however, it metabolizes 25 % of all medications in the human liver [71]. The primarily hepatic expression of CYP2D6 governs first-pass metabolism after oral drug administration, whereas the low level of its intestinal expression does not appear to be important. CYP2D6 is important for the metabolism of many drugs, including antipsychotics and antidepressants. Unlike other CYPs, CYP2D6 is not inducible, and thus genetic mutations are largely responsible for the interindividual variation in enzyme expression and activity. To date, more than 151 variant alleles of CYP2D6 gene (http://www.cypalleles.ki.se/cyp2d6.htm) and 443 SNPs in CYP2D6 upstream sequence, introns, and exons (http://www.ncbi.nlm.nih.gov/snp) have been found. CYP2D6*1 is referred to as the wild type. Race-ethnicity is an important factor that may influence drug response through gene variants. Significantly decreased capacity to metabolize CYP2D6 substrates occurs in about 8 % of Caucasians, 3–8 % of blacks and African-Americans, and 6 % of Asians [72]. The CYP2D6 UM phenotype has been observed in 1–10 % of Caucasians, 0–2 % of East Asians, 2 % of blacks and African-Americans, and 10–29 % of North Africans/Middle Easterners and 1 % of Mexicans [51].

CYP3A4 has the highest abundance in the human liver (40 %) and metabolizes more than 50 % of clinical drugs [73]. CYP3A4 gene is located on chromosome 7q22.1. To date, more than 45 variant alleles of CYP3A4 gene (http://www.cypalleles.ki.se/cyp3a4.htm) and 1176 SNPs in CYP3A4 upstream sequence, introns, and exons (http://www.ncbi.nlm.nih.gov/snp) have been identified. CYP3A4*1A is referred to as the wild type. The CYP3A4*20 polymorphism, which results in a premature stop codon and lack of enzyme activity, is prevalent in 26 % of African-Americans, 22 % of Asians, and 6 % of Caucasians [63].

Of the 32 neuropsychiatric drugs listed in FDA-approved pharmacogenomic biomarkers in drug labeling, 10 have information related to dosing, precautions, or warnings (http://www.fda.gov/drugs/scienceresearch/researchareas/pharmacogenetics/ucm083378.htm). Dosage changes for known poor metabolizers of CYP2D6 or CYP2C19 are outlined for aripiprazole, atomoxetine, citalopram, clobazam, iloperidone, pimozide, and tetrabenazine.

Case Study

Mr. A was a 31-year-old man with the diagnosis of chronic schizophrenia. He smoked regularly (12 cigarettes/day). A review of medical records indicated that the patient had shown an incomplete response to trials of at least 6 weeks with the antipsychotics haloperidol (20 mg/day), sulpiride (1000 mg/day), and risperidone (6 mg/day). The antipsychotic drug was then switched to clozapine, and the dose was gradually increased up to 850 mg/day with no significant side effects. However, despite the high clozapine dose and established compliance, plasma clozapine concentration (220 ng/ml) remained below the minimum therapeutic concentration threshold (350 ng/ml). The caffeine metabolic ratio, an in vivo CYP1A2 activity probe, was 17.8 which revealed ultrarapid metabolizing activity. Genotyping result showed that the patient was homozygous for the *CYP1A2*1F* allele. After two weeks of concurrent treatment with fluvoxamine 50 mg/day, the caffeine metabolic ratio decreased to 9.2 and plasma clozapine level increased to 510 ng/ml. The Positive and Negative Syndrome Scale (PANSS) scores also decreased from 87 to 65. This prospective case study suggests that ultrarapid CYP1A2 activity may delay therapeutic response to clozapine on conventional dose titration regimens. It appears to be worthwhile to evaluate the CYP1A2 phenotype using caffeine metabolism or, alternatively, genotype for CYP1A2*1F in smokers, to ascertain the pharmacokinetic basis of treatment resistance to clozapine. Concurrent administration of fluvoxamine and clozapine may increase plasma clozapine level significantly.

16.6.1.1 Aripiprazole

Aripiprazole is metabolized by CYP2D6 and CYP3A4 to its active metabolite dehydroaripiprazole [74]. The mean concentration/dose ratios of aripiprazole and the sum of aripiprazole and dehydroaripiprazole were significantly higher in patients with mutated alleles for CYP2D6 than in those without mutated alleles [75–77]. It is recommended that CYP2D6 PMs typically need 30–40 % lower doses of aripiprazole to achieve a similar steady-state serum concentration as EMs [78]. A study of 89 psychiatric patients in Japanese patients with schizophrenia prospectively evaluated the concentration/dose ratios of aripiprazole and dehydroaripiprazole in those with CYP2D6 wild type or CYP2D6*10 alleles [75]. These data demonstrate that the CYP2D6*10 alleles may lead to significantly elevated levels of aripiprazole and dehydroaripiprazole in Asian patients.

16.6.1.2 Asenapine

Asenapine has multiple inactive metabolites, produced via direct glucuronidation (primarily via UGT1A4), demethylation, and oxidative metabolism (primarily via CYP1A2) [11]. Notably, asenapine is an inhibitor of CYP2D6. Caution is required when coadministering asenapine with drugs that are substrates of CYP2D6 [11].

16.6.1.3 Clozapine

Clozapine is metabolized via the hepatic microsomal enzyme system into two principle metabolites: N-desmethylclozapine and clozapine N-oxide [79]. N-Desmethylclozapine is catalyzed by CYP1A2, CYP3A4, CYP2C9, and CYP2C19, and clozapine N-oxide is catalyzed by CYP2D6, CYP3A4, CYP1A2, and flavin-containing monooxygenase 3 (FMO3) [80]. The contribution of CYP1A2, CYP2C19, CYP3A4, CYP2C9, and CYP2D6 is estimated to amount to 30 %, 24 %, 22 %, 12 %, and 6 %, respectively, with regard to the N-demethylation of clozapine [81]. Resistance to clozapine treatment due to low plasma drug levels has been reported in smokers with CYP1A2*1F (−163C>A) genotype [82, 83]. CYP1A2 variants CYP1A2*1C and CYP1A2*1D, suggested to cause low enzyme activity, seem to be associated with higher serum clozapine concentrations and an increased risk of developing insulin and lipid elevations and insulin resistance [84].

16.6.1.4 Lurasidone

Lurasidone is metabolized predominantly by CYP3A4, yielding two nonmajor, active metabolites (ID-14283 and ID-14326) and two major, nonactive metabolites (ID-20219 and ID-20220) [85]. Till now, there are no published cases or studies evaluating lurasidone in healthy persons or patients with CYP3A4 variants.

16.6.1.5 Olanzapine

Olanzapine is metabolized to its 10- and 4′-N-glucuronides, 4′-N-desmethylolanzapine (CYP1A2), and olanzapine N-oxide (FMO3). The 10-N-glucuronide is the most abundant metabolite, but formation of 4′-N-desmethylolanzapine is correlated with the clearance of olanzapine [86]. Studies of patients with schizophrenia reported no significant correlation between CYP2D6 polymorphisms and plasma olanzapine levels [54, 87]. Moreover, The CYP1A2*1D and CYP1A2*1F polymorphisms might also have a significant impact on olanzapine serum concentrations [88, 89]. Patients with the CYP3A43 AA genotype (rs472660) have high clearance of olanzapine, subtherapeutic blood levels, and more psychotic symptoms and were more likely to discontinue treatment [90].

16.6.1.6 Paliperidone

Paliperidone is the active metabolite of risperidone (9-OH-risperidone), and renal excretion is the major route of elimination [91]. Therefore, paliperidone is a useful alternative for patients that have moderate to severe hepatic impairment or are taking medications that inhibit hepatic metabolism.

16.6.1.7 Quetiapine

Quetiapine is predominantly metabolized by CYP3A4 and results in four metabolites: 7-hydroxyl, sulfoxide, N-desalkyl, and O-desalkyl products [92]. CYP2D6 is involved in the 7-hydroxylation of quetiapine. Quetiapine has no effect on the in vitro activity of CYP1A2, CYP2C9, CYP2C19, CYP2D6, and CYP3A4 at clinically relevant concentrations [93]. Carriers of the CYP3A4*22 allele had 2.5-fold higher serum levels of quetiapine than did wild-type patients [94].

16.6.1.8 Risperidone

Risperidone is metabolized by CYP2D6 to 9-OH-risperidone (paliperidone) [95]. The risperidone/9-OH-risperidone ratio was strongly associated with the CYP2D6 genotype [96, 97]. Currently there is insufficient data to allow estimation of dose adjustment for PMs, IMs, or UMs receiving risperidone.

16.6.1.9 Ziprasidone

Ziprasidone is extensively metabolized in the liver by aldehyde oxidase and CYP3A4 [98]. Approximately two-thirds of the initial metabolism of ziprasidone results from generation of S-methyldihydroziprasidone by aldehyde oxidase, and one-third results in ziprasidone sulfoxide. These metabolites undergo further degradation by CYP3A4. Till now, there are no published cases or studies evaluating ziprasidone in healthy persons or patients with CYP genetic variants.

16.6.2 Dosage Adjustments: Regulatory Package Insert

16.6.2.1 Aripiprazole

Aripiprazole is metabolized by multiple pathways involving the CYP2D6 and CYP3A4 enzymes, but not CYP1A enzymes. Thus, no dosage adjustment is required for smokers. After oral administration of aripiprazole to healthy subjects, a strong inhibitor of CYP2D6 (quinidine) increased aripiprazole AUC by 107 %, while Cmax was unchanged. The AUC and Cmax of dehydroaripiprazole, the active metabolite, decreased by 32 % and 47 %, respectively. After oral administration of aripiprazole to healthy subjects, a strong inhibitor of CYP3A4 (ketoconazole) increased aripiprazole AUC and Cmax by 63 % and 37 %, respectively. The AUC and Cmax of dehydroaripiprazole increased by 77 % and 43 %, respectively. After oral administration of aripiprazole to healthy subjects, following concomitant administration of carbamazepine, an inducer of CYP3A4, the geometric means of Cmax and AUC for aripiprazole were 68 % and 73 % lower, respectively, compared to when oral aripiprazole (30 mg) was administered alone. Similarly, for dehydroaripiprazole the geometric means of Cmax and AUC after carbamazepine coadministration were 69 % and 71 % lower, respectively, than those following treatment with oral aripiprazole alone. No dosage adjustment of aripiprazole is recommended for elderly patients, patients with renal impairment, gender, race, or smoking status (aripiprazole package insert).

16.6.2.2 Asenapine

The risks of using asenapine in combination with other drugs have not been extensively evaluated. Two notable drug-drug interactions are evident: asenapine (an inhibitor of CYP2D6) can increase plasma levels of paroxetine, and fluvoxamine (a CYP1A2 inhibitor) can increase plasma levels of asenapine [11]. Coadministration of a single 20 mg dose of paroxetine (a CYP2D6 substrate and inhibitor) during treatment with 5 mg asenapine twice daily in healthy male subjects resulted in an almost twofold increase in paroxetine exposure. The therapeutic dose of fluvoxamine would be expected to cause a greater increase in asenapine plasma concentrations (asenapine package insert).

16.6.2.3 Clozapine

Clozapine is a substrate for many CYP isoenzymes, in particular 1A2 and 3A4. Caution is called for in patients receiving concomitant treatment with other drugs which are either inhibitors or inducers of these enzymes. Elevated serum levels of clozapine have been reported in patients receiving the drug in combination with fluoxetine, paroxetine, sertraline (up to twofold), or fluvoxamine (up to tenfold). Concomitant administration of inducers of CYP3A4 (e.g., phenytoin, carbamazepine, rifampicin, St John's wort) may reduce the plasma levels of clozapine. Concomitant administration of highly protein-bound drugs, such as warfarin and digoxin, may lead to adverse effects as a result of changes in plasma levels of clozapine due to competition for protein binding sites. Tobacco smoke, a known inducer of CYP450 1A2, may decrease the plasma levels of clozapine. In cases of sudden cessation of tobacco smoking, the plasma clozapine concentration may be increased, thus leading to an increase in adverse effects (clozapine package insert).

16.6.2.4 Lurasidone

Lurasidone is contraindicated with strong CYP3A4 inhibitors (e.g., ketoconazole) and strong CYP3A4 inducers. Lurasidone should be started at a dose of 20 mg/day, and the dose should not exceed 40 mg/day if coadministered with moderate CYP3A4 inhibitors. Grapefruit, grapefruit juice, and products containing grapefruit extract should be avoided during treatment with lurasidone because of the potential to inhibit CYP3A4. Lurasidone should be administered with food (at least 350 calories independent of fat content). The Cmax of lurasidone is increased approximately threefold, and the AUC is increased approximately twofold in the presence of food. Dosage adjustments are not recommended on the basis of age, gender, smoking status, and race. Dose adjustment is recommended in moderate and severe hepatic and renal impairment patients (lurasidone package insert).

16.6.2.5 Olanzapine

Inducers of CYP1A2, including tobacco smoke and carbamazepine, decrease olanzapine concentrations [86]. Carbamazepine therapy (200 mg bid) causes an approximately 50 % increase in the clearance of olanzapine [99]. Fluvoxamine, a CYP1A2 inhibitor, decreases the clearance of olanzapine. An elderly, nonsmoking woman prescribed fluvoxamine comedication is estimated to reach a 4.6-fold higher olanzapine concentration than a young male smoker coadministered with carbamazepine [100].

16.6.2.6 Paliperidone

Paliperidone is not expected to cause clinically important pharmacokinetic interactions with drugs that are metabolized by cytochrome P450 isozymes. On initiation of strong inducers of both CYP3A4 and P-gp (e.g., carbamazepine, rifampin, or St John's wort), it may be necessary to increase the dose of paliperidone. No dose adjustment is required in patients with mild or moderate hepatic impairment. Paliperidone has not been studied in patients with severe hepatic impairment. Use of paliperidone is not recommended in patients with moderate or severe renal impairment (creatinine clearance $<$50 mL/min). Dose reduction is recommended for patients with mild renal impairment (creatinine clearance $\geq$50 mL/min to < 80 mL/min). Because elderly patients are more likely to have decreased renal function, adjust dose based on renal function (paliperidone package insert).

16.6.2.7 Risperidone

Carbamazepine and other CYP3A4 inducers decrease plasma concentrations of risperidone. Increase the risperidone dose up to twofold of the patient's usual dose. Dose adjustment is not recommended for risperidone during coadministration of CYP3A4 inhibitors (e.g., ranitidine, cimetidine, erythromycin). The dose of risperidone should be adjusted when used in combination with CYP2D6 inhibitors and enzyme inducers. Fluoxetine, paroxetine, and other CYP2D6 enzyme inhibitors increase plasma concentrations of risperidone [101]. Reduce the initial dose of risperidone. Chronic administration of clozapine with risperidone may decrease the clearance of risperidone (risperidone package insert).

16.6.2.8 Quetiapine

Coadministration of strong CYP3A4 inhibitors (e.g., ketoconazole, ritonavir) is suggested to reduce quetiapine dose to one-sixth of original dose. Concomitant use of strong CYP3A4 inducers (e.g., carbamazepine, phenytoin, rifampin) should increase quetiapine dose up to fivefold. When CYP3A4 inducer is discontinued, the quetiapine dose should be reduced to the original level within 7–14 days (quetiapine fumarate package insert) [102].

16.6.2.9 Ziprasidone

Coadministration of carbamazepine 200 mg twice daily resulted in a decrease of approximately 36 % in the AUC of ziprasidone [103]. This effect may be greater when higher doses of carbamazepine are administered. Ketoconazole, a potent inhibitor of CYP3A4, at a dose of 400 mg QD for 5 days, increased the AUC and Cmax of ziprasidone by about 35–40 % [104]. The absorption of ziprasidone is increased up to twofold in the presence of food. Dosage modifications for age, smoking status, or gender are not recommended.

The AUC increased by 26 % in the cirrhotic group compared with the matched control group [105].

16.6.3 Monitoring Recommendations and Patient Safety

In psychopharmacology, treatment with antipsychotic drugs is often suboptimal, mainly because of the high interindividual variability in pharmacokinetic properties. Differences in absorption, distribution, metabolism, and excretion of drugs due to age, diseases, concomitant medication, or genetic peculiarities can result in no or poor response to treatment or can cause serious adverse effects and toxicity [106]. For antipsychotics, optimal dose titration should be guided by measuring plasma concentrations. Therapeutic drug monitoring (TDM) is a valid tool for tailoring the dosage of antipsychotic drugs [107]. In case of pharmacokinetic interactions, the plasma levels of the affected drug will change. Combination treatment with a drug known for its interaction potential is the indication for TDM. In elderly patients, TDM is particularly recommended; these patients with reduced elimination capacity and receiving several kinds of medications may have a higher risk of developing side effects.

When using TDM to guide antipsychotic therapy, it is assumed that there is a relationship between plasma concentrations and clinical effects. It is also assumed that there is a plasma concentration range of the drug which is associated with maximal effectiveness and safety, the "therapeutic window." For many antipsychotic agents, the therapeutic reference range is not merely based on pharmacokinetic and pharmacodynamic studies but also on in vivo receptor binding studies using imaging techniques [108, 109]. Positron emission tomography (PET) of molecular drug targets in the brain shows the associations between brain target occupancy, plasma concentrations, and clinical effects and adverse reactions [108].

16.6.4 Special Populations

Determining the appropriate dosage of antipsychotic drug requires the integration of several factors, including potential drug-drug interactions. Moreover, physicians should take into account certain factors inherent to the patients. For example, elder people tend to metabolize drugs slower than younger people and women slower than men. Comorbid medical conditions which impair hepatic function, such as cirrhosis, would decrease the rate of drug metabolism. Further, cytochrome P450 enzymes are polymorphic, and ethnic differences exist that influence the metabolism of drugs. For example, about 5–10 % of Caucasians are poor metabolizers of CYP2D6, while about 20 % of Chinese and Japanese are poor metabolizers of CYP2C19 [110].

16.6.4.1 Elderly Patients

Aging is characterized by progressive impairment of functional capacities of all system organs, reduction in homeostatic mechanisms, and altered response to receptor stimulation. These age-related physiologic changes influence both the pharmacokinetics and pharmacodynamics of drugs in elderly patients. Pharmacokinetic and pharmacodynamic changes as well as polypharmacy and comorbidities may alter significantly the effect of medication with advancing age [111]. Hepatic clearance can be reduced by up to 30 %. Among these, phase I metabolism is more likely to be impaired than phase II metabolism. However, there are no age-related changes in the CYP activities. Elderly patients with dementia are frequently treated with antipsychotic drugs to control behavioral and psychological symptoms of dementia (BPSD). The use of first-generation antipsychotics (FGAs) in the elderly patients is strongly limited by severe and intolerable side effects [112]. SGAs show an efficacy superior to placebo in randomized studies in BPSD treatment, with a better tolerability profile versus FGAs [113]. For this population, the appropriate dose of antipsychotics should be lower than the young population. However, in recent years, the use of antipsychotics has been widely debated for concerns about safety in elderly patients affected with dementia and the possible risks for stroke and sudden death [114, 115]. Drug regulatory agencies issued specific recommendations for underlining that treatment of BPSD with antipsychotics is "off-label." In fact, elderly patients are at increased risk of adverse events due to atypical antipsychotic drugs because of age-related changes in pharmacokinetics and pharmacodynamics and current medical conditions, polypharmacy, and potential drug interactions. US Food and Drug Administration black box warnings have clearly shown the potential risks of their use (e.g., cerebrovascular accidents, risk of sudden death). Before prescribing an antipsychotic drug, the following factors should be seriously considered: the presence of cardiovascular diseases, QTc interval on electrocardiogram, electrolytic imbalances, familiar history for torsades de pointes, concomitant treatments, and use of drugs able to lengthen QTc [113].

16.6.4.2 Children and Adolescents

Antipsychotic drugs are used for the treatment of various psychiatric disorders in children and adolescents, including psychosis, physical aggression, mania, irritable mood, and Tourette's disorder [116]. In the last two decades, there has been a general increase in psychotropic drug prescribing in children and adolescent in many countries [117]. Much of the information about the efficacy and safety of antipsychotics in this population is extrapolated from adult studies; in particular, little is known about the long-term effects of these drugs on the development of the central nervous system. Children appear to be at higher risk than adults for a number of adverse effects, such as extrapyramidal symptoms and metabolic and endocrine abnormalities [118].

16.6.4.3 Pregnancy and Breast-Feeding

Pharmacotherapy during pregnancy is often complicated by pregnancy-related pharmacokinetic changes and the need for dose adjustments. Pregnancy-associated changes in absorption, distribution, metabolism, and excretion may result in decreased drug concentrations and possible treatment effects, particularly in late pregnancy. Mechanisms include changes in gastrointestinal motility and pH impacting absorption, expansion of total body water and plasma volume, decreased concentrations of drug binding proteins affecting distribution, changes in drug metabolism rates by cytochrome P450 (CYP) and other metabolizing and transport enzymes, and changes in hepatic and renal blood flow and increased glomerular filtration rate affecting urinary excretion [119, 120]. The activities of CYP isoenzymes CYP3A4, CYP2D6, and CYP2C9 and uridine 5′-diphosphate glucuronosyltransferase are increased during pregnancy, whereas activities of CYP1A2 and CYP2C19 are decreased [121]. These various changes fluctuate according to different patterns throughout the time frame of pregnancy. These physiologic changes may have additive, synergistic, or competing effects on overall drug exposure.

However, a number of methodological and ethical challenges arise when wishing to conduct research on antipsychotic medication during pregnancy. Information about the effects of antipsychotics in pregnancy usually comes from nonrandomized, prospective, and observational studies and, more often, single case reports or small case series studies [122, 123]. When investigated collectively, antipsychotic medications have been associated with a statistically significant increase in the risk of birth defects as a whole [124]. However, most SGAs appear to increase risk of gestational metabolic complications and babies large for gestational age and with mean birth weight significantly heavier as compared with those exposed to FGAs [123]. Given the lack of data regarding longer term outcomes for children exposed to antipsychotic medication in pregnancy, ensuring there is appropriate ongoing monitoring of infant and child development is optimal [125].

The passage of a drug into breast milk is influenced by many factors including its volume of distribution, molecular weight, lipid/water solubility, relative affinity for plasma and milk proteins, the pH of blood and milk, and blood flow to the breast [126]. The safety of SGAs remains to be established and none are currently recommended during lactation. Olanzapine [127], quetiapine [128], and risperidone [129] achieve very low levels in infant plasma, with no evident adverse effects, suggesting that these agents may be safe. However, clozapine achieves relatively high concentrations in breast milk and infant serum, and agranulocytosis and somnolence have been reported in breast-fed infants [130]. Therefore, clozapine should be contraindicated during breast-feeding.

References

1. Guo JJ et al (2012) Exposure to potentially dangerous drug-drug interactions involving antipsychotics. Psychiatr Serv 63(11):1080–1088
2. Cascorbi I (2011) P-glycoprotein: tissue distribution, substrates, and functional consequences of genetic variations. Handb Exp Pharmacol 201:261–283
3. Linnet K, Ejsing TB (2008) A review on the impact of P-glycoprotein on the penetration of drugs into the brain. Focus on psychotropic drugs. Eur Neuropsychopharmacol 18(3):157–169
4. Akamine Y et al (2012) Psychotropic drug-drug interactions involving P-glycoprotein. CNS Drugs 26(11):959–973

5. Moons T et al (2011) Relationship between P-glycoprotein and second-generation antipsychotics. Pharmacogenomics 12(8):1193–1211
6. DeVane CL (2002) Clinical significance of drug binding, protein binding, and binding displacement drug interactions. Psychopharmacol Bull 36(3):5–21
7. Benet LZ, Hoener BA (2002) Changes in plasma protein binding have little clinical relevance. Clin Pharmacol Ther 71(3):115–121
8. Caley CF, Cooper CK (2002) Ziprasidone: the fifth atypical antipsychotic. Ann Pharmacother 36(5):839–851
9. Linnet K (2002) Glucuronidation of olanzapine by cDNA-expressed human UDP-glucuronosyltransferases and human liver microsomes. Hum Psychopharmacol 17(5):233–238
10. Vermeir M et al (2008) Absorption, metabolism, and excretion of paliperidone, a new monoaminergic antagonist, in humans. Drug Metab Dispos 36(4):769–779
11. Citrome L (2014) Asenapine review, part I: chemistry, receptor affinity profile, pharmacokinetics and metabolism. Expert Opin Drug Metab Toxicol 10(6):893–903
12. Kennedy WK et al (2013) Clinically significant drug interactions with atypical antipsychotics. CNS Drugs 27(12):1021–1048
13. Spina E, de Leon J (2007) Metabolic drug interactions with newer antipsychotics: a comparative review. Basic Clin Pharmacol Toxicol 100(1):4–22
14. Mauri MC et al (2007) Clinical pharmacokinetics of atypical antipsychotics: a critical review of the relationship between plasma concentrations and clinical response. Clin Pharmacokinet 46(5):359–388
15. Sheehan JJ et al (2010) Atypical antipsychotic metabolism and excretion. Curr Drug Metab 11(6):516–525
16. Urichuk L et al (2008) Metabolism of atypical antipsychotics: involvement of cytochrome p450 enzymes and relevance for drug-drug interactions. Curr Drug Metab 9(5):410–418
17. Prior TI, Baker GB (2003) Interactions between the cytochrome P450 system and the second-generation antipsychotics. J Psychiatry Neurosci 28(2):99–112
18. Murray M (2006) Role of CYP pharmacogenetics and drug-drug interactions in the efficacy and safety of atypical and other antipsychotic agents. J Pharm Pharmacol 58(7):871–885
19. Rowland A et al (2013) The UDP-glucuronosyltransferases: their role in drug metabolism and detoxification. Int J Biochem Cell Biol 45(6):1121–1132
20. Desai HD et al (2001) Smoking in patients receiving psychotropic medications: a pharmacokinetic perspective. CNS Drugs 15(6):469–494
21. Zevin S, Benowitz NL (1999) Drug interactions with tobacco smoking. An update. Clin Pharmacokinet 36(6):425–438
22. Haslemo T et al (2006) The effect of variable cigarette consumption on the interaction with clozapine and olanzapine. Eur J Clin Pharmacol 62(12):1049–1053
23. Lowe EJ, Ackman ML (2010) Impact of tobacco smoking cessation on stable clozapine or olanzapine treatment. Ann Pharmacother 44(4):727–732
24. Wu TH et al (2008) Pharmacokinetics of olanzapine in Chinese male schizophrenic patients with various smoking behaviors. Prog Neuropsychopharmacol Biol Psychiatry 32(8):1889–1893
25. Shimoda K et al (1999) Lower plasma levels of haloperidol in smoking than in nonsmoking schizophrenic patients. Ther Drug Monit 21(3):293–296
26. Eugster HP et al (1993) Caffeine, estradiol, and progesterone interact with human CYP1A1 and CYP1A2. Evidence from cDNA-directed expression in Saccharomyces cerevisiae. Drug Metab Dispos 21(1):43–49
27. Hagg S et al (2000) Effect of caffeine on clozapine pharmacokinetics in healthy volunteers. Br J Clin Pharmacol 49(1):59–63
28. de Leon J (2004) Atypical antipsychotic dosing: the effect of smoking and caffeine. Psychiatr Serv 55(5):491–493
29. Hanley MJ et al (2011) The effect of grapefruit juice on drug disposition. Expert Opin Drug Metab Toxicol 7(3):267–286

30. Yasui N et al (1999) Lack of significant pharmacokinetic interaction between haloperidol and grapefruit juice. Int Clin Psychopharmacol 14(2):113–118
31. Lane HY et al (2001) Lack of CYP3A4 inhibition by grapefruit juice and ketoconazole upon clozapine administration in vivo. Drug Metabol Drug Interact 18(3–4):263–278
32. Lane HY et al (2001) Repeated ingestion of grapefruit juice does not alter clozapine's steady-state plasma levels, effectiveness, and tolerability. J Clin Psychiatry 62(10):812–817
33. Schmidt LE, Dalhoff K (2002) Food-drug interactions. Drugs 62(10):1481–1502
34. Disanto AR, Golden G (2009) Effect of food on the pharmacokinetics of clozapine orally disintegrating tablet 12.5 mg: a randomized, open-label, crossover study in healthy male subjects. Clin Drug Investig 29(8):539–549
35. Gandelman K et al (2009) The impact of calories and fat content of meals on oral ziprasidone absorption: a randomized, open-label, crossover trial. J Clin Psychiatry 70(1):58–62
36. Lincoln J et al (2010) How sequential studies inform drug development: evaluating the effect of food intake on optimal bioavailability of ziprasidone. J Psychiatr Pract 16(2):103–114
37. Preskorn S et al (2013) Effect of food on the pharmacokinetics of lurasidone: results of two randomized, open-label, crossover studies. Hum Psychopharmacol 28(5):495–505
38. Chew ML et al (2008) Anticholinergic activity of 107 medications commonly used by older adults. J Am Geriatr Soc 56(7):1333–1341
39. Kannankeril PJ, Roden DM (2007) Drug-induced long QT and torsade de pointes: recent advances. Curr Opin Cardiol 22(1):39–43
40. Roden DM (2004) Drug-induced prolongation of the QT interval. N Engl J Med 350(10):1013–1022
41. France NP, Della Pasqua O (2015) The role of concentration-effect relationships in the assessment of QTc interval prolongation. Br J Clin Pharmacol 79(1):117–131
42. Flanagan RJ, Dunk L (2008) Haematological toxicity of drugs used in psychiatry. Hum Psychopharmacol 23(Suppl 1):27–41
43. Chang S-C, Lu M-L (2012) Metabolic and cardiovascular adverse effects associated with treatment with antipsychotic drugs. J Exp Clin Med 4(2):103–107
44. Citrome L, Volavka J (2005) Consensus development conference on antipsychotic drugs and obesity and diabetes: response to consensus statement. J Clin Psychiatry 66(8):1073–1074
45. Rummel-Kluge C et al (2010) Head-to-head comparisons of metabolic side effects of second generation antipsychotics in the treatment of schizophrenia: a systematic review and meta-analysis. Schizophr Res 123(2–3):225–233
46. Correll CU et al (2007) Does antipsychotic polypharmacy increase the risk for metabolic syndrome? Schizophr Res 89(1–3):91–100
47. Huang MC et al (2009) Prevalence of metabolic syndrome among patients with schizophrenia or schizoaffective disorder in Taiwan. Acta Psychiatr Scand 120(4):274–280
48. Mizuno Y et al (2014) Pharmacological strategies to counteract antipsychotic-induced weight gain and metabolic adverse effects in schizophrenia: a systematic review and meta-analysis. Schizophr Bull 40(6):1385–1403
49. Wang LJ et al (2013) Adjunctive effects of aripiprazole on metabolic profiles: comparison of patients treated with olanzapine to patients treated with other atypical antipsychotic drugs. Prog Neuropsychopharmacol Biol Psychiatry 40:260–266
50. Crettol S et al (2014) Pharmacogenomics in psychiatry: from therapeutic drug monitoring to genomic medicine. Clin Pharmacol Ther 95(3):254–257
51. Ravyn D et al (2013) CYP450 pharmacogenetic treatment strategies for antipsychotics: a review of the evidence. Schizophr Res 149(1–3):1–14
52. Stingl JC et al (2014) Relevance of UDP-glucuronosyltransferase polymorphisms for drug dosing: a quantitative systematic review. Pharmacol Ther 141(1):92–116
53. Ghotbi R et al (2010) Carriers of the UGT1A4 142T>G gene variant are predisposed to reduced olanzapine exposure–an impact similar to male gender or smoking in schizophrenic patients. Eur J Clin Pharmacol 66(5):465–474

54. Nozawa M et al (2008) The relationship between the response of clinical symptoms and plasma olanzapine concentration, based on pharmacogenetics: Juntendo University Schizophrenia Projects (JUSP). Ther Drug Monit 30(1):35–40
55. Erickson-Ridout KK et al (2012) Glucuronidation of the second-generation antipsychotic clozapine and its active metabolite N-desmethylclozapine. Potential importance of the UGT1A1 A(TA)(7)TAA and UGT1A4 L48V polymorphisms. Pharmacogenet Genomics 22(8):561–576
56. Samer CF et al (2013) Applications of CYP450 testing in the clinical setting. Mol Diagn Ther 17(3):165–184
57. Carrillo JA et al (2000) Evaluation of caffeine as an in vivo probe for CYP1A2 using measurements in plasma, saliva, and urine. Ther Drug Monit 22(4):409–417
58. Shirley KL et al (2003) Correlation of cytochrome P450 (CYP) 1A2 activity using caffeine phenotyping and olanzapine disposition in healthy volunteers. Neuropsychopharmacology 28(5):961–966
59. Paz E et al (2008) Evaluation of three dosing models for the prediction of steady-state trough clozapine concentrations. Clin Biochem 41(7–8):603–606
60. Gunes A, Dahl ML (2008) Variation in CYP1A2 activity and its clinical implications: influence of environmental factors and genetic polymorphisms. Pharmacogenomics 9(5):625–637
61. Relling MV et al (1992) Racial and gender differences in N-acetyltransferase, xanthine oxidase, and CYP1A2 activities. Clin Pharmacol Ther 52(6):643–658
62. Rasmussen BB et al (2002) The interindividual differences in the 3-demthylation of caffeine alias CYP1A2 is determined by both genetic and environmental factors. Pharmacogenetics 12(6):473–478
63. McGraw J, Waller D (2012) Cytochrome P450 variations in different ethnic populations. Expert Opin Drug Metab Toxicol 8(3):371–382
64. Tay JK et al (2007) Functional polymorphisms of the cytochrome P450 1A2 (CYP1A2) gene and prolonged QTc interval in schizophrenia. Prog Neuropsychopharmacol Biol Psychiatry 31(6):1297–1302
65. Romkes M et al (1991) Cloning and expression of complementary DNAs for multiple members of the human cytochrome P450IIC subfamily. Biochemistry 30(13):3247–3255
66. Miners JO, Birkett DJ (1998) Cytochrome P4502C9: an enzyme of major importance in human drug metabolism. Br J Clin Pharmacol 45(6):525–538
67. Flockhart DA (1995) Drug interactions and the cytochrome P450 system. The role of cytochrome P450 2C19. Clin Pharmacokinet 29(Suppl 1):45–52
68. Gardiner SJ, Begg EJ (2006) Pharmacogenetics, drug-metabolizing enzymes, and clinical practice. Pharmacol Rev 58(3):521–590
69. Desta Z et al (2002) Clinical significance of the cytochrome P450 2C19 genetic polymorphism. Clin Pharmacokinet 41(12):913–958
70. Xie HG et al (2001) Molecular basis of ethnic differences in drug disposition and response. Annu Rev Pharmacol Toxicol 41:815–850
71. Ingelman-Sundberg M et al (2007) Influence of cytochrome P450 polymorphisms on drug therapies: pharmacogenetic, pharmacoepigenetic and clinical aspects. Pharmacol Ther 116(3):496–526
72. Cascorbi I (2003) Pharmacogenetics of cytochrome p4502D6: genetic background and clinical implication. Eur J Clin Invest 33(Suppl 2):17–22
73. Zhou SF (2008) Drugs behave as substrates, inhibitors and inducers of human cytochrome P450 3A4. Curr Drug Metab 9(4):310–322
74. Swainston Harrison T, Perry CM (2004) Aripiprazole: a review of its use in schizophrenia and schizoaffective disorder. Drugs 64(15):1715–1736
75. Suzuki T et al (2014) Effects of genetic polymorphisms of CYP2D6, CYP3A5, and ABCB1 on the steady-state plasma concentrations of aripiprazole and its active metabolite, dehydroaripiprazole, in Japanese patients with schizophrenia. Ther Drug Monit 36(5):651–655

76. Hendset M et al (2014) Serum concentrations of risperidone and aripiprazole in subgroups encoding CYP2D6 intermediate metabolizer phenotype. Ther Drug Monit 36(1):80–85
77. Suzuki T et al (2011) Effects of the CYP2D6*10 allele on the steady-state plasma concentrations of aripiprazole and its active metabolite, dehydroaripiprazole, in Japanese patients with schizophrenia. Ther Drug Monit 33(1):21–24
78. Hendset M et al (2007) Impact of the CYP2D6 genotype on steady-state serum concentrations of aripiprazole and dehydroaripiprazole. Eur J Clin Pharmacol 63(12):1147–1151
79. Jann MW et al (1993) Pharmacokinetics and pharmacodynamics of clozapine. Clin Pharmacokinet 24(2):161–176
80. Linnet K, Olesen OV (1997) Metabolism of clozapine by cDNA-expressed human cytochrome P450 enzymes. Drug Metab Dispos 25(12):1379–1382
81. Olesen OV, Linnet K (2001) Contributions of five human cytochrome P450 isoforms to the N-demethylation of clozapine in vitro at low and high concentrations. J Clin Pharmacol 41(8):823–832
82. Eap CB et al (2004) Nonresponse to clozapine and ultrarapid CYP1A2 activity: clinical data and analysis of CYP1A2 gene. J Clin Psychopharmacol 24(2):214–219
83. Ozdemir V et al (2001) Treatment-resistance to clozapine in association with ultrarapid CYP1A2 activity and the C→A polymorphism in intron 1 of the CYP1A2 gene: effect of grapefruit juice and low-dose fluvoxamine. J Clin Psychopharmacol 21(6):603–607
84. Melkersson KI et al (2007) Impact of CYP1A2 and CYP2D6 polymorphisms on drug metabolism and on insulin and lipid elevations and insulin resistance in clozapine-treated patients. J Clin Psychiatry 68(5):697–704
85. Chiu YY et al (2014) Lurasidone drug-drug interaction studies: a comprehensive review. Drug Metabol Drug Interact 29(3):191–202
86. Callaghan JT et al (1999) Olanzapine. Pharmacokinetic and pharmacodynamic profile. Clin Pharmacokinet 37(3):177–193
87. Thomas P et al (2008) Correlates of response to Olanzapine in a North Indian Schizophrenia sample. Psychiatry Res 161(3):275–283
88. Czerwensky F et al (2014) The CYP1A2*1D and *1F polymorphisms have a significant impact on olanzapine serum concentrations. Ther Drug Monit 37(2):152–160
89. Laika B et al (2010) Pharmacogenetics and olanzapine treatment: CYP1A2*1F and serotonergic polymorphisms influence therapeutic outcome. Pharmacogenomics J 10(1):20–29
90. Bigos KL et al (2011) Genetic variation in CYP3A43 explains racial difference in olanzapine clearance. Mol Psychiatry 16(6):620–625
91. Citrome L (2012) Oral paliperidone extended-release: chemistry, pharmacodynamics, pharmacokinetics and metabolism, clinical efficacy, safety and tolerability. Expert Opin Drug Metab Toxicol 8(7):873–888
92. Grimm SW et al (2006) Effects of cytochrome P450 3A modulators ketoconazole and carbamazepine on quetiapine pharmacokinetics. Br J Clin Pharmacol 61(1):58–69
93. DeVane CL, Nemeroff CB (2001) Clinical pharmacokinetics of quetiapine: an atypical antipsychotic. Clin Pharmacokinet 40(7):509–522
94. van der Weide K, van der Weide J (2014) The influence of the CYP3A4*22 polymorphism on serum concentration of quetiapine in psychiatric patients. J Clin Psychopharmacol 34(2):256–260
95. Mannens G et al (1993) Absorption, metabolism, and excretion of risperidone in humans. Drug Metab Dispos 21(6):1134–1141
96. Scordo MG et al (1999) Cytochrome P450 2D6 genotype and steady state plasma levels of risperidone and 9-hydroxyrisperidone. Psychopharmacology (Berl) 147(3):300–305
97. Yasui-Furukori N et al (2003) Effects of CYP2D6 genotypes on plasma concentrations of risperidone and enantiomers of 9-hydroxyrisperidone in Japanese patients with schizophrenia. J Clin Pharmacol 43(2):122–127
98. Beedham C et al (2003) Ziprasidone metabolism, aldehyde oxidase, and clinical implications. J Clin Psychopharmacol 23(3):229–232

99. Lucas RA et al (1998) A pharmacokinetic interaction between carbamazepine and olanzapine: observations on possible mechanism. Eur J Clin Pharmacol 54(8):639–643
100. Gex-Fabry M et al (2003) Therapeutic drug monitoring of olanzapine: the combined effect of age, gender, smoking, and comedication. Ther Drug Monit 25(1):46–53
101. Ereshefsky L et al (1995) Antidepressant drug interactions and the cytochrome P450 system. The role of cytochrome P450 2D6. Clin Pharmacokinet 29(Suppl 1):10–18; discussion 18–9
102. Nemeroff CB et al (2002) Quetiapine: preclinical studies, pharmacokinetics, drug interactions, and dosing. J Clin Psychiatry 63(Suppl 13):5–11
103. Miceli JJ et al (2000) The effect of carbamazepine on the steady-state pharmacokinetics of ziprasidone in healthy volunteers. Br J Clin Pharmacol 49(Suppl 1):65S–70S
104. Miceli JJ et al (2000) The effects of ketoconazole on ziprasidone pharmacokinetics–a placebo-controlled crossover study in healthy volunteers. Br J Clin Pharmacol 49(Suppl 1):71S–76S
105. Everson G et al (2000) The pharmacokinetics of ziprasidone in subjects with normal and impaired hepatic function. Br J Clin Pharmacol 49(Suppl 1):21S–26S
106. Patteet L et al (2012) Therapeutic drug monitoring of common antipsychotics. Ther Drug Monit 34(6):629–651
107. Hiemke C et al (2011) AGNP consensus guidelines for therapeutic drug monitoring in psychiatry: update 2011. Pharmacopsychiatry 44(6):195–235
108. Grunder G et al (2011) Therapeutic plasma concentrations of antidepressants and antipsychotics: lessons from PET imaging. Pharmacopsychiatry 44(6):236–248
109. Hiemke C (2008) Therapeutic drug monitoring in neuropsychopharmacology: does it hold its promises? Eur Arch Psychiatry Clin Neurosci 258(Suppl 1):21–27
110. Yang J et al (2012) Metabolic capabilities of cytochrome P450 enzymes in Chinese liver microsomes compared with those in Caucasian liver microsomes. Br J Clin Pharmacol 73(2):268–284
111. Trifiro G, Spina E (2011) Age-related changes in pharmacodynamics: focus on drugs acting on central nervous and cardiovascular systems. Curr Drug Metab 12(7):611–620
112. Alexopoulos GS et al (2004) Using antipsychotic agents in older patients. J Clin Psychiatry 65(Suppl 2):5–99; discussion 100–102; quiz 103–4
113. Gareri P et al (2014) Use and safety of antipsychotics in behavioral disorders in elderly people with dementia. J Clin Psychopharmacol 34(1):109–123
114. Shin JY et al (2013) Risk of ischemic stroke with the use of risperidone, quetiapine and olanzapine in elderly patients: a population-based, case-crossover study. J Psychopharmacol 27(7):638–644
115. Ray WA et al (2009) Atypical antipsychotic drugs and the risk of sudden cardiac death. N Engl J Med 360(3):225–235
116. Findling RL et al (2005) Use of antipsychotics in children and adolescents. J Clin Psychiatry 66(Suppl 7):29–40
117. Almandil NB, Wong IC (2011) Review on the current use of antipsychotic drugs in children and adolescents. Arch Dis Child Educ Pract Ed 96(5):192–196
118. Vitiello B et al (2009) Antipsychotics in children and adolescents: increasing use, evidence for efficacy and safety concerns. Eur Neuropsychopharmacol 19(9):629–635
119. Deligiannidis KM et al (2014) Pharmacotherapy for mood disorders in pregnancy: a review of pharmacokinetic changes and clinical recommendations for therapeutic drug monitoring. J Clin Psychopharmacol 34(2):244–255
120. McCormack SA, Best BM (2014) Obstetric pharmacokinetic dosing studies are urgently needed. Front Pediatr 2:9
121. Anderson GD (2006) Using pharmacokinetics to predict the effects of pregnancy and maternal-infant transfer of drugs during lactation. Expert Opin Drug Metab Toxicol 2(6):947–960
122. Nulman I (2014) The effects of the new antipsychotic medications on mothers and babies. J Popul Ther Clin Pharmacol 21(3):e542–e547

123. Gentile S (2010) Antipsychotic therapy during early and late pregnancy. A systematic review. Schizophr Bull 36(3):518–544
124. Habermann F et al (2013) Atypical antipsychotic drugs and pregnancy outcome: a prospective, cohort study. J Clin Psychopharmacol 33(4):453–462
125. Galbally M et al (2014) Antipsychotic drugs in pregnancy: a review of their maternal and fetal effects. Ther Adv Drug Saf 5(2):100–109
126. Llewellyn A, Stowe ZN (1998) Psychotropic medications in lactation. J Clin Psychiatry 59(Suppl 2):41–52
127. Gardiner SJ et al (2003) Transfer of olanzapine into breast milk, calculation of infant drug dose, and effect on breast-fed infants. Am J Psychiatry 160(8):1428–1431
128. Lee A et al (2004) Excretion of quetiapine in breast milk. Am J Psychiatry 161(9):1715–1716
129. Ilett KF et al (2004) Transfer of risperidone and 9-hydroxyrisperidone into human milk. Ann Pharmacother 38(2):273–276
130. Menon SJ (2008) Psychotropic medication during pregnancy and lactation. Arch Gynecol Obstet 277(1):1–13

Chapter 17
Clinically Significant Interactions with Mood Stabilisers

David Taylor and Kalliopi Vallianatou

Abstract Mood stabilisers are associated with a wide range of clinically significant drug-drug interactions. The glucuronidation of lamotrigine is inhibited by valproate and induced by oral contraceptives, carbamazepine and phenytoin. Lamotrigine induces the glucuronidation of quetiapine. Valproate is an inhibitor of CYP2C9 and glucuronosyltransferase enzymes and increases plasma levels of some benzodiazepines, tricyclic antidepressants and lamotrigine. Valproate's metabolism is inhibited by aspirin and erythromycin and induced by carbapenem antibiotics. Carbamazepine is involved in innumerable interactions largely because of its potent ability to induce the activity of CYP3A4 and, to a lesser degree, CYP1A2 enzymes. Carbamazepine thus lowers plasma levels of many drugs including many analgesics, antipsychotics, benzodiazepines, antidepressants and antimicrobial agents. The metabolism of carbamazepine is inhibited by diltiazem, verapamil, danazol, isoniazid and ticlodipine. Lithium is largely renally excreted, a process that is inhibited by NSAIDs, thiazide and loop diuretics, ACE inhibitors and some calcium channel blockers. Lithium may give rise to neurotoxicity when combined with antipsychotics or antidepressants.

Keywords Pharmacokinetics • Metabolism • Valproate • Valprioc acid • Divalproex • Lamotrigine • Carbamazepine • Lithium

---

Search Details We searched PubMed and Embase in January 2015 using the search terms "metabolism", "pharmacokinetic" and "interaction" with the following drug names: "valproate", "valproic", "divalproex", "lamotrigine", "carbamazepine" and "lithium". We also referred official European Medicines Association Summaries of Product Characteristics for all drugs listed (accessed online January 30, 2015). Reference sections for all retrieved papers were scrutinised for further relevant papers.

D. Taylor, PhD, FFRPS, FRPharmS (✉)
Pharmacy Department, Maudsley Hospital, Denmark Hill, London, UK
e-mail: david.taylor@slam.nhs.uk

K. Vallianatou, MPharm, MRPharmS
Pharmacy Department, South London and Maudsley NHS Foundation Trust, Maudsley Hospital, Denmark Hill, London, UK
e-mail: david.taylor@slam.nhs.uk

M. Jann et al. (eds.), *Applied Clinical Pharmacokinetics and Pharmacodynamics of Psychopharmacological Agents*,
DOI 10.1007/978-3-319-27883-4_17

17.1 Lamotrigine

The metabolism of lamotrigine does not involve any CYP enzymes, so its interaction potential is limited. Lamotrigine is largely directly conjugated with glucuronic acid forming an inactive 2-*N*-glucuronide [1]. This reaction is catalysed by glucuronosyltransferase 1A4 (UGT1A4) [2]. Competition for this pathway may result in the altered metabolism of other drugs (or more likely their metabolites) that utilise this metabolic route.

17.1.1 Evidence for the Absence of Interaction

Lamotrigine was initially marketed as an add-on treatment for seizure disorders. As such, its interaction potential, especially with other anticonvulsants, was of great importance. As a consequence, there is a small body of literature demonstrating lamotrigine's failure to interact with drugs with which it might be given. For example, lamotrigine has been shown [3] not to affect handling of oxcarbazepine in a prospective study of 47 participants. Likewise, oxcarbazepine has no effect on lamotrigine plasma levels, although the combination of the two drugs was less well tolerated than either drug alone. In another study of 14 healthy volunteers [4], no interaction was found for the co-administration of lamotrigine 50 mg and olanzapine 5 mg, except for the fact that olanzapine seemed to increase time to peak concentration of lamotrigine. The doses used in this study are effectively subtherapeutic, but another prospective study in 43 healthy subjects found essentially no interaction when daily doses of 200 mg lamotrigine and 15 mg olanzapine were given [5].

An analysis of plasma concentrations of risperidone and its major metabolite, 9-hydroxy risperidone, in real-life patients [6] showed no difference in parent/metabolite concentration ratios for people receiving lamotrigine (as confirmed by plasma concentrations) and those not receiving lamotrigine. The authors concluded that lamotrigine had no effect on the conversion of risperidone to 9-hydroxy risperidone (presumably via CYP2D6 and CYP3A4). Similarly, there seemed to be no interaction between lamotrigine and sertraline in a 51 patient observational study [7]. Bupropion, whose metabolites are extensively glucuronidated, does not seem to affect lamotrigine pharmacokinetics [8]. Similarly, maximum daily doses (30 mg) of aripiprazole had no effect on lamotrigine handling in an 18-subject study [9].

17.1.2 Valproate

The interaction between valproic acid and its chemical congeners and lamotrigine is widely recognised: dosing recommendations for lamotrigine are altered substantially for patients co-prescribed valproate. Valproate and lamotrigine share glucuronidation via UGT as a major metabolite pathway, and the interaction is thought to result from competitive inhibition of this enzyme group. The extent of the interaction was first quantified in a crossover study of 18 volunteer subjects who received valproate (as divalproex) and three doses of lamotrigine: 50 mg, 100 mg and 150 mg/day [10]. Using previously obtained data on lamotrigine pharmacokinetics, the co-administration of valproate appeared to be increased from around 26 h to around 70 h, and clearance values were proportionality decreased. The use of lamotrigine however increased the clearance of valproate and caused a 25 % decrease in plasma concentration of valproate. The nature of this bidirectional interaction is inconsistent with competitive inhibition but might be explained by lamotrigine's induction of UGT function occurring in the context of competition for the enzyme.

Later studies have added to our understanding of the nature of this interaction. The reduction in lamotrigine clearance is seemingly independent of valproate dose or plasma level of valproate [11]. Also, Rowland and co-workers [12] using microsomal liver samples showed that the glucuronidation of lamotrigine was metabolised by UGT1A4 and by another glucuronosyltransferase UGT2B7. Valproate, a known substrate of UGT2B7, was shown not to affect the function of UGT1A4. The authors concluded that valproate decreased lamotrigine clearance via inhibition of UGT2B7. The increased clearance of valproate associated with lamotrigine co-administration might then, one assumes, be related to lamotrigine's induction of UGT1A4.

In practice, co-administration of valproate should provoke a halving of the lamotrigine dose. Valproate doses are not usually adjusted, but plasma level monitoring is recommended.

17.1.3 *Oral Contraceptives*

Combined oral contraceptives are recognised as potent inducers of UGT enzymes. An interaction with lamotrigine was first reported in 2001 [13]: seven cases were described in which lamotrigine plasma concentrations were reduced by an average of 49 % and where adverse consequences (e.g. seizures) were apparent. A later prospective study [14] using lamotrigine 300 mg/day in 18 healthy subjects demonstrated that co-administration of ethinylestradiol 30 μg + levonorgestrel 150 μg (Microgynon 30) reduced maximum plasma concentration of lamotrigine by 39 % and area under the curve by 52 %. The presumed mechanism was induction of the UGT system. A further study in patients receiving lamotrigine for seizure disorders [15] revealed that withdrawal of oral contraceptives rapidly led to a near doubling of lamotrigine plasma concentrations and a reduction of 2-N-glucuronide generation.

In practice, patients receiving oral contraceptives on starting lamotrigine should ultimately receive double the standard dose of lamotrigine for the condition being treated. Those receiving lamotrigine whose oral contraceptives are withdrawn should have their lamotrigine dose halved (in decrements over 1–2 weeks).

17.1.4 Quetiapine

Two observational studies have suggested that lamotrigine reduces quetiapine plasma concentrations; both used therapeutic drug monitoring (TDM) data from real-life patients. In the first study [16], co-administration of lamotrigine in 144 patients was associated with a 17 % reduction in expected quetiapine plasma concentration. In the second [17], concentration/dose ratio was reduced by 58 % in 22 patients. Lamotrigine's induction of UGT was suggested as an explanation for the reduction in plasma levels of quetiapine. Dose adjustment is probably not required in practice.

17.1.5 Carbamazepine

TDM data suggest that carbamazepine increases the clearance of lamotrigine by 30–50 % [18] (n = 184). Although carbamazepine is a potent inducer of CYP enzymes, the mechanism for this interaction is not known. Lamotrigine itself seems to increase plasma concentrations of carbamazepine's major metabolite, carbamazepine-10,11-epoxide, an interaction associated with clinical toxicity (nausea, diplopia, etc.) [19]. Carbamazepine concentrations were not affected. The authors suggested that lamotrigine inhibits epoxide hydrolase, the enzyme that converts the 10,11 epoxide to 10,11-dihydroxide.

17.1.6 Phenytoin

Phenytoin was first shown to increase lamotrigine clearance in 1986 [20]. The extent of this increase is around 125 % [18], although higher estimates (e.g. 160 % [21]) have been made. On withdrawal of phenytoin, lamotrigine clearance returns to normal only after complete cessation of phenytoin [21]. In practice, lamotrigine dose should be adjusted when phenytoin is added (increase dose by 25–50 %) or withdrawn (decrease dose by 25–50 %).

17.1.7 Lopinavir/Ritonavir (Kaletra)

One study of 24 healthy volunteers showed that Kaletra substantially increases the clearance of lamotrigine, probably via induction of glucuronidation [22]. When given with Kaletra, lamotrigine doses should be increased by 200 %.

17.2 Valproate

The pharmacokinetic characteristics of valproate have been widely studied but much remains to be clarified in respect to the mechanisms of drug-drug interactions in which it is involved. Valproate is poorly absorbed and has variable plasma protein binding and multiple metabolic routes of elimination [23]. Interactions result from competition for plasma protein binding and from valproate's capacity to inhibit numerous metabolic pathways, including CYP2C9 [24] and UGT [10].

17.2.1 Aspirin

Valproate's interaction with aspirin is complex, involving both metabolic inhibition and protein binding displacement. Competition for plasma protein (albumin) binding sites causes displacement of both drugs and an increase in free plasma concentrations [25]. Aspirin inhibits beta-oxidation and slows conversion of valproate to its major metabolites (valproate (E)-2-ene; 3-ketovalproate) while accelerating glucuronidation [26]. The net effect is a substantial increase in valproate activity, largely because of increased concentrations of free (and therefore active) valproate in the blood. Standard blood tests, which measure total valproate, will not reveal changes in free valproate.

The dose at which aspirin begins to exert its effects on valproate pharmacokinetics is not known [25]. Aspirin should therefore be avoided in patients receiving valproate.

17.2.2 Carbamazepine

Early reports suggested an interaction between valproate and carbamazepine, but both increases and decreases of carbamazepine plasma concentrations were described [27]. In vitro experiments using perfused rat liver later demonstrated that valproate inhibited the metabolism of carbamazepine to carbamazepine-10,11-epoxide, although the mechanism of this effect was not elucidated [28]. In contrast, a later study in human volunteers demonstrated that valproate had no effect on parent carbamazepine concentrations but potently reduced clearance of carbamazepine-10,11-epoxide [29]. The presumed mechanism was valproate's inhibition of the enzyme epoxide hydrolase. The known pharmacological activity of the epoxide metabolite of carbamazepine means that any change to its pharmacokinetics is likely to have clinical relevance. However, a further study in human volunteers with epilepsy confirmed a selective increase in epoxide metabolite concentrations induced by valproate but in the absence of any clear deterioration in performance on a battery of cognitive performance tests [30]. Most recently, a human volunteer study confirmed that valproate increased plasma concentrations of carbamazepine-10,11-epoxide but also showed that valproate inhibited both the conversion of the epoxide metabolite to its trans-diol derivative (via epoxide hydrolase) and the glucuronidation of carbamazepine-10,11-trans-diol (via glucuronosyltransferase) [31].

A further complication is that carbamazepine and valproate compete for plasma protein binding with valproate winning out – free carbamazepine fraction increased from 23.5 to 29.5 % in one study [32]. Further still, carbamazepine has been reported to reduce valproate concentrations by as much as 40 % [33] (although "enzyme induction" was the only mechanism suggested).

Carbamazepine and valproate are widely prescribed together, but close monitoring is required. This monitoring, at the very least, should include observation of the patient for the emergence or worsening of adverse effects and, ideally, should include monitoring of plasma levels (free and total) of the two drugs and carbamazepine-10,11-epoxide.

17.2.3 Quetiapine

One prospective study has examined the potential for interaction between valproate and quetiapine [34]. In 33 patients with schizophrenia or bipolar disorder, the addition of valproate reduced peak quetiapine concentrations (Cmax) by 17 % (but area under the curve AUC was unchanged), whereas the addition of quetiapine to divalproex treatment reduced both Cmax and AUC of valproic acid by 11 %. The authors concluded that combination treatment with quetiapine and valproate resulted in only non-significant changes.

Since the publication of this study demonstrating the safety of this combination, a handful of apparent adverse interactions have been reported. Two patients developed delirium when quetiapine was added to ongoing valproate [35], and two further patients developed hyper-ammonaemia (a known adverse effect of valproate) while taking the combination [36]. The first of these reports suggests a pharmacodynamic interaction, and the second does not conclusively implicate quetiapine as a causative factor. Nonetheless, clearly some caution is required when co-prescribing quetiapine and valproate.

17.2.4 Benzodiazepines

Benzodiazepines generally have complex metabolic pathways which involve both CYP enzymes (especially CYP3A4) and glucuronidation. Lorazepam has a much simpler metabolic route involving only glucuronidation. A dual study of human volunteers and perfused rat liver showed that valproate reduced lorazepam glucuronidation by around 40 % with a corresponding increase in lorazepam plasma concentrations [37]. Interestingly, despite this substantial effect, valproate concentrations were low, averaging only 33ug/ml. It has also been suggested that valproate inhibits clonazepam metabolism [38], but this is disputed [39].

Valproate and benzodiazepines share glucuronidation as a primary (valproate; lorazepam) or terminal (most benzodiazepines and their active metabolites) route of elimination. Prolongation of the effects of benzodiazepines may occur when co-administered with valproate.

17.2.5 Tricyclic Antidepressants

Like benzodiazepines, tricyclics are metabolised primarily by CYP-mediated hepatic Phase I reactions but ultimately cleared by glucuronidation. Again, as with benzodiazepines, many of the metabolites are pharmacologically active, and inactivation occurs only via glucuronidation. Case reports describe increased plasma levels of amitriptyline [40], nortriptyline [40, 41] and clomipramine [42, 43] resulting from the addition of valproate. A similar interaction was observed in a prospective study of amitriptyline and valproate: parent and metabolite plasma concentrations were substantially increased [44]. The authors suggested that valproate's inhibition of hydroxylation might be responsible for the rises seen, but inhibition of glucuronidation is also possible and perhaps more likely. Inhibition of CYP2C enzymes has also been suggested as the mechanism for this interaction [42].

The co-administration of valproate and tricyclic drugs is not contraindicated, but when valproate is added to established tricyclic treatment, a reduction in dose of the tricyclic should be considered, and plasma levels may be useful to guide dose adjustment.

17.2.6 Carbapenems

Carbapenems (e.g. meropenem, imipenem) are broad-spectrum antibiotics used for serious sepsis and in cystic fibrosis. Numerous case reports, beginning in 1997 [45] and continuing over nearly two decades [46, 47], describe massive reductions (up to 90 %) in valproate plasma concentrations after co-administration of carbapenems. In a retrospective analysis [48], an average reduction in valproate levels of 66 % occurred within 24 h of meropenem initiation.

The probable mechanism of this interaction is the induction of the glucuronidation of valproate [48], but numerous other routes have been proposed, including the inhibition of hydrolysis of valproate glucuronide back to valproate, enhanced renal clearance of valproate glucuronide and alterations in valproate distribution [46, 47, 49]. Whatever the mechanism of interaction, this is clearly a very significant interaction. The use of carbapenems is usually unavoidable, so when used alongside valproate, the dose of valproate may well need to be substantially increased almost immediately. Dose increases are best guided by plasma levels, but it is important to note that the possible nature of this interaction may mean that plasma concentration/tissue concentration ratios are significantly altered.

17.2.7 Others

Valproate should be used cautiously with *clozapine* because of the potential for increased CNS effects [50] and inhibition of clozapine metabolism [51]. *Erythromycin* may inhibit valproate metabolism causing a substantial rise in valproate plasma concentration [52]. Valproate appears to lower plasma concentrations of *olanzapine* by around 50 % [53] although the mechanism is not known. The antitubercular drug *isoniazid* inhibits valproate metabolism to a substantial degree causing toxic valproate concentrations [54]. Valproate inhibits the metabolism of *phenobarbital* [55] and creases the metabolism of the immunosuppressant drug mycophenolate [56] (the plasma concentrations of which are critical to clinical efficacy). Again, in these latter cases, the mechanism of interaction has not been determined.

17.3 Carbamazepine

Carbamazepine is involved in innumerable interactions, largely because of its potent ability to induce CYP3A4 function [57]. A great many drugs have their metabolism enhanced by the co-administration of carbamazepine, and a handful of drugs inhibit the metabolism of carbamazepine usually but not exclusively via CYP3A4 inhibition [58]. There are relatively few pharmacodynamic interactions. The two tables below described known pharmacokinetic and pharmacodynamic interactions involving carbamazepine (Tables 17.1 and 17.2).

17.4 Lithium

Lithium is a monovalent cation given orally in the form of various lithium salts. Lithium tablets are manufactured as either immediate release preparations which reach a peak plasma lithium concentration 1–3 h post-administration or sustained-release preparations that peak 4–12 h post-administration [110]. Lithium concentrations in the brain peak a further 24 h later owing to the relatively lower permeability of the blood-brain barrier. Its terminal elimination half-life ranges from 18 to 36 h. Lithium concentration measured in the plasma may be twice the concentration in red blood cells and the cerebrospinal fluid [111].

Table 17.1 Summary of interactions – carbamazepine

Interacting drug	Nature of interaction	Mechanism	Reference
Acetazolamide	Risk of SIADH. Acetazolamide increases CBZ concentrations	Not known	[57]
Analgesics			
Fentanyl	Some evidence that CBZ increases fentanyl requirements during surgery	Not known	[59]
Methadone	CBZ reduces serum trough concentration by 60 %	? CYP3A4 induction	[60]
Propoxyphene	CBZ concentrations increased by 50–100 %	Not known	[61]
Antibacterials			
Erythromycin	No effect of CBZ on erythromycin, but erythromycin increases CBZ concentrations two- to threefold	?CYP3A4 inhibition	[62]
Clarithromycin	CBZ concentrations increased at least twofold	?CYP3A4 inhibition	[63, 64]
Anticoagulants			
Warfarin	Warfarin doses need to be reduced by at least 50 % when CBZ added	?CYP3A4 induction	[65–67]
Antidepressants			
Amitriptyline	Plasma concentrations of parent drug and nortriptyline reduced by up to 50 %	? CYP3A4 induction	[68]
Imipramine	CBZ reduces imipramine levels by 42 % and desipramine (metabolite) by 24 % but increases free fractions.	CYP3A4 and ? UGT induction	[69]
Mirtazapine	Substantial decrease (~60 %) in mirtazapine concentration	CYP3A4 induction	[70]
Moclobemide	CBZ reduces moclobemide concentrations by 41 %	CYP3A4 induction	[71]
SSRIs	Sertraline concentrations substantially reduced by CBZ	CYP3A4 induction	[72, 73]
	Fluoxetine decrease CBZ clearance by ~30 %	? CYP3A4 inhibition	
	Fluvoxamine doubles CBZ concentrations	?CYP3A4 inhibition	
Trazodone	Trazodone inhibits CBZ metabolism. Effect of CBZ on trazodone unknown	CYP3A4 inhibition	[74, 75]
Antiepileptics			

(continued)

Table 17.1 (continued)

Interacting drug	Nature of interaction	Mechanism	Reference
Levetiracetam	Toxicity may occur when levetiracetam is co-administered. Not thought to be a pharmacokinetic interaction	Pharmacodynamic	[76]
Phenobarbital	Phenobarbital may decrease CBZ concentrations	Not known	[77]
Topiramate	CBZ reduces topiramate concentrations by ~40 % but co-administration may lead to toxicity	?CYP3A4 induction	[78]
Valproate	See Sect. 17.3		
Antipsychotics			
Haloperidol	Plasma concentrations of haloperidol reduced by 40 %	CYP3A4 induction	[79]
Loxapine	CBZ concentrations increased by loxapine	Not known	[80]
Olanzapine	CBZ reduces peak plasma concentrations and half-life. AUC decreased by a third	CYP3A4 induction	[81]
Paliperidone	Dose-dependent decrease in paliperidone concentrations ranging from 45 to 66 %	CYP3A4; p-glycoprotein induction	[82]
Quetiapine	Quetiapine plasma levels may be reduced to zero by the co-administration of CBZ	CYP3A4 induction	[83]
Risperidone	CBZ halves risperidone plasma concentrations and has a similar effect on 9-hydroxyrisperidone	?CYP3A4 induction	[84]
Antivirals			
Efavirenz	CBZ substantially decreases efavirenz exposure, and efavirenz substantially decreases exposure of CBZ	? CYP3A4 induction	[85]
Indinavir	Plasma concentrations of indinavir reduced by around 75 %	CYP3A4 induction	[86]
Benzodiazepines			
Alprazolam	Plasma concentrations of alprazolam reduced by ~80 %	CYP3A4 induction	[87]
Clobazam	CBZ enhances metabolism of clobazam to norclobazam	CYP3A4 induction	[88]
Clonazepam	Bidirectional interaction: CBZ clearance decreased by ~20 %; clonazepam clearance increased by ~20 %	CYP3A4 induction ? competition for CYP3A4	[89]

Table 17.1 (continued)

Interacting drug	Nature of interaction	Mechanism	Reference
Midazolam	Massive (>90 %) reduction in plasma levels	CYP3A4 induction	[90]
Calcium channel blockers	Diltiazem increases CBZ concentrations by >100 %. Similar effect seen with verapamil	Unknown	[57, 91, 92]
Ciclosporin	CBZ reduces concentration of ciclosporin by around 50 %	? CYP3A4 induction	[93]
Danazol	CBZ and CBZ-epoxide concentrations increased by danazol. CBZ concentrations doubled	Inhibition of epoxide-trans-diol pathway	[94, 95]
Fluconazole	Fluconazole increases CBZ concentrations by around 100 %	CYP3A4 inhibition	[96]
Isoniazid	CBZ toxicity reported	Not known	[97, 98]
Isotretinoin	CBZ and CBZ-epoxide concentrations reduced by isotretinoin	? increased metabolism and/or decreased absorption	[99]
Ivabradine	CBZ reduces bioavailability by around 80 %. Peak concentrations reduced by 77 %	CYP3A4 induction	[100]
Muscle relaxants	CBZ shortens action of rocuronium	? CYP3A4 induction	[101]
Oestrogens	Plasma concentrations reduced by ~40 %. Breakthrough bleeding and ovulation occur	? CYP3A4 induction	[102]
Prednisolone	CBZ increases prednisolone clearance by ~30 %	? CYP3A4 induction	[103]
Progestogens	Levonorgestrel concentrations reduced by ~35 %	? CYP3A4 induction	[102]
Tacrolimus	CBZ reduces tacrolimus concentrations by ~50 %	CYP3A4 induction	[104]
Theophylline	CBZ reduces theophylline concentration	? CYP3A4 induction	[105, 106]
Ticlopidine	Ticlopidine may inhibit CBZ metabolism	Not known	[107]
Zolpidem	Bioavailability of zolpidem reduced by 57 % by 400 mg carbamazepine. Half-life of zolpidem decreased from 2.3 to 1.6 h	CYP3A4 induction	[108]

? presumed mechanism; no or limited experimental evidence

Table 17.2 Carbamazepine – interactions with other drugs [57, 109]

Carbamazepine is thought to decrease plasma concentrations of the following:	
Acetaminophen (paracetamol)	Praziquantel
Apixaban	Propranolol
Bosutinib	Ritonavir
Bupropion	Rivaroxaban
Busulfan	Quinine
Chloramphenicol	Quinidine
Clopidogrel	Simvastatin
Codeine	St John's Wort
Crizotinib	Thyroxine
Cyclophosphamide	Tibolone
Dabigatran	Tipranavir
Darunavir	Ulipristal
Disopyramide	Vitamin D derivatives
Doxycycline	
Dronedarone	
Etoposide	
Fingolimod	
Flunarizine	
Griseofulvin	
Imatinib	
Itraconazole	
Ketoconazole	
Lapatinib	
Lopinavir	
Metronidazole	
Metyrapone	
Nevirapine	
Ondansetron	
Pethidine (meperidine)	

Lithium does not bind to proteins and is distributed unevenly into different body compartments. It is not metabolised by the liver but is excreted almost exclusively via the kidneys. The lithium cation is filtered through the glomeruli, but 80 % of this is reabsorbed in the proximal tubules together with sodium [110]. Excretion of lithium correlates with renal function (its clearance is about 25 % of creatinine clearance values [112]). Therefore most pharmacokinetic drug interactions with lithium involve changes in distribution or elimination and are often associated with changes in sodium balance [111].

17.4.1 Antipsychotics

The combination of lithium with an antipsychotic drug during the initial phase of a manic episode when one of the agents alone is insufficient is common in clinical practice. This combination may be continued in the longer term for prophylaxis of recurring manic or depressive episodes. There are several reports that pronounced extrapyramidal side effects (EPSEs) and severe neurotoxicity (including irreversible brain damage) have developed with the combined use of lithium and various antipsychotics [113–117]. Other authors have not detected any evidence of neurotoxicity with the combination of lithium and an antipsychotic [118]. However, it is noteworthy that in the later reports of safe use, the lithium levels and the antipsychotic dose were considerably lower. Nevertheless, neurotoxicity with the use of lithium in combination with various antipsychotics, e.g. chlorpromazine, thioridazine, fluphenazine and newer ones olanzapine, risperidone and clozapine, has been reported [119–122]. Maintaining lithium levels below 1 mmol/L has been suggested as a method to reduce the risk of neurotoxicity.

One study reports higher amisulpride blood concentrations when lithium was added to amisulpride [123], and another study found reduced chlorpromazine concentrations when lithium was also used [124]. A few patients have experienced seizures with lithium and clozapine in combination [125]. Finally, caution is needed with the combination of lithium and clozapine because of the risk of lithium masking clozapine-induced agranulocytosis [126].

17.4.2 Thiazides

Thiazide diuretics appear to have the greatest potential to increase lithium concentrations to a clinically significant degree [127]. Cases describing increased lithium levels with the concurrent use of lithium and bendroflumethiazide and hydrochorthiazide have been described in the literature [128–130]. Studies looking at drug levels commonly report a 20–40 % rise in lithium plasma levels when thiazide diuretics are added to lithium treatment. A case report described a twofold rise in lithium levels in a 45-year-old woman who was prescribed bendroflumethiazide 5 mg daily for mild ankle oedema while on 1.6 g/day lithium carbonate [128].

It is thought that the mechanism of this interaction is related to the site of action of thiazide diuretics. They inhibit the sodium-chloride transporter in the distal tubule of the nephron resulting in an increased sodium loss in the urine [131]. As a compensatory mechanism after a few days, increased sodium reabsorption occurs in the proximal tubule which automatically leads to increased lithium reabsorption and consequently increased lithium levels [132]. The rise in lithium levels and toxicity has been observed commonly within the first 10 days of concurrent use although later toxicity has also been reported (e.g. after 19 days and up to 3 months) [133].

If a thiazide diuretic has to be prescribed for a patient on lithium, then the dose of the latter should first be reduced and frequency of plasma level monitoring increased. An empirical reduction of 40–70 % of lithium dosage has been proposed [134, 135] when thiazides are introduced and lithium levels rechecked in 5–6 days monitored closely thereafter. Upon withdrawal of the diuretic, the frequency of plasma level monitoring should be increased again to determine the correct dose of lithium.

17.4.3 Loop Diuretics

The result of the interaction between loop diuretics and lithium is unpredictable. A study looking at the effect of furosemide 40 mg/day for 14 days on 6 healthy volunteers taking lithium 300 mg three times per day did not find any significant changes in mean lithium plasma levels, though one of the subjects experienced marked lithium toxicity symptoms as her level rose from 0.44 to 0.71 mmol/L [136]. A nested case-control study looked into the association between hospitalisation for lithium toxicity and the use of interacting drugs such as diuretics, non-steroidal anti-inflammatory drugs (NSAIDs) and angiotensin-converting inhibitors (ACEIs) in the elderly. The concurrent use of loop diuretics was associated with a 70 % increase in the risk of hospitalisation for lithium toxicity [137]. The authors noted that older patients may be more likely to develop sodium imbalance which could result in increased lithium reabsorption in the proximal tubule. Confounding factors such as sodium-restricting diets, fluid or electrolyte imbalance in patients receiving loop diuretics can affect the assessment of the interaction between lithium and a loop diuretic. In a double blind, placebo-controlled crossover study, 13 healthy volunteers received lithium 300 mg twice daily with hydrochlorothiazide 25 mg twice/day or furosemide 20 mg twice/day or placebo at weeks 2, 4 and 6. The lithium levels after 5 days of hydrochlorthiazide treatment increased by 23.3 %, while no difference was noted after furosemide use [138]. Authors noted that the effect of thiazide diuretics might be dose-dependent; hence, the low thiazide dose used may explain the modest increase in lithium levels seen here with the hydrochlorothiazide compared to other reports. These findings, however, are consistent with those of previous studies despite the small sample size and low lithium doses [138].

Although lithium dose adjustment might not be required when a loop diuretic is added to a lithium-treated patient, frequent monitoring of lithium plasma levels is recommended [127, 133].

17.4.4 Potassium-Sparing Diuretics

The evidence for the interaction between potassium-sparing diuretics such as amiloride, spironolactone or triamterene with lithium is very limited. Amiloride did not produced notable increase in lithium plasma levels in two studies [139, 140]. In fact, amiloride has been valuable in treating lithium-induced diabetes insipidus. It reduced urine volume and increased urine osmolality in patients with vasopressin-resistant lithium-induced polyuria [140]. Evidence for triamterene and eplerenone is very sparse. In a study with 8 healthy volunteers, triamterene increased lithium excretion [141] to a small extent.

Spironolactone when added to lithium treatment was observed to slightly increase lithium levels in one study [142], while lithium excretion was slightly increased in another [143]. Since outcomes of these studies seem contradictory and inconclusive, monitoring of lithium levels would be advisable.

17.4.5 Carbonic Anhydrase Inhibitors and Osmotic Diuretics

Carbonic anhydrase inhibitor diuretics such as acetazolamide were found to increase lithium excretion leading to reduced plasma levels. This is probably owing to inhibition of sodium reabsorption in the proximal and distal renal tubules [127]. Osmotic diuretics (e.g. mannitol) similarly enhance lithium excretion (a 36 % increase reported) with corresponding reduced plasma concentrations [127, 143].

Herbal diuretic use resulted in life-threatening lithium toxicity in a case report when taken by a patient on lithium as an over-the-counter medication for weight loss [144]. Patients on lithium should be appropriately counselled on possibility of herbal-drug interactions.

17.4.6 Angiotensin-Converting Enzyme Inhibitors (ACEIs)

Numerous case reports have been published describing the development of lithium toxicity following the addition of angiotensin-converting enzyme inhibitors (ACEIs) to lithium-treated patients [145–147]. The development of toxicity seems to be gradual in onset with symptoms typically manifesting 2–5 weeks after beginning of treatment with an ACEI [127, 148]. A retrospective, longitudinal, case-control study of 20 hypertensive patients already stabilised on lithium examined the impact of ACEI (captopril, enalapril or lisinopril) initiation on lithium plasma levels. An overall 26 % decrease in lithium clearance was observed, which corresponded to an average of 35 % increase in lithium plasma levels. Four (20 %) of the patients presented with symptoms suggestive of lithium toxicity and required dose reduction or treatment discontinuation [147]. There was significant correlation between increased age and greater reduction in lithium clearance values, which is consistent with the average age of 54 years of patients affected in most case reports. The mechanism of the interaction cannot be attributed to drug equilibration since its time course is delayed. One of the theories implicates fluid depletion due to lithium-induced natriuresis and reduced thirst stimulation by ACEIs. The normal compensatory mechanism that would maintain glomerular filtration in such cases by constricting the efferent renal arterioles is blocked by ACEIs. Hence, lithium excretion is reduced.

The previously mentioned study, assessing the risk of hospitalisation for lithium toxicity due to the use of interacting drugs with lithium in the elderly, found that patients started on ACEIs were four times more likely to be hospitalised [137]. The combination of ACEIs with lithium should be ideally discouraged in the elderly considering their additional risk factors (reduced renal function, etc.).

If an ACEI is absolutely indicated, it has been recommended that lithium concentrations are closely monitored (e.g. every 1–2 weeks) for at least a month or two [133, 147]. Lithium dose reduction may be needed.

17.4.7 Angiotentsin II (AT II) Receptor Antagonists

Information about the interaction between lithium and AT II receptor antagonists comes only from case reports. Losartan and valsartan [149, 150] were found to induce lithium toxicity when added to lithium treatment. Lithium concentrations were increased by 75 % in a 77-year-old, and toxicity was evident 11 days after the combination started [149].

Angiotensin II receptor antagonists inhibit the reabsorption of sodium and water in the proximal tubule which is normally mediated by angiotensin II [149]. They also block aldosterone secretion (to a lesser extent than ACEIs) which results in increased sodium loss in the distal tubule [149]. The resulting natriuresis triggers lithium reabsorption into the circulation with consequent lithium toxicity. The time course of lithium toxicity was found to be delayed, as with ACEIs. Although the interaction between AT II receptor antagonists with lithium might be less likely compared with ACEIs, caution is recommended. More frequent lithium concentration monitoring (e.g. on weekly basis) for at least a month would be prudent [133, 149].

17.4.8 Non-steroidal Anti-inflammatory Drugs (NSAIDs)

There is a plethora of evidence that concomitant use of NSAIDs with lithium results in elevated lithium concentrations and that a decrease in lithium levels is seen on NSAID discontinuation [151]. Numerous NSAIDs have been implicated including diclofenac, ibuprofen, indomethacin, ketoprofen, mefenamic acid, naproxen, niflumic acid, piroxicam and celecoxib [133]. There is a great variability between different NSAIDs in regard to the effect on lithium plasma level as well as variability between individuals taking the same NSAID [127]. For example, two controlled studies reported a 20–59 % increase in lithium levels, on average, when indomethacin was added to lithium [152, 153]. The effect of indomethacin on lithium levels appears to be greater compared with other NSAIDs and greater in psychiatric patients versus healthy controls [152]. In many cases, lithium concentrations were increased within a week of starting the NSAID though in some, lithium intoxication was suspected only after almost a month of combined treatment [154]. Elderly patients are already at greater risk of lithium toxicity and interacting medications add a further risk.

Sulindac appears to have inconsistent effects on lithium levels in the literature with some reporting a reduction, some an increase and some no effect on lithium levels upon sulindac co-administration [155–158].

Several hypotheses regarding the mechanism of the interaction between lithium and NSAIDs have been postulated. NSAIDs inhibit the production of prostaglandins by the kidney resulting in reduced blood flow and so a decrease in renal excretion of lithium [151]. The sodium retention often seen with NSAIDs possibly as a result of reduced renal prostaglandins would be anticipated to increase lithium reabsorption as well [127].

If an NSAID (or a COX-2 inhibitor) must be used in a lithium-treated patient, this should be prescribed only for regular daily use and not 'as needed' (prn) [159]. The lithium plasma concentration should be closely monitored (initially every few days) [133] and lithium dose adjusted over the first few weeks. One study group proposed twice a week monitoring of lithium levels until the magnitude of the interaction is assessed [157]. Dose reduction of lithium may be needed.

NSAIDs are widely available over the counter; therefore, it is essential that patients are educated on the risks of concomitant use with lithium.

17.4.9 Aspirin

While aspirin also reduces the synthesis of renal prostaglandins, it has not been observed to affect lithium levels to a significant extend [127]. As with NSAIDs, monitoring of lithium levels is advisable if patients have concomitant fever or cold as this can result in altered fluid and sodium balances.

17.4.10 Calcium Channel Blockers (CCBs)

Case reports describe the development of neurotoxicity (consisting of ataxia, dysarthria, tremor) with the addition of verapamil and diltiazem to lithium-treated patients even though in some, the lithium levels remained unchanged [160, 161]. A prospective study that evaluated the pharmacokinetic effect of nifedipine (20 mg/day for 6–12 weeks) on lithium found a 30 % reduction in lithium clearance [162].

Patients with bipolar disorder are reported to have higher intracellular calcium [163], and calcium channel blockers such as verapamil and nimodipine have been studied for the management of refractory bipolar disorder [164, 165]. It is thought that lithium may also act as a calcium antagonist potentiating the action of CCBs in the brain [127]. Thus, the resultant neurotoxicity seems be due to a pharmacodynamic interaction between lithium and CCBs. Although reports of uneventful concurrent use of lithium and CCBs can be found in the literature [165], extreme caution should be exercised when CCBs are added and particularly with those having a greater effect on cardiac conduction such as verapamil or diltiazem.

17.4.11 Antiepileptics

There is some evidence that the combination of lithium and carbamazepine can result in increased incidence of neurotoxicity (such as dizziness, confusion, ataxia, somnolence) in spite of lithium plasma concentrations being within the therapeutic range. This interaction appears to be pharmacodynamic [166]. An isolated case report of interstitial nephritis with acute renal failure induced by carbamazepine resulted in toxic lithium concentrations [167]. Renal failure is a rare side effect of carbamazepine [168]. Hence, caution is required when combined with lithium. In addition, carbamazepine commonly causes hyponatraemia [168] which can trigger lithium reabsorption and lithium toxicity.

Three case reports of lithium toxicity with phenytoin and lithium combination are inconclusive due to complicating factors including the absence of a clear temporal relationship [127].

17.4.12 Xanthines

The limited evidence available for the concurrent use of aminophylline or theophylline with lithium suggests that the renal excretion of lithium is accelerated resulting in significant reduction in lithium plasma levels. A study in 10 healthy volunteers (20–37 years old) evaluated the effect of different doses of theophylline on lithium clearance and concentration. Lithium clearance was increased on average by 30 % when theophylline is added [169]. A more pronounced effect on lithium clearance was seen with higher theophylline levels. Adverse effects reported with the combination included polyuria, polydipsia and fatigue. Similarly, increases in lithium clearance have been observed with the addition of aminophylline [143] as a result of a direct blockade of sodium reabsorption at the proximal tubule. Importantly, care is required when a patient on lithium discontinues treatment with theophylline or aminophylline since lithium levels may rise and toxicity could ensue [127].

A moderate consumption of caffeine would not seem to require any lithium dose adjustment; however, withdrawal of caffeine should be done cautiously due to risk of toxicity as lithium levels may rise [133].

17.4.13 Antidepressants

The augmentation of antidepressant treatment with lithium is a common choice in the treatment of refractory depression. The combination of lithium with serotonin reuptake inhibitors has been beneficial and generally well tolerated. Symptoms suggestive of enhanced serotoninergic effect or serotonin syndrome have been described in various case reports with lithium and SSRIs [170, 171]. A study evaluating the potential pharmacokinetic interaction between venlafaxine and lithium found no clinically significant effect, but a case report describes the incidence of excessive somnolence due to pharmacodynamic interaction [172].

Serotonin syndrome and symptoms similar to neuroleptic malignant syndrome have been reported with the combination of a tricyclic antidepressant and lithium [173, 174].

17.4.14 Sodium Intake and Lithium

Higher sodium intake has been observed to reduce both the therapeutic effects of lithium and its concentration. Administration of lithium during low sodium intake has resulted in the appearance of toxic side effects [175]. Since the body does not distinguish between lithium and sodium ions, the sodium reabsorption triggered by low sodium intake might be accompanied by increased lithium retention leading to higher plasma levels. By the same mechanism in reverse, higher sodium intake has resulted in reduced therapeutic effect of the lithium [175].

Patients should be advised to avoid antacids containing sodium and restriction in their dietary sodium without informed advice and close lithium renal monitoring [133].

Lithium is contraindicated in patients with low sodium levels (e.g. in those dehydrated or on low sodium diets) and should be used cautiously with drugs affecting electrolyte balance (e.g. corticosteroids) [176].

17.4.15 Methyldopa

A few case reports have described symptoms of toxicity (e.g. confusion, restlessness, tremor, rigid movements) following the use of methyldopa with lithium [177, 178]. The mechanism of this interaction though unclear might involve an enhanced effect of lithium on the central nervous system by methyldopa and possibly lithium retention due to increased sodium reabsorption caused by methyldopa. Of note, methyldopa might cause psychiatric side effects and is contraindicated in depression [179].

17.4.16 Antibacterials

Increased lithium concentration to toxic concentrations with consequent nephrotoxicity following the addition of metronidazole has been described in three case reports [180, 181]. The impaired kidney function described was prolonged. However, in another case report, the concurrent use of these two drugs was well tolerated [180]. Lithium dose reduction should be considered (depending on the baseline lithium level) if metronidazole must be used concurrently. Close monitoring of lithium concentration, creatinine, electrolyte and urine osmolality [180, 181] is advised.

Toxicity and raised lithium levels by more than threefold was reported following the addition of tetracycline [182].

It should be noted though that in some cases, it might not be the interaction with the actual antibiotic that results in a rise in lithium levels but the associated possible dehydration during an infection. Monitoring of lithium levels and patient's mental state would be prudent.

17.4.17 Neuromuscular Blockers

Limited evidence suggest prolonged neuromuscular blockade after the use of neuromuscular blockers (e.g. pancuronium, suxomethonium) in patients on lithium [183, 184].

References

1. Rambeck B, Wolf P (1993) Lamotrigine clinical pharmacokinetics. Clin Pharmacokinet 25:433–443
2. Magdalou J, Herber R, Bidault R et al (1992) In vitro N-glucuronidation of a novel antiepileptic drug, lamotrigine, by human liver microsomes. J Pharmacol Exp Ther 260:1166–1173
3. Theis JG, Sidhu J, Palmer J et al (2005) Lack of pharmacokinetic interaction between oxcarbazepine and lamotrigine. Neuropsychopharmacology 30:2269–2274
4. Jann MW, Hon YY, Shamsi SA et al (2006) Lack of pharmacokinetic interaction between lamotrigine and olanzapine in healthy volunteers. Pharmacotherapy 26:627–633
5. Sidhu J, Job S, Bullman J et al (2006) Pharmacokinetics and tolerability of lamotrigine and olanzapine coadministered to healthy subjects. Br J Clin Pharmacol 61:420–426
6. Castberg I, Spigset O (2006) Risperidone and lamotrigine: no evidence of a drug interaction. J Clin Psychiatry 67:1159
7. Christensen J, Sandgaard AP, Sidenius P et al (2012) Lack of interaction between sertraline and lamotrigine in psychiatric patients: a retrospective study. Pharmacopsychiatry 45:119–121
8. Odishaw J, Chen C (2000) Effects of steady-state bupropion on the pharmacokinetics of lamotrigine in healthy subjects. Pharmacotherapy 20:1448–1453
9. Schieber FC, Boulton DW, Balch AH et al (2009) A non-randomized study to investigate the effects of the atypical antipsychotic aripiprazole on the steady-state pharmacokinetics of lamotrigine in patients with bipolar I disorder. Hum Psychopharmacol 24:145–152
10. Anderson GD, Yau MK, Gidal BE et al (1996) Bidirectional interaction of valproate and lamotrigine in healthy subjects. Clin Pharmacol Ther 60:145–156
11. Kanner AM, Frey M (2000) Adding valproate to lamotrigine: a study of their pharmacokinetic interaction. Neurology 55:588–591

12. Rowland A, Elliot DJ, Williams JA et al (2006) In vitro characterization of lamotrigine N2-glucuronidation and the lamotrigine-valproic acid interaction. Drug Metab Dispos 34:1055–1062
13. Sabers A, Buchholt JM, Uldall P et al (2001) Lamotrigine plasma levels reduced by oral contraceptives. Epilepsy Res 47:151–154
14. Sidhu J, Job S, Singh S et al (2006) The pharmacokinetic and pharmacodynamic consequences of the co-administration of lamotrigine and a combined oral contraceptive in healthy female subjects. Br J Clin Pharmacol 61:191–199
15. Christensen J, Petrenaite V, Atterman J et al (2007) Oral contraceptives induce lamotrigine metabolism: evidence from a double-blind, placebo-controlled trial. Epilepsia 48:484–489
16. Castberg I, Skogvoll E, Spigset O (2007) Quetiapine and drug interactions: evidence from a routine therapeutic drug monitoring service. J Clin Psychiatry 68:1540–1545
17. Andersson ML, Bjorkhem-Bergman L, Lindh JD (2011) Possible drug-drug interaction between quetiapine and lamotrigine – evidence from a Swedish TDM database. Br J Clin Pharmacol 72:153–156
18. Weintraub D, Buchsbaum R, Resor SR Jr et al (2005) Effect of antiepileptic drug comedication on lamotrigine clearance. Arch Neurol 62:1432–1436
19. Warner T, Patsalos PN, Prevett M et al (1992) Lamotrigine-induced carbamazepine toxicity: an interaction with carbamazepine-10,11-epoxide. Epilepsy Res 11:147–150
20. Binnie CD, van Emde Boas W, Kasteleijn-Nolste-Trenite DG et al (1986) Acute effects of lamotrigine (BW430C) in persons with epilepsy. Epilepsia 27:248–254
21. Anderson GD, Gidal BE, Messenheimer JA et al (2002) Time course of lamotrigine de-induction: impact of step-wise withdrawal of carbamazepine or phenytoin. Epilepsy Res 49:211–217
22. van der Lee MJ, Dawood L, ter Hofstede HJ et al (2006) Lopinavir/ritonavir reduces lamotrigine plasma concentrations in healthy subjects. Clin Pharmacol Ther 80:159–168
23. DeVane CL (2003) Pharmacokinetics, drug interactions, and tolerability of valproate. Psychopharmacol Bull 37(Suppl 2):25–42
24. Gunes A, Bilir E, Zengil H et al (2007) Inhibitory effect of valproic acid on cytochrome P450 2C9 activity in epilepsy patients. Basic Clin Pharmacol Toxicol 100:383–386
25. Sandson NB, Marcucci C, Bourke DL et al (2006) An interaction between aspirin and valproate: the relevance of plasma protein displacement drug-drug interactions. Am J Psychiatry 163:1891–1896
26. Abbott FS, Kassam J, Orr JM et al (1986) The effect of aspirin on valproic acid metabolism. Clin Pharmacol Ther 40:94–100
27. Levy RH (1984) Variability in level-dose ratio of valproate: monotherapy versus polytherapy. Epilepsia 25(Suppl 1):S10–S13
28. Chang SL, Levy RH (1985) Inhibition of epoxidation of carbamazepine by valproic acid in the isolated perfused rat liver. J Pharmacokinet Biopharm 13:453–466
29. Pisani F, Caputo M, Fazio A et al (1990) Interaction of carbamazepine-10,11-epoxide, an active metabolite of carbamazepine, with valproate: a pharmacokinetic study. Epilepsia 31:339–342
30. McKee PJ, Blacklaw J, Butler E et al (1992) Variability and clinical relevance of the interaction between sodium valproate and carbamazepine in epileptic patients. Epilepsy Res 11:193–198
31. Bernus I, Dickinson RG, Hooper WD et al (1997) The mechanism of the carbamazepine-valproate interaction in humans. Br J Clin Pharmacol 44:21–27
32. Mattson GF, Mattson RH, Cramer JA (1982) Interaction between valproic acid and carbamazepine: an in vitro study of protein binding. Ther Drug Monit 4:181–184
33. Panesar SK, Orr JM, Farrell K et al (1989) The effect of carbamazepine on valproic acid disposition in adult volunteers. Br J Clin Pharmacol 27:323–328
34. Winter HR, Devane CL, Figueroa C et al (2007) Open-label steady-state pharmacokinetic drug interaction study on co-administered quetiapine fumarate and divalproex sodium in

patients with schizophrenia, schizoaffective disorder, or bipolar disorder. Hum Psychopharmacol 22:469–476
35. Huang CC, Wei IH (2010) Unexpected interaction between quetiapine and valproate in patients with bipolar disorder. Gen Hosp Psychiatry 32:446.e1–2
36. Halaby A, Haddad R, Naja WJ (2013) Hyperammonemia induced by interaction of valproate and quetiapine. Curr Drug Saf 8:284–286
37. Anderson GD, Gidal BE, Kantor ED et al (1994) Lorazepam-valproate interaction: studies in normal subjects and isolated perfused rat liver. Epilepsia 35:221–225
38. Watson WA (1979) Interaction between clonazepam and sodium valproate. N Engl J Med 300:678–679
39. Browne TR (1979) Reply to Watson WA – interaction between clonazepam and sodium valproate. N Engl J Med 300:679
40. Vandel S, Bertschy G, Jounet JM et al (1988) Valpromide increases the plasma concentrations of amitriptyline and its metabolite nortriptyline in depressive patients. Ther Drug Monit 10:386–389
41. Fu C, Katzman M, Goldbloom DS (1994) Valproate/nortriptyline interaction. J Clin Psychopharmacol 14:205–206
42. Fehr C, Grunder G, Hiemke C et al (2000) Increase in serum clomipramine concentrations caused by valproate. J Clin Psychopharmacol 20:493–494
43. DeToledo JC, Haddad H, Ramsay RE (1997) Status epilepticus associated with the combination of valproic acid and clomipramine. Ther Drug Monit 19:71–73
44. Bertschy G, Vandel S, Jounet JM et al (1990) Valpromide-amitriptyline interaction. Increase in the bioavailability of amitriptyline and nortriptyline caused by valpromide. Encéphale 16:43–45
45. Nagai K, Shimizu T, Togo A et al (1997) Decrease in serum levels of valproic acid during treatment with a new carbapenem, panipenem/betamipron. J Antimicrob Chemother 39:295–296
46. Muzyk AJ, Candeloro CL, Christopher EJ (2010) Drug interaction between carbapenems and extended-release divalproex sodium in a patient with schizoaffective disorder. Gen Hosp Psychiatry 32:560.e1–3
47. Taha FA, Hammond DN, Sheth RD (2013) Seizures from valproate-carbapenem interaction. Pediatr Neurol 49:279–281
48. Spriet I, Goyens J, Meersseman W et al (2007) Interaction between valproate and meropenem: a retrospective study. Ann Pharmacother 41:1130–1136
49. Omoda K, Murakami T, Yumoto R et al (2005) Increased erythrocyte distribution of valproic acid in pharmacokinetic interaction with carbapenem antibiotics in rat and human. J Pharm Sci 94:1685–1693
50. Costello LE, Suppes T (1995) A clinically significant interaction between clozapine and valproate. J Clin Psychopharmacol 15:139–141
51. Taylor D (1997) Pharmacokinetic interactions involving clozapine. Br J Psychiatry 171:109–112
52. Redington K, Wells C, Petito F (1992) Erythromycin and valproate interaction. Ann Intern Med 116:877–878
53. Bergemann N, Kress KR, Bu-Tair F et al (2006) Valproate lowers plasma concentration of olanzapine. J Clin Psychopharmacol 26:432–434
54. Jonville AP, Gauchez AS, Autret E et al (1991) Interaction between isoniazid and valproate: a case of valproate overdosage. Eur J Clin Pharmacol 40:197–198
55. Kapetanovic IM, Kupferberg HJ, Porter RJ et al (1981) Mechanism of valproate-phenobarbital interaction in epileptic patients. Clin Pharmacol Ther 29:480–486
56. Annapandian VM, John GT, Mathew BS et al (2009) Pharmacokinetic interaction between sodium valproate and mycophenolate in renal allograft recipients. Transplantation 88:1143–1145

57. Spina E, Pisani F, Perucca E (1996) Clinically significant pharmacokinetic drug interactions with carbamazepine. An update. Clin Pharmacokinet 31:198–214
58. Dresser GK, Spence JD, Bailey DG (2000) Pharmacokinetic-pharmacodynamic consequences and clinical relevance of cytochrome P450 3A4 inhibition. Clin Pharmacokinet 38:41–57
59. Tempelhoff R, Modica PA, Spitznagel EL Jr (1990) Anticonvulsant therapy increases fentanyl requirements during anaesthesia for craniotomy. Can J Anaesth 37:327–332
60. Kuhn KL, Halikas JA, Kemp KD (1989) Carbamazepine treatment of cocaine dependence in methadone maintenance patients with dual opiate-cocaine addiction. NIDA Res Monogr 95:316–317
61. Dam M, Christiansen J (1977) Interaction of propoxyphene with carbamazepine. Lancet 2:509
62. Wroblewski BA, Singer WD, Whyte J (1986) Carbamazepine-erythromycin interaction. Case studies and clinical significance. JAMA 255:1165–1167
63. O'Connor NK, Fris J (1994) Clarithromycin-carbamazepine interaction in a clinical setting. J Am Board Fam Pract 7:489–492
64. Albani F, Riva R, Baruzzi A (1993) Clarithromycin-carbamazepine interaction: a case report. Epilepsia 34:161–162
65. Herman D, Locatelli I, Grabnar I et al (2006) The influence of co-treatment with carbamazepine, amiodarone and statins on warfarin metabolism and maintenance dose. Eur J Clin Pharmacol 62:291–296
66. Ross JR, Beeley L (1980) Interaction between carbamazepine and warfarin. Br Med J 280:1415–1416
67. Kendall AG, Boivin M (1981) Warfarin-carbamazepine interaction. Ann Intern Med 94:280
68. Jerling M, Bertilsson L, Sjoqvist F (1994) The use of therapeutic drug monitoring data to document kinetic drug interactions: an example with amitriptyline and nortriptyline. Ther Drug Monit 16:1–12
69. Szymura-Oleksiak J, Wyska E, Wasieczko A (2001) Pharmacokinetic interaction between imipramine and carbamazepine in patients with major depression. Psychopharmacology (Berl) 154:38–42
70. Sitsen J, Maris F, Timmer C (2001) Drug-drug interaction studies with mirtazapine and carbamazepine in healthy male subjects. Eur J Drug Metab Pharmacokinet 26:109–121
71. Rakic Ignjatovic A, Miljkovic B, Todorovic D et al (2009) Moclobemide monotherapy vs. combined therapy with valproic acid or carbamazepine in depressive patients: a pharmacokinetic interaction study. Br J Clin Pharmacol 67:199–208
72. Khan A, Shad MU, Preskorn SH (2000) Lack of sertraline efficacy probably due to an interaction with carbamazepine. J Clin Psychiatry 61:526–527
73. Martinelli V, Bocchetta A, Palmas AM et al (1993) An interaction between carbamazepine and fluvoxamine. Br J Clin Pharmacol 36:615–616
74. Sanchez-Romero A, Mayordomo-Aranda A, Garcia-Delgado R et al (2011) Probable interaction between trazodone and carbamazepine. Pharmacopsychiatry 44:158–159
75. Romero AS, Delgado RG, Pena MF (1999) Interaction between trazodone and carbamazepine. Ann Pharmacother 33:1370
76. Sisodiya SM, Sander JW, Patsalos PN (2002) Carbamazepine toxicity during combination therapy with levetiracetam: a pharmacodynamic interaction. Epilepsy Res 48:217–219
77. Sennoune S, Iliadis A, Bonneton J et al (1996) Steady state pharmacokinetics of carbamazepine-phenobarbital interaction in patients with epilepsy. Biopharm Drug Dispos 17:155–164
78. Mack CJ, Kuc S, Mulcrone SA et al (2002) Interaction of topiramate with carbamazepine: two case reports and a review of clinical experience. Seizure 11:464–467
79. Iwahashi K, Miyatake R, Suwaki H et al (1995) The drug-drug interaction effects of haloperidol on plasma carbamazepine levels. Clin Neuropharmacol 18:233–236

80. Collins DM, Gidal BE, Pitterle ME (1993) Potential interaction between carbamazepine and loxapine: case report and retrospective review. Ann Pharmacother 27:1180–1187
81. Lucas RA, Gilfillan DJ, Bergstrom RF (1998) A pharmacokinetic interaction between carbamazepine and olanzapine: observations on possible mechanism. Eur J Clin Pharmacol 54:639–643
82. Yasui-Furukori N, Kubo K, Ishioka M et al (2013) Interaction between paliperidone and carbamazepine. Ther Drug Monit 35:649–652
83. Nickl-Jockschat T, Paulzen M, Schneider F et al (2009) Drug interaction can lead to undetectable serum concentrations of quetiapine in the presence of carbamazepine. Clin Neuropharmacol 32:55
84. Ono S, Mihara K, Suzuki A et al (2002) Significant pharmacokinetic interaction between risperidone and carbamazepine: its relationship with CYP2D6 genotypes. Psychopharmacology (Berl) 162:50–54
85. Ji P, Damle B, Xie J et al (2008) Pharmacokinetic interaction between efavirenz and carbamazepine after multiple-dose administration in healthy subjects. J Clin Pharmacol 48:948–956
86. Hugen PW, Burger DM, Brinkman K et al (2000) Carbamazepine – indinavir interaction causes antiretroviral therapy failure. Ann Pharmacother 34:465–470
87. Furukori H, Otani K, Yasui N et al (1998) Effect of carbamazepine on the single oral dose pharmacokinetics of alprazolam. Neuropsychopharmacology 18:364–369
88. Levy RH, Lane EA, Guyot M et al (1983) Analysis of parent drug-metabolite relationship in the presence of an inducer. Application to the carbamazepine-clobazam interaction in normal man. Drug Metab Dispos 11:286–292
89. Yukawa E, Satou M, Nonaka T et al (2002) Pharmacoepidemiologic investigation of clonazepam relative clearance by mixed-effect modeling using routine clinical pharmacokinetic data in Japanese patients. J Clin Pharmacol 42:81–88
90. Backman JT, Olkkola KT, Ojala M et al (1996) Concentrations and effects of oral midazolam are greatly reduced in patients treated with carbamazepine or phenytoin. Epilepsia 37:253–257
91. Ahmad S (1990) Diltiazem-carbamazepine interaction. Am Heart J 120:1485–1486
92. Brodie MJ, MacPhee GJ (1986) Carbamazepine neurotoxicity precipitated by diltiazem. Br Med J (Clin Res Ed) 292:1170–1171
93. Soto Alvarez J, Sacristan Del Castillo JA, Alsar Ortiz MJ (1991) Effect of carbamazepine on cyclosporin blood level. Nephron 58:235–236
94. Kramer G, Theisohn M, von Unruh GE et al (1986) Carbamazepine-danazol drug interaction: its mechanism examined by a stable isotope technique. Ther Drug Monit 8:387–392
95. Zielinski JJ, Lichten EM, Haidukewych D (1987) Clinically significant danazol-carbamazepine interaction. Ther Drug Monit 9:24–27
96. Tsouli S, Maranis S, Kyritsis AP (2011) Fluconazole-carbamazepine interaction in a patient with bipolar disorder. Psychiatry Clin Neurosci 65:112
97. Block SH (1982) Carbamazepine-isoniazid interaction. Pediatrics 69:494–495
98. Wright JM (1983) Carbamazepine-isoniazid interaction. Pediatrics 71:139
99. Marsden JR (1988) Effect of isotretinoin on carbamazepine pharmacokinetics. Br J Dermatol 119:403–404
100. Vlase L, Neag M, Popa A et al (2011) Pharmacokinetic interaction between ivabradine and carbamazepine in healthy volunteers. J Clin Pharm Ther 36:225–229
101. Spacek A, Neiger FX, Krenn CG et al (1999) Rocuronium-induced neuromuscular block is affected by chronic carbamazepine therapy. Anesthesiology 90:109–112
102. Davis AR, Westhoff CL, Stanczyk FZ (2011) Carbamazepine coadministration with an oral contraceptive: effects on steroid pharmacokinetics, ovulation, and bleeding. Epilepsia 52:243–247
103. Olivesi A (1986) Modified elimination of prednisolone in epileptic patients on carbamazepine monotherapy, and in women using low-dose oral contraceptives. Biomed Pharmacother 40:301–308

104. Wada K, Takada M, Sakai M et al (2009) Drug interaction between tacrolimus and carbamazepine in a Japanese heart transplant recipient: a case report. J Heart Lung Transplant 28:409–411
105. Rosenberry KR, Defusco CJ, Mansmann HC Jr et al (1983) Reduced theophylline half-life induced by carbamazepine therapy. J Pediatr 102:472–474
106. Mitchell EA, Dower JC, Green RJ (1986) Interaction between carbamazepine and theophylline. N Z Med J 99:69–70
107. Brown RI, Cooper TG (1997) Ticlopidine-carbamazepine interaction in a coronary stent patient. Can J Cardiol 13:853–854
108. Vlase L, Popa A, Neag M et al (2011) Pharmacokinetic interaction between zolpidem and carbamazepine in healthy volunteers. J Clin Pharmacol 51:1233–1236
109. British Medical Association and Royal Pharmaceutical Society of Great Britain (2014) British national formulary, 68th edn. BMJ Group and Pharmaceutical Press, London
110. Malhi GS, Tanious M (2011) Optimal frequency of lithium administration in the treatment of bipolar disorder: clinical and dosing considerations. CNS Drugs 25:289–298
111. Ward ME, Musa MN, Bailey L (1994) Clinical pharmacokinetics of lithium. J Clin Pharmacol 34:280–285
112. Price LH, Heninger GR (1994) Lithium in the treatment of mood disorders. N Engl J Med 331:591–598
113. Keitner GI, Rahman S (1984) Reversible neurotoxicity with combined lithium-haloperidol administration. J Clin Psychopharmacol 4:104–105
114. Sandyk R, Hurwitz MD (1983) Toxic irreversible encephalopathy induced by lithium carbonate and haloperidol. A report of 2 cases. S Afr Med J 64:875–876
115. Cohen WJ, Cohen NH (1974) Lithium carbonate, haloperidol, and irreversible brain damage. JAMA 230:1283–1287
116. Coffey CE, Ross DR (1980) Treatment of lithium/neuroleptic neurotoxicity during lithium maintenance. Am J Psychiatry 137:736–737
117. Tharoor H, Deora S, Chauhan A et al (2007) Lithium-neuroleptic combination leading to permanent neurological sequelae. German J Psychiatry 10:18–20
118. Goldney RD, Spence ND (1986) Safety of the combination of lithium and neuroleptic drugs. Am J Psychiatry 143:882–884
119. Prakash R, Kelwala S, Ban TA (1982) Neurotoxicity with combined administration of lithium and a neuroleptic. Compr Psychiatry 23:567–571
120. Bailine SH, Doft M (1986) Neurotoxicity induced by combined lithium-thioridazine treatment. Biol Psychiatry 21:834–837
121. Swanson CL Jr, Price WA, McEvoy JP (1995) Effects of concomitant risperidone and lithium treatment. Am J Psychiatry 152:1096
122. Swartz CM (2001) Olanzapine-lithium encephalopathy. Psychosomatics 42:370
123. Bergemann N, Bu-Tair F, Kress KR et al (2007) Increase in plasma concentration of amisulpride after addition of concomitant lithium. J Clin Psychopharmacol 27:546–549
124. Rivera-Calimlim L, Kerzner B, Karch FE (1978) Effect of lithium on plasma chlorpromazine levels. Clin Pharmacol Ther 23:451–455
125. Garcia G, Crismon ML, Dorson PG (1994) Seizures in two patients after the addition of lithium to a clozapine regimen. J Clin Psychopharmacol 14:426–428
126. Kanaan RA, Kerwin RW (2006) Lithium and clozapine rechallenge: a restrospective case analysis. J Clin Psychiatry 67:756–760
127. Finley PR, Warner MD, Peabody CA (1995) Clinical relevance of drug interactions with lithium. Clin Pharmacokinet 29:172–191
128. Petersen V, Hvidt S, Thomsen K et al (1974) Effect of prolonged thiazide treatment on renal lithium clearance. Br Med J 3:143–145
129. Poust RI, Mallinger AG, Mallinger J et al (1976) Effect of chlorothiazide on the pharmacokinetics of lithium in plasma and erythrocytes. Psychopharmacol Commun 2:273–284
130. Helms PM (1982) Lithium-hydrochlorothiazide interaction? Am J Psychiatry 139:1082

131. Davies DL, Wilson GM (1975) Diuretics: mechanism of action and clinical application. Drugs 9:178–226
132. Amdisen A (1982) Lithium and drug interactions. Drugs 24:133–139
133. Pharmaceutical Press (2015) Stockley's drug interactions. https://www.medicinescomplete.com/
134. Himmelhoch JM, Forrest J, Neil JF et al (1977) Thiazide-lithium synergy in refractory mood swings. Am J Psychiatry 134:149–152
135. Himmelhoch JM, Poust RI, Mallinger AG et al (1977) Adjustment of lithium dose during lithium-chlorothiazide therapy. Clin Pharmacol Ther 22:225–227
136. Jefferson JW, Kalin NH (1979) Serum lithium levels and long-term diuretic use. JAMA 241:1134–1136
137. Juurlink DN, Mamdani MM, Kopp A et al (2004) Drug-induced lithium toxicity in the elderly: a population-based study. J Am Geriatr Soc 52:794–798
138. Crabtree BL, Mack JE, Johnson CD et al (1991) Comparison of the effects of hydrochlorothiazide and furosemide on lithium disposition. Am J Psychiatry 148:1060–1063
139. Kosten TR, Forrest JN (1986) Treatment of severe lithium-induced polyuria with amiloride. Am J Psychiatry 143:1563–1568
140. Batlle DC, von Riotte AB, Gaviria M et al (1985) Amelioration of polyuria by amiloride in patients receiving long-term lithium therapy. N Engl J Med 312:408–414
141. Wetzels JF, van Bergeijk JD, Hoitsma AJ et al (1989) Triamterene increases lithium excretion in healthy subjects: evidence for lithium transport in the cortical collecting tubule. Nephrol Dial Transplant 4:939–942
142. Baer L, Platman SR, Kassir S et al (1971) Mechanisms of renal lithium handling and their relationship to mineralocorticoids: a dissociation between sodium and lithium ions. J Psychiatr Res 8:91–105
143. Thomsen K, Schou M (1968) Renal lithium excretion in man. Am J Physiol 215:823–827
144. Pyevich D, Bogenschutz MP (2001) Herbal diuretics and lithium toxicity. Am J Psychiatry 158:1329
145. Correa FJ, Eiser AR (1992) Angiotensin-converting enzyme inhibitors and lithium toxicity. Am J Med 93:108–109
146. Douste-Blazy P, Rostin M, Livarek B et al (1986) Angiotensin converting enzyme inhibitors and lithium treatment. Lancet 1:1448
147. Finley PR, O'Brien JG, Coleman RW (1996) Lithium and angiotensin-converting enzyme inhibitors: evaluation of a potential interaction. J Clin Psychopharmacol 16:68–71
148. Lehmann K, Ritz E (1995) Angiotensin-converting enzyme inhibitors may cause renal dysfunction in patients on long-term lithium treatment. Am J Kidney Dis 25:82–87
149. Leung M, Remick RA (2000) Potential drug interaction between lithium and valsartan. J Clin Psychopharmacol 20:392–393
150. Blanche P, Raynaud E, Kerob D et al (1997) Lithium intoxication in an elderly patient after combined treatment with losartan. Eur J Clin Pharmacol 52:501
151. Phelan KM, Mosholder AD, Lu S (2003) Lithium interaction with the cyclooxygenase 2 inhibitors rofecoxib and celecoxib and other nonsteroidal anti-inflammatory drugs. J Clin Psychiatry 64:1328–1334
152. Frolich JC, Leftwich R, Ragheb M et al (1979) Indomethacin increases plasma lithium. Br Med J 1:1115–1116
153. Reimann IW, Diener U, Frolich JC (1983) Indomethacin but not aspirin increases plasma lithium ion levels. Arch Gen Psychiatry 40:283–286
154. Monji A, Maekawa T, Miura T et al (2002) Interactions between lithium and non-steroidal antiinflammatory drugs. Clin Neuropharmacol 25:241–242
155. Jones MT, Stoner SC (2000) Increased lithium concentrations reported in patients treated with sulindac. J Clin Psychiatry 61:527–528
156. Furnell MM, Davies J (1985) The effect of sulindac on lithium therapy. Drug Intell Clin Pharm 19:374–376
157. Ragheb M, Powell AL (1986) Lithium interaction with sulindac and naproxen. J Clin Psychopharmacol 6:150–154

158. Ragheb MA, Powell AL (1986) Failure of sulindac to increase serum lithium levels. J Clin Psychiatry 47:33–34
159. Taylor D, Paton C, Kapur S (2015) Maudsley prescribing guidelines in psychiatry, 12th edn. Wiley Blackwell, Oxford/London
160. Wright BA, Jarrett DB (1991) Lithium and calcium channel blockers: possible neurotoxicity. Biol Psychiatry 30:635–636
161. Dubovsky SL, Franks RD, Allen S (1987) Verapamil: a new antimanic drug with potential interactions with lithium. J Clin Psychiatry 48:371–372
162. Bruun NE, Ibsen H, Skott P et al (1988) Lithium clearance and renal tubular sodium handling during acute and long-term nifedipine treatment in essential hypertension. Clin Sci (Lond) 75:609–613
163. Dubovsky SL, Christiano J, Daniell LC et al (1989) Increased platelet intracellular calcium concentration in patients with bipolar affective disorders. Arch Gen Psychiatry 46:632–638
164. Pazzaglia PJ, Post RM, Ketter TA et al (1993) Preliminary controlled trial of nimodipine in ultra-rapid cycling affective dysregulation. Psychiatry Res 49:257–272
165. Mallinger AG, Thase ME, Haskett R et al (2008) Verapamil augmentation of lithium treatment improves outcome in mania unresponsive to lithium alone: preliminary findings and a discussion of therapeutic mechanisms. Bipolar Disord 10:856–866
166. Spina E, Perucca E (2002) Clinical significance of pharmacokinetic interactions between antiepileptic and psychotropic drugs. Epilepsia 43(Suppl 2):37–44
167. Mayan H, Golubev N, Dinour D et al (2001) Lithium intoxication due to carbamazepine-induced renal failure. Ann Pharmacother 35:560–562
168. Novartis Pharmaceuticals UK Limited (2014) Summary of product characteristics. Tegretol tablets 100mg, 200mg, 400mg. https://www.medicines.org.uk/emc/medicine/1328
169. Perry PJ, Calloway RA, Cook BL et al (1984) Theophylline precipitated alterations of lithium clearance. Acta Psychiatr Scand 69:528–537
170. Evans M, Marwick P (1990) Fluvoxamine and lithium: an unusual interaction. Br J Psychiatry 156:286
171. Sobanski T, Bagli M, Laux G et al (1997) Serotonin syndrome after lithium add-on medication to paroxetine. Pharmacopsychiatry 30:106–107
172. Adan-Manes J, Novalbos J, Lopez-Rodriguez R et al (2006) Lithium and venlafaxine interaction: a case of serotonin syndrome. J Clin Pharm Ther 31:397–400
173. Fava S, Galizia AC (1995) Neuroleptic malignant syndrome and lithium carbonate. J Psychiatry Neurosci 20:305–306
174. Kojima H, Terao T, Yoshimura R (1993) Serotonin syndrome during clomipramine and lithium treatment. Am J Psychiatry 150:1897
175. Demers RG, Heninger GR (1971) Sodium intake and lithium treatment in mania. Am J Psychiatry 128:100–104
176. Sanofi (2014) Summary of product characteristics. Priadel 400mg prolonged release tablets. https://www.medicines.org.uk/
177. Yassa R (1986) Lithium-methyldopa interaction. CMAJ 134:141–142
178. Osanloo E, Deglin JH (1980) Interaction of lithium and methyldopa. Ann Intern Med 92:433–434
179. Actavis UK Ltd (2012) Summary of product characteristics. Methyldopa tablets BP 500mg. https://www.medicines.org.uk/
180. Ayd FJ Jr (1982) Metronidazole-induced lithium intoxication. Int Drug Ther Newsl 17:15–16
181. Teicher MH, Altesman RI, Cole JO et al (1987) Possible nephrotoxic interaction of lithium and metronidazole. JAMA 257:3365–3366
182. McGennis AJ (1978) Lithium carbonate and tetracycline interaction. Br Med J 1:1183
183. Borden H, Clarke MT, Katz H (1974) The use of pancuronium bromide in patients receiving lithium carbonate. Can Anaesth Soc J 21:79–82
184. Hill GE, Wong KC, Hodges MR (1976) Potentiation of succinylcholine neuromuscular blockade by lithium carbonate. Anesthesiology 44:439–442

Chapter 18
Clinically Significant Interactions with Antidepressants

Y.W. Francis Lam

Abstract Depression is one of the most frequent and severe mental disorders, and concurrent medical conditions commonly coexist in depressed patients. This presents numerous potentials for interactions between antidepressants and other non-psychotropics prescribed for the same patient. Many selective serotonin reuptake inhibitors and selective serotonin and norepinephrine reuptake inhibitors possess various extent of inhibition towards different cytochrome P-450 isoenzymes, which constitute the primary mechanism of reported antidepressant drug interactions in the literature. Most of the antidepressants are also metabolized by the cytochrome P-450 enzyme system. As such, modulation of their hepatic elimination can occur with concurrently administered substrates, inhibitors, or inducers of the same cytochrome P-450 isoenzyme. In addition, the basal enzyme activity and genetic polymorphism affecting specific cytochrome P-450 isoenzyme can affect the magnitude and clinical significance of the cytochrome P-450-mediated drug-antidepressant interaction. In addition to drug-metabolizing enzymes, uptake and efflux drug transporters that are present at many biological membranes, including the blood-brain barrier, the intestinal epithelial cells, the hepatocytes, and the renal tubular cells, can also affect systemic exposure and central nervous system penetration of most antidepressants, and hence pharmacological response. Although cytochrome P-450-mediated drug interactions still constitute the majority of the reported literature data, more recent studies have focused on these drug transporters in mediating drug interactions, including the antidepressants. In contrast to pharmacokinetic interactions, pharmacodynamic drug interactions involving the antidepressants mostly are derived from case reports and less well documented. Nevertheless, the more relevant and clinically significant pharmacodynamic interactions will also be reviewed.

Y.W.F. Lam, PharmD, FCCP
Department of Pharmacology, University of Texas Health Science Center San Antonio, San Antonio, TX, USA

College of Pharmacy, University of Texas, Austin, TX, USA
e-mail: lamf@unthscsa.edu

M. Jann et al. (eds.), *Applied Clinical Pharmacokinetics and Pharmacodynamics of Psychopharmacological Agents*,
DOI 10.1007/978-3-319-27883-4_18

Keywords Antidepressants • Pharmacokinetics • Pharmacodynamics • Transporters • Cytochrome P-450 • Tricyclics • Selective serotonin reuptake inhibitors • Monoamine oxidase inhibitors • Serotonin-norepinephrine reuptake inhibitors

18.1 Introduction

Depression commonly coexists with other medical disorders, and it is not uncommon for depressed patients treated concurrently with antidepressants and other non-psychotropics. As such, the potentials for drug interactions among these medications are high and potentially clinically significant [1]. The aim of this chapter is to review the pharmacokinetic and pharmacodynamic interactions between antidepressants and non-psychotropics.

As a result of relative selectivity in their interaction with specific receptor accounting for their different mechanisms of action and pharmacological effects, the newer antidepressants such as selective serotonin reuptake inhibitors and selective serotonin and norepinephrine reuptake inhibitors have fewer pharmacodynamic interactions, when compared to older antidepressants such as the tricyclic antidepressants and the monoamine oxidase inhibitors. However, they are more likely to cause drug interaction involving altered drug metabolism via cytochrome P-450 enzymes modulation.

18.2 Pharmacokinetic Drug Interactions

Most of the newer antidepressants are metabolized by the cytochrome P-450 isoenzymes (Table 18.1). Nevertheless, as a result of their wide therapeutic index, the effect of altered systemic drug concentrations mediated by enzyme modulation, whether by inhibition or induction, is usually not of clinical significance. On the other hand, with their ability to inhibit different cytochrome P-450 isoenzymes (Table 18.1), the newer antidepressants can cause clinically significant drug interactions. The effect of selective serotonin reuptake inhibitors on metabolism of other drugs is reviewed elsewhere [2]. Available literature suggests that paroxetine and fluoxetine are potent inhibitors of CYP2D6 compared to other selective serotonin reuptake inhibitors with much less inhibitory effect, such as fluvoxamine, sertraline, and venlafaxine [3, 4], whereas fluvoxamine is a dual inhibitor with potent inhibitory effect towards CYP1A2 and CYP2C19.

The differential enzyme inhibitory effects of selective serotonin reuptake inhibitors have been advocated as a determinant for selection of specific drug to minimize drug interaction potential. However, the magnitude of inhibitory effect is proportional to the dose of the inhibitor, as illustrated in the study by Nichols et al. with O-desvenlafaxine, the active metabolite of venlafaxine [5]. The effects of multiple

Table 18.1 Cytochrome P-450 isoenzymes that either mediate the metabolism of or are modulated by antidepressants

	CYP isoforms responsible for metabolism	CYP isoforms modulated (inhibited or induced)
Bupropion	CYP2B6	CYP2D6 (inhibition, ++)
Citalopram, escitalopram	CYP2C19, 2D6, 3A4	CYP2D6 (inhibition, +)
Duloxetine	CYP2D6, 1A2	CYP2D6 (inhibition, ++)
Fluoxetine	CYP2C9, 2C19, 2D6, 3A4	CYP1A2 (inhibition, +) CYP2C9 (inhibition, ++) CYP2C19 (inhibition, +) CYP2D6 (inhibition, +++) CYP3A4 (inhibition, +)
Fluvoxamine	CYP1A2, 2D6	CYP1A2 (inhibition, +++) CYP2C9 (inhibition, ++) CYP2C19 (inhibition, +++) CYP2D6 (inhibition, +) CYP3A4 (inhibition, ++)
Mirtazapine	CYP1A2, 2D6, 3A4	None reported
Nefazodone	CYP3A4	CYP2D6 (inhibition, +) CYP3A4 (inhibition, +++)
Paroxetine	CYP2D6, 3A4	CYP1A2 (inhibition, +) CYP2C9 (inhibition, +) CYP2C19 (inhibition, +) CYP2D6 (inhibition, +++) CYP3A4 (inhibition, +)
Sertraline	CYP2C9, 2C19, 2D6, 3A4	CYP1A2 (inhibition, +) CYP2C9 (inhibition, +) CYP2C19 (inhibition, +) CYP2D6 (inhibition, ++) CYP3A4 (inhibition, +)
Venlafaxine	CYP2D6, 3A4	CYP2D6 (inhibition, +)

daily dosing of 100 or 400 mg desvenlafaxine on desipramine pharmacokinetics were investigated in healthy volunteers [5]. The lower-dosage regimen resulted in 25 % and 17 % increases in Cmax and AUC of desipramine, respectively, whereas the higher-dose regimen increased the Cmax and AUC of desipramine by 52 % and 90 %, respectively. Although the geometric least squares mean ratios and 90 % confidence intervals (CI) for desipramine AUC (117, 90 % CI 110–125 %) in the absence and presence of concurrent 100 mg of desvenlafaxine implied AUC bioequivalence between the two treatment arms and a study conclusion that low-dose desvenlafaxine is a relatively weak inhibitor of CYP2D6, patients receiving a higher dose, e.g., for management of obsessive compulsive disorders, or those receiving additional CYP2D6 inhibitors (e.g., bupropion is most often combined with a selective serotonin reuptake inhibitor) could be at increased risk of adverse effects associated with higher concentrations of the affected drugs.

In addition, the inhibitory effect can be modulated by the basal metabolic capacity and/or genetic capacity of the patients. As shown in the study by Azuma et al., the magnitude of inhibition is much more with CYP2D6 extensive metabolizers than in intermediate metabolizers [6]. We have previously showed that the potent inhibitory effect of the CYP2D6 substrate paroxetine was minimal in an ultrarapid metabolizer of CYP2D6 (with a genotype of *CYP2D6*2 × 2/*9*), as the subject eliminated paroxetine at an exceeding rapid rate, resulting in undetectable concentration after chronic dosing of 10 mg per day for 8 days and lack of any inhibitory effect towards CYP2D6 [7]. Genetic polymorphism in CYP2C19 was also shown to influence efficacy and side effects of citalopram. After analyzing the samples in non-Hispanic Whites from the Sequenced Treatment Alternatives to Relieve Depression (STAR*D) trial, Mrazek et al. reported that CYP2C19 poor metabolizer were more likely to experience remission ($P=0.03$) as well as having a trend of lower tolerance ($P=0.06$) [8]. As such, this potential impact on efficacy and tolerance could also occur with CYP2C19 extensive metabolizer or ultrarapid metabolizer receiving concurrent citalopram and CYP2C19 inhibitor such as omeprazole [9].

18.2.1 Antidepressants and Antiviral Agents

The use of pegylated interferon alpha (peg-interferon alpha) in the management of patients with hepatitis C virus has been reported to result in psychiatric symptoms including depressed mood [10, 11], and it is not uncommon to have antidepressants prescribed concurrently with directly acting antiviral agents such as telaprevir and boceprevir, which is part of a standard triple therapy consisting also of peg-interferon alpha and ribavirin. Currently, only escitalopram has level 1 evidence for treatment or prevention of depression in patients undergoing HCV treatment [11].

Metabolism of the directly acting antiviral agents is metabolized by the cytochrome P-450 enzymes, and hence, the potential of drug interaction exists with antidepressant therapy. Chronic dosing of telaprevir 750 mg every 8 h reduced multiple-dose escitalopram (10 mg daily) AUC by 35 %, whereas multiple dosing of boceprevir 800 mg three times per day caused a 21 % decrease in escitalopram AUC after a single 10 mg dose. The precise mechanism of the interaction is not clear, although it could be related to the induction of CYP2C19 and/or CYP3A4 responsible for escitalopram metabolism. The results of the two pharmacokinetic reports suggest that the escitalopram dosing might need to be higher in patients receiving concurrent therapy with either agent. Alternatively, antidepressants that are more selectively metabolized by CYP2D6 could be used as alternate antidepressants, since neither telaprevir nor boceprevir appear to possess CYP2D6 modulation effect. Likewise, reduction in systemic exposure of other SSRIs such as paroxetine and fluoxetine had also been reported with concurrent administration of HIV protease inhibitors. Even though there is no data to suggest reduced exposure leads to decreased efficacy, clinicians need to be aware of such interaction potential.

Lorenzini et al. recently described a case of serotonin syndrome as a result of drug-drug interaction in a 46-year-old patient with depression and coinfected with human immunodeficiency virus and hepatitis C virus [12]. The patient was initially admitted to the hospital for treatment of peritonitis and evaluation as a liver transplant candidate. Her depression had been treated with escitalopram 10 mg twice daily for 5 years. Ten days after being admitted to the hospital, she was started on 40 mg esomeprazole daily for the management of gastroesophageal reflux. Three days later, she was also started on a regimen of antiretroviral drugs consisting of darunavir 600 mg twice daily, ritonavir 100 mg twice daily, and a combination pill of 200 mg emtricitabine and 245 mg tenofovir. Four days after the addition of the antiretroviral regimens, the patient presented with nausea and confusion, and based on the presence of diaphoresis, mydriasis, myoclonus, deep tendon hyperreflexia and rigidity, she was diagnosed with serotonin syndrome and escitalopram was discontinued. The patient's clinical course improved 1 day after discontinuance of the antidepressant.

To elucidate the mechanistic basis of the clinical course, determination of the patient's escitalopram concentrations, CYP2C19 and CYP2D6 genotypes, as well as CYP2C19, CYP2D6, and CYP3A4/5 metabolic phenotypes, were performed, since all three isoenzymes contribute to escitalopram elimination [13]. The availability of two blood samples (1 at 3 days prior to initiation of esomeprazole and another 1 at 2 days after starting esomeprazole) for laboratory determination of escitalopram concentrations showed a dramatic difference in values: 52 nmol/L and 619 nmol/L, respectively (normal range: 40–250 nmol/L). Twelve hours after receiving her last dose of the antidepressant, the patient's escitalopram concentration remained elevated at 695 nmol/L. Serial concentration measurements over the next 5 days showed a prolonged elimination half-life of 67–69 h compared to the usual range of 27–33 h. In addition, DNA analysis revealed the patient having the genotypes of *CYP2C19*1/*2* and *CYP2D6*5/*10* and metabolic phenotyping results corresponding to that for a CYP2C19 intermediate metabolizer, a CYP2D6 poor metabolizer, as well as one with reduced CYP3A4/5 activity.

This unfortunate case illustrates the complexity of a drug-drug interaction in the presence of genetic deficiency in metabolic enzyme activity. The patient's CYP2C19 enzyme activity was much lower due to both the presence of the CYP2C19 inhibitor esomeprazole [14] and the defective *CYP2C19*2* allele. The elimination of escitalopram is further impaired by low CYP3A4 activity in the presence of ritonavir [15] and low CYP2D6 activity as a result of genetic polymorphism. The end result was a doubling in escitalopram elimination half-life with significantly elevated concentrations. Since escitalopram is commonly used to treat depression in this patient population [11] who commonly receive CYP2C19 and CYP3A4 modulators (proton pump inhibitors and ritonavir-based boosted antiretroviral regimen, respectively), clinicians need to be highly alert of these drug interactions.

18.2.2 Antidepressants and Tamoxifen

The antiestrogen tamoxifen is an important and effective endocrine therapy for patients with estrogen-receptor-positive breast cancer. It is essentially a prodrug, requiring conversion to active metabolites, in particular endoxifen, for its therapeutic effect. The metabolic conversion is mediated by CYP isoenzymes, with

CYP2D6 playing a vital role in the formation of endoxifen [16]. Not surprisingly, drug-induced CYP2D6 modulation could affect significantly the amount of endoxifen formed in individual patients, and potentially the therapeutic effect of tamoxifen in breast cancer [17, 18].

Both SSRIs and SNRIs are commonly prescribed to patients receiving tamoxifen therapy, not only for treating depressive symptoms but also for managing hot flashes, a common consequential occurrence with tamoxifen treatment that could affect the patient's adherence to the tamoxifen regimen. Not surprisingly, potent CYP2D6 inhibitors such as fluoxetine and paroxetine resulted in the greatest effect, with up to 66 % reduction in the amount of endoxifen concentration [19], and reportedly associated with decreased tamoxifen efficacy [20]. Consequently, it seems prudent to avoid the concurrent use of potent CYP2D6 inhibitors in tamoxifen-treated patients, as is recommended by *clinical guideline as well as regulatory agency*. When antidepressant treatment is warranted, weaker CYP2D6 inhibitors such as citalopram and venlafaxine should be considered to achieve the therapeutic objective of managing hot flashes with minimal influence on the amount of endoxifen [19].

18.2.3 Antidepressants with Beta-Blockers

With growing evidence of increased mortality and negative clinical outcomes in patients with chronic heart failure and concomitant depression [21], there is an increased trend of using antidepressants in this patient cohort [22]. Patients with heart failure are commonly prescribed beta-blockers, and it is important to take into consideration the potential interaction between potent CYP2D6 inhibitors and beta-blockers that are primarily metabolized by CYP2D6, e.g., metoprolol [23–27], carvedilol [28], and nebivolol [29]. On the other hand, the importance of CYP2D6 inhibition would depend on the overall contribution of the enzyme to the elimination of the affected drug. Even though propranolol also depends on CYP2D6 for metabolism, other metabolic enzymes and pathway, such as CYP1A2 and glucuronidation, are more important for its elimination, so the significance of CYP2D6-mediated drug interaction is much less. On the other hand, one would expect the potent CYP1A2 inhibitory effect of fluvoxamine to increase propranolol plasma concentration and pharmacological effect.

18.2.4 Antidepressants with Immunosuppressants

Patients with end-stage heart failure could be candidates for heart transplantation. Although depression occurrence appeared to decrease during the first year after heart transplantation, it often reappears in the following year necessitating initiation or continuation of antidepressant treatment [21]. The use of antidepressants in posttransplantation patients also poses drug interaction potential with immunosuppressants for the prevention of organ rejection. Immunosuppressants such as cyclosporine, sirolimus, and tacrolimus are primarily metabolized by CYP3A4; therefore, concurrent use of antidepressants that are substrates or inhibitor of this CYP isoenzyme could result in higher plasma concentrations of these immunosuppressants and potentially drug-related toxicities and even possibly increased incidence of infections. Fortunately, the common practice of therapeutic drug monitoring of immunosuppressant therapy with necessary dosage adjustment minimizes the occurrence of clinically significant drug interaction. Based on differential inhibitory effect on CYP3A4 [30], nefazodone would be the antidepressant most likely to cause significant drug interaction and should be avoided.

18.2.5 Antidepressants with Statins

Many diabetic patients have abnormal lipid profile and are managed with statins. In the setting of concurrent diabetes and depression, the clinical course of diabetes has been suggested to worsen [31, 32], possibly due to decreased desire on the part of the patient to adhere to proper dietary modification, exercise, lifestyle changes, and medication adherence. The antidepressant of choice may be limited by the undesirable weight gain associated with the tricyclic antidepressants and mirtazapine [33–35]. On the other hand, the SSRIs are safe but possess drug interaction potential that could increase adverse effect associated with statin use.

Most statins with the exception of fluvastatin, pravastatin, and rosuvastatin are primarily metabolized by CYP3A4. Therefore, antidepressant with potent CYP3A4 inhibitory effect would decrease statin metabolism and increase its associated adverse effects. Although the incidence of statin-induced severe adverse event like rhabdomyolysis is rare, the risk is significantly increased in the presence of CYP3A4 inhibition. While it is a common occurrence that drug interaction usually occurs when the inhibitor is added to a regimen of the affected drug, Karnik and Maldonado [36] reported an interesting case in which the addition of simvastatin to a patient stabilized on nefazodone resulted in rhabdomyolysis. The patient had been treated with nefazodone 150 mg twice daily for years with no side effects. However, after she had taken 40 mg of simvastatin for a month, she presented to the hospital with clinical picture and laboratory profile consistent with rhabdomyolysis. Withholding of both medications resulted in greater than 60 % decrease in creatine kinase and 30–40 % decreases in serum transaminases over 3 days. The nefazodone regimen was restarted, and the patient was referred to the primary care physician for alternative lipid-lowering therapy. This case not only demonstrated a predictable drug interaction between the CYP3A4 substrate simvastatin and the inhibitor nefazodone, but it also illustrated the concept of the drug inhibition magnitude is dose dependent, as the patient had been receiving 20 mg daily of simvastatin with nefazodone with no evidence of drug interaction or occurrence of side effect. Other than CYP-mediated inhibition as the most likely mechanism of the drug interaction, there could also be modulation of organic anion transporting polypeptide-mediated uptake of the statin into the hepatocyte, as simvastatin is a well-known substrate of the organic anion transporting polypeptide. However, as indicated in the following section, there is very little information on drug interaction between antidepressants and substrates of drug uptake transporters.

18.3 Antidepressant Interactions with Drug Transporters

Drug transporters are present at many biological membranes, including the blood-brain barrier, the intestinal epithelial cells, the hepatocytes, and the renal tubular cells. These drug transporters are broadly divided into two classes: the efflux transporters (also known as adenosine triphosphate-binding cassette [ABC] transporters, and multidrug resistance [MDR] transporters), and the uptake transporters (also known as solute-linked carrier [SLC] transporters). The well-characterized and well-studied efflux transporters are ABCB1 (also known as P-glycoprotein [Pgp] or MDR1), ABCC1 (multidrug resistance-associated protein 1 [MRP1]), ABBC2 (multidrug resistance-associated protein 2 [MRP2]), and ABCG2 (breast cancer resistance protein [BRCP]). The better-known uptake transporters are organic anion transporting polypeptides (OATPs), organic cation transporters (OCTs), and organic anion transporters (OATs).

18.3.1 ABCB1

As is the case for the cytochrome drug-metabolizing enzymes, drugs that interact with ABC transporters can be classified as substrates, inducers, or inhibitors. Based on in vitro measurements and animal studies comparing brain concentrations of antidepressants in knockout versus wild-type mice such as those conducted for venlafaxine [37–39], the antidepressants that have been identified as substrates for ABCC1 are listed in Table 18.2, as opposed to those with more conflicting data such as citalopram and fluoxetine. SSRIs such as paroxetine and sertraline have been reported to inhibit ABCB1 [40], and paroxetine have been shown in a case report to inhibit ABCB1 in the blood-brain barrier, resulting in digitalis toxicity with occurrence of symptoms such as delirium, disorientations, and visual hallucinations [41]. The beta-blocker carvedilol is a substrate for ABCB1 [42]; however, in contrast to the predictable effect of paroxetine and sertraline on the metabolism of carvedilol, their impact on its transport has not been studied.

The presence of ABCB1 on the intestinal epithelial cells can impair drug absorption of orally administered drugs. St. John's wort (*Hypericum perforatum*) is increasingly being used as a natural remedy for management of mild to moderate depression [43], and clinical studies have shown the therapeutic effect of the extracts of *Hypericum perforatum*. Available evidence suggests that hyperforin, one of the main constituents of St. John's wort, induces the activation of the pregnane X receptor, which eventually leads to increasing expression of different genes including

Table 18.2 Selected examples of substrates and modulators of ABCB1

Selected pharmacological classes	
Anticancer drugs	Doxorubicin, imatinib, methotrexate, paclitaxel, vinblastine, vincristine
Antidepressants	Amitriptyline, nortriptyline, paroxetine, venlafaxine
Antipsychotics	Risperidone
Antiretroviral drugs	Amprenavir, indinavir, lopinavir, nelfinavir, ritonavir, saquinavir
Cardiovascular drugs	Amiodarone, digoxin, diltiazem, verapamil
Beta-blockers	Carvedilol
Selected inhibitors	Amiodarone, cyclosporine, nifedipine, verapamil
Selected inducers	Rifampin, St. John's wort

ABCB1, *CYP3A4*, and *CYP2C9*. As a result of its ability to induce ABCB1 as well as cytochrome P-450 isoenzymes such as CYP3A4, CYP1A2, and CYP2C9 [44–46], St. John's wort has the potential to interact with, resulting in reduced absorption and lower systemic availability of a wide range of medications, including digoxin (ABCB1 induction) [47], cyclosporine with resultant organ rejection after transplantation (ABCB1 and CYP3A4 induction) [48], warfarin with resultant decreased international normalized ratio (CYP2C9, CYP3A4, and CYP1A2 induction) [46, 49, 50], the anticancer drug imatinib (CYP3A4 induction) [51], and antiretroviral agents such as indinavir (ABCB1 and CYP3A4 induction) [52].

In addition, literature data from a PET study using labeled verapamil suggests increased ABCB1 activity in depressed patients receiving antidepressants relative to healthy controls [53], although the increased activity could be due to the drug treatment and not to the disease per se. Nevertheless, ABCB1-mediated efflux of antidepressants and/or concurrent administration of ABCB1 modulators could influence the systemic absorption, as well as the amount of specific antidepressant substrate crossing the blood-brain barrier and be of clinical relevance in the treatment of depression. For example, the ABCB1 inhibitor itraconazole had been shown to increases the bioavailability of paroxetine [54]. Likewise, it is intriguing regarding the possibility that concurrent administration of ABCB1 inhibitor or substrate (e.g., risperidone) could affect the expression of, or compete for, ABCB1 at the blood-brain barrier and increase antidepressant concentrations [55] (e.g., sertraline) or augment their therapeutic effect in treatment-resistant patients [56]. However, currently, there is little clinical evidence to support the relevance of modulation of efflux transporters at the blood-brain barrier [57].

18.3.2 *OATPs*

In contrast to ABCB1, human OATPs are uptake transporters that facilitate hepatic uptake of drugs into the hepatocytes for metabolism or biliary secretion, and they were discovered much more recently. A total of 11 OATP transporters have been characterized and grouped into six families, with OATP1A2, OATP1A1, OATP1B3, and OATP2B1 as the most studied [58]. Compared to ABCB1, only a few substrates have been identified for OATPs [59], none of which is psychotropic, despite the findings that OATP1A2 and OATP1C1 are present in the brain [60, 61].

18.3.3 OCTs

Three OCTs have been identified in humans: OCT1 (also known as human OCT1 [hOCT1]), OCT2 (also known as human OCT2 [hOCT2]), and OCT3 (also known as human OCT3 [hOCT3]), all of which belong to the SLC22A family. OCT1 and OCT2 are primarily expressed in the hepatocytes and the kidney, respectively, whereas OCT3 is expressed in the intestinal epithelium, in addition to being expressed in hepatocyte and the kidney, albeit to a lesser extent. Interestingly, literature data suggest that OCT2 and OCT3 are expressed in the brain [62] and the monoamines are also transported by the OCTs [63–65], in addition to being transported by high-affinity neuronal plasma membrane transporters (e.g., serotonin transporters and norepinephrine transporters).

Despite the above findings [62–65], very little is known about whether there is any interaction between psychotropics and the human OCTs. As a first step to elucidate potential modulation of human OCTs by psychotropics, Haenisch et al. recently conducted an in vitro study to evaluate extent of inhibitory effect of different antidepressants and antipsychotic drugs at the three human OCTs. The results indicated that for antidepressants, desipramine, fluoxetine, nefazodone, and trimipramine showed appreciable inhibitory effect at OCT1, and despite relatively low OCT1 expression in the brain, there exist the potentials for these antidepressants to interfere with OCT-mediated transport of drugs such as metformin. Among the antidepressants studied, bupropion and nefazodone showed modest inhibitory effect at OCT2 and OCT3, respectively, and suggest that at clinically relevant doses, these two antidepressants could interfere with drug transport mediated by these two OCTs [66]. The clinical significance of these findings is currently unknown, and in vivo and human drug interaction studies are needed in the future to substantiate these in vitro findings.

18.4 Pharmacodynamic Drug Interactions

Pharmacodynamic interactions independent of pharmacokinetic mechanism usually involve synergistic or antagonistic effect at the receptor level, for example, between selective serotonin reuptake inhibitors and drugs that affect serotonergic neurotransmission and between SNRIs (such as duloxetine, venlafaxine) with those affecting both serotonergic and noradrenergic neurotransmission. Not surprisingly, tertiary amine tricyclic antidepressants and mirtazapine have higher incidence of pharmacodynamic interactions based on their action at multiple receptors and transporters. Likewise, MAOIs can interact with multiple drugs that affect noradrenergic, dopaminergic, and serotonergic neurotransmission.

However, given the potential consequence of antidepressant pharmacodynamic interactions, including hypertensive crisis or serotonin syndrome, the evaluation of such interactions in humans is not as straightforward as pharmacokinetic drug-drug interactions with measurable endpoint such as change in concentration of the affected drug. In addition, the occurrence of potentially serious adverse event also poses an ethical concern. For these reasons, literature reports on pharmacodynamic drug-drug interactions are frequently based on case reports with explanation based on extrapolation from mechanisms of action of the interacting drugs.

18.4.1 Serotonin Syndrome

One of the most significant risks associated with antidepressant use is overstimulation of serotonergic neurons as a result of drug-drug interaction. The serotonin syndrome is a serious condition that potentially can result in fatality. It is usually caused by increased serotonin stimulation [67]. The most common pharmacological intervention that results in serotonin syndrome is the concurrent use of drugs that enhance central serotonergic activity, most commonly among selective serotonin reuptake inhibitors, serotonin/norepinephrine reuptake inhibitors, and tricyclic antidepressants (Table 18.3). Although the reversible selective monoamine oxidase inhibitor moclobemide had been reported to produce a fatal case of serotonin syndrome when administered together with citalopram in a patient [68], a recent phase IV multicenter retrospective cohort study reported no increase in toxicity when rasagiline, a selective monoamine oxidase type B inhibitor was combined with a variety of different antidepressants [69]. Similarly, although the FDA had issued an alert on the combination of

Table 18.3 Selected examples of medications with serotonergic properties that may precipitate serotonin syndrome

Selected pharmacological classes	
Analgesics	Fentanyl, meperidine, tramadol
Antibiotics	Linezolid, tedizolid (approved in 2014)
Antitussive agents and cold products	Dextromethorphan, ephedrine, pseudoephedrine, phenylephrine
Monoamine oxidase inhibitors	Phenelzine, selegiline (oral formulation), tranylcypromine
Selective serotonin reuptake inhibitors	Citalopram, escitalopram, fluvoxamine, fluoxetine, paroxetine, sertraline
Serotonin norepinephrine reuptake inhibitors	Duloxetine, venlafaxine
Tricyclic antidepressants	Amitriptyline, clomipramine, desipramine, doxepin, imipramine, nortriptyline
Other antidepressants	Bupropion, St. John's wort

triptans with either selective serotonin reuptake inhibitors or serotonin/norepinephrine reuptake inhibitors, triptans have no known effects at the 5-HT_2 receptors, and the role of triptans, if any, in causing serotonin syndrome, has not been established. A literature review of the purported evidence suggested that the combination has been taken by millions of patients without any known adverse consequences related to the serotonin syndrome [70].

The oxazolidinone antibiotic linezolid is currently used for the treatment of infections with susceptible strains of methicillin-resistant *Staphylococcus aureus* or vancomycin-resistant *Enterococcus*. In addition to its antibacterial property, linezolid also exhibits mild reversible nonselective inhibition of monoamine oxidase and actually was originally discovered as a psychotropic agent with antidepressant effects. After its approval in the United States, several reports of serotonin syndrome have emerged [71, 72]. Taylor et al. conducted a retrospective study and reported a 3 % incidence of serotonin toxicity in patients treated with a combination of linezolid and selective serotonin reuptake inhibitors or venlafaxine. The time course of the drug interaction in most patients had an onset of symptoms that ranged from less than 24 h to 3 weeks of co-administration and resolution of symptoms that ranged from 1 to 5 days once one or both of the drugs were discontinued [73]. Another report described the occurrence of serotonin syndrome with concurrent administration of linezolid 600 mg twice daily and 150 mg daily of venlafaxine in an 85-year-old patient with an infected total hip joint prosthesis [74]. Given the low incidence of this drug interaction [73], linezolid co-administration with serotonergic drugs probably should not be considered an absolute contraindication. However, clinicians need to be aware of the potential adverse effects when considering the utility of this MAOI antibiotic for patients with susceptible pathogens.

Concurrent administration of serotonergic antidepressants and atypical antipsychotics is a common practice for managing psychotic depression, and serotonin syndrome has been reported in elderly patients with coexisting depression and psychosis in a 69-year-old male patient who received a combination regimen of trazodone, risperidone, and sertraline and a 72-year-old female patient treated with phenelzine and quetiapine. In both patients, symptoms disappeared within 24 h of discontinuation of the psychotropics that were implicated in the occurrence of the serotonin syndrome [75].

It is not uncommon for chronic pain and depression to coexist in the same patient, and tramadol is sometimes preferred in place of more potent analgesics. Tramadol also possesses serotonergic properties and concurrent administration of a selective serotonin reuptake inhibitor and tramadol could potentially result in increased serotonin stimulation and precipitate the serotonin syndrome. A total of nine case reports of serotonin syndrome occurring with co-administration of tramadol and therapeutic doses of selective serotonin reuptake inhibitors (citalopram, fluoxetine, paroxetine, and sertraline) have been published over a span of about 12 years. The tramadol dosage regimens documented in these case reports ranged from 50 mg daily for a few days to 400 mg per day on a chronic basis [76].

In addition to acting on the opioid receptor, tramadol also inhibits the reuptake of serotonin and norepinephrine. Nevertheless, the magnitude of inhibition of the serotonin reuptake transporter by tramadol is weak. Therefore, by itself, tramadol likely have a low potential to cause serotonin toxicity. Given that tramadol is metabolized by the cytochrome P-450 isoenzyme CYP2D6, the activity of which is variably inhibited by different SSRIs, the potential exists for a pharmacokinetic interaction involving CYP2D6 inhibition and/or the presence of poor metabolizer status for CYP2D6. A study showed that paroxetine, the most potent CYP2D6 inhibitor of the available selective serotonin reuptake inhibitors [4], produced a 37 % increase in systemic exposure of tramadol with a corresponding 67 % decrease in the extent of formation of M1 metabolite of tramadol [77]. The resultant decrease in tramadol metabolism would result in enhanced serotonergic activity within the brain and potentially serotonin syndrome. Indeed, a patient who carries two mutations affecting the *CYP2D6* gene and *CYP2C19* gene with corresponding low enzyme activities and prescribed concurrent citalopram (10 mg/day) and tramadol (50 mg/day) was reported to have increased concentrations of both drugs and exhibit the serotonin syndrome [78].

Therefore, if concurrent drug administration with tramadol is needed for a patient, a selective serotonin reuptake inhibitor with the least CYP2D6 inhibitory effect, for example, citalopram, sertraline, and venlafaxine, should be considered, as well as using lower dose of tramadol. Likewise, a patient who does not benefit from appropriate analgesic dosage regimen of tramadol could be a poor metabolizer of CYP2D6, and alternative analgesic might be necessary to avoid the potential of serotonin syndrome secondary to accumulation of tramadol.

Increased serotonergic activity can also occur as a sole result of pharmacokinetic drug-drug interaction. Four HIV-infected patients receiving a combination of fluoxetine (20–40 mg per day) and antiretroviral agents (protease inhibitors and non-nucleoside reverse transcriptase inhibitors) were evaluated for symptoms consistent with serotonin syndrome at an HIV outpatient clinic. After dose reduction or discontinuance of the fluoxetine regimen, the symptoms disappeared and all patients improved clinically. The occurrence of the syndrome was attributed to be increased fluoxetine concentrations secondary to inhibition of its metabolism by the antiretroviral regimens [79].

18.4.2 Hypertensive Crisis

Another well-described drug-drug interaction involves the monoamine oxidase inhibitors and the sympathomimetic amines, which could result in hypertensive crisis similar to the cheese reaction that occurred with a combination of monoamine oxidase inhibitors and aged cheese or other products containing the pressor agent tyramine (red wine, fermented foods) (Fig. 18.1) [80]. In general, direct-acting sympathomimetic agents such as α-adrenergic agonists and β-adrenergic agonists are considered less dangerous for this drug-drug interaction than indirect-acting sympathomimetic agents such as ephedrine and pseudoephedrine. Given the pharmacological profile of linezolid, Cantarinin et al. had demonstrated in a placebo-controlled,

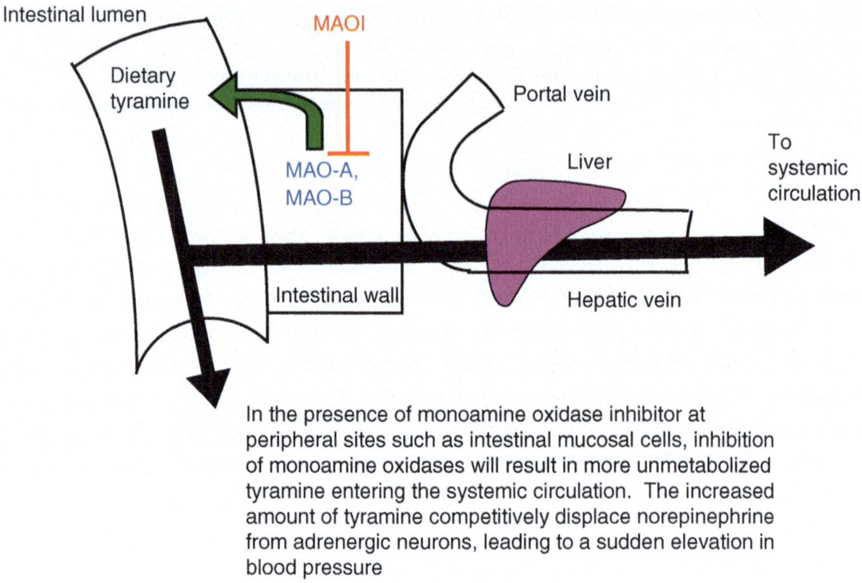

Fig. 18.1 Mechanism of cheese reaction resulting from tyramine ingestion and monoamine oxidase inhibitor administration

three-period crossover study its capacity to elicit a pressor response similar to that of moclobemide. In 12 healthy volunteers, single dose of 600 mg linezolid and 300 mg of moclobemide produced a significantly greater pressor activity than placebo [81]. The transdermal formulation of selegiline, an inhibitor of monoamine oxidase type B, had been shown to provide antidepressant effect without the harmful pressor consequences and could be used as an alternative when therapy with a monoamine oxidase inhibitor is desired [82]. Similarly, to avoid significant increases in blood pressure in linezolid-treated patients who require a decongestant product, topical nasal decongestants such as oxymetazoline should be considered instead of systemic decongestants-containing compounds such as pseudoephedrine.

18.5 Summary

With coexisting medical conditions and an increasing number of medications for their management, the potential of drug-drug interactions encountered in clinical setting continues to be a major concern. Depression is common among patients with different medical diseases such as cancer, AIDS, and cardiovascular disorders. This chapter outlines the pharmacological basis of the relevant pharmacokinetic and pharmacodynamic interactions reported in the literature. While not every potential interaction is clinically significant, understanding the pharmacokinetic and pharmacodynamic mechanisms would enable a clinician to anticipate such event and take the appropriate step to either prevent or minimize the adverse consequences.

References

1. Sinclair LI, Davies SJ, Parton G, Potokar JP (2010) Drug-drug interactions in general hospital and psychiatric hospital in-patients prescribed psychotropic medications. Int J Psychiatry Clin Pract 14:212–219
2. Ereshefsky L, Riesenman C, Lam YW (1996) Serotonin selective reuptake inhibitor drug interactions and the cytochrome P450 system. J Clin Psychiatry 57(Suppl 8):17–24; discussion 25
3. Alfaro CL, Lam YW, Simpson J, Ereshefsky L (1999) CYP2D6 status of extensive metabolizers after multiple-dose fluoxetine, fluvoxamine, paroxetine, or sertraline. J Clin Psychopharmacol 19:155–163
4. Alfaro CL, Lam YW, Simpson J, Ereshefsky L (2000) CYP2D6 inhibition by fluoxetine, paroxetine, sertraline, and venlafaxine in a crossover study: intraindividual variability and plasma concentration correlations. J Clin Pharmacol 40:58–66
5. Nichols AI, Abell M, Chen Y, Behrle JA, Frick G, Paul J (2013) Effects of desvenlafaxine on the pharmacokinetics of desipramine in healthy adults. Int Clin Psychopharmacol 28:99–105
6. Azuma J, Hasunuma T, Kubo M, Miyatake M, Koue T, Higashi K, Fujiwara T, Kitahara S, Katano T, Hara S (2012) The relationship between clinical pharmacokinetics of aripiprazole and CYP2D6 genetic polymorphism: effects of CYP enzyme inhibition by coadministration of paroxetine or fluvoxamine. Eur J Clin Pharmacol 68:29–37
7. Lam YW, Gaedigk A, Ereshefsky L, Alfaro CL, Simpson J (2002) CYP2D6 inhibition by selective serotonin reuptake inhibitors: analysis of achievable steady-state plasma concentrations and the effect of ultrarapid metabolism at CYP2D6. Pharmacotherapy 22:1001–1006
8. Mrazek DA, Biernacka JM, O'Kane DJ, Black JL, Cunningham JM, Drews MS, Snyder KA, Stevens SR, Rush AJ, Weinshilboum RM (2011) CYP2C19 variation and citalopram response. Pharmacogenet Genomics 21:1–9
9. Ogilvie BW, Yerino P, Kazmi F, Buckley DB, Rostami-Hodjegan A, Paris BL, Toren P, Parkinson A (2011) The proton pump inhibitor, omeprazole, but not lansoprazole or pantoprazole, is a metabolism-dependent inhibitor of CYP2C19: implications for coadministration with clopidogrel. Drug Metab Dispos 39:2020–2033
10. de Knegt RJ, Bezemer G, Van Gool AR, Drenth JP, Hansen BE, Droogleever Fortuyn HA, Weegink CJ, Hengeveld MW, Janssen HL (2011) Randomised clinical trial: escitalopram for the prevention of psychiatric adverse events during treatment with peginterferon-alfa-2a and ribavirin for chronic hepatitis C. Aliment Pharmacol Ther 34:1306–1317
11. Schaefer M, Sarkar R, Knop V, Effenberger S, Friebe A, Heinze L, Spengler U, Schlaepfer T, Reimer J, Buggisch P, Ockenga J, Link R, Rentrop M, Weidenbach H, Fromm G, Lieb K, Baumert TF, Heinz A, Discher T, Neumann K, Zeuzem S, Berg T (2012) Escitalopram for the prevention of peginterferon-alpha2a-associated depression in hepatitis C virus-infected patients without previous psychiatric disease: a randomized trial. Ann Intern Med 157:94–103
12. Lorenzini KI, Calmy A, Ambrosioni J, Assouline B, Daali Y, Fathi M, Rebsamen M, Desmeules J, Samer CF (2012) Serotonin syndrome following drug-drug interactions and CYP2D6 and CYP2C19 genetic polymorphisms in an HIV-infected patient. AIDS 26:2417–2418
13. Sangkuhl K, Klein TE, Altman RB (2011) PharmGKB summary: citalopram pharmacokinetics pathway. Pharmacogenet Genomics 21:769–772
14. Rocha A, Coelho EB, Sampaio SA, Lanchote VL (2010) Omeprazole preferentially inhibits the metabolism of (+)-(S)-citalopram in healthy volunteers. Br J Clin Pharmacol 70:43–51
15. Sevrioukova IF, Poulos TL (2010) Structure and mechanism of the complex between cytochrome P4503A4 and ritonavir. Proc Natl Acad Sci U S A 107:18422–18427
16. Binkhorst L, van Gelder T, Mathijssen RH (2012) Individualization of tamoxifen treatment for breast carcinoma. Clin Pharmacol Ther 92:431–433
17. Binkhorst L, van Gelder T, Loos WJ, de Jongh FE, Hamberg P, Moghaddam-Helmantel IM, de Jonge E, Jager A, Seynaeve C, van Schaik RH, Verweij J, Mathijssen RH (2012) Effects of CYP induction by rifampicin on tamoxifen exposure. Clin Pharmacol Ther 92:62–67

18. Stearns V, Johnson MD, Rae JM, Morocho A, Novielli A, Bhargava P, Hayes DF, Desta Z, Flockhart DA (2003) Active tamoxifen metabolite plasma concentrations after coadministration of tamoxifen and the selective serotonin reuptake inhibitor paroxetine. J Natl Cancer Inst 95:1758–1764
19. Borges S, Desta Z, Li L, Skaar TC, Ward BA, Nguyen A, Jin Y, Storniolo AM, Nikoloff DM, Wu L, Hillman G, Hayes DF, Stearns V, Flockhart DA (2006) Quantitative effect of CYP2D6 genotype and inhibitors on tamoxifen metabolism: implication for optimization of breast cancer treatment. Clin Pharmacol Ther 80:61–74
20. Goetz MP, Knox SK, Suman VJ, Rae JM, Safgren SL, Ames MM, Visscher DW, Reynolds C, Couch FJ, Lingle WL, Weinshilboum RM, Fritcher EG, Nibbe AM, Desta Z, Nguyen A, Flockhart DA, Perez EA, Ingle JN (2007) The impact of cytochrome P450 2D6 metabolism in women receiving adjuvant tamoxifen. Breast Cancer Res Treat 101:113–121
21. Rutledge T, Reis VA, Linke SE, Greenberg BH, Mills PJ (2006) Depression in heart failure a meta-analytic review of prevalence, intervention effects, and associations with clinical outcomes. J Am Coll Cardiol 48:1527–1537
22. Gottlieb SS, Kop WJ, Thomas SA, Katzen S, Vesely MR, Greenberg N, Marshall J, Cines M, Minshall S (2007) A double-blind placebo-controlled pilot study of controlled-release paroxetine on depression and quality of life in chronic heart failure. Am Heart J 153:868–873
23. Parker RB, Soberman JE (2011) Effects of paroxetine on the pharmacokinetics and pharmacodynamics of immediate-release and extended-release metoprolol. Pharmacotherapy 31:630–641
24. Stout SM, Nielsen J, Welage LS, Shea M, Brook R, Kerber K, Bleske BE (2011) Influence of metoprolol dosage release formulation on the pharmacokinetic drug interaction with paroxetine. J Clin Pharmacol 51:389–396
25. McCollum DL, Greene JL, McGuire DK (2004) Severe sinus bradycardia after initiation of bupropion therapy: a probable drug-drug interaction with metoprolol. Cardiovasc Drugs Ther 18:329–330
26. Walley T, Pirmohamed M, Proudlove C, Maxwell D (1993) Interaction of metoprolol and fluoxetine. Lancet 341:967–968
27. Onalan O, Cumurcu BE, Bekar L (2008) Complete atrioventricular block associated with concomitant use of metoprolol and paroxetine. Mayo Clin Proc 83:595–599
28. Stout SM, Nielsen J, Bleske BE, Shea M, Brook R, Kerber K, Welage LS (2010) The impact of paroxetine coadministration on stereospecific carvedilol pharmacokinetics. J Cardiovasc Pharmacol Ther 15:373–379
29. Lindamood C, Ortiz S, Shaw A, Rackley R, Gorski JC (2011) Effects of commonly administered agents and genetics on nebivolol pharmacokinetics: drug-drug interaction studies. J Clin Pharmacol 51:575–585
30. Lam YW, Alfaro CL, Ereshefsky L, Miller M (2003) Pharmacokinetic and pharmacodynamic interactions of oral midazolam with ketoconazole, fluoxetine, fluvoxamine, and nefazodone. J Clin Pharmacol 43:1274–1282
31. Hofmann M, Kohler B, Leichsenring F, Kruse J (2013) Depression as a risk factor for mortality in individuals with diabetes: a meta-analysis of prospective studies. PLoS One 8:e79809
32. van Dooren FE, Nefs G, Schram MT, Verhey FR, Denollet J, Pouwer F (2013) Depression and risk of mortality in people with diabetes mellitus: a systematic review and meta-analysis. PLoS One 8:e57058
33. Leucht C, Huhn M, Leucht S (2012) Amitriptyline versus placebo for major depressive disorder. Cochrane Database Syst Rev (12):CD009138
34. Serretti A, Mandelli L (2010) Antidepressants and body weight: a comprehensive review and meta analysis. J Clin Psychiatry 71:1259–1272
35. Watanabe N, Omori IM, Nakagawa A, Cipriani A, Barbui C, Churchill R, Furukawa TA (2011) Mirtazapine versus other antidepressive agents for depression. Cochrane Database Syst Rev (12):CD006528

36. Karnik NS, Maldonado JR (2005) Antidepressant and statin interactions: a review and case report of simvastatin and nefazodone-induced rhabdomyolysis and transaminitis. Psychosomatics 46:565–568
37. Bachmeier C, Levin GM, Beaulieu-Abdelahad D, Reed J, Mullan M (2013) Effect of venlafaxine and desvenlafaxine on drug efflux protein expression and biodistribution in vivo. J Pharm Sci 102:3838–3843
38. Bachmeier CJ, Beaulieu-Abdelahad D, Ganey NJ, Mullan MJ, Levin GM (2011) Induction of drug efflux protein expression by venlafaxine but not desvenlafaxine. Biopharm Drug Dispos 32:233–244
39. Ehret MJ, Levin GM, Narasimhan M, Rathinavelu A (2007) Venlafaxine induces P-glycoprotein in human Caco-2 cells. Hum Psychopharmacol 22:49–53
40. Weiss J, Dormann SM, Martin-Facklam M, Kerpen CJ, Ketabi-Kiyanvash N, Haefeli WE (2003) Inhibition of P-glycoprotein by newer antidepressants. J Pharmacol Exp Ther 305:197–204
41. Yasui-Furukori N, Kaneko S (2006) Digitalis intoxication induced by paroxetine co-administration. Lancet 367:788
42. Bachmakov I, Werner U, Endress B, Auge D, Fromm MF (2006) Characterization of beta-adrenoceptor antagonists as substrates and inhibitors of the drug transporter P-glycoprotein. Fundam Clin Pharmacol 20:273–282
43. Eliason BC, Kruger J, Mark D, Rasmann DN (1997) Dietary supplement users: demographics, product use, and medical system interaction J Am Board Fam Pract. J Am Board Fam Pract 10:265–271
44. Durr D, Stieger B, Kullak-Ublick GA, Rentsch KM, Steinert HC, Meier PJ, Fattinger K (2000) St John's Wort induces intestinal P-glycoprotein/MDR1 and intestinal and hepatic CYP3A4. Clin Pharmacol Ther 68:598–604
45. Roby CA, Anderson GD, Kantor E, Dryer DA, Burstein AH (2000) St John's Wort: effect on CYP3A4 activity. Clin Pharmacol Ther 67:451–457
46. Wang Z, Gorski JC, Hamman MA, Huang SM, Lesko LJ, Hall SD (2001) The effects of St John's wort (Hypericum perforatum) on human cytochrome P450 activity. Clin Pharmacol Ther 70:317–326
47. Johne A, Brockmoller J, Bauer S, Maurer A, Langheinrich M, Roots I (1999) Pharmacokinetic interaction of digoxin with an herbal extract from St John's wort (Hypericum perforatum). Clin Pharmacol Ther 66:338–345
48. Barone GW, Gurley BJ, Ketel BL, Abul-Ezz SR (2001) Herbal supplements: a potential for drug interactions in transplant recipients. Transplantation 71:239–241
49. Yue QY, Bergquist C, Gerden B (2000) Safety of St John's wort (Hypericum perforatum). Lancet 355:576–577
50. Jiang X, Williams KM, Liauw WS, Ammit AJ, Roufogalis BD, Duke CC, Day RO, McLachlan AJ (2004) Effect of St John's wort and ginseng on the pharmacokinetics and pharmacodynamics of warfarin in healthy subjects. Br J Clin Pharmacol 57:592–599
51. Smith P, Bullock JM, Booker BM, Haas CE, Berenson CS, Jusko WJ (2004) The influence of St. John's wort on the pharmacokinetics and protein binding of imatinib mesylate. Pharmacotherapy 24:1508–1514
52. Piscitelli SC, Burstein AH, Chaitt D, Alfaro RM, Falloon J (2000) Indinavir concentrations and St John's wort. Lancet 355:547–548
53. de Klerk OL, Willemsen AT, Roosink M, Bartels AL, Hendrikse NH, Bosker FJ, den Boer JA (2009) Locally increased P-glycoprotein function in major depression: a PET study with [11C] verapamil as a probe for P-glycoprotein function in the blood-brain. Int J Neuropsychopharmacol 12:895–904
54. Yasui-Furukori N, Saito M, Niioka T, Inoue Y, Sato Y, Kaneko S (2007) Effect of itraconazole on pharmacokinetics of paroxetine: the role of gut transporters. Ther Drug Monit 29:45–48

55. Wang JS, DeVane CL, Gibson BB, Donovan JL, Markowitz JS, Zhu HJ (2006) Population pharmacokinetic analysis of drug-drug interactions among risperidone, bupropion, and sertraline in CF1 mice. Psychopharmacology (Berl) 183:490–499
56. Clarke G, O'Mahony SM, Cryan JF, Dinan TG (2009) Verapamil in treatment resistant depression: a role for the P-glycoprotein transporter? Hum Psychopharmacol 24:217–223
57. Kalvass JC, Polli JW, Bourdet DL, Feng B, Huang SM, Liu X, Smith QR, Zhang LK, Zamek-Gliszczynski MJ, International TC (2013) Why clinical modulation of efflux transport at the human blood-brain barrier is unlikely: the ITC evidence-based position. Clin Pharmacol Ther 94:80–94
58. Hagenbuch B, Meier PJ (2004) Organic anion transporting polypeptides of the OATP/ SLC21 family: phylogenetic classification as OATP/ SLCO superfamily, new nomenclature and molecular/functional properties. Pflugers Archy 447:653–665
59. Kalliokoski A, Niemi M (2009) Impact of OATP transporters on pharmacokinetics. Br J Pharmacol 158:693–705
60. Gao B, Hagenbuch B, Kullak-Ublick GA, Benke D, Aguzzi A, Meier PJ (2000) Organic anion-transporting polypeptides mediate transport of opioid peptides across blood-brain barrier. J Pharmacol Exp Ther 294:73–79
61. Lee W, Glaeser H, Smith LH, Roberts RL, Moeckel GW, Gervasini G, Leake BF, Kim RB (2005) Polymorphisms in human organic anion-transporting polypeptide 1A2 (OATP1A2): implications for altered drug disposition and central nervous system drug entry. J Biol Chem 280:9610–9617
62. Amphoux A, Vialou V, Drescher E, Bruss M, Mannoury La Cour C, Rochat C, Millan MJ, Giros B, Bonisch H, Gautron S (2006) Differential pharmacological in vitro properties of organic cation transporters and regional distribution in rat brain. Neuropharmacology 50:941–952
63. Bacq A, Balasse L, Biala G, Guiard B, Gardier AM, Schinkel A, Louis F, Vialou V, Martres MP, Chevarin C, Hamon M, Giros B, Gautron S (2012) Organic cation transporter 2 controls brain norepinephrine and serotonin clearance and antidepressant response. Mol Psychiatry 17:926–939
64. Baganz N, Horton R, Martin K, Holmes A, Daws LC (2010) Repeated swim impairs serotonin clearance via a corticosterone-sensitive mechanism: organic cation transporter 3, the smoking gun. J Neurosci 30:15185–15195
65. Baganz NL, Horton RE, Calderon AS, Owens WA, Munn JL, Watts LT, Koldzic-Zivanovic N, Jeske NA, Koek W, Toney GM, Daws LC (2008) Organic cation transporter 3: keeping the brake on extracellular serotonin in serotonin-transporter-deficient mice. Proc Natl Acad Sci U S A 105:18976–18981
66. Haenisch B, Drescher E, Thiemer L, Xin H, Giros B, Gautron S, Bonisch H (2012) Interaction of antidepressant and antipsychotic drugs with the human organic cation transporters hOCT1, hOCT2 and hOCT3. Naunyn Schmiedebergs Arch Pharmacol 385:1017–1023
67. Sternbach H (1991) The serotonin syndrome. Am J Psychiatry 148:705–713
68. Dams R, Benijts TH, Lambert WE, Van Bocxlaer JF, Van Varenbergh D, Van Peteghem C, De Leenheer AP (2001) A fatal case of serotonin syndrome after combined moclobemide-citalopram intoxication. J Anal Toxicol 25:147–151
69. Panisset M, Chen JJ, Rhyee SH, Conner J, Mathena J, STACCATO Study Investigators (2014) Serotonin toxicity association with concomitant antidepressants and rasagiline treatment: retrospective study (STACCATO). Pharmacotherapy 34:1250–1258
70. Wenzel RG, Tepper S, Korab WE, Freitag F (2008) Serotonin syndrome risks when combining SSRI/SNRI drugs and triptans: is the FDA's alert warranted? Ann Pharmacother 42:1692–1696
71. Clark DB, Andrus MR, Byrd DC (2006) Drug interactions between linezolid and selective serotonin reuptake inhibitors: case report involving sertraline and review of the literature. Pharmacotherapy 26:269–276

72. Huang V, Gortney JS (2006) Risk of serotonin syndrome with concomitant administration of linezolid and serotonin agonists. Pharmacotherapy 26:1784–1793
73. Taylor JJ, Wilson JW, Estes LL (2006) Linezolid and serotonergic drug interactions: a retrospective survey. Clin Infect Dis 43:180–187
74. Jones SL, Athan E, O'Brien D (2004) Serotonin syndrome due to co-administration of linezolid and venlafaxine. J Antimicrob Chemother 54:289–290
75. Kohen I, Gordon ML, Manu P (2007) Serotonin syndrome in elderly patients treated for psychotic depression with atypical antipsychotics and antidepressants: two case reports. CNS Spectr 12:596–598
76. Nelson EM, Philbrick AM (2012) Avoiding serotonin syndrome: the nature of the interaction between tramadol and selective serotonin reuptake inhibitors. Ann Pharmacother 46:1712–1716
77. Laugesen S, Enggaard TP, Pedersen RS, Sindrup SH, Brosen K (2005) Paroxetine, a cytochrome P450 2D6 inhibitor, diminishes the stereoselective O-demethylation and reduces the hypoalgesic effect of tramadol. Clin Pharmacol Ther 77:312–323
78. Mahlberg R, Kunz D, Sasse J, Kirchheiner J (2004) Serotonin syndrome with tramadol and citalopram. Am J Psychiatry 161:1129
79. DeSilva KE, Le Flore DB, Marston BJ, Rimland D (2001) Serotonin syndrome in HIV-infected individuals receiving antiretroviral therapy and fluoxetine. AIDS 15:1281–1285
80. Asatoor AM, Levi AJ, Milne MD (1963) Tranylcypromine and cheese. Lancet 2:733–734
81. Cantarini MV, Painter CJ, Gilmore EM, Bolger C, Watkins CL, Hughes AM (2004) Effect of oral linezolid on the pressor response to intravenous tyramine. Br J Clin Pharmacol 58:470–475
82. Azzaro AJ, Vandenberg CM, Blob LF, Kemper EM, Sharoky M, Oren DA, Campbell BJ (2006) Tyramine pressor sensitivity during treatment with the selegiline transdermal system 6 mg/24 h in healthy subjects. J Clin Pharmacol 46:933–944

Chapter 19
Clinically Significant Interactions with Benzodiazepines

Jose Valdes, Douglas L. Boggs, Angela A. Boggs, and Jose A. Rey

Abstract Benzodiazepines are a class of lipophilic compounds used for a variety of indications including anxiety disorders, insomnia, epilepsy, musculoskeletal disorders, and as sedatives during surgery. The chemical nucleus of each benzodiazepine as well as their pharmacodynamic activity is identical. However, alterations to this basic structure lead to numerous benzodiazepines with different pharmacokinetic properties and lipid solubility resulting in agents with differing rates of elimination, concentrations, volumes of distribution, and potencies. In this chapter we will review the varied kinetics of available benzodiazepines and discuss the metabolic pathways leading to excretion of these medications. This review includes the enzymes (Phase I and Phase II) responsible for metabolism of the parent compound and their intermediates. We also review the pharmacologic and pharmacokinetic activity of the intermediate metabolites. Furthermore we will identify pharmacokinetic interactions of benzodiazepines including: drug-drug interactions, P-gylcoprotein interactions, protein-binding interactions, and food/herbal interactions. Other factors that may require alterations in benzodiazepine dosing such as weight, sex, age, smoking status, genetic polymorphisms, and pharmacokinetic

J. Valdes, PharmD, BCPP (✉)
Department of Pharmacy Practice, Neurology and Neuropsychiatry, College of Pharmacy, Nova Southeastern University, Palm Beach Gardens, FL, USA
e-mail: josevald@nova.edu

D.L. Boggs, PharmD, BCPP
Department of Psychiatry, School of Medicine, Yale University, New Haven, CT, USA
e-mail: Douglas.boggs@yale.edu

A.A. Boggs, PharmD, BCPP
Department of Pharmacy, VA Connecticut Healthcare System, Newington, CT, USA
e-mail: Douglas.boggs@yale.edu

J.A. Rey, PharmD, BCPP
Department of Pharmacy Practice, College of Pharmacy, Nova Southeastern University, Fort Lauderdale, FL, USA
e-mail: joserey@nova.edu

M. Jann et al. (eds.), *Applied Clinical Pharmacokinetics and Pharmacodynamics of Psychopharmacological Agents*,
DOI 10.1007/978-3-319-27883-4_19

interactions will similarly be discussed. Finally we will identify the clinical monitoring that is required for individuals being prescribed benzodiazepines including respiratory depression, sedation, and withdrawal. The goal of this chapter is to give the reader a background of the factors that should be considered when choosing or monitoring the available benzodiazepines in clinical practice.

Keywords Benzodiazepines • Pharmacokinetics • Metabolism • Drug interactions

19.1 Background

Early into the 1930s, a young pharmacist and postgraduate student by the name of Leo Sternbach synthesized several heptoxdiazine compounds in an attempt at developing synthetic dyes. Unbeknownst to him, these compounds Dr. Sternbach would revisit approximately three decades later, would serendipitously lead to the first anxiolytic benzodiazepine introduced for clinical use (Librium) and then one of the best-selling prescription drugs of all time (Valium) three years later [1]. Benzodiazepines are a class of lipophilic compounds used for a variety of indications including anxiety disorders, insomnia, epilepsy, musculoskeletal disorders, and as sedatives during surgery. The chemical nuclei of all benzodiazepines are identically composed of a seven-membered 1,4-diazepam ring, leading to similar effects of promoting binding of γ-aminobutyric (GABA) at the $GABA_A$ receptors allosterically. Several additions/substitutions to this basic structure at the benzene and/or diazepine ring (such as a nitro or halogen group in the seven position for sedative effects) lead to a number of compounds with different pharmacokinetic properties and lipid solubility resulting in agents with differing rates of elimination, concentrations, volumes of distribution, potencies, presence of active metabolites, duration of action, and time to onset of clinical effect [2]. Due to the fact that benzodiazepines can vary so greatly, the unique profile of the benzodiazepine should be considered when selecting the optimal agent for a particular patient. In this chapter we will review the pharmacokinetic properties of the different benzodiazepines as well as highlight interactions with other agents.

19.2 Pharmacokinetics of Benzodiazepines

Upon ingestion, benzodiazepines are rapidly and extensively absorbed from the GI tract, except for clorazepate due to decarboxylation in gastric secretions. Bioavailabilities vary between agents from approximately 80 to 100 % (except for midazolam which is metabolized by CYP3A5 in the intestinal epithelial tissue reducing bioavailability by up to 50 %) and times to peak concentration ranging from minutes to hours [3]. The length of time for the onset of action is determined by the rate of absorption from the GI tract, as opposed to the duration of action, which is determined by the rate of elimination and clearance as well as rate and extent of drug distribution. As benzodiazepines equilibrate with brain tissue after crossing the blood brain barrier due to their lipophilicity, a constant brain to plasma ratio is maintained. Concentrations in the serum reflect a proportion of concentration of benzodiazepine in the brain. This proportion is created due to the extent of receptor occupancy, which dictates the behavioral effect [4]. Following a dose of a benzodiazepine as it is absorbed and distributed from the plasma to other compartments (e.g., fat, skeletal muscle, liver), the two principal metabolic pathways of benzodiazepines convert the dose into a less lipophilic compound. Either hepatic microsomal oxidation and subsequent *N*-dealkylation or aliphatic hydroxylation and glucuronide conjugation ensure most metabolites become water soluble to allow for excretion through the kidneys and elimination from the body. While some benzodiazepines can be directly conjugated to inactive metabolites (Phase II reactions), the majority undergo initial modification by oxidation in hepatocytes through the cytochrome P450 (CYP) enzyme system (phase I reactions). Most benzodiazepines are metabolized via the CYP3A4 or CYP2C19 enzymes (see Fig. 19.1); however other cytochromes play a role in the metabolism of benzodiazepines as well (e.g., CYP1A2, CYP2D6, CYP2C9, CYP3A5) [5]. The metabolism of a benzodiazepine is complicated by its lipophilicity and therefore must follow two-compartment disposition kinetics resulting in two half-lives. The initial half-life (alpha) is the rate at which the medication moves from central to peripheral compartments; the second (longer) half-life (beta) is the rate of metabolism and excretion of the medication. Multiple doses of benzodiazepines can lead to accumulation, which can especially occur in benzodiazepines that have active metabolites with longer half-lives than the parent compound. The accumulation of benzodiazepines depends on the time of administration and the alpha and beta half-lives of each benzodiazepine and pharmacologically active metabolites [6]. Due to the differences in the pharmacokinetics and pharmacodynamics of the various benzodiazepines, one must consider multiple factors prior to prescribing or recommending a medication to achieve the desired effect and to maximize patient safety. Some factors to consider are potency (which can vary by as much as 20-fold), oral absorption rates, duration of action/half-life, and drug interactions which can increase or decrease serum levels significantly [3].

19.3 Benzodiazepines Metabolized by Primarily Phase I Reactions

Alprazolam (Niravam, Xanax, Xanax XR) (8-chloro-1-methyl-6-phenyl-4*H*-[1, 2, 4]triazolo [4,3-a] [1, 4] benzodiazepine) is a fast-acting benzodiazepine (duration approximately 5–11 h for immediate release and extended release, respectively) with an onset of 1–2 h [7]. Alprazolam (half-life: 8–15 h) is primarily metabolized by oxidation through the CYP3A family into two hydroxylated metabolites: 4-hydroxyalprazolam and α-hydroxyalprazolam [8]. CYP3A4 is thought to be responsible for

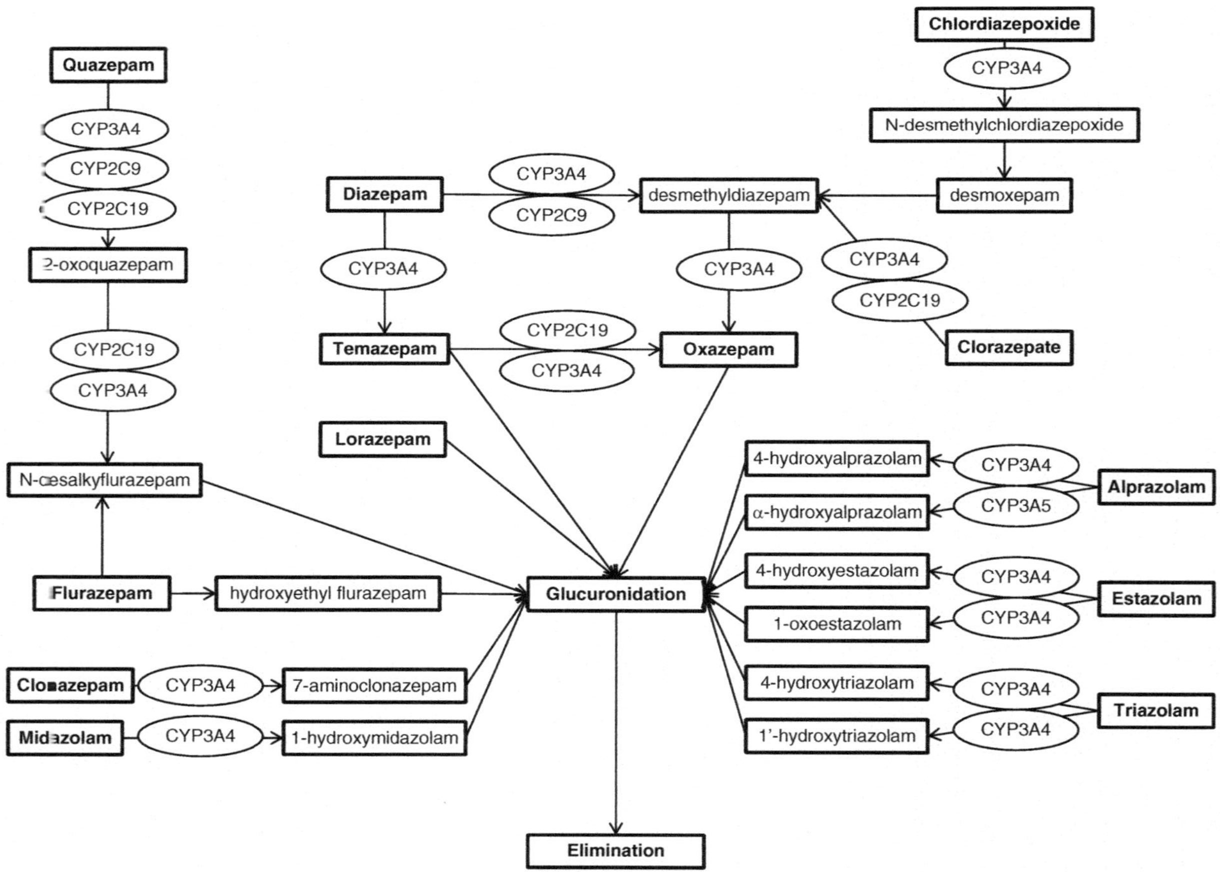

Fig. 19.1 Benzodiazepine Metabolic Pathways

the conversion to 4-hydroxyalprazolam, and CYP3A5 is involved in metabolism to α-hydroxyalprazolam [9]. However, recently some controversy exists whether CYP3A5 displays or contributes to any clinically relevant metabolism of alprazolam [10]. The metabolites 4-hydroxyalprazolam and α-hydroxyalprazolam have low relative potencies for the $GABA_A$ receptor, are metabolized quickly, and found in such low concentrations relative to the alprazolam that they are thought to contribute little to the pharmacologic properties of the parent drug. Both 4-hydroxyalprazolam and α-hydroxyalprazolam undergo conjugation in order to be excreted in the urine.

Chlordiazepoxide (Librium) (7-chloro-4-hydroxy-*N*-methyl-5-phenyl-3*H*-[1, 4] benzodiazepine-2-imine) is the oldest clinically used benzodiazepine. Pharmacokinetic studies have not progressed much to give a better understanding of how the body metabolizes this medication. Chlordiazepoxide is a fast-acting (0.5–2 h) benzodiazepine with a half-life of 6–28 h [11]. The parent compound is pharmacologically active as well as its four metabolites (desmethylchlordiazepoxide, demoxepam (half-life: 28–63 h), desmethyldiazepam (nordiazepam) (half-life: 30–200 h), and oxazepam (half-life: 5–15 h). However it also has several inactive metabolites as well [12]. The metabolism of desmethyldiazepam and oxazepam will be covered below in the diazepam and oxazepam sections, respectively. Initially chlordiazepoxide undergoes CYP450-mediated demethylation to desmethylchlordiazepoxide, then hydrolysis to demoxepam. Demoxepam is broken down into several metabolites, but the only other pharmacologically active metabolite is desmethyldiazepam, which is converted to oxazepam and undergoes conjugation directly (see below). Since chlordiazepoxide has several active metabolites, accumulation of the metabolites occurs, and it can take 2–3 weeks to reach steady state. For instance, in single-dose studies, demoxepam is in very low concentrations, but after repeated administration of chlordiazepoxide, the concentrations of demoxepam are greatly increased [12]. Caution needs to be taken particularly with the elderly and those with hepatic impairment as intermediate long-lasting metabolites can accumulate over time [13].

Clonazepam (Klonopin) (5-(2-chlorophenyl)-7-nitro-1,3-dihydro-1,4-benzodiazepin-2-one) is fast acting (20–40 min) with a half-life of 19–60 h. While clonazepam has no active metabolites, its half-life is fairly long lasting. Clonazepam undergoes nitroreduction to form 7-aminoclonazepam through CYP3A4. 7-aminoclonazepam is then removed by acetylation from *N*-acetyltransferase-2 (NAT2), hydroxylation, and glucuronidation [14–16]. Though many perceive clonazepam to be safe with regard to reducing the addiction potential of benzodiazepines due to its long half-life, addiction medicine specialist have found it is also frequently abused as a street drug [17]. In a study of reimbursement claims in Haute-Garonne, France, to evaluate the frequency of "doctor shopping" for benzodiazepines to describe abuse potential, the authors concluded that clonazepam and alprazolam fell in the category of intermediate abuse potential versus benzodiazepines like diazepam and clorazepate were of high abuse potential [18].

Clorazepate (Tranxene) (7-chloro-2-oxo-5-phenyl-1,3-dihydro-1, 4-benzodiazepine-3-carboxylic acid) is an intermediate-acting (1–2 h) benzodiazepine with rapid absorption (second only to diazepam) and with long-lasting effects due to its large half-life. Clorazepate is decarboxylated by CYP3A4 and CYP2C19 to desmethyldiazepam which has a half-life of 30–200 h and causes the majority of clinical effects. Desmethyldiazepam is then converted to oxazepam which has a reduced half-life of 5–15 h. The metabolism of desmethyldiazepam and oxazepam will be covered below in the diazepam and oxazepam sections respectfully. Studies suggest clorazepate is converted to desmethyldiazepam within a couple of hours of administration [19–21].

Diazepam (Diastat AcuDial, Diastat Pediatric, Valium) (7-chloro-1,3-dihydro-1-methyl-5-phenyl-2*H*-[1,4]benzodiazepine-2-one) is the second benzodiazepine introduced into the market. Diazepam is a highly lipophilic benzodiazepine with a very fast onset of 15 min (less with IV formulations) and a long duration of action due to its active metabolites, which largely contribute to the majority of pharmacologic effects. Diazepam's three active metabolites are desmethyldiazepam, temazepam, and oxazepam with the half-lives of 30–200 h, 8–20 h, and 5–15 h, respectively [22]. Temazepam and oxazepam undergo conjugation and are eliminated at a similar rate at which they are generated (discussed below). Diazepam has two major metabolic pathways *N*-demethylation to form desmethyldiazepam by CYP3A4 and CYP2C19 or CYP3A4 hydroxylation to temazepam (discussed below) [23, 24]. CYP2D1 can cause the formation of 4-hydroxydiazepam, but in humans the fraction is negligible. Other CYP enzymes including CYP2B6, CYP2C9, and CYP3A5 may also be involved in the formation of desmethyldiazepam [25]. The major route of metabolism for desmethyldiazepam is hydroxylation by CYP3A4 to oxazepam (discussed below).

Estazolam (ProSom) (8-chloro-6-phenyl-4H-[1,2,4]triazolo[4,3-a][1,4]benzodiazepine) is a rapidly absorbed intermediate-acting benzodiazepine with a time to onset of 0.5–2 h and a half-life of 10–24 h. The majority of estazolam is metabolized into two metabolites, 4-hydroxyestazolam by hydroxylation CYP3A4 (major) and conversion to 1-oxoestazolam (minor). Both metabolites undergo conjugation and are excreted in the urine. Neither metabolite is thought to contribute significantly to the pharmacological effects of estazolam due to their low potencies and low concentrations [26].

Flurazepam (Dalmane) (7-chloro-1-[2-(diethylamino)ethyl]-5-[2-fluorophenyl)-2,3dihydro -1*H*-[1,4]benzodiazepine-2-one) is absorbed quickly and is a long-acting benzodiazepine with a very fast onset of action in 15–20 min peaking at 3–6 h and a duration of action of 7–8 h. Flurazepam has a half-life of approximately 2 h; however, several metabolites have been identified including hydroxyethylflurazepam (half-life 2–4 h) and desalkylflurazepam (40–250 h). The metabolism of flurazepam is most likely mediated via oxidative CYP450 enzymes, but the specific enzymes have not been identified in the literature. The effects of flurazepam are almost extensively due to desalkylflurazepam due to its long half-life [27–29].

Midazolam (Versed) (8-chloro-6-(2-fluorophenyl)-1-methyl-4*H*-imidazo [1,5-a] [1,4] benzodiazepine) is quickly absorbed and very fast acting with an oral onset of action of 10–20 min and intravenous onset in as little as 3 min which makes it an ideal medication given intravenously for preanesthesia prior to surgery. Midazolam is metabolized rapidly and almost exclusively by CYP3A4 in the intestines and in the liver resulting in a half-life of 2–6 h. Hydroxylation by CYP3A4 results in the major metabolite 1'-hydroxymidazolam, which has similar pharmacologic activity as the parent compound and a half-life of approximately one hour, and the minor metabolite 4-hydroymidazolam [30]. 1'-hydroxymidazolam concentrations are roughly two-thirds of midazolam and most likely contribute to the pharmacologic activity of midazolam [31]. A secondary phase II pathway causes midazolam to undergo N2-glucuronidation catalyzed by UGT1A4, which produces a minor metabolite that may be more important in the presence of a CYP3A4 inhibitor [32]. Both 1'-hydroxymidazolam and 4-hydroymidazolam undergo further hydroxylation by CYP3A4 to another inactive metabolite 1',4-dihydroxymidazolam. 1'-hydroxymidazolam can also undergo N2-glucuronidation from UGT1A4 or O-glucuronidation from UGT2B4 or UGT2B7 [30].

Quazepam (Doral) (7-chloro-5-(2-fluorophenyl)-1-(2,2,2-trifluoroethyl)-3H-1,4-benzodiazepine-2-thione) is a rapidly absorbed benzodiazepine with a fast onset of action (20–60 min) and a long duration of action (7–10 h) due to its distribution half-life of approximately 2 h and its even longer elimination half-life. Quazepam is quickly metabolized by substitution of a sulfur group with oxygen to yield the pharmacologically active 2-oxoquazepam (half-life: 10–35 h) by CYP3A4, CYP 2C9, and CYP2C19. 2-oxoquazepam is then converted by CYP3A4 or CYP2C9 to pharmacologically active desalkylflurazepam (also known as *N*-desmethyl-2-oxoquazepam with a half-life of 40–250 h) or inactive 3-hydroxy-2-oxoquazepam in about equal amounts [33, 34].

Triazolam (Halcion) (8-chloro-6-(2-chlorophenyl)-1-methyl-4*H*-[1,2,4]triazolo [4,3-a][1,4] benzodiazepine) is a very short-acting benzodiazepine with a half-life of 1.5–5 h and a very fast onset of action that produces hypnotic effects within 15–30 min making it an effective sleep aid. Triazolam is extensively metabolized through hydroxylation by CYP3A4 (and possibly CYP3A5) into two inactive metabolites 4-hydroxytriazolam or 1'-hydroxytriazolam. Both metabolites then undergo conjugation in order to be excreted in the urine [35, 36].

19.4 Benzodiazepines Metabolized Primarily by Phase II Reactions

Lorazepam (Ativan) (7-chloro-5-(2-chlorophenyl)-3-hydroxy-1,3-dihydro-1,4-benzodiazepin-2-one) is an intermediate-acting benzodiazepine, which can take 30–60 min to take effect if given orally or fast acting 20–30 min if given intramuscularly; however IV onset is very fast 2–3 min, supporting its use as a sedative and treatment for status epilepticus. Lorazepam with a half-life of approximately 10–20 h is directly inactivated to 3-*O*-glucuronide and excreted in the urine [37]. The majority of transformation is thought to be due to UDP-glucuronosyltransferase (UGT) 2B15. No noticeable effects have been noted in lorazepam kinetics when administered with medications that alter UGT2B15 metabolism [38]. More recently other UGT enzymes have been identified that may assist in metabolism (e.g., UGT2B4, 1A7, 2B7, 1A10, and 2B15). Interestingly the UGT enzymes show preference to specific enantiomers of lorazepam. While UGT2B4, 2B7, and 2B15 metabolize both the (R) and (S)-enantiomers, (R)-lorazepam was additionally metabolized by UGT1A7 and 1A10 [39].

Oxazepam (Serax) (7-chloro-3-hydroxy-5-phenyl-1,3-dihydro-1,4-benzodiazepin-2-one) is a slow-acting benzodiazepine due to its slow absorption from the GI tract. Onset of action can be expected between 60 and 120 min and half-life approximately 5–15 h. Oxazepam is a metabolite of several other benzodiazepines (e.g., diazepam, temazepam, clorazepate, chlordiazepoxide). Oxazepam has a chiral center and is formulated as a racemic (*S*)-enantiomer and (*R*)-enantiomer of which the (*S*)-enantiomer is thought to have the majority of the pharmacologic effects. Both enantiomers are directly inactivated to 3-*O*-glucuronide and excreted in the urine directly by UGT1A9, 2B7, and 2B15 enzymes. The majority of transformation of the (*S*)-enantiomer is due to UGT 2B15 while the (*R*)–enantiomer is metabolized by UGT 1A9 and UGT 2B7 [40–42].

Temazepam (Restoril) (7-chloro-3-hydroxy-1-methyl-5-phenyl-3H-1,4-benzodiazepin-2-one) is an intermediate-acting benzodiazepine with an onset of action of 30–60 min and a half-life of 8–15 h for the parent compound. The majority of temazepam is converted to 3-*O*-glucuronide by UGT1A9, 2B7, and 2B15 after which the metabolite is then excreted in the urine. A smaller portion undergoes demethylation by CYP3A4 and CYP2C19 to oxazepam (see above) which will then also be converted to 3-*O*-glucuronide by UGT1A9, 2B7, and 2B15 [23, 43].

19.4.1 Benzodiazepine Drug Interactions

According to the Centers for Disease Control, 48.5 %, 21.7 %, and 10.6 % of persons are using at least one, three or more, or five or more prescription drugs in the past 30 days, respectively [44]. Additionally, it is estimated that 1 in every 20 people between the ages of 18 and 80 will have received a prescription for a benzodiazepine [45]. One study focusing on VA patients found that of 13,745 patients receiving a benzodiazepine, 45.3 % were identified to have a major interaction with the concomitant use of another medication [46]. Considering the amount of major interactions of benzodiazepines with other medications, it is imperative that healthcare workers be aware of the potential for dangerous combinations. When prescribing or recommending a benzodiazepine for a particular person, one must be certain to ask about any other medications being taken including prescription medications, over the counter products, herbals, dietary supplements, as well as history of alcohol use, smoking, and history of liver/kidney dysfunction. In addition to obtaining an accurate history to reduce the risk of prescribing a benzodiazepine that interacts with another medication or product, understanding and maintaining a working knowledge of potential interactions is essential. Table 19.1 provides a summary of pharmacokinetic and metabolic parameters to consider when prescribing or recommending the use of benzodiazepines.

19.4.2 P-Glycoprotein Interactions

First discovered in the investigation of multidrug-resistant tumors, the overexpression of p-glycoprotein correlated with resistance to several chemotherapeutic agents used against the tumors. This leads to research into p-glycoproteins which determined its ability to transport a wide range of compounds and determine the extent of its expression (highly) in epithelial and endothelial tissues of the gut, blood–brain barrier, and important drug-clearing organs such as the liver and the kidney. P-glycoprotein is certainly significant in the distribution and elimination of drugs, though transport activity can be saturable and subject to a variety of interactions with substrates and inhibitors. Few clinically relevant interactions between drugs have been reported to be attributable solely to p-glycoprotein, due to overlapped metabolism through other mechanisms (e.g., CYP enzymes) [47]. At least four benzodiazepines interact with p-glycoprotein, bromazepam, chlordiazepoxide, diazepam, and flurazepam, though all but flurazepam appear to behave as activators of p-glycoprotein ATPase activity (enhancing transport from the membrane bilayer to the exterior) which did not show interference with daunorubicin [48]. Flurazepam, however, is also an inhibitor of p-glycoprotein and did significantly inhibit the efflux of daunorubicin by approximately 80 % (concentration dependent) [49]. Though 80 % inhibition blocks almost all transport of daunorubicin, the concentration required to inhibit accumulation of daunorubicin is higher than the serum concentration range after human consumption and thus may not play a major role in clinical situations.

19.4.3 Protein-Binding Interactions

There is considerable variability between the benzodiazepines and the degree of protein binding, ranging from 80 % with alprazolam to nearly 99 % with diazepam. Benzodiazepines primarily bind to albumin; however triazolobenzodiazepines may bind to alpha glycoproteins to some degree. Binding of benzodiazepines to proteins will decrease the concentration of unbound (free) drug, which will decrease the

Table 19.1 Pharmacokinetic and metabolic parameters of benzodiazepines

Medication	T_{max} (h)	Half-life (h)	Metabolism	Active metabolite(s)	Active metabolite half-life (h)	Metabolite metabolism	Rate of onset
Alprazolam	1–2	8–15	3A4, 3A5(?)	None	–	–	60–120 min
Chlordiazepoxide	1–4	6–28	3A4	*N*-desmethylchlordiazepoxide	10–18 h	Hydrolysis	30 – 120 min
				Demoxepam	28–63		–
				Desmethyldiazepam	30–200	3A4	–
				Oxazepam	5–15	UGT2B15(ma), UGT1A9(mi), UGT2B7(mi)	–
Clonazepam	1–4	19–60	3A4	None	–	–	20–40 min
Clorazepate	0.5–2	1–2	3A4 and 2C19	Desmethyldiazepam	30–200	3A4	60–120 min
				Oxazepam	5–15	UGT2B15(ma), UGT1A9(mi), UGT2B7(mi)	–
Diazepam	0.5–1.5	20–70	3A4 and 2C19	Desmethyldiazepam	30–200	3A4	15 min
				Temazepam	9–12	Glucuronidation(ma), 3A4(mi), 2C19(mi)	–
				Oxazepam	5–15	UGT2B15(ma), UGT1A9(mi), UGT2B7(mi)	–
Estazolam	1.5–2.5	10–24	3A4	None	–	–	0.5 – 2 h
Flurazepam	1–2	1–2		*N*-desalkylflurazepam	40–250		15 – 20 min
Lorazepam	1–5	10–20	UGT2B15(ma)	None	–	–	30 – 60 min
Midazolam	0.5–1	1.5–2.5	3A4(ma), UGT1A4(mi)	1'-hydroxymidazolam	1	3A4, UGT1A4, UGT2B4, UGT2B7	10–20 min

(continued)

Oxazepam	2–4	5–15	UGT2B15(ma), UGT1A9(mi), UGT2B7(mi)	None	–	–	60–120 min
Quazepam	2–3	1–2	3A4, 2C9, 2C19	2-oxoquazepam	10–35	3A4, 2C9	20–60 min
				Desalkylflurazepam	40–250		–
Temazepam	2–3	8–15	UGT2B15(ma), UGT1A9(mi), UGT2B7(mi), 3A4(mi), 2C19(mi)	Oxazepam	5–15	UGT2B15(ma), UGT1A9(mi), UGT2B7(mi)	30–60 min
Triazolam	1–4	1.5–5	3A4, 3A5(?)	None	–	–	15–30 min

Metabolism is conducted by the cytochrome P450 (CYP) system unless otherwise reported, *ma* major route of metabolism, *mi* minor route of metabolism, *UGT* glucuronosyltransferase intensity of action and prolong their effects by slowing elimination [50]. While interactions with other medications can increase the free fraction of benzodiazepines, their high therapeutic index is most likely of little clinical importance [51]. However, people with hypoalbuminemia (e.g., elderly, malnutrition, cirrhosis, renal insufficiency, severe burns) have enhanced pharmacodynamic effects resulting in higher levels of free drug and increased frequency/intensity of adverse effects [52]. Overall, the interactions of highly protein-bound drugs with benzodiazepines are based on the competition for binding sites on plasma proteins and generally do not have a large clinical effect.

19.4.4 Other Interactions

Weight Over one-third of adults and just over a sixth of children in the United States are obese with a stable prevalence over the years [53]. Several alterations, both pathologically and physiologically, have been associated with obesity. However the impact on drug dosing, distribution, metabolism, and elimination remains largely unknown. Benzodiazepines being highly lipophilic compounds, one must consider the volume of distribution in obese subjects, which is generally higher than in nonobese subjects. This will cause benzodiazepines to have a higher volume of distribution [54]. The increase in volume of distribution can lead to prolonged effects [55], but the clinical significance in healthy individuals is minimal when considering the metabolism of the benzodiazepine. In 90 % of obese patients, there are histological abnormalities in liver tissue presenting as fatty infiltrates. This can result in altered enzyme activity of phase I (e.g., oxidation, reduction, and hydrolysis using CYP enzymes) or phase II systems (e.g., glucuronidation, *N*-acetylmethylation, and sulfate conjugation via uridine diphosphate glucuronosyltransferase (UGT) enzymes). With regard to phase I metabolism in obese subjects, studies showed clearance of drugs metabolized via CYP3A4 (e.g., midazolam, triazolam, alprazolam) was consistently lower, while CYP2E1 clearance showed higher activity compared to nonobese patients. Though triazolam clearance was significantly lower, midazolam and alprazolam lacked power for significance. CYP2E1 metabolism correlated with total body weight and degree of liver steatosis. Diazepam clearance via CYP2D6 enzymes in obese individuals showed a higher clearance compared to nonobese individuals with no difference in desmethyldiazepam clearance. Other CYP enzymes (CYP1A2, 2C9, and 2C19) showed a trend of increased clearance versus nonobese subjects; however the trend was not significant [56]. Overall, clearance of medications with renal and phase I metabolism is not significantly affected in obese individuals [54]. Phase II systems in obesity did show a significant difference compared to nonobese subjects when evaluating the clearance of oxazepam and lorazepam in both groups. Clearance was found to be significantly higher in obese patients for oxazepam and lorazepam compared to nonobese patients, due to an increased conjugating capacity in proportion to total body weight. With regard to elimination, obese patients showed an increase of 62 % in their estimated glomerular filtration rate (eGFR) irrespective of hypertension. Obese children did not differ compared to nonobese children with respect to eGFR [56].

Sex Another important consideration is the difference of sex on the metabolism of benzodiazepines. Pharmacokinetic differences in women can be affected due to partly having lower body weight, lower gastric emptying times, less intestinal enzymatic activity, and/or decreased GFR (10–25 % differences after adjusting for body size) [57]. Due to benzodiazepines lipophilic properties, women may have larger volumes of distribution and longer durations of action due to having larger fat stores compared to men. With regard to metabolism and metabolic rates, studies are conflicting between men and women using benzodiazepines and therefore cannot be commented on. Women taking oral contraceptives however have been found to show a decreased clearance of benzodiazepines, specifically diazepam. It was also postulated that oral contraceptives can reduce the absorption rate of diazepam as well; however no difference has been found for triazolam which is also extensively metabolized via oxidation. Overall, several benzodiazepines are metabolized through the CYP3A system, which has statistically significant differences in men and women. These differences however have not translated into significant clinical differences of benzodiazepines [58]. While nonbenzodiazepine hypnotics have shown significant clinical effects in females, higher blood levels, and prolonged effects [59], these differences have not been consistently seen in females with benzodiazepines [60].

Age Benzodiazepines are a widely used class of medicine which increases in use as we age. In fact, 2.6% of people between 18 and 35 years old use a benzodiazepine compared to 8.7% of people between the ages of 65 and 80. Not only are older patients receiving more benzodiazepines than younger patients but they also receive it for longer periods of time. Of people 65–80 years old who use benzodiazepines, 31.4% received prescriptions for long-term use versus 14.7% of people between the ages of 18 and 35 [45]. Elderly individuals are generally more susceptible to the adverse effects of benzodiazepines and have decreased clearance due to a variety of reasons including decreased oxidative metabolism which yields active metabolites and overall decreased efficiency of the liver and kidneys. When benzodiazepines are required in the elderly, it is generally recommended to use only those that undergo phase II conjugation metabolism (lorazepam, oxazepam, temazepam). Though renal insufficiency could impair excretion of the metabolites from conjugation, the metabolites are inactive and have been demonstrated to have no clinical consequences. When other benzodiazepines are used especially those with active metabolites with long half-lives such as diazepam, low doses should be started, and patients should be monitored closely for side effects due to an increased risk of accumulation [50]. In children, drug metabolism is variable and depends on the biotransformation pathway of the benzodiazepine used. Though CYP450 enzymes are low at birth, by ages 2–3 years CYP metabolism exceeds adult values and then decreases over time to reach adult levels by puberty. Glucuronidation is also low in neonates, which will prolong the half-life of clorazepate, but will reach adult levels by ages

3–4 years. Diazepam clearance is also reduced due to the minimized capacity of hydroxylation in infants [3].

Smoking Smoking can lead to enhanced elimination of medications through inducing CYP450 enzymes, especially CYP1A2 which represents the metabolism of approximately 5 % of all drugs [56]. While benzodiazepines are not generally substrates of CYP1A2 some studies have shown increased metabolism of some benzodiazepines, although these results are not consistent [61, 62]. In general it is possible that smoking results in increased metabolism but likely does not substantially change pharmacokinetic parameters of most benzodiazepines, although the package insert for alprazolam reports a 50 % decrease in concentrations in smokers. Nicotine may also have an effect as a CNS stimulant which may attenuate sedation as seen in smokers compared to nonsmokers using benzodiazepines [63].

19.4.5 Food and Herbals

Due to benzodiazepines being highly lipophilic, they generally have fast absorption times as well as bioavailabilities. Interactions that exist with food and herbal supplements are due to inhibition/induction of various CYP enzymes. Grapefruit juice is a classic example of a food that inhibits the CYP3A4 enzyme system [64]. Interacting specifically with diazepam, midazolam, quazepam, and triazolam, grapefruit juice increases the AUC and Cmax of the benzodiazepines and can last up to 72 h after a single glass [65, 66]. Interestingly alprazolam concentrations are not sensitive to grapefruit, although it is metabolized by CYP3A4 [65]. Echinacea has also been shown to cause a decrease in the plasma concentration of midazolam via CYP3A enzyme induction [67]. Taking a benzodiazepine concomitantly with kava can increase central nervous system side effects. In one case report, a 54-year-old man was found in a semicomatose state after using alprazolam and kava, cimetidine, and terazosin [68]. Studies of St. John's wort reducing the effectiveness of alprazolam, midazolam, and quazepam via CYP3A4 induction have also been published, with the theoretical possibility for the same effects on clonazepam, diazepam, and triazolam [69–71].

19.4.6 Pharmacokinetic Drug Interactions

The majority of pharmacokinetic drug interactions are due to inhibition or induction of CYP450 enzymes, specifically CYP3A4 or CYP2C19. As shown in Fig. 19.1, these enzymes metabolize many benzodiazepines and their active metabolites. When given in the presence of enzymatic inhibitors, benzodiazepines could have higher peak levels and effects that are longer lasting. In the presence of inducers, higher doses of the benzodiazepine may be needed to have the intended clinical effect. Since many psychotropic medications interact with the CYP450 system, it is important to evaluate the other medications before starting a benzodiazepine, especially those that are metabolized through phase I reactions. Since lorazepam, oxazepam, and temazepam primarily are metabolized by phase II reactions and have no active metabolites, they are likely to not have significant drug interactions.

19.4.7 Pharmacodynamic Interactions

Pharmacodynamic interactions involve either inhibition or enhancement of the clinical effects of the drug. The most important pharmacodynamic drug interactions with benzodiazepines involve the concomitant use of other CNS depressants including antipsychotics, barbiturates, phenytoin, sedative antihistamines, opioids, and alcohol. Combination with these substances can lead to increased sedation, motor impairment, and respiratory depression. Respiratory depression is especially dangerous when opioid agonists or alcohol is combined with benzodiazepines as it can result in death [72, 73]. Another combination that is dangerous is the combination of intramuscular olanzapine and parenteral benzodiazepines due to their association with excessive sedation, respiratory depression, and death [74].

19.4.8 Case Presentation

A 19-year-old male college student diagnosed with generalized anxiety disorder has been taking clorazepate 15 mg twice a day for the last year. The patient has reported at previous appointments effectiveness with clorazepate and denied side effects. A month later the patient returns to clinic complaining of daytime sedation, dizziness, and an inability to focus on schoolwork. He has not been able to take clorazepate during the day for fear of having a car accident while driving. He also reports increased anxiety since he is unable to take clorazepate and requests a change in medication since finals week is starting soon, and daily anxiety is making it increasingly difficult to go to class, focus on school work, and sleep at night. As you review the patient's current medication regimen, you discover the patient was started on omeprazole 20 mg/day for gastroesophageal reflux disease (GERD) 3 weeks ago and was told to discontinue in another week.

19.4.8.1 Case Discussion

Omeprazole is a strong inhibitor of CYP2C19 and CYP3A4 [75]. The benzodiazepine clorazepate is a substrate of CYP2C19 and CYP3A4 (see above). The addition of omeprazole significantly impaired the ability of CZYP2C19 and CYP3A4 to metabolize clorazepate. The result of this drug interaction was an increase in clorazepate blood levels, which increased side effects of clorazepate such as sedation, decreased concentration, and dizziness reported by the patient above. You eventually recognized the significance of the drug interaction with the addition of omeprazole to clorazepate and recommended switching omeprazole to pantoprazole, a proton pump inhibitor that does not cause 2C19 inhibition.

19.4.9 Genetic Polymorphisms

It is now recognized that one reason why some medications may have an effect in one person and have a different effect on another is due to the genetic variation each person has. This genetic variation has been shown to play a role in the way we metabolize medications especially via phase I and phase II reactions [76]. Specific genes encode each UGT and CYP enzyme, making them susceptible to genetic variability. In fact, the nomenclature for UGT and CYP enzymes tell you exactly which gene they can be found in (i.e., CYP indicating cytochrome P450, followed by a number indicating the gene family, followed by a letter indicating the subfamily, followed by another number indicating the gene) [76]. When a person inherits a genetic allele from each parent, they can inherit a wild-type or a variant allele. Polymorphisms occur when one or both wild-type alleles are replaced by a variant which results in people who are "poor metabolizers" (two variant alleles) or patients with reduced enzyme activity (a wild-type and a variant allele). Alternatively when a person obtains multiple copies of wild-type allele, a polymorphism occurs, resulting in "ultra-rapid" or "rapid" metabolizers due to the excess enzyme activity seen [77]. Though genetic testing is not routinely performed in patients (prospective trials needed to demonstrate improved outcomes and cost effectiveness), a keen observer may suspect a patient of being a rapid, reduced, or poor metabolizer of an agent based on their response to therapy or by using information from large-scale studies to determine risks associated with certain ethnicities (e.g., Asians and HLA-B* 1502 testing) [76].

19.5 Phase I

Only a few CYP450 are significantly involved in the metabolism of benzodiazepines including CYP3A4/5 and CYP 2C19 (see above).

CYP 3A4/5 Represents the metabolism of approximately 50 % of all drugs, with the majority metabolized via CYP3A4 [56]. However data on the impact on benzodiazepine metabolism due to CYP3A4/5 polymorphisms is mixed. With over 40 different variants of CYP3A4 and 14 variants of CYP3A5, most are nonfunctional and have a minimal role in predicting metabolic activity [78]. Of functional significance, only a few CYP3A4 (e.g., CYP3A4*8, CYP 3A4*11, CYP3A4*12, and CYP 3A4*13) and CYP3A5 variants (e.g., CYP3A5*3, CYP3A5*5, CYP3A5*6, and CYP3A5*7) have been identified.

The only benzodiazepines reported to have significant pharmacokinetic differences related to CYP3A4/5 polymorphisms are alprazolam and midazolam [79–81]. Due to the limited impact on CYP3A-mediated drug metabolism in vivo, and because pharmacokinetic effects did not significantly change behavioral effects, clinical relevance of testing for polymorphisms of CYP3A4/5 is unknown [82].

CYP2C19 Represents the metabolism of approximately 10 % of all drugs [56]. At least seven variant alleles have been identified that inactivate CYP2C19 (CYP2C10*2 – CYP2C19*8), with the two most important being CYP2C19*2 (accounts for up to 85 % of poor metabolizers in Caucasian and Japanese subjects) and CYP2C19*3 (accounts for up to 25 % of poor metabolizers in Japanese subjects). The frequency of poor metabolizers is thought to be especially high among Asians (15–30 %) while relatively low among Caucasians (3–6 %) [83, 84]. Several benzodiazepines are partially metabolized through CYP2C19 (see above). Significant differences comparing poor metabolizers to extensive (normal) metabolizers have been seen with diazepam, desmethyldiazepam, and quazepam leading to longer half-lives and lower clearances [76, 85, 87]. In one study, diazepam was found to have an effect on the emergence from general anesthesia in patients with CYP2C19 polymorphisms, concluding that CYP2C19 polymorphisms can have a significant and clinical effect [88].

19.6 Phase II Reactions

UGT enzymes catalyze the conjugation of various endogenous and exogenous compounds and are considered the most important of the phase II processes, responsible for the metabolism of ~50 % of all drugs. At least 19 human UGTs (classified in three families as UGT1A, UGT2A, and UGT2B) have been identified to date. Similar to the CYP450 enzymes, UGT enzymes can be polymorphic, and people are described as either poor metabolizers or extensive metabolizers. The most significant UGTs with respect to drug metabolism are UGT1A1, UGT1A3, UGT1A4, UGT1A6, UGT1A9, UGT2B7, and UGT2B15, with some evidence suggesting UGT2B4, UGT2B10, and UGT2B17 may contribute to glucuronidation [39]. While most benzodiazepines are metabolized by CYP enzymes first then UGTs, lorazepam and oxazepam are metabolized solely by glucuronidation. Of the UGTs, UGT2B15 is the most significant, as UGT2B7 is a poor glucuronidator of s-oxazepam, and polymorphic variation may not affect metabolism [89].

19.7 UGT2B15

Genetic polymorphisms have been shown to change pharmacokinetic parameters in lorazepam; however no noticeable effects have been noted in lorazepam kinetics when administered with medications that alter UGT2B15 metabolism [38]. Additionally both lorazepam and s-oxazepam have resulted in increased concentrations in the presence of UGT2B15*2 allele (approximately 50 %), but the clinical importance is still questionable [38, 90].

19.7.1 Dosage Adjustments (Per Package Insert)

Alprazolam

Elderly or debilitating disease:

- Immediate release: Starting dose 0.25 mg PO every 8–12 h
- Extended release: Starting dose 0.5 mg PO daily

Renal dosing: No adjustment provided in package insert; use with caution
Hepatic dosing:

- Immediate release: Initial dose of 0.25 mg two to three times a day titrated as needed and tolerated
- Extended release: Initial doses of 0.5 mg PO titrated as needed and tolerated

Chlordiazepoxide

Elderly: Not drug of choice due to prolonged sedation (long-acting metabolite and increased risk of falls/fractures; if used 5 mg two to four times daily is recommended
Renal dosing:

- CrCl <10 mL/min: 50 % of recommended dose [91]
- Peritoneal dialysis: 50 % of recommended dose [91]

Hepatic dosing: No adjustment provided in package insert; use with caution

Clonazepam

Elderly: Start on low doses and monitor
Hepatic dosing: No adjustment provided in package insert; use with caution
Renal dosing: No adjustment provided in package insert; use with caution

Clorazepate

Elderly: Use is not recommended in the elderly; if used, initiate at 7.5 mg one to two times a day
Hepatic dosing: No adjustment provided in package insert; use with caution
Renal dosing: No adjustment provided in package insert; use with caution

Diazepam

Elderly: Use oral over intramuscular, absorption orally is more reliable.

- Oral: 2–2.5 mg one to two times a day, titrated as needed and tolerated
- Rectal gel: Consider using reduced dose due to increased half-life in the elderly and debilitated patients

Hepatic dosing: Half-life prolonged, decrease dose by 50 %
Renal dosing: No adjustment provided in package insert; use with caution

Estazolam

Elderly: 0.5–1 mg at bed time. Initiate at lower doses for small elderly or debilitated patients
Hepatic dosing: No adjustment provided in package insert; use with caution
Renal dosing: No adjustment provided in package insert; use with caution

Flurazepam

Elderly: 15 mg orally at bed time
Hepatic dosing: No adjustment provided in package insert; use with caution
Renal dosing: No adjustment provided in package insert; use with caution

Lorazepam

Geriatric: Initial dose not to exceed 2 mg

- 1–2 mg orally daily in divided doses; avoid doses greater than 3 mg a day
- Intramuscular/intravenous: Reduce the initial dose for adults by 50 % and titrate as needed and tolerated

Hepatic dosing:

PO: Use with caution in severe impairment, may require lower doses
IM/IV: Caution in mild/moderate; not recommended in severe impairment

Renal dosing:

PO: No dosage adjustment needed [91]
IV/IM: Caution in mild/moderate (risk of propylene glycol toxicity); not recommended in severe impairment

Midazolam

Elderly: Reduce dose by 20–50 % in patients receiving opioids or other CNS depressants, in the elderly, chronically ill, or debilitated.
Hepatic dosing: No adjustment provided in package insert; use with caution; patients with any degree of hepatic impairment or hepatic encephalopathy likely to be sensitive to its effects
Renal dosing: No adjustment provided in package insert; use with caution; active metabolite may not be eliminated easily and may accumulate.

Oxazepam

Elderly: Initial dose of 10 mg orally three times a day; titrate slowly to 15 mg three to four times a day as needed and tolerated
Hepatic dosing: No adjustment provided in package insert; use with caution
Renal dosing: No adjustment provided in package insert; use with caution

Quazepam

Elderly: Initial dosing at 7.5 mg orally at bedtime
Hepatic dosing: No adjustment provided in package insert; use with caution
Renal dosing: No adjustment provided in package insert; use with caution

Temazepam

Elderly/debilitated: 7.5 mg orally at bed time
Hepatic dosing: No adjustment provided in package insert; use with caution
Renal dosing: No adjustment provided in package insert; use with caution

Triazolam

Elderly/debilitated: Initial dose of 0.125 mg orally at bed time. Max dose of 0.25 mg daily
Hepatic dosing: No adjustment provided in package insert; use with caution
Renal dosing: No adjustment provided in package insert; use with caution

19.7.2 Monitoring Recommendations

Respiratory Benzodiazepines do not effect respiration in normal subjects. However, they can reduce upper airway muscle tone and decrease response to hypoxia. Benzodiazepines are not indicated for use in obstructive sleep apnea (OSA) [92]. At least one study found temazepam does not significantly increase respiratory disturbance compared to placebo, suggesting the effects on OSA are modest [93]. Benzodiazepines should be given cautiously with other central nervous system depressants as they can have synergistic effects on decreasing respiration [73].

Sedation/Motor Impairment Benzodiazepines are often used as sedative hypnotics causing sedation. Though sedation is the intended effect, it may continue into the morning (hangover phenomenon) and cause significant impairment. Furthermore if benzodiazepines are being used as anxiolytics, sedation and lack of coordination could lead to serious consequences such as motor vehicle accidents or falls [94]. Falls could be very serious in the elderly and therefore long-term therapy is generally discouraged [95]. It is important to monitor patients for these side effects when first starting medication.

Withdrawal Benzodiazepines can cause physiological dependence and stopping them abruptly can cause a withdrawal syndrome. Symptoms of withdrawal include sleep disturbances, irritability, anxiety, hand tremor, sweating, difficulty concentrating, nausea, vomiting, palpitations, headache, and muscular pain. In severe cases seizures and psychotic symptoms can occur [96, 97]. The half-life of the benzodiazepine and the active metabolite correspond to the time at which withdrawal symptoms start relative to the last dose of medication.

References

1. Ban TA (2006) The role of serendipity in drug discovery. Dialogues Clin Neurosci 8(3):335–344
2. Hayer E, Adams D (1998) Sedative hypnotics. In: Quitkin F, Adams D, Bowden C et al (eds) Current psychotherapeutic drugs. American Psychiatric Press Inc, Washington DC
3. Riss J, Cloyd J, Gates J, Collins S (2008) Benzodiazepines in epilepsy: pharmacology and pharmacokinetics. Acta Neurol Scand 118(2):69–86
4. Greenblatt DJ, Miller LG, Shader RI (1990) Neurochemical and pharmacokinetic correlates of the clinical action of benzodiazepine hypnotic drugs. Am J Med 88(3A):18S–24S
5. Mandrioli R, Mercolini L, Raggi MA (2008) Benzodiazepine metabolism: an analytical perspective. Curr Drug Metab 9(8):827–844
6. Greenblatt DJ, Harmatz JS, Shader RI (1991) Clinical pharmacokinetics of anxiolytics and hypnotics in the elderly. Therapeutic considerations (Part I). Clin Pharmacokinet 21(3):165–177
7. Xanax [package insert] (2013) Pfizer, New York. http://labeling.pfizer.com/ShowLabeling.aspx?id=547. Date Accessed: May 2015
8. Greenblatt DJ, Wright CE (1993) Clinical pharmacokinetics of alprazolam. Therapeutic implications. Clin Pharmacokinet 24(6):453–471
9. Gorski JC, Jones DR, Hamman MA, Wrighton SA, Hall SD (1999) Biotransformation of alprazolam by members of the human cytochrome P4503A subfamily. Xenobiotica Fate Foreign Compounds Biol Syst 29(9):931–944
10. Molanaei H, Stenvinkel P, Qureshi AR et al (2012) Metabolism of alprazolam (a marker of CYP3A4) in hemodialysis patients with persistent inflammation. Eur J Clin Pharmacol 68(5):571–577
11. Baskin SI, Esdale A (1982) Is chlordiazepoxide the rational choice among benzodiazepines? Pharmacotherapy 2(2):110–119
12. Greenblatt DJ, Shader RI, Franke K, Harmatz JS (1978) Pharmacokinetics of chlordiazepoxide and metabolites following single and multiple oral doses. Int J Clin Pharmacol Biopharm 16(10):486–493
13. Vozeh S (1981) Pharmacokinetic of benzodiazepines in old age. Schweiz Med Wochenschr 111(47):1789–1793
14. Greenblatt DJ, Blaskovich PD, Nuwayser ES, Harmatz JS, Chen G, Zinny MA (2005) Clonazepam pharmacokinetics: comparison of subcutaneous microsphere injection with multiple-dose oral administration. J Clin Pharmacol 45(11):1288–1293
15. Crevoisier C, Delisle MC, Joseph I, Foletti G (2003) Comparative single-dose pharmacokinetics of clonazepam following intravenous, intramuscular and oral administration to healthy volunteers. Eur Neurol 49(3):173–177
16. Seree EJ, Pisano PJ, Placidi M, Rahmani R, Barra YA (1993) Identification of the human and animal hepatic cytochromes P450 involved in clonazepam metabolism. Fundam Clin Pharmacol 7(2):69–75
17. Longo LP, Johnson B (2000) Addiction: Part I. Benzodiazepines--side effects, abuse risk and alternatives. Am Fam Physician 61(7):2121–2128

18. Pradel V, Delga C, Rouby F, Micallef J, Lapeyre-Mestre M (2010) Assessment of abuse potential of benzodiazepines from a prescription database using 'doctor shopping' as an indicator. CNS Drugs 24(7):611–620
19. Greenblatt DJ, Divoll MK, Soong MH, Boxenbaum HG, Harmatz JS, Shader RI (1988) Desmethyldiazepam pharmacokinetics: studies following intravenous and oral desmethyldiazepam, oral clorazepate, and intravenous diazepam. J Clin Pharmacol 28(9):853–859
20. Frey HH, Scherkl R (1988) Clorazepate, correlation between metabolism and anticonvulsant activity. Eur J Pharmacol 158(3):213–216
21. Greenblatt DJ (1978) Determination of desmethyldiazepam in plasma by electron-capture GLC: application to pharmacokinetic studies of clorazepate. J Pharm Sci 67(3):427–429
22. Greenblatt DJ, Shader RI, Divoll M, Harmatz JS (1981) Benzodiazepines: a summary of pharmacokinetic properties. Br J Clin Pharmacol 11(Suppl 1):11S–16S
23. Ono S, Hatanaka T, Miyazawa S et al (1996) Human liver microsomal diazepam metabolism using cDNA-expressed cytochrome P450s: role of CYP2B6, 2C19 and the 3A subfamily. Xenobiotica Fate Foreign Compounds Biol Syst 26(11):1155–1166
24. Schmider J, Greenblatt DJ, von Moltke LL, Shader RI (1996) Relationship of in vitro data on drug metabolism to in vivo pharmacokinetics and drug interactions: implications for diazepam disposition in humans. J Clin Psychopharmacol 16(4):267–272
25. Beischlag TV, Kalow W, Mahon WA, Inaba T (1992) Diazepam metabolism by rat and human liver in vitro: inhibition by mephenytoin. Xenobiotica Fate Foreign Compounds Biol Syst 22(5):559–567
26. Miura M, Otani K, Ohkubo T (2005) Identification of human cytochrome P450 enzymes involved in the formation of 4-hydroxyestazolam from estazolam. Xenobiotica Fate Foreign Compounds Biol Syst 35(5):455–465
27. Greenblatt DJ, Divoll M, Harmatz JS, MacLaughlin DS, Shader RI (1981) Kinetics and clinical effects of flurazepam in young and elderly noninsomniacs. Clin Pharmacol Ther 30(4):475–486
28. Miller LG, Greenblatt DJ, Abernethy DR et al (1988) Kinetics, brain uptake, and receptor binding characteristics of flurazepam and its metabolites. Psychopharmacology (Berl) 94(3):386–391
29. Chan K, Jones RD (1993) Simultaneous determination of flumazenil, midazolam and metabolites in human biological fluids by liquid chromatography. J Chromatogr 619(1):154–160
30. Ziegler WH, Schalch E, Leishman B, Eckert M (1983) Comparison of the effects of intravenously administered midazolam, triazolam and their hydroxy metabolites. Br J Clin Pharmacol 16(Suppl 1):63S–69S
31. Johnson TN, Rostami-Hodjegan A, Goddard JM, Tanner MS, Tucker GT (2002) Contribution of midazolam and its 1-hydroxy metabolite to preoperative sedation in children: a pharmacokinetic-pharmacodynamic analysis. Br J Anaesth 89(3):428–437
32. Klieber S, Hugla S, Ngo R et al (2008) Contribution of the N-glucuronidation pathway to the overall in vitro metabolic clearance of midazolam in humans. Drug Metab Dispos Biol Fate Chem 36(5):851–862
33. Kato K, Yasui-Furukori N, Fukasawa T et al (2003) Effects of itraconazole on the plasma kinetics of quazepam and its two active metabolites after a single oral dose of the drug. Ther Drug Monit 25(4):473–477
34. Miura M, Ohkubo T (2004) In vitro metabolism of quazepam in human liver and intestine and assessment of drug interactions. Xenobiotica Fate Foreign Compounds Biol Syst 34(11–12):1001–1011
35. Perloff MD, von Moltke LL, Court MH, Kotegawa T, Shader RI, Greenblatt DJ (2000) Midazolam and triazolam biotransformation in mouse and human liver microsomes: relative contribution of CYP3A and CYP2C isoforms. J Pharmacol Exp Ther 292(2):618–628

36. Patki KC, Von Moltke LL, Greenblatt DJ (2003) In vitro metabolism of midazolam, triazolam, nifedipine, and testosterone by human liver microsomes and recombinant cytochromes p450: role of cyp3a4 and cyp3a5. Drug Metab Dispos Biol Fate Chem 31(7):938–944
37. Greenblatt DJ, Shader RI, Franke K et al (1979) Pharmacokinetics and bioavailability of intravenous, intramuscular, and oral lorazepam in humans. J Pharm Sci 68(1):57–63
38. Chung JY, Cho JY, Yu KS et al (2005) Effect of the UGT2B15 genotype on the pharmacokinetics, pharmacodynamics, and drug interactions of intravenous lorazepam in healthy volunteers. Clin Pharmacol Ther 77(6):486–494
39. Uchaipichat V, Suthisisang C, Miners JO (2013) The glucuronidation of R- and S-lorazepam: human liver microsomal kinetics, UDP-glucuronosyltransferase enzyme selectivity, and inhibition by drugs. Drug Metab Dispos Biol Fate Chem 41(6):1273–1284
40. Court MH, Duan SX, Guillemette C et al (2002) Stereoselective conjugation of oxazepam by human UDP-glucuronosyltransferases (UGTs): S-oxazepam is glucuronidated by UGT2B15, while R-oxazepam is glucuronidated by UGT2B7 and UGT1A9. Drug Metab Dispos Biol Fate Chem 30(11):1257–1265
41. Alvan G, Odar-Cederlof I (1978) The pharmacokinetic profile of oxazepam. Acta Psychiatr Scand Suppl 274:47–55
42. Greenblatt DJ, Divoll M, Harmatz JS, Shader RI (1980) Oxazepam kinetics: effects of age and sex. J Pharmacol Exp Ther 215(1):86–91
43. Locniskar A, Greenblatt DJ (1990) Oxidative versus conjugative biotransformation of temazepam. Biopharm Drug Dispos 11(6):499–506
44. CDC/NCHS, National Health and Nutrition Examination Survey (2013) http://www.cdc.gov/nchs/data/hus/hus13.pdf – 092, 2015
45. Olfson M, King M, Schoenbaum M (2015) Benzodiazepine use in the United States. JAMA Psychiatry 72(2):136–142
46. French DD, Chirikos TN, Spehar A, Campbell R, Means H, Bulat T (2005) Effect of concomitant use of benzodiazepines and other drugs on the risk of injury in a veterans population. Drug Saf 28(12):1141–1150
47. Fenner KS, Troutman MD, Kempshall S et al (2009) Drug-drug interactions mediated through P-glycoprotein: clinical relevance and in vitro-in vivo correlation using digoxin as a probe drug. Clin Pharmacol Ther 85(2):173–181
48. Lima SA, Cordeiro-da-Silva A, de Castro B, Gameiro P (2008) Benzodiazepine-mediated structural changes in the multidrug transporter P-glycoprotein: an intrinsic fluorescence quenching analysis. J Membr Biol 223(3):117–125
49. Lima SA, Tavares J, Gameiro P, de Castro B, Cordeiro-da-Silva A (2008) Flurazepam inhibits the P-glycoprotein transport function: an insight to revert multidrug-resistance phenotype. Eur J Pharmacol 581(1–2):30–36
50. Rational Use of Benzodiazepines (1996) World Health Organization
51. Patsalos PN, Perucca E (2003) Clinically important drug interactions in epilepsy: general features and interactions between antiepileptic drugs. Lancet Neurol 2(6):347–356
52. Greenblatt DJ, Koch-Weser J (1974) Clinical toxicity of chlordiazepoxide and diazepam in relation to serum albumin concentration: a report from the Boston Collaborative Drug Surveillance Program. Eur J Clin Pharmacol 7(4):259–262
53. Ogden CL, Carroll MD, Kit BK, Flegal KM (2014) Prevalence of childhood and adult obesity in the United States, 2011–2012. JAMA 311(8):806–814
54. Hanley MJ, Abernethy DR, Greenblatt DJ (2010) Effect of obesity on the pharmacokinetics of drugs in humans. Clin Pharmacokinet 49(2):71–87
55. Augustin P, Desmard M, Arapis K, Fournier P, Ribeiro-Parenti L, Montravers P (2013) Prolonged benzodiazepine coma as a complication of morbid obesity. Obes Surg 23(9):1452–1453
56. Brill MJ, Diepstraten J, van Rongen A, van Kralingen S, van den Anker JN, Knibbe CA (2012) Impact of obesity on drug metabolism and elimination in adults and children. Clin Pharmacokinet 51(5):277–304

57. Whitley H, Lindsey W (2009) Sex-based differences in drug activity. Am Fam Physician 80(11):1254–1258
58. Greenblatt DJ, von Moltke LL (2008) Gender has a small but statistically significant effect on clearance of CYP3A substrate drugs. J Clin Pharmacol 48(11):1350–1355
59. Greenblatt DJ, Harmatz JS, Singh NN et al (2014) Gender differences in pharmacokinetics and pharmacodynamics of zolpidem following sublingual administration. J Clin Pharmacol 54(3):282–290
60. Greenblatt DJ, Harmatz JS, von Moltke LL et al (2000) Comparative kinetics and response to the benzodiazepine agonists triazolam and zolpidem: evaluation of sex-dependent differences. J Pharmacol Exp Ther 293(2):435–443
61. Ochs HR, Greenblatt DJ, Knuchel M (1985) Kinetics of diazepam, midazolam, and lorazepam in cigarette smokers. Chest 87(2):223–226
62. Schein JR (1995) Cigarette smoking and clinically significant drug interactions. Ann Pharmacother 29(11):1139–1148
63. Lucas C, Martin JL (2013) Smoking and drug interactions. Aust Prescr 36:102–104
64. Andersen V, Pedersen N, Larsen NE, Sonne J, Larsen S (2002) Intestinal first pass metabolism of midazolam in liver cirrhosis – effect of grapefruit juice. Br J Clin Pharmacol 54(2):120–124
65. Yasui N, Kondo T, Furukori H et al (2000) Effects of repeated ingestion of grapefruit juice on the single and multiple oral-dose pharmacokinetics and pharmacodynamics of alprazolam. Psychopharmacology (Berl) 150(2):185–190
66. Dahan A, Altman H (2004) Food-drug interaction: grapefruit juice augments drug bioavailability--mechanism, extent and relevance. Eur J Clin Nutr 58(1):1–9
67. Penzak SR, Robertson SM, Hunt JD et al (2010) Echinacea purpurea significantly induces cytochrome P450 3A activity but does not alter lopinavir-ritonavir exposure in healthy subjects. Pharmacotherapy 30(8):797–805
68. Almeida JC, Grimsley EW (1996) Coma from the health food store: interaction between kava and alprazolam. Ann Intern Med 125(11):940–941
69. Dresser GK, Schwarz UI, Wilkinson GR, Kim R (2001) St. John's wort induces intestinal and hepatic CYP3A4 and P-glycoprotein in healthy volunteers. Clin Pharmacol Ther 2001;69:P23
70. Markowitz JS, Donovan JL, DeVane CL et al (2003) Effect of St John's wort on drug metabolism by induction of cytochrome P450 3A4 enzyme. JAMA 290(11):1500–1504
71. Kawaguchi A, Ohmori M, Tsuruoka S et al (2004) Drug interaction between St John's Wort and quazepam. Br J Clin Pharmacol 58(4):403–410
72. Tanaka E (2002) Toxicological interactions between alcohol and benzodiazepines. J Toxicol Clin Toxicol 40(1):69–75
73. Reynaud M, Petit G, Potard D, Courty P (1998) Six deaths linked to concomitant use of buprenorphine and benzodiazepines. Addiction 93(9):1385–1392
74. Naso AR (2008) Optimizing patient safety by preventing combined use of intramuscular olanzapine and parenteral benzodiazepines. Am J Health-Syst Pharm AJHP Off J Am Soc Health-Syst Pharm 65(12):1180–1183
75. Li XQ, Andersson TB, Ahlstrom M, Weidolf L (2004) Comparison of inhibitory effects of the proton pump-inhibiting drugs omeprazole, esomeprazole, lansoprazole, pantoprazole, and rabeprazole on human cytochrome P450 activities. Drug Metab Dispos Biol Fate Chem 32(8):821–827
76. Fukasawa T, Yasui-Furukori N, Aoshima T, Suzuki A, Tateishi T, Otani K (2004) Single oral dose pharmacokinetics of quazepam is influenced by CYP2C19 activity. Ther Drug Monit 26(5):529–533
77. Lynch T, Price A (2007) The effect of cytochrome P450 metabolism on drug response, interactions, and adverse effects. Am Fam Phys 76(3):391–396
78. Eiselt R, Domanski TL, Zibat A et al (2001) Identification and functional characterization of eight CYP3A4 protein variants. Pharmacogenetics 11(5):447–458

79. Park JY, Kim KA, Park PW et al (2006) Effect of CYP3A5*3 genotype on the pharmacokinetics and pharmacodynamics of alprazolam in healthy subjects. Clin Pharmacol Ther 79(6):590–599
80. Wong M, Balleine RL, Collins M, Liddle C, Clarke CL, Gurney H (2004) CYP3A5 genotype and midazolam clearance in Australian patients receiving chemotherapy. Clin Pharmacol Ther 75(6):529–538
81. Yu KS, Cho JY, Jang IJ et al (2004) Effect of the CYP3A5 genotype on the pharmacokinetics of intravenous midazolam during inhibited and induced metabolic states. Clin Pharmacol Ther 76(2):104–112
82. He P, Court MH, Greenblatt DJ, Von Moltke LL (2005) Genotype-phenotype associations of cytochrome P450 3A4 and 3A5 polymorphism with midazolam clearance in vivo. Clin Pharmacol Ther 77(5):373–387
83. Goldstein JA, Ishizaki T, Chiba K et al (1997) Frequencies of the defective CYP2C19 alleles responsible for the mephenytoin poor metabolizer phenotype in various Oriental, Caucasian, Saudi Arabian and American black populations. Pharmacogenetics 7(1):59–64
84. Goldstein JA, de Morais SM (1994) Biochemistry and molecular biology of the human CYP2C subfamily. Pharmacogenetics 4(6):285–299
85. Bertilsson L, Henthorn TK, Sanz E, Tybring G, Sawe J, Villen T (1989) Importance of genetic factors in the regulation of diazepam metabolism: relationship to S-mephenytoin, but not debrisoquine, hydroxylation phenotype. Clin Pharmacol Ther 45(4):348–355
86. Qin XP, Xie HG, Wang W et al (1999) Effect of the gene dosage of CgammaP2C19 on diazepam metabolism in Chinese subjects. Clin Pharmacol Ther 66(6):642–646
87. Sohn DR, Kusaka M, Ishizaki T et al (1992) Incidence of S-mephenytoin hydroxylation deficiency in a Korean population and the interphenotypic differences in diazepam pharmacokinetics. Clin Pharmacol Ther 52(2):160–169
88. Inomata S, Nagashima A, Itagaki F et al (2005) CYP2C19 genotype affects diazepam pharmacokinetics and emergence from general anesthesia. Clin Pharmacol Ther 78(6):647–655
89. de Leon J (2003) Glucuronidation enzymes, genes and psychiatry. Int J Neuropsychopharmacol/Off Sci J Coll Internationale Neuropsychopharmacologicum 6(1):57–72
90. He X, Hesse LM, Hazarika S et al (2009) Evidence for oxazepam as an in vivo probe of UGT2B15: oxazepam clearance is reduced by UGT2B15 D85Y polymorphism but unaffected by UGT2B17 deletion. Br J Clin Pharmacol 68(5):721–730
91. Aronoff G, Bennett W, Berns J et al (2007) Drug prescribing in renal failure: dosing guidelines for adults and children, 5th edn. American College of Physicians, Philadelphia
92. Norton JR, Ward DS, Karan S et al (2006) Differences between midazolam and propofol sedation on upper airway collapsibility using dynamic negative airway pressure. Anesthesiology 104(6):1155–1164
93. Camacho ME, Morin CM (1995) The effect of temazepam on respiration in elderly insomniacs with mild sleep apnea. Sleep 18(8):644–645
94. Barbone F, McMahon AD, Davey PG et al (1998) Association of road-traffic accidents with benzodiazepine use. Lancet 352(9137):1331–1336
95. Leipzig RM, Cumming RG, Tinetti ME (1999) Drugs and falls in older people: a systematic review and meta-analysis: I. Psychotropic drugs. J Am Geriatr Soc 47(1):30–39
96. Petursson H (1994) The benzodiazepine withdrawal syndrome. Addiction 89(11):1455–1459
97. Rickels K, Schweizer E, Case WG, Greenblatt DJ (1990) Long-term therapeutic use of benzodiazepines. I. Effects of abrupt discontinuation. Arch Gen Psychiatry 47(10):899–907

Chapter 20
Clinical Significant Interactions with Opioid Analgesics

Tony K.L. Kiang and Mary H.H. Ensom

This chapter summarizes the pharmacokinetic drug interactions of select opioid agents, focusing on underlying molecular mechanisms (e.g., known metabolic interactions at the enzymatic and transporter levels, such as cytochrome P450 [CYP450], uridine 5'-diphospho-glucuronosyltransferases [UGT], and drug transporters) and drawing a connection to pharmacodynamic interactions in clinical studies. The majority of data has focused on drug metabolism, and there are *in vitro* data to support the *in vivo* observations. Many opioids (e.g., codeine) are metabolized by enzymes that are known to exhibit genetic polymorphism, and this additional (gene-drug interaction) factor must be considered. Most data on opioids have focused on their classical analgesic properties, effects on pain threshold, and adverse effects such as somnolence, nausea/vomiting, gastrointestinal motility, or miosis. Additional atypical adverse effects such QT_C prolongation (e.g., associated with methadone) or serotonin syndrome (e.g., associated with tramadol) must be considered and can be manifested by pharmacokinetic-associated pharmacodynamic interactions. Information on pharmacokinetic-mediated pharmacodynamic interactions is relatively scarce in the literature compared to the available pharmacokinetic data. The available human data for opioids only represent a small fraction of all the possible drug interactions but one may use various *in vitro* or *in silico* approaches to aid the prediction of pharmacokinetic interactions. Evidence that a significant pharmacokinetic interaction is associated with a pharmacodynamic interaction must be appropriately weighted based on limitations in the design of existing studies. This chapter concludes with a proposed clinical decision-making algorithm that may be used to ascertain the clinical significance of pharmacokinetic-mediated pharmacodynamic interactions with opioid analgesics.

T.K.L. Kiang, BSc (Pharm), ACPR, PhD • M.H.H. Ensom, PharmD (✉)
Faculty of Pharmaceutical Sciences, The University of British Columbia,
Vancouver, BC, Canada
e-mail: mary.ensom@ubc.ca

M. Jann et al. (eds.), *Applied Clinical Pharmacokinetics and Pharmacodynamics of Psychopharmacological Agents*,
DOI 10.1007/978-3-319-27883-4_20

Search Terms: Drug interactions, Cytochrome P450 [CYP450], Uridine 5'-diphospho-glucuronosyltransferases [UGT], Drug transporters, Pharmacokinetics, Pharmacodynamics, Genetic polymorphism, Reaction phenotyping, Decision-making algorithm

20.1 Background

Opioid analgesics are the cornerstone of pain management therapy in cancer [1], noncancer [2], and postoperative pain management [3]. The utility of opioid drugs in both acute and chronic pain is underscored by their prominent positions on the widely used World Health Organization analgesic ladder for management of moderate and severe pain [4]. The pharmacology of opioid analgesics has been discussed in Chap. 10. The current chapter will summarize the pharmacokinetic drug interactions of select opioid agents, focusing on the underlying molecular mechanisms (e.g., known metabolic interactions at the enzymatic and transporter levels, such as cytochrome P450 [CYP450], uridine 5'-diphospho-glucuronosyltransferases [UGT], and drug transporters) and drawing a connection to pharmacodynamic interactions in clinical studies. Despite the fact that it is impossible to have experimental data on every single drug-drug interaction in humans, our mechanistic approach using the information already known at the molecular/enzymatic level can aid clinicians in predicting potential drug-drug interactions that will likely occur for a given opioid drug. We also propose an algorithm that may allow clinicians to systematically determine the significance of the observed clinical interactions.

Drug interactions mediated by pharmacokinetic changes can occur via absorption, distribution, metabolism, and excretion. The majority of the research on opioid pharmacokinetic interactions has focused on metabolism (and to a lesser degree, on transport) since most of the opioids are biotransformed singularly or in combination by various phase I (e.g., CYP450) and/or phase II (e.g., UGT) enzymes and/or phase III (e.g., p-glycoprotein [pgp]) systems [5, 6] and thus are subjected to drug interactions mediated by and/or genetic polymorphisms [7] associated with these enzymes and/or transporters. In general, phase I or II drug metabolism usually mediates the deactivation reaction (e.g., hydromorphone) but sometimes can lead to bioactivation (e.g., codeine) and the production of pharmacologically more potent metabolites. Interacting drugs can act as either inducers (e.g., rifampin for CYP3A4) or inhibitors (e.g., quinidine for CYP2D6) and, depending on the nature of metabolism (e.g., deactivation or bioactivation), can either enhance or decrease the therapeutic effects or pharmacological side effects of opioid drugs (and vice versa). On the other hand, phase III systems are responsible for the transport of drugs across lipophilic membranes (e.g., pgp transporter at the blood-brain barrier), are primarily responsible for decreasing drug concentrations at the tissue of interest, and, like phase I or II metabolic pathways, are also subjected to induction and inhibition. Phase III transporters are by convention not classified as metabolism enzymes, but for the purpose of this chapter, the phrases "metabolism" and "biotransformation" will be used to denote all phase I–III processes. Moreover, genetic polymorphisms associated with metabolism enzymes can lead to phenotypic changes that result in increased metabolism (e.g., ultrarapid metabolizer phenotype for CYP2D6) or diminished metabolism (e.g., poor metabolizer status for CYP2D6). Considering all of these elements of drug metabolism and transport, it is not difficult to see that one can potentially encounter several layers of complexity while assessing drug-drug interactions associated with opioids. Therefore, the primary focus of this chapter will be on understanding the molecular basis (i.e., reaction phenotyping of opioid agents, formation of inactive or active metabolites, and known effects of genetic polymorphisms) responsible for the pharmacokinetic drug-drug interactions and the associated pharmacodynamic changes, which will serve as the foundation for interpreting clinical drug interactions. Evidence supporting other modes of drug interactions (e.g., absorption or protein binding displacement) will be summarized as well. Mechanisms of interactions mediated by opioids' pharmacodynamic effects on receptor binding or neurotransmitter release are outlined in Chap. 10, and will not be reviewed further here.

20.2 Methodology

One can classify opioids by chemical class or receptor binding activity (i.e., agonist vs. partial agonist) [8] (see Chap. 10). However, for the purpose of this chapter, only opioids that are commonly used in the clinical setting will be reviewed: morphine, codeine, oxycodone, hydromorphone, methadone, fentanyl, and tramadol as these are often itemized on the World Health Organization analgesic ladder. A search of PubMed, Embase, and Google Scholar was conducted (English and human articles only, no time limit) using various combinations of the following terms: individual opioids listed above, pharmacokinetics, pharmacodynamics, drug-drug interactions, CYP450, UGT, transporters, pharmacogenomics, pharmacogenetics, and polymorphism. Reference lists of selected citations were also manually reviewed and pertinent articles extracted. The chapter will be structured per individual opioid drug, as follows:

I. Metabolism-mediated pharmacokinetic and pharmacodynamic interactions
   (a) Reaction phenotyping and clinical pharmacokinetic and pharmacodynamic interactions
   (b) Genetic polymorphism
II. Assessing the clinical significance of pharmacokinetic and pharmacodynamic interactions
   (a) Clinical decision-making algorithm

20.3 Metabolism/Transport-Mediated Pharmacokinetic and Pharmacodynamic Interactions

20.3.1 Morphine

20.3.1.1 Reaction Phenotyping and Clinical Pharmacokinetic and Pharmacodynamic Interactions

Morphine is primarily metabolized by UGT enzymes and is a substrate of p-glycoprotein [9]. Various UGT enzymes are capable of catalyzing the conjugation of morphine [10], but the principal UGT enzyme appears to be hepatic UGT2B7 [11] by virtue of its higher affinity toward morphine compared to other UGT enzymes [10]. However, a comprehensive reaction phenotyping study, which is needed to determine the relative contribution of specific UGT enzymes toward the conjugation of morphine, is still lacking in the literature. The conjugation of morphine leads to the production of morphine-6-glucuronide (M-6-G) and morphine-3-glucuronide (M-3-G). M-6-G appears to be equipotent compared to morphine [12], whereas M-3-G appears to be therapeutically inert but may be associated with toxic effects [13]. The area under the concentration-time curve (AUC) ratios between M-6-G or M-3-G and morphine is often used in clinical drug interaction studies to delineate the effects of interacting drugs on morphine metabolism. Under normal conditions, more M-3-G is produced compared to M-6-G, and their plasma exposure values far exceed that of morphine [14]. Based on these data, drugs that are capable of inducing or inhibiting UGT2B7 (e.g., Tables 20.1 and 20.2 [10]) can potentially affect the disposition of morphine and hence its pharmacodynamic effects in the clinic.

Few studies have examined the effects of coadministered drugs on the disposition of morphine in humans (Table 20.1). Overall, morphine pharmacokinetics is minimally altered in the presence of UGT substrates or inhibitors, as evident by the lack of effects on the clearance or exposure of morphine and/or its glucuronides when propranolol [15], ranitidine [16], or travafloxacin [17] was given concurrently in humans. Despite an apparent morphine-sparing effect and the maintenance of sustained M-6-G concentrations (in the presence of reduced morphine dose) by diclofenac in patients receiving morphine patient-controlled analgesia [18], that particular study was not designed to determine, mechanistically, diclofenac's effects on morphine glucuronidation. Moreover, despite the fact that the clearance and exposure of morphine were increased in the presence of rifampin, a potent UGT inducer [19], the formation of morphine glucuronide also decreased; therefore, the apparently significant pharmacokinetic interaction could not be explained by an effect of rifampin on morphine glucuronidation alone. In addition to hepatic metabolism, studies are also available on the effects of cimetidine, used as a modulator of hepatic blood flow [20] and gabapentin [21], an inhibitor of renal excretion, and neither found a significant effect on the pharmacokinetics of morphine in humans

Table 20.1 *In vivo* pharmacokinetic interactions associated with opioid agents in humans

Interacting drug/gene	Summary effects on opioid pharmacokinetics	Reference
Morphine (drug)		
Cimetidine	No effect on clearance or AUC of morphine. Morphine glucuronide not measured	Mojaverian et al. [20]
Diclofenac	Potentially morphine-sparing effect (same concentration of M-6-G glucuronide despite reduced morphine patient-controlled analgesic dose)	Tighe et al. [18]
Gabapentin	No effect on any measured pharmacokinetic parameters (including AUC and clearance) of morphine and M-3-G	Eckhardt et al. [21]
Propranolol	No effect on plasma or urinary concentrations of morphine or morphine glucuronide	Brunk et al. [15]
Quinidine	Increased plasma morphine concentration and AUC, decreased plasma glucuronide/morphine ratio	Kharasch et al. [9]
Ranitidine	No effect on the serum AUC or urinary M-3-G to M-6-G ratio, but decreased serum M-3-G to M-6-G ratio	Aasmundstad and Storset [16]
Rifampin	Increased clearance, decreased AUC of morphine. Decreased clearance of morphine glucuronides	Fromm et al. [19]
Travafloxacin	No effect on any measured pharmacokinetic parameters (including AUC and half-life) of morphine and M-3-G	Vincent et al. [17]
Valspodar	No effect on any measured pharmacokinetic parameters (including AUC and clearance) of morphine. Increased AUC and maximum concentration of M-3-G	Drewe et al. [22]
Morphine (gene)		
−802A>T (UGT) – UGT2B7*2	No effect on M-3-G/morphine or M-6-G/morphine ratio in cancer patients	Holthe et al. [26] Holthe et al. [25]
−840A>G (UGT)	Decreased M-6-G or M-3-G/morphine ratio	Darbari et al. [27]

(continued)

Table 20.1 (continued)

Interacting drug/gene	Summary effects on opioid pharmacokinetics	Reference
−161C>T (UGT)	Decreased M-6-G/morphine ratio and M-6-G or M-3-G concentrations	Saywer et al. [28]
−842G>A (UGT)	Decreased plasma morphine concentration. No effects on glucuronide concentrations in preterm newborns	Matic et al. [29]
Codeine (drug)		
Diclofenac	No effects on the pharmacokinetics of codeine. No change in the concentrations of codeine-6-glucuronide	Ammon et al. [34]
Quinidine	In extensive metabolizers. Decreased morphine in plasma	Sindrup et al. [36]
Quinidine	Decreased morphine concentration in plasma and cerebrospinal fluid	Sindrup et al. [38]
Quinidine	In extensive metabolizers. Decreased the O-demethylation of codeine. More prominent decrease in Caucasians compared to Chinese. Diminished the formation of morphine or morphine glucuronides	Caraco et al. [39]
Quinidine	Decreased plasma morphine	Kathiramalainathan et al. [37]
Quinidine, fluoxetine	Decreased the O-demethylation of dextromethorphan (maker substrate for CYP2D6)	Fernandes et al. [40]
Rifampin	Increased clearance through glucuronidation (increased glucuronide metabolites and norcodeine), decreased formation of morphine	Caraco et al. [41]
Codeine (gene)		
Extensive vs. poor metabolizer of sparteine (CYP2D6 substrate)	Lack of detection of morphine in plasma in poor metabolizers	Sindrup et al. [49]
Extensive vs. poor metabolizer of debrisoquine (CYP2D6 substrate)	Lower exposure of morphine in plasma in poor metabolizers and reduced clearance through the O-demethylation (i.e., CYP2D6) pathway	Yue et al. [52]
Extensive vs. poor metabolizer of dextromethorphan (CYP2D6 substrate)	Increased partial clearance of codeine to morphine in plasma of extensive metabolizers	Chen et al. [53]
Extensive vs. poor metabolizer of sparteine (substrate for CYP2D6)	Lack of detection of plasma morphine or M-6-G in poor metabolizers	Poulsen et al. [50]
Extensive vs. poor metabolizers of sparteine	Higher plasma concentrations and amount of morphine excreted in urine in extensive metabolizers	Mikus et al. [54]

Table 20.1 (continued)

Interacting drug/gene	Summary effects on opioid pharmacokinetics	Reference
Extensive vs. poor metabolizer of CYP2D6 (genotyped)	Only trace formation of morphine in plasma of poor metabolizers. Percentage of morphine converted from codeine in extensive metabolizers (3.9 %) much greater than poor metabolizers (0.17 %)	Eckhardt et al. [55]
Extensive vs. poor metabolizer of sparteine (CYP2D6 substrate)	Lack of detection of plasma morphine or M-6-G in poor metabolizers	Poulsen et al. [51]
Ultrarapid vs. extensive vs. poor metabolizers (genotyped)	Higher plasma exposure of morphine in ultrarapid compared to extensive and poor metabolizers. Lower ratio of morphine to codeine (and their respective glucuronides) in urine	Kirchheiner et al. [56]
Oxycodone (drug)		
Clarithromycin	Increased plasma exposure of oxycodone and decreased that of noroxycodone (age-independent effect)	Liukas et al. [58]
Grapefruit juice	Increased plasma exposure of oxycodone, decreased noroxycodone/oxycodone ratio. Increased plasma exposure of oxymorphone	Nieminen et al. [59]
Itraconazole	Increased plasma exposure of oxycodone (after oral or intravenous dosing) and noroxymorphone, but decreased that of noroxycodone	Saari et al. [61]
Ketoconazole (as CYP3A4 inhibitor) and quinidine (as CYP2D6 inhibitor)	Quinidine increased plasma exposure of noroxycodone and decreased the exposure of oxymorphone. Ketoconazole had opposite effects	Samer et al. [64]
Ketoconazole (as CYP3A4 inhibitor) and paroxetine (as CYP2D6 inhibitor)	Ketoconazole increased exposure of oxycodone, whereas paroxetine had no effect, compared to placebo	Kummer et al. [60]
Miconazole (oral gel) (as a mixed CYP3A4 and CYP2D6 inhibitor)	Increased plasma exposure of oxycodone and noroxycodone but decreased that of oxymorphone	Gronlund et al. [68]
Paroxetine (as CYP2D6 inhibitor) and/or itraconazole (as CYP3A4 inhibitor) – oral oxycodone	Paroxetine decreased plasma exposure of oxymorphone but not oxycodone. Paroxetine and itraconazole together increased plasma exposure of oxycodone	Gronlund et al. [66]
Paroxetine (as CYP2D6 inhibitor) and/or itraconazole (as CYP3A4 inhibitor) – intravenous oxycodone	Paroxetine did not affect the exposure of oxycodone Paroxetine and itraconazole together increased plasma exposure of oxycodone	Gronlund et al. [67]

(continued)

Table 20.1 (continued)

Interacting drug/gene	Summary effects on opioid pharmacokinetics	Reference
Rifampin	Decreased plasma exposure of oxycodone, oxymorphone and increased noroxycodone/oxycodone ratio (both oral and intravenous dosing)	Nieminen et al. [70]
Ritonavir or lopinavir/ritonavir	Increased plasma exposure of oxycodone, decreased plasma exposure of noroxycodone, and increased plasma exposure of oxymorphone (only with lopinavir/ritonavir)	Nieminen et al. [62]
St. John's wort (CYP3A4 inducer)	Decreased plasma exposure of oxycodone	Nieminen et al. [71]
Telithromycin (as inhibitors for both CYP2D6 and CYP3A4)	Increased plasma exposure of oxycodone and decreased plasma exposure of noroxycodone. No effects on the pharmacokinetics of oxymorphone	Gronlund et al. [69]
Voriconazole	Increased plasma exposure of oxycodone. Increased plasma oxymorphone/oxycodone ratio, decreased noroxycodone/oxycodone ratio	Hagelberg et al. [63]
Quinidine	No effect on oxycodone concentrations, increased plasma noroxycodone concentrations, decreased formation (lack of detection) of plasma oxymorphone	Heiskanen et al. [65]
Oxycodone (gene)		
CYP2D6 extensive vs. poor metabolizers	Significantly increased plasma oxymorphone/oxycodone ratio in extensive metabolizers	Zwisler et al. [73]
CYP2D6 extensive vs. poor metabolizers	Significantly increased plasma oxymorphone/oxycodone ratio in extensive metabolizers in postoperative patients (intravenous oxycodone)	Zwisler et al. [74]
CYP2D6 ultrarapid vs. extensive vs. poor metabolizers	Increased oxymorphone and decreased noroxycodone plasma concentration in ultrarapid metabolizers of CYP2D6	Samer et al. [64]
CYP2D6 ultrarapid vs. extensive vs. intermediate vs. poor metabolizers	Increased oxymorphone/oxycodone ratio dependent on CYP2D6 metabolizer phenotype status (ultrarapid > extensive > intermediate > poor)	Stamer et al. [72]
Hydromorphone (gene)		
−802A > T (UGT) – UGT2B7*2	No effect on various pharmacokinetic parameters of hydromorphone, or H3G (including exposure)	Vandenbossche et al. [81]
Fentanyl (drug)		
Itraconazole	No effects on the pharmacokinetics (including clearance) of fentanyl (given intravenously) in plasma	Palkama et al. [85]

Table 20.1 (continued)

Interacting drug/gene	Summary effects on opioid pharmacokinetics	Reference
Parecoxib or troleandomycin	No effects on the pharmacokinetics (including exposure) of intravenously administered fentanyl in plasma by parecoxib. Troleandomycin decreased clearance of fentanyl in plasma	Ibrahim et al. [87]
Rifampin, troleandomycin, or grapefruit juice	Rifampin decreased exposure and increased clearance of fentanyl in plasma (given as oral lozenge) whereas troleandomycin had opposite effects. Rifampin increased whereas troleandomycin decreased the exposure of norfentanyl in plasma. Grapefruit juice had no effects	Kharasch et al. [86]
Ritonavir	Decreased clearance and increased exposure in plasma of intravenously administered fentanyl	Olkkola et al. [88]
Voriconazole and fluconazole	Decreased fentanyl (given intravenously) clearance (voriconazole and fluconazole) and increased fentanyl exposure (voriconazole) in plasma. Both voriconazole and fluconazole decreased exposure of norfentanyl in plasma	Saari et al. [89]
Tramadol (drug)		
Escitalopram	Decreased plasma exposure of M1 metabolite	Noehr-Jensen et al. [94]
Methadone (CYP2D6 inhibition) or buprenorphine	Decreased urinary ratio of M1/tramadol from methadone compared to buprenorphine-treated subjects. No difference in M2/tramadol or tramadol concentrations in urine between two treatments	Coller et al. [95]
Paroxetine (CYP2D6 inhibition)	Increased plasma exposure of tramadol. Decreased plasma exposure of M1 metabolite	Laugesen et al. [96]
Paroxetine	Increased urinary tramadol/M1 ratio	Nielsen et al. [97]
Rifampin (CYP3A4 induction)	Decreased plasma exposure of tramadol and M1 metabolite (oral and intravenously administered tramadol)	Saarikoski et al. [98]
Ticlopidine (CYP2D6 inhibitor) and itraconazole (CYP3A4 inhibitor)	Ticlopidine increased plasma exposure of tramadol and decreased exposure of M1 metabolite. Itraconazole had no effects	Hagelberg et al. [99]
Tramadol (gene)		
CYP2D6 extensive vs. poor metabolizers	Increased plasma M1 concentrations in extensive metabolizers (not detectable in poor metabolizers)	Poulsen et al. [100]

(continued)

Table 20.1 (continued)

Interacting drug/gene	Summary effects on opioid pharmacokinetics	Reference
CYP2D6 extensive vs. poor metabolizers	Increased plasma exposure of M1 metabolite and decreased exposure of tramadol in extensive metabolizers	Pedersen et al. [101]
CYP2D6 extensive vs. poor metabolizers	Detectable plasma M1 concentrations only in extensive metabolizers	Enggaard et al. [102]
CYP2D6 ultrarapid vs. extensive vs. intermediate metabolizers	Increased tramadol plasma clearance in ultrarapid and extensive metabolizers vs. intermediate metabolizers	Gan et al. [106]
CYP2D6 extensive vs. poor metabolizers	Increased plasma exposure of M1 metabolite, decreased exposure of tramadol in extensive metabolizers	Garcia-Quetglas et al. [103]
CYP2D6 ultrarapid vs. extensive vs. intermediate vs. poor metabolizers	Plasma exposure of the M1 metabolite dependent on phenotype status (ultrarapid > extensive > intermediate > poor)	Stamer et al. [105]
CYP2D6 extensive vs. poor metabolizers	Increased plasma concentration of M1 metabolite in extensive metabolizers	Halling et al. [104]
CYP2D6 ultrarapid vs. extensive metabolizers	Increased plasma exposure of M1 metabolite but decreased exposure of tramadol in ultrarapid metabolizers	Kirchheiner et al. [107]
Methadone (drug)		
Amprenavir (PI)	Decreased both S- and R-methadone plasma exposure (higher magnitude of decrease in S- compared to R-isoform)	Hendrix et al. [126]
Atazanavir (PI)	No change in S- or R-methadone plasma concentrations	Friedland et al. [135]
Delavirdine (NNRTI)	Increased plasma methadone exposure	McCance-Katz et al. [145]
Dolutegravir (INI)	No effect on R-, S-, or total methadone plasma exposure	Song et al. [140]
Fluconazole (CYP3A4 inhibitor)	Increased methadone exposure in plasma	Cobb et al. [121]
Fosamprenavir-ritonavir (PI)	Decreased plasma exposure of S-methadone > R-methadone	Cao et al. [149]
Indinavir (PI)	No effect on plasma exposure of methadone (despite significant inhibitory effects on CYP3A4 substrate marker exposure)	Kharasch et al. [136]
Lamivudine/zidovudine (NRTI)	No effect on plasma exposure of methadone	Rainey et al. [150]
Lersivirine (NNRTI)	No effect on R- or S-methadone plasma exposure	Vourvahis et al. [146]
Lopinavir-ritonavir vs. ritonavir (PI)	Lopinavir-ritonavir decreased plasma exposure of methadone. No effect by ritonavir	McCance-Katz et al. [127]
Lopinavir-ritonavir (PI)	Decreased plasma exposure of methadone	Clarke et al. [128]

Table 20.1 (continued)

Interacting drug/gene	Summary effects on opioid pharmacokinetics	Reference
Lopinavir-ritonavir (PI)	Decreased plasma concentrations of methadone (despite significant inhibitory effects toward CYP3A4 substrate marker exposure)	Kharasch and Stubbert [129]
Nelfinavir (PI)	Decreased plasma exposure of R- and S-methadone (more reduction with S-isomer), despite significant inhibitory effects on CYP3A4 substrate maker exposure	Kharasch et al. [130]
Nelfinavir (PI)	Decreased plasma exposure of methadone	McCance-Katz et al. [131]
Nelfinavir (PI)	Decreased plasma exposure of R- and S-methadone	Hsyu et al. [132]
Nevirapine (NNRTI)	Decreased plasma exposure of R- and total methadone	Stocker et al. [142]
Nevirapine (NNRTI)	Decreased plasma exposure of methadone	Arroyo et al. [143]
Nevirapine (NNRTI)	Decreased plasma exposure of methadone	Clarke et al. [144]
Paroxetine (CYP2D6 inhibitor)	Increased plasma concentrations of both R- and S-methadone in CYP2D6 extensive metabolizers. Increased plasma concentration of S-methadone in poor CYP2D6 metabolizers	Begre et al. [123]
Quetiapine (CYP2D6 inhibitor)	Increased plasma R-methadone/dose ratio (extensive CYP2D6 metabolizers > intermediate metabolizers > poor metabolizers)	Uehlinger et al. [124]
Rifampin (CYP3A4 inducer), troleandomycin (CYP3A4 inhibitor), grapefruit juice (intestinal CYP3A4 inhibitor)	Rifampin increased clearance of oral and intravenous methadone. Troleandomycin and grapefruit juice had no effects on methadone clearance	Kharasch et al. [114]
Raltegravir (INI)	No effect on plasma methadone exposure	Anderson et al. [141]
Saquinavir/Ritonavir (PI)	Decreased plasma exposure of methadone	Jamois et al. [133]
Saquinavir/ritonavir (PI)	Decreased S- or R-methadone plasma exposure	Gerber et al. [134]
Saquinavir/ritonavir (PI)	No effect on S- or R-methadone plasma exposure	Shelton et al. [137]
Sertraline	Increased plasma methadone/dose ratio in the first 6 weeks of treatment. No difference by week 12	Hamilton et al. [125]
Tenofovir (NRTI)	No effect on plasma exposure of methadone (R-, S-, or total)	Smith et al. [138]

(continued)

Table 20.1 (continued)

Interacting drug/gene	Summary effects on opioid pharmacokinetics	Reference
Voriconazole (CYP3A4 inhibitor)	Increased both R- and S-methadone exposure in plasma	Liu et al. [122]
Zidovudine (NRTI)	No effect on plasma exposure of methadone	Schwartz et al. [139]
Methadone (gene)		
ABCB1 3435TT (reduced pgp activity)	Decreased R-methadone plasma concentration-dose ratio	Uehlinger et al. [124]
CYP2D6 ultrarapid vs. extensive vs. poor metabolizers	Increased concentrations to dose-to-weight ratios of R-methadone in plasma (poor metabolizer > ultrarapid metabolizer)	Eap et al. [147]
CYP3A4 activity CYP2B6*6/*6 CYP2D6 ultrarapid vs. extensive vs. intermediate vs. poor metabolizer ABCB1 3435TT (reduced pgp activity)	Lower CYP3A activity led to increased trough R- and S-methadone plasma concentration CYP2B6*6*6 phenotype led to increased plasma S-methadone concentration CYP2D6 extensive metabolizers had decreased R- and S-methadone plasma concentration vs. extensive and intermediate metabolizers ABCB1 3435TT decreased trough R- and S-methadone plasma concentrations	Crettol et al. [148]

CYP cytochrome P450, *ECG* electrocardiogram, *INI* integrase inhibitors, *NNRTI* non-nucleoside reverse transcriptase inhibitors, *NRTI* nucleoside reverse transcriptase inhibitors, *pgp* p-glycoprotein, *PI* protease inhibitors, *UGT* uridine 5'-diphospho-glucuronosyltransferases

(Table 20.1). On the other hand, inconsistent findings were obtained with pgp inhibitors, valspodar [22] which did not affect morphine pharmacokinetics compared to quinidine [9] which apparently increased the absorption (decreased intestinal efflux) of morphine in humans (Table 20.1).

In general, studies that have characterized the pharmacodynamic effects of morphine have shown little influence by the interacting drug, whereas those that have demonstrated an apparent pharmacological effect were potentially confounded by other factors (Table 20.2). All of these negative findings should be interpreted with caution, however, as these studies had relatively small sample sizes and except for diclofenac, which is a known potent inhibitor of UGT2B7 [10], the potency or specificity of other putative UGT modulators has not been well characterized. As well, the case of rifampin further highlights the complexity of all combined metabolic processes in humans: that one should also consider other metabolic pathways being affected by the modulator rather than only taking into consideration a single process (i.e., glucuronidation) by itself. Alternatively, one might hypothesize that morphine, being a high extraction drug, may be relatively insensitive to changes in its intrinsic clearance (i.e., as a result of enzyme modulation) than hepatic blood flow, which may explain the general lack of pharmacokinetic interactions reported for morphine in the literature.

20.3.1.2 Genetic Polymorphism

As morphine is primarily conjugated by UGT2B7, polymorphism in this specific metabolizing enzyme that results in altered phenotype can potentially result in significant pharmacokinetic alterations. The available literature illustrates a mixed picture, however, where only certain genetic polymorphisms are associated with altered glucuronide to morphine ratios in humans (Table 20.1). *In vitro* studies using microsomes containing polymorphic -802A>T variant (UGT2B7*2) show little difference in the formation of morphine glucuronide compared to the wild type [23, 24]. These *in vitro* observations are supported by the lack of an effect by UGT2B7*2 variants in the glucuronide/morphine plasma ratios in cancer patients [25, 26]. On the other hand, patients with sickle cell disease possessing the -840A>G allele as a hetero- or homozygote had a significantly reduced morphine glucuronide/morphine ratio [27], subjects with the -161C>T allele (which is also in complete linkage disequilibrium with UGT2B7*2) had decreased M-6-G/morphine ratios and reduced morphine glucuronide concentrations compared to the wild type [28], and preterm newborns with the -842G>A allele showed decreased morphine concentrations and increased M-3-G/morphine ratios [29]. It has to be noted, however, that these genetic studies are of relatively small sample sizes and only association in nature; and it remains to be clarified whether these pharmacokinetic variations are translated to clinically relevant pharmacodynamic effects.

20.3.2 Codeine

20.3.2.1 Reaction Phenotyping and Clinical Pharmacokinetic and Pharmacodynamic Interactions

Codeine is a weak analgesic that requires further activation to morphine to exert its pharmacological effects. The hepatic enzyme responsible for the activation of codeine is CYP2D6 [30], although this pathway constitutes only a small portion of codeine clearance as most of codeine is deactivated by UGT2B7, UGT2B4 [24] and CYP3A4 [31] in the formation of inactive glucuronide metabolites and norcodeine, respectively. Given the influence of concurrent bioactivation and deactivation pathways, pharmacokinetic drug-drug interactions involving codeine are dependent on the combined effects of the modulators toward all of these enzyme pathways. For example, a CYP3A4 modulator, although not directly responsible for the bioactivation of codeine, can also affect the CYP2D6 bioactivation pathway indirectly by enhancing or reducing the availability of codeine. This scenario was demonstrated in a case report where an individual with ultrarapid CYP2D6 genotype (i.e., enhanced codeine activation) taking CYP3A4 inhibitors (i.e., reduced codeine deactivation) exhibited codeine intoxication, presumably a result of additive effects of two concurrent drug-drug interactions on two separate codeine metabolic pathways [32]. The complexity of codeine metabolism highlighting the interplay between

Table 20.2 *In vivo* pharmacodynamic interactions (mediated by pharmacokinetic changes) associated with opioid agents in humans

Interacting drug/gene	Summary effects on opioid pharmacodynamics	Reference
Morphine (drug)		
Cimetidine	No effects on the duration of miosis associated with morphine	Mojaverian et al. [20]
Diclofenac	Morphine-sparing effect, although the analgesic effect from diclofenac itself was difficult to control	Tighe et al. [18]
Gabapentin	Increased analgesic effect of morphine (cold pressor test, although the analgesic effect of gabapentin itself was difficult to control)	Eckhardt et al. [21]
Quinidine	Increased morphine-induced miosis	Kharasch et al. [9]
Rifampin	Significantly decreased the analgesic effects of morphine (cold pressor test)	Fromm et al. [19]
Travafloxacin	No change on adverse effects associated with morphine	Vincent et al. [17]
Valspodar	No effects on adverse events associated with morphine	Drewe et al. [22]
Codeine (drug)		
Diclofenac	No change in the findings from cold pressor test	Ammon et al. [34]
Quinidine	In extensive metabolizers. No difference in pin-prick or tolerance pain thresholds	Sindrup et al. [36]
Quinidine	In extensive metabolizers. Decreases in codeine therapeutic effects only observed in Caucasians but not in the Chinese	Caraco et al. [39]
Quinidine, fluoxetine	No effect on codeine dependence	Fernandes et al. [40]
Quinidine	Decreased positive ("high") and negative ("nausea") effects	Kathiramalainathan et al. [37]
Rifampin	Decreased respiratory and psychomotor but no change in miotic effects in extensive metabolizers. Opposite effects in poor metabolizers	Caraco et al. [41]
Codeine (gene)		
Extensive vs. poor metabolizer of sparteine (CYP2D6 substrate)	Increased pricking pain threshold only in extensive metabolizers	Sindrup et al. [49]

Table 20.2 (continued)

Interacting drug/gene	Summary effects on opioid pharmacodynamics	Reference
Extensive vs. poor metabolizer of sparteine (CYP2D6 substrate)	Extensive metabolizers responded to codeine (pain reduction and tolerance threshold), whereas codeine had no effects in poor metabolizers	Poulsen et al. [50]
Extensive vs. poor metabolizers of sparteine	Reduced gastric motility only in extensive metabolizers	Mikus et al. [54]
Extensive vs. poor metabolizer of CYP2D6 (genotyped)	Analgesic effect only evident (cold pressor test) in extensive metabolizers. Incidence of side effects (from visual analogue scale) comparable between the two phenotypes	Eckhardt et al. [55]
Extensive vs. poor metabolizer of sparteine (CYP2D6 substrate)	No difference between the two CYP2D6 phenotypes with respect to postoperative pain	Poulsen et al. [51]
Ultrarapid vs. extensive vs. poor metabolizers (genotyped)	Higher incidence of sedation in ultrarapid compared to extensive metabolizers	Kirchheiner et al. [56]
Oxycodone (drug)		
Clarithromycin	No difference in behavioral/ocular/or analgesic pharmacodynamic effects	Liukas et al. [58]
Grapefruit juice	No effects on analgesia. Increased deteriorating effect and self-rated performance	Nieminen et al. [59]
Itraconazole	Increased alertness, and deterioration of performance, but no change in heat pain or cold pain threshold	Saari et al. [61]
Ketoconazole (as CYP3A4 inhibitor) and paroxetine (as CYP2D6 inhibitor)	Ketoconazole increased analgesic efficacy, pupil dilation, nausea, drowsiness, and pruritus. Paroxetine had no effect	Kummer et al. [60]
Ketoconazole (as CYP3A4 inhibitor) and quinidine (as CYP2D6 inhibitor)	Quinidine decreased whereas ketoconazole increased pain threshold. Ketoconazole treatment also increased side effect measures of oxycodone	Samer et al. [64]
Miconazole (oral gel)	No pharmacodynamics interaction observed (analgesia, drowsiness, pleasantness, pupil size, cold pain threshold, and the digit symbol substitution test (a psychomotor measure))	Gronlund et al. [68]

(continued)

Table 20.2 (continued)

Interacting drug/gene	Summary effects on opioid pharmacodynamics	Reference
Paroxetine (as CYP2D6 inhibitor) and/or itraconazole (as CYP3A4 inhibitor)	Paroxetine alone had no effects on subjective drug effects, drowsiness, or deterioration of performance. Paroxetine and itraconazole together significantly increased these effects	Gronlund et al. [66]
Paroxetine (as CYP2D6 inhibitor) and/or itraconazole (as CYP3A4 inhibitor) – intravenous oxycodone	No change in pharmacodynamic effects by paroxetine alone or in combination with itraconazole	Gronlund et al. [67]
Rifampin	Decreased self-reported drowsiness, drug effect, deterioration of performance, miosis (intravenous), and heterotropia (oral). Decreased the analgesic effects of oral oxycodone only	Nieminen et al. [70]
Ritonavir or lopinavir/ritonavir	Increased self-reported drug effect, nausea/vomiting. No effects on analgesia	Nieminen et al. [62]
St. John's wort (CYP3A4 inducer)	Decreased self-reported drug effect. No effects on analgesia	Nieminen et al. [71]
Telithromycin (as inhibitors for both CYP2D6 and CYP3A4)	Increased self-rated drug effect but decreased self-rated performance and pupil size. Increased heat pain threshold and cold pain analgesia. No effects on heat pain analgesia or tactile sensitivity	Gronlund et al. [69]
Voriconazole	Increased subjective drug effects, heterophoria, and miosis. No effects on analgesia. Effects on adverse events not quantifiable	Hagelberg et al. [63]
Quinidine	No effects on psychomotor or subjective drug effects. No effects on adverse events	Heiskanen et al. [65]
Oxycodone (gene)		
CYP2D6 extensive vs. poor metabolizers	Increased pain tolerance thresholds and pain reduction (cold pressor test) in extensive metabolizers	Zwisler et al. [73]
CYP2D6 extensive vs. poor metabolizers	No difference between metabolizer phenotypes on intravenous oxycodone analgesic effects in postoperative patients	Zwisler et al. [74]

Table 20.2 (continued)

Interacting drug/gene	Summary effects on opioid pharmacodynamics	Reference
CYP2D6 ultrarapid vs. extensive vs. poor metabolizers	Greater effects of oxycodone on cold pressor test, subjective pain threshold, and pupil size in ultrarapid versus extensive or the poor metabolizers of CYP2D6. Side effect measures more likely observed in ultrarapid metabolizers	Samer et al. [64]
CYP2D6 ultrarapid vs. extensive vs. intermediate vs. poor metabolizers	Ultrarapid and extensive metabolizers required reduced oxycodone consumption but only compared to poor metabolizers. No difference in pain scores	Stamer et al. [72]
Hydromorphone (gene)		
–802A>T (UGT) – UGT2B7*2	No effect on adverse events	Vandenbossche et al. [81]
Fentanyl (drug)		
Parecoxib or troleandomycin	Troleandomycin, but not parecoxib, had an effect on pupil diameter on intravenously administered fentanyl	Ibrahim et al. [87]
Itraconazole	No change in pharmacodynamic effects (therapeutic effect, drowsiness, nausea, itching – via visual analogue scale)	Palkama et al. [85]
Tramadol (drug)		
Escitalopram (CYP2D6 inhibition)	No change in response to cold pressor test	Noehr-Jensen et al. [94]
Paroxetine (CYP2D6 inhibition)	Decreased analgesic effects of tramadol compared to tramadol alone	Laugesen et al. [96]
Tramadol (gene)		
CYP2D6 extensive vs. poor metabolizers	Increased pain thresholds and analgesic effects (cold pressor test) in extensive metabolizers	Poulsen et al. [100]
CYP2D6 extensive vs. poor metabolizers	Decreased analgesia response rate in poor metabolizers	Stamer et al. [101]
CYP2D6 extensive vs. poor metabolizers	Increased analgesic effects (cold pressor test) in extensive metabolizers. Increased pain tolerance thresholds to nerve stimulation in poor metabolizers	Enggaard et al. [102]
CYP2D6 ultrarapid vs. extensive vs. intermediate metabolizers	More adverse events observed in intermediate metabolizers	Gan et al. [106]

(continued)

Table 20.2 (continued)

Interacting drug/gene	Summary effects on opioid pharmacodynamics	Reference
CYP2D6 ultrarapid vs. extensive metabolizers	Increased pain threshold and pain tolerance in ultrarapid metabolizers. Increased miotic effects and higher incidence of nausea in ultrarapid metabolizers	Kirchheiner et al. [107]
Methadone (drug)		
Amprenavir (PI)	No effect on analgesia, withdrawal, or dose change	Hendrix et al. [126]
Atazanavir (PI)	No effect on methadone withdrawal	Friedland et al. [135]
Delavirdine (NNRTI)	No effect on cognitive deficits, opioid withdrawal, or adverse effects	McCance-Katz et al. [145]
Dolutegravir (INI)	No effect on adverse events, ECG, vital signs	Song et al. [140]
Fluconazole	No effect on opioid overdose	Cobb et al. [121]
Fosamprenavir-ritonavir (PI)	No effect on withdrawal, adverse events, or dosage change	Cao et al. [149]
Lersivirine (NNRTI)	No effect on methadone withdrawal	Vourvahis et al. [146]
Lopinavir-ritonavir (PI)	No effect on methadone withdrawal or dose adjustment	Clarke et al. [128]
Nelfinavir (PI)	No effect on methadone-induced miosis	Kharasch et al. [130]
Nelfinavir (PI)	No effect on methadone withdrawal	McCance-Katz et al. [131]
Nelfinavir (PI)	No effect on withdrawal or adverse event rate	Hsyu et al. [132]
Nevirapine (NNRTI)	Induced withdrawal symptoms in 90 % of subjects	Arroyo et al. [143]
Nevirapine (NNRTI)	Induced withdrawal symptoms in 6 out of 8 subjects	Clarke et al. [144]
Raltegravir (INI)	No change in adverse events	Anderson et al. [141]
Saquinavir/Ritonavir (PI)	No effect on adverse events, ECG, vital signs	Jamois et al. [133]
Saquinavir/ritonavir (PI)	No effect on withdrawal or dose requirement	Gerber et al. [134]
Saquinavir/ritonavir (PI)	No effect on sedation or dose requirement	Shelton et al. [137]
Sertraline (CYP2B6, CYP2D6, and CYP3A4 inhibitor)	No effect on adverse events associated with methadone. Methadone dose adjustment not required	Hamilton et al. [125]

Table 20.2 (continued)

Interacting drug/gene	Summary effects on opioid pharmacodynamics	Reference
Tenofovir (NRTI)	No change in opioid withdrawal effects and miotic effects	Smith et al. [138]
Voriconazole	No effect on opioid withdrawal or overdose	Liu et al. [122]
Methadone (gene)		
CYP2D6 ultrarapid vs. extensive vs. poor metabolizers	No difference in treatment outcome	Eap et al. [151]

CYP cytochrome P450, *ECG* electrocardiogram, *INI* integrase inhibitors, *NNRTI* non-nucleoside reverse transcriptase inhibitors, *NRTI* nucleoside reverse transcriptase inhibitors, *PI* protease inhibitors

various metabolic pathways is also demonstrated in a model-based simulation clinical study [33]. With respect to real clinical drug interaction data, few studies are available in the literature and most have focused on drug modulators that affect known enzymatic pathways (i.e., CYP2D6, UGT2B7, UGT2B4, and CYP3A4) associated with codeine metabolism. For the glucuronidation pathway, diclofenac, a potent UGT2B7 inhibitor [10], did not affect the pharmacokinetics of codeine in human subjects as evident by similar elimination rates or maximum concentration of codeine-6-glucuronide in the experimental versus the control group [34] (Table 20.1). The lack of pharmacokinetic drug interaction also did not translate to altered pharmacodynamic effect because the addition of diclofenac to codeine did not change the results of a cold pressor test (although it was difficult to tease out diclofenac's own analgesic effects) in these human subjects (Table 20.2). Of interest is that the lack of an observed pharmacokinetic interaction was in contradiction to the *in vitro* observation in liver tissue homogenates where diclofenac inhibited the formation of codeine-6-glucuronide in a potent manner (Ki = 7.9 μM), suggesting that *in vitro* findings do not always correlate with the *in vivo* situation [35].

With respect to the CYP2D6 bioactivation pathway, studies conducted with quinidine or fluoxetine, putative inhibitors of CYP2D6, reported decreased plasma morphine concentrations in extensive metabolizers [36–39], decreased morphine concentrations in cerebrospinal fluid [38], reduced O-demethylation of codeine with corresponding reduction in plasma morphine glucuronide concentrations (an effect more prominent in Caucasians than in Chinese) [39], and decreased O-demethylation of dextromethorphan (a marker substrate for CYP2D6) [40] in human subjects coadministered codeine and quinidine/fluoxetine compared to controls taking codeine alone. These data strongly suggest that the functional inhibition of CYP2D6 activity will translate to significant pharmacokinetic interactions with codeine, resulting in reduced formation of morphine and morphine-6-glucuronide. In light of this knowledge, irrespective of the lack of available human data, one could still predict that potent and selective inhibitors of CYP2D6 will likely interact with codeine bioactivation if administered concurrently. Various lists of CYP2D6 inhibitors have been compiled by many authors, and readers are directed to these references for further details (e.g., http://www.fda.gov/Drugs/DevelopmentApprovalProcess/DevelopmentResources/DrugInteractionsLabeling/ucm093664.htm). CYP2D6 is not subjected to enzyme induction. However, other metabolic pathways of codeine (e.g., CYP3A4 and UGT2B7) can be subjected to enzyme induction, which can indirectly affect the metabolism of codeine through the CYP2D6 pathway. This was demonstrated in a study by Caraco et al. (1997) where subjects treated with rifampin showed increased formation of both codeine glucuronide and norcodeine (inactive metabolites), while the formation of morphine was significantly decreased presumably due to the shunting of codeine metabolism through these inactivation pathways [41].

While clinically significant pharmacokinetic interactions were observed when potent CYP2D6 inhibitors were coadministered with codeine, the corresponding pharmacodynamic effects were not always apparent. For example, despite significantly decreased plasma morphine concentrations [36] or demonstrated reduction in the O-demethylation of dextromethorphan (marker substrate for CYP2D6), the coadministration of quinidine in human subjects taking codeine did not change the results of the pin-prick/tolerance pain threshold tests or have any effects on physical codeine dependence in the test subjects [36, 40]. On the other hand, a significant reduction of morphine or morphine glucuronide concentrations in the presence of quinidine did lead to decreased therapeutic and positive ("high") or negative ("nausea") effects of codeine in certain studies [37]. Similarly, in extensive codeine metabolizers, patients administered codeine and rifampin had significantly decreased respiratory and psychomotor, but no change in miotic effects [41], presumably associated with reduced formation of morphine. An interesting observation is that an apparent opposite pharmacodynamic effect (i.e., decreased miotic effect in the absence of attenuated respiratory or psychomotor effects) of codeine in the presence of rifampin was observed in the same study but only in the cohort of poor (codeine) metabolizers [41]. The latter observation seems to suggest a differential pattern of codeine bioactivation/deactivation which may be dependent on an individual's CYP2D6 phenotype status, a concept that will be discussed further below.

20.3.2.2 Genetic Polymorphism

The importance of CYP2D6 in the bioactivation of codeine has fueled significant interests in understanding the effects of CYP2D6 genetic polymorphism on codeine pharmacokinetics or pharmacodynamics in humans. A survey of the literature finds several alarming reports of codeine-related fatalities or severe adverse events potentially secondary to genetic polymorphism of CYP2D6 leading to a higher conversion rate of codeine to morphine [32, 42–46]. A case report where an infant died of suspected morphine overdose secondary to the breastfeeding mother (who was later determined to be an ultrarapid metabolizer) ingesting codeine (prescribed within the typical dose limit) highlights the importance of the CYP2D6 gene and codeine pharmacokinetic/pharmacodynamic interaction [47]. Many CYP2D6 alleles are known but the functional status of every single one has not been characterized. In short, alleles can be designated as null functioning (e.g., CYP2D6*4, *5, or *6), reduced functioning (CYP2D6*10 or *41), or full functioning (*CYP2D6*1 or *2). Based on allele combinations, an individual can be categorized into one of several CYP2D6 metabolic activity phenotypes [48]: poor metabolizer (lacking any functioning allele), intermediate metabolizer (one normal and one reduced functioning allele), extensive metabolizer (at least one full- or two reduced-functioning alleles), and ultrarapid metabolizer (duplication of full-functioning alleles) (48). Although the percentage of individuals in each CYP2D6 phenotype category varies between ethnicity, the majority of humans will be classified as either extensive or intermediate metabolizers. Pharmacokinetic or pharmacodynamic interactions will likely be observed on the two ends of the spectrum, where poor metabolizers would not be able to convert codeine to morphine leading to therapy failure, whereas ultrarapid metabolizers will convert a higher percentage of codeine to morphine leading to toxicity.

Clinical data supporting a pharmacokinetic interaction between CYP2D6 phenotype status and codeine metabolism are clearly evident in the literature. Many studies have compared the effects of extensive versus poor metabolizer status in humans and reported either a lack of detection of plasma morphine [49–51], absence of morphine-6-glucuronide [50, 51], or reduced formation or exposure to morphine in plasma and urine [52–55] in poor metabolizers taking codeine compared to extensive metabolizers. Moreover, the effects of ultrarapid metabolizer phenotype on codeine metabolism have also been compared to individuals categorized as extensive or poor metabolizers, where significantly higher morphine exposure in plasma and lower total morphine/codeine ratios in urine were also observed for these patients with duplicate functional CYP2D6 alleles [56] (Table 20.1). These clinically significant pharmacokinetic interactions have also been correlated with significant interactions on the pharmacodynamic level, where only extensive metabolizers are responsive to codeine's analgesic effects (Table 20.2). Likewise, extensive or ultrarapid metabolizers of CYP2D6 are also more prone to adverse pharmacodynamic effects of codeine, as demonstrated by a significant reduction in gastric motility (i.e., constipation effect of the opioid) and increased incidence of sedation [54, 56] On the other hand, a lack of difference in codeine's therapeutic effect on postoperative pain [51] or adverse reactions [55] has also been reported when comparing extensive versus poor metabolizers, but the evidence favoring a significant interaction (presented above) certainly outweighs that of the null effect, and clinical genotyping may be warranted to optimize codeine therapy [48].

20.3.3 *Oxycodone*

20.3.3.1 Reaction Phenotyping and Clinical Pharmacokinetic and Pharmacodynamic Interactions

Oxycodone exerts its analgesic activity directly (i.e., is not a prodrug), is deactivated by CYP3A4 (N-demethylation) in the formation of the inert noroxycodone, and is bioactivated by CYP2D6 (O-demethylation) in the formation of the relatively more potent oxymorphone in humans [57]. The formation of noroxycodone is the predominant pathway in human liver microsomes and constitutes to a large extent the total intrinsic clearance of oxycodone [57]. Based on this mechanistic information, one can predict drug-drug interactions with CYP3A4, and potentially CYP2D6, modulators.

The available clinical data in the literature support a prominent role of CYP3A4 in mediating pharmacokinetic drug-drug interactions with oxycodone. Various inhibitors of CYP3A4 (i.e., clarithromycin [58], grapefruit juice [59], ketoconazole [60], itraconazole [61], ritonavir or lopinavir/ritonavir [62], voriconazole [63]) have been shown to significantly increase the plasma exposure of oxycodone or reduce the formation of noroxycodone. The data support a shunting effect where the inhibition of CYP3A4-mediated N-demethylation enhances the O-demethylation of oxycodone through the CYP2D6 pathway (i.e., grapefruit juice [59], ritonavir or lopinavir/ritonavir [62], voriconazole [63]). On the other hand, CY2D6 inhibitors, when used alone, are only able to reduce the exposure of noroxymorphone with little effects on that of oxycodone, as demonstrated in studies that have used quinidine [64, 65] and paroxetine [60, 66, 67]. The observation of a relatively minor and possibly insignificant role of CYP2D6 in mediating oxycodone drug-drug interactions is supported by the fact that only the coadministration of both CYP2D6 and CYP3A4 inhibitors can have an effect on the pharmacokinetics of oxycodone, as shown in studies using miconazole [68], paroxetine with itraconazole [66, 67], and telithromycin [69] (Table 20.1). Supporting a major role of CYP3A4 in mediating pharmacokinetic drug interactions with oxycodone, inducers of this enzyme have also been demonstrated to significantly reduce the plasma exposure of oxycodone and increase that of the inactive metabolite, noroxycodone/rifampin [70], and St. John's wort [71] (Table 20.1).

Despite significant clinical pharmacokinetic drug-drug interactions observed with CYP3A4 modulators and oxycodone, the pharmacodynamic effects from the interactions were less apparent. Some CYP3A4 modulators produced pharmacokinetic interactions in the absence of pharmacodynamic effects (e.g., clarithromycin [58] miconazole [68], paroxetine with ketoconazole [67]), whereas others only generated mixed pharmacodynamic effects (e.g., grapefruit juice [59], rifampin [70], ritonavir [62], St. John's wort [71], and telithromycin [69], voriconazole [63] (Table 20.2)). However, the relative importance of CYP3A4 and CYP2D6 in mediating pharmaco dynamic drug interactions is consistent with the pattern observed for pharmacokinetic interactions where modulators of CYP3A4 are more likely to be associated with significant pharmacodynamic interactions compared to CYP2D6 modulators (e.g., paroxetine and quinidine; Tables 20.1 and 20.2). It is unclear why there is a lack of robust pharmacokinetic-pharmacodynamic relationship in oxycodone drug interactions, but one might hypothesize that the small samples used in these studies and/or the semiquantitative nature of some pharmacodynamic tests (e.g., self-rated drug effect) may have contributed to some false-negative findings. Nevertheless, taken together, the overall evidence supports the prediction of significant pharmacokinetic-pharmacodynamic drug interactions of oxycodone with strong CYP3A4 inducers or inhibitors. Many authors have published various lists of CYP3A4 modulators, and readers are directed to these references for further details (e.g., http://www.fda.gov/Drugs/DevelopmentApprovalProcess/DevelopmentResources/DrugInteractionsLabeling/ucm093664.htm).

20.3.3.2 Genetic Polymorphism

All of the investigations on the pharmacogenetics of oxycodone have focused on the minor, but bioactivating, CYP2D6 pathway because no functional polymorphic phenotypes have yet been identified for oxycodone's major metabolic pathway (CYP3A4). The available data in the literature indicate that the plasma oxymorphone/oxycodone ratio is clearly dependent on CYP2D6 metabolizer status where ultrarapid metabolizers produce more oxymorphone than extensive metabolizers [64, 72], and in turn have higher catalytic activity compared to the poor metabolizers [73, 74] (Table 20.1). However, consistent with the observation made on the CYP2D6 drug modulators, genetic polymorphism of CYP2D6 has little or at best mixed impact on the pharmacodynamics of oxycodone (Table 20.2); thus, more studies are needed to increase this body of knowledge. The clinical significance of CYP2D6 polymorphism on oxycodone drug effects remains to be proven.

20.3.4 Hydromorphone

20.3.4.1 Reaction Phenotyping and Clinical Pharmacokinetic and Pharmacodynamic Interactions

Hydromorphone is relatively more potent than morphine and primarily metabolized by UGT enzymes in the formation of therapeutically inactive metabolites. The primary enzymes responsible for the conjugation of hydromorphone have been identified as hepatic UGT1A3 [75] and UGT2B7 [76], and the major metabolite generated is hydromorphone-3-glucuronide (H3G), the plasma concentration of which can be many fold higher than hydromorphone in humans [77]. Like its parent compound, H3G has been demonstrated to be more potent than its counterpart, morphine-3-glucuronide [78], and induce neurotoxic side effects [13] in various animal models. However, the presence of these adverse effects of H3G remains to be determined in humans, and preliminary reports have demonstrated a lack of correlation between plasma H3G concentrations and untoward side effects (e.g., myoclonus) in patients given hydromorphone [79].

Unlike morphine, few or no drug interaction studies associated with hydromorphone metabolism have been reported in the literature. However, various substrates, inhibitors, and inducers of human hepatic UGT1A3 and UGT2B7 have been identified [10] *in vitro*, which can potentially mediate pharmacokinetic interactions with hydromorphone *in vivo*. Despite the lack of human data, the clinical significance of the effects of these putative modulators on hydromorphone metabolism may be predicted using data obtained from *in vitro* models (e.g., human liver microsomal systems or primary cultures of hepatocytes) in an approach that may minimize drug testing in humans yet generate meaningful clinical drug interaction data [80].

20.3.4.2 Genetic Polymorphism

Similar to a general lack of metabolism-mediated pharmacokinetic interaction data for hydromorphone in the literature, little is available on the impact of genetic polymorphism in humans. In a study in Taiwanese patients, individuals with UGT2B7*2 genotype (a -802A>T genetic variant that results in reduced catalytic activity) exhibited similar pharmacokinetic parameters (exposure and maximum concentration) of hydromorphone and H3G in plasma compared to wild-type patients [81]. The H3G/hydromorphone ratio also did not change, supporting a lack of genetic effect on the metabolism of hydromorphone in these subjects. The lack of pharmacokinetic gene-drug interaction also translated to null pharmacodynamic effects, where UGT2B7 genotype did not impact the incidence of adverse events associated with hydromorphone. These negative findings are consistent with those observed for morphine [25, 26] and may suggest that UGT2B7*2 genetic polymorphism has little impact toward opioid metabolism, in general. However, the effects of other polymorphic alleles of UGT2B7 or UGT1A3 (which is also known to exhibit polymorphism [10]) on the metabolism of hydromorphone remain to be determined.

20.3.5 Fentanyl

20.3.5.1 Reaction Phenotyping and Clinical Pharmacokinetic and Pharmacodynamic Interactions

Fentanyl is a versatile opioid as it can be administered by various routes and is often used in the treatment of cancer and non-cancer pain [82]. Fentanyl is extensively metabolized primarily by hepatic CYP3A4 in the production of norfentanyl, as demonstrated in experiments conducted in human liver microsomes [83, 84], and the metabolite is considered therapeutically inert. Because it is catalyzed primarily by CYP3A4, fentanyl may be subjected to various drug-drug interactions known to take place with this isoenzyme. All of the clinical studies in the literature, to the best of our knowledge, have focused on the effects of CYP3A4 modulators on the pharmacokinetics of fentanyl and the findings are somewhat inconsistent: itraconazole (a potent inhibitor) [85], grapefruit juice [86], and parecoxib [87] (the latter 2 agents are relatively weaker inhibitors of CYP3A4) had little effects on the clearance, whereas troleandomycin, ritonavir, fluconazole, and voriconazole (potent inhibitors of CYP3A4) significantly reduced the plasma exposure and/or clearance of intravenously or orally administered (as a lozenge) fentanyl in human subjects [86, 88, 89]. Consistent with the trend that the significance of interacting effects on fentanyl may be dependent on the potency of the CYP3A4 modulator, rifampin, a strong CYP3A4 inducer, was also shown to clearly increase the clearance and reduce the exposure of fentanyl in plasma [86] (Table 20.1). Not all interaction studies mentioned above have discussed pharmacodynamics effects, but those that have reported such effects are generally in agreement with the pharmacokinetic (or lack of) interactions observed: that troleandomycin, but not parecoxib, modulated the effects of fentanyl on pupil diameter [87], whereas itraconazole had little influence on fentanyl's therapeutic and adverse (drowsiness, nausea, pruritus) effects [85] (Table 20.2). Moreover, case reports are available in the literature that seem to favor a pharmacokinetic-mediated pharmacodynamic interaction, such as the manifestation of delirium after coadministration of diltiazem (a known CYP3A4 inhibitor) and the reduction of fentanyl transdermal patch's therapeutic efficacy when rifampin is given concurrently [90]. The inconsistencies observed in the literature of CYP3A4 modulators might be explained by the fact that these inhibitors or inducers may have also affected other (minor) metabolic pathways known to metabolize fentanyl [91], (e.g., resulting in mixed patterns of drug interactions that can be rationalized only if the investigators had determined the pharmacokinetics of all possible metabolites of fentanyl). Alternatively, fentanyl is considered a relatively high extraction drug; thus, its clearance is more dependent on hepatic blood flow than intrinsic hepatic clearance (i.e., metabolism-mediated clearance). This theory, as suggested by Ibrahim et al [87], might explain our observation that only strong modulators (i.e., those presented above) have an effect on the pharmacokinetics or pharmacodynamic of fentanyl in humans.

20.3.5.2 Genetic Polymorphism

Since no functional genetic polymorphisms have been identified for CYP3A4, the primary isoenzyme responsible for the deactivation of fentanyl, little or no known pharmacogenomic data are available in the literature.

20.3.6 Tramadol

20.3.6.1 Reaction Phenotyping and Clinical Pharmacokinetic and Pharmacodynamic Interactions

Tramadol is marketed as a racemic mixture and exerts its analgesic action via mu-receptor binding and norepinephrine/serotonin reuptake inhibition [8]. Tramadol is primarily metabolized by CYP2D6 (O-demethylation) and CYP3A4

(N-demethylation) in the formation of active M1 and inactive M2 metabolites, respectively, as demonstrated *in vitro* in human liver microsomes and c-DNA-expressed CYP450 enzymes [92]. The M1 metabolite is relatively more potent than tramadol, as evident by its much higher affinity toward mu-receptor binding [93]. The majority of the clinical drug interaction data in the literature have focused on the effects of CYP2D6 modulators on the disposition of tramadol. Relatively weak inhibitors of CYP2D6 such as escitalopram [94] and strong inhibitors such as methadone [95] or paroxetine [96, 97] were capable of decreasing the plasma exposure or urinary recovery of the M1 metabolite while increasing that of tramadol (Table 20.1). Stronger inhibition of M1 metabolite formation was translated to reduced analgesic effects in humans [96], whereas escitalopram did not change the subjects' responses to the cold pressor test [95] (Table 20.2). On the other hand, fewer data were available on the effects of CYP3A4 modulators toward the disposition of tramadol in humans. Rifampin pretreatment was shown to reduce the plasma exposure of both the parent and the active M1 metabolite in patients administered oral or intravenous tramadol [98], supporting the result of enzyme induction and possibly enhanced metabolism through the CYP3A4 pathway (no M2 metabolite data were collected in support of this theory in the study). Itraconazole, as a relatively potent CYP3A4 inhibitor, had no additional effects to tramadol or M1 metabolite plasma exposure when used in combination with ticlopidine, an inhibitor of CYP2D6 [99]. Unfortunately, neither study assessed pharmacodynamic outcomes; thus, a correlation could not be established with (or lack of) changes observed on the pharmacokinetics of tramadol. More data are certainly needed to ascertain the contributions of CYP3A4 and CYP2D6 toward the pharmacokinetic and pharmacodynamic drug-drug interactions associated with tramadol.

20.3.6.2 Genetic Polymorphism

No functional genetic polymorphisms have been identified for CYP3A4; thus, the clinical literature data on tramadol pharmacogenomics have focused only on the role of the polymorphic CYP2D6. Various studies have reported the effects of CYP2D6 metabolizer phenotype on the pharmacokinetics of tramadol and found increased plasma exposure of the M1 metabolite (which corresponded with decreased exposure of the parent drug) in extensive metabolizers compared to poor metabolizers administered tramadol [100–104]. The pharmacokinetic effects were more prominent in ultrarapid metabolizers where further increases in plasma M1 metabolite exposure were observed compared to extensive or intermediate metabolizers [105–107] (Table 20.1). These pharmacokinetic changes also corresponded with pharmacodynamic effects, where the degree of analgesia or level of pain threshold appears to be dependent on the presence of functional CYP2D6 alleles (i.e., ultrarapid > extensive > poor metabolizers) (Table 20.2). On the other hand, the extent of adverse events observed is less apparent, where some studies reported more adverse events with intermediate metabolizers (vs. ultrarapid) [106] and others reported the opposite [107]. One may hypothesize that tramadol and its M1 metabolite may each lead to a range of side effects, and the discrepancy observed with respect to CYP2D6 metabolizer status and adverse events might be attributed to pharmacokinetic changes observed with either the parent or the metabolite. Overall, the literature clearly supports a pharmacokinetic-pharmacodynamic interaction mediated by CYP2D6 genetic polymorphism. This, taken together with drug interaction data using CYP2D6 inhibitors discussed above, suggests that the coadministration of CYP2D6 modulators can be predicted to lead to significant drug interactions in the clinic. Various lists of CYP2D6 inhibitors have been compiled by many authors, and readers are directed to these references for further details (e.g., http://www.fda.gov/Drugs/DevelopmentApprovalProcess/DevelopmentResources/DrugInteractionsLabeling/ucm093664.htm).

20.3.7 Methadone

20.3.7.1 Reaction Phenotyping and Clinical Pharmacokinetic and Pharmacodynamic Interactions

Methadone is a racemic mixture of R- and S-enantiomers that exhibit differential activity toward mu-receptor binding. The R-form exhibits a higher affinity toward the opioid receptor [108] and hence exhibits greater analgesic effects. The S-enantiomer has antagonistic activity toward N-methyl-D-aspartate receptors and is an uptake inhibitor of norepinephrine and serotonin neurotransmitters [109, 110], which are responsible for pharmacological drug-drug interactions with other serotonin modulators such as the selective serotonin reuptake inhibitor class of antidepressants. Methadone is unique in that it has an extremely long half-life [111] and is one of the principal therapies in opioid withdrawal/maintenance regimens widely used to manage heroin addictions [112]. Methadone is extensively metabolized in the liver to inactive N-demethylated metabolites, and *in vitro* reaction phenotyping studies have determined CYP2B6 [113–115] and CYP3A4 [116–118] to be the principal enzymes. Other CYP450 enzymes (e.g., CYP2D6 and CYP2C9) have also been identified but the relative contributions of these isoenzymes to the overall metabolism of methadone still remain to be determined [113, 119, 120]. Moreover, CYP2B6, but not CYP3A4, catalyzes methadone in a regioselective manner [115, 119], an effect that can potentially result in different concentrations of R- or S-methadone and complicates the interpretation of results from drug interaction studies.

Methadone is subjected to potential clinically significant drug-drug interactions, primarily mediated by CYP2D6 and CYP3A4 modulators. Clinical studies have described mixed effects of classical CYP3A4 inhibitors on the pharmacokinetics of methadone, where fluconazole [121] and voriconazole [122] both increased methadone exposure in plasma, but troleandomycin [114] and grapefruit juice [114] had little effects (Table 20.1). However, significant pharmacokinetic interactions from fluconazole or voriconazole did not translate to pharmacodynamic effects because the coadministration of either drug was not associated with signs of methadone overdose or withdrawal in test subjects (Table 20.2). Confirming a role of CYP3A4 in methadone metabolism, rifampin, a potent CYP3A4 inducer, was shown to increase the clearance of methadone [114] (Table 20.1), but correlation to pharmacodynamic effects was not established in that particular study. Moreover, studies with CYP2D6 inhibitors or mixed CYP2D6/CYP3A4 inhibitors have also reported significant drug-drug interactions, where paroxetine [123] increased the plasma concentrations of both racemic forms of methadone in patients genotyped as CYP2D6 extensive metabolizers, quetiapine [124] elevated the plasma R-methadone/dose ratio in a finding that was also dependent on CYP2D6 metabolizer phenotype, and sertraline, a mixed CYP2D6/3A4 inhibitor [125], also elevated methadone concentration/dose ratio in the plasma (Table 20.1). Other than a lack of correlation between sertraline's pharmacokinetic effects and adverse events associated with methadone, the other studies did not attempt to correlate pharmacokinetic interactions with pharmacodynamic changes (Table 20.2).

Clinical drug interactions between methadone and HIV antiviral agents have received significant interest because of the overlapping patient populations that would require the two types of therapies. Overall, most of the literature focuses on protease inhibitors (PIs) (Table 20.1), where mixed findings toward the pharmacokinetics of methadone have been reported. In general, PIs are substrates for CYP3A4 and theoretically should compete with the metabolism competitively and elevate the plasma concentrations of methadone. The opposite effects, however, were observed in clinical studies where amprenavir [126], lopinavir-ritonavir [127–129], nelfinavir [130–132], and saquinavir/ritonavir [133, 134] have all been shown to decrease plasma exposure of total, R-, or S-methadone in human subjects (Table 20.1). On the other hand, a lack of effect on the pharmacokinetics of methadone has also been demonstrated for several protease inhibitors, despite control experiments demonstrating significant inhibition toward CYP3A4 in situ: atazanavir [135], indinavir [136], and saquinavir/ritonavir [137]. These observations support a drug interaction pattern that is unlikely mediated by CYP3A4 inhibition, but rather induction by PI toward other metabolic pathways of methadone (e.g., CYP2D6 or CYP2B6) in humans. Molecular studies (e.g., using *in vitro* experimental models that can be subjected to drug induction experiments such as cultured human hepatocytes) are still needed to support this theory. The majority of pharmacokinetic changes mediated by PI are not correlated with altered pharmacodynamic effects of methadone (e.g., withdrawal, adverse events, requirement for dose adjustment, laboratory testing, electrocardiogram (ECG) readings) (Table 20.2).

Data are also available on the nucleoside reverse transcriptase inhibitors (NRTIs) where neither tenofovir nor zidovudine affected the plasma exposure of the two enantiomers of methadone [138, 139] (Table 20.1). Likewise, integrase inhibitors (INIs) dolutegravir [140] and raltegravir [141] also had little effects on the plasma exposure of methadone. With respect to pharmacodynamic effects, none of these antiviral agents were associated with altered withdrawal, miosis, or abnormal laboratory values (e.g., ECG readings) when coadministered with methadone. These observations are consistent with the general lack of metabolism-mediated drug interactions associated with the NRTIs and INIs in the literature. On the other hand, significant pharmacokinetic changes were observed for non-nucleoside reverse transcriptase inhibitors (NNRTIs) which were consistent with their metabolic properties: that the inductive effects of nevirapine toward CYP3A4 may have resulted in decreased plasma exposure [142–144], the inhibitory effects of delavirdine toward CYP3A4 contributed to increased plasma exposure [145], and a general lack of metabolic-interaction effects of lersivirine resulted in no change [146] in the plasma exposure of methadone in humans (Table 20.1). The coadministration of nevirapine should be cautioned since two studies have demonstrated increased withdrawal symptoms when combined with methadone (Table 20.2).

20.3.7.2 Genetic Polymorphism

Only a few studies are available in the literature examining the effects of genetic polymorphisms on methadone metabolism (Table 20.1) and there appear to be significant interacting effects by CYP2D6 metabolizer status [147, 148], CYP2B6 polymorphism [148], or ABCB1 polymorphism [124, 148]. However, more pharmacokinetic studies are needed to support these observations and to correlate with pharmacodynamic effects, where information is still fairly sparse (Table 20.2).

20.4 Assessing the Clinical Significance of Pharmacokinetic and Pharmacodynamic Interactions: Clinical Decision-Making Algorithm

We have provided an extensive overview on the pharmacokinetic-pharmacodynamic drug-drug interactions associated with a selection of opioid drugs that are commonly used in the clinic today. We propose that the following clinical decision-making algorithm, modified from what we have developed previously [152], can be used to ascertain the clinical significance of pharmacokinetic-mediated pharmacodynamic interactions with opioid analgesics:

1. Does the effector drug and its metabolites possess pharmacokinetic properties (i.e., absorption, distribution, metabolism, elimination) that can be subjected to drug interaction? *The majority of data on opioids has focused on drug metabolism, and there are in vitro data to support the in vivo observations. Moreover, many opioids* (e.g., *codeine) are metabolized by enzymes that are known to exhibit genetic polymorphism and this additional (gene-drug interaction) factor must be considered.*
2. Does the effector drug and its metabolites possess pharmacodynamic properties that can be subjected to drug interaction? *The majority of data on opioids has focused on their classical analgesic properties, effects on pain threshold, and adverse effects such as somnolence, nausea/vomiting, gastrointestinal motility, or miosis. Additional atypical adverse effects such* QT_C *prolongation* (e.g., *associated with methadone) or serotonin syndrome* (e.g., *associated with tramadol)*

must be considered and can be manifested by pharmacokinetic-associated pharmacodynamic interactions.

3. Does the interacting drug possess pharmacokinetic or pharmacodynamic properties that can subject an opioid agent to drug interactions? *The same considerations discussed for points 1) and 2) above also apply here.*
4. Is there evidence that the combination has caused statistically significant changes in drug pharmacokinetics in humans? *The evidence must be appropriately weighted based on limitations in study design* (e.g., *nature of experimental model, generalizability of the data to the real clinical situation, etc.). The available human data for opioids only represent a small fraction of all the possible drug interactions but one may use various in vitro or in silico approaches to aid the prediction of pharmacokinetic interactions.*
5. Is there evidence that a significant pharmacokinetic interaction is associated with a pharmacodynamic interaction? *The evidence must be appropriately weighted based on limitations in study design. Information on pharmacokinetic-mediated pharmacodynamic interactions is relatively scarce in the literature compared to the available pharmacokinetic data.*

References

1. Portenoy RK, Ahmed E (2014) Principles of opioid use in cancer pain. J Clin Oncol 32(16):1662–1670
2. Cheung CW, Qiu Q, Choi SW, Moore B, Goucke R, Irwin W (2014) Chronic opioid therapy for chronic non-cancer pain: a review and comparison of treatment guidelines. Pain Physician 17(5):401–414
3. de Leon-Casasola O (2014) A review of the literature on multiple factors involved in postoperative pain course and duration. Postgrad Med 126(4):42–52
4. Miller E (2004) The world health organization analgesic ladder. J Midwifery Womens Health 49(6):542–545
5. Overholser BR, Foster DR (2011) Opioid pharmacokinetic drug-drug interactions. Am J Manag Care 17(Suppl 11):S276–S287
6. Smith HS (2009) Opioid metabolism. Mayo Clin Proc 84(7):613–624
7. Rollason V, Samer C, Piquet V, Dayer P, Desmeules J (2008) Pharmacogenetics of analgesics: toward the individualization of prescription. Pharmacogenomics 9(7):905–933
8. Trescot AM, Datta S, Lee M, Hansen H (2008) Opioid pharmacology. Pain Physician 11(2 Suppl):S133–S153
9. Kharasch ED, Hoffer C, Whittington D, Sheffels P (2003) Role of P-glycoprotein in the intestinal absorption and clinical effects of morphine. Clin Pharmacol Ther 74(6):543–554
10. Kiang TK, Ensom MH, Chang TK (2005) UDP-glucuronosyltransferases and clinical drug-drug interactions. Pharmacol Ther 106(1):97–132
11. Coffman BL, Rios GR, King CD, Tephly TR (1997) Human UGT2B7 catalyzes morphine glucuronidation. Drug Metab Dispos 25(1):1–4
12. Kilpatrick GJ, Smith TW (2005) Morphine-6-glucuronide: actions and mechanisms. Med Res Rev 25(5):521–544
13. Smith MT (2000) Neuroexcitatory effects of morphine and hydromorphone: evidence implicating the 3-glucuronide metabolites. Clin Exp Pharmacol Physiol 27(7):524–528

14. Osborne R, Joel S, Trew D, Slevin M (1990) Morphine and metabolite behavior after different routes of morphine administration: demonstration of the importance of the active metabolite morphine-6-glucuronide. Clin Pharmacol Ther 47(1):12–19
15. Brunk SF, Delle M, Wilson WR (1974) Effect of propranolol on morphine metabolism. Clin Pharmacol Ther 16(6):1039–1044
16. Aasmundstad TA, Storset P (1998) Influence of ranitidine on the morphine-3-glucuronide to morphine-6-glucuronide ratio after oral administration of morphine in humans. Hum Exp Toxicol 17(6):347–352
17. Vincent J, Hunt T, Teng R, Robarge L, Willavize SA, Friedman HL (1998) The pharmacokinetic effects of coadministration of morphine and trovafloxacin in healthy subjects. Am J Surg 176(6A Suppl):32S–38S
18. Tighe KE, Webb AM, Hobbs GJ (1999) Persistently high plasma morphine-6-glucuronide levels despite decreased hourly patient-controlled analgesia morphine use after single-dose diclofenac: potential for opioid-related toxicity. Anesth Analg 88(5):1137–1142
19. Fromm MF, Eckhardt K, Li S, Schanzle G, Hofmann U, Mikus G et al (1997) Loss of analgesic effect of morphine due to coadministration of rifampin. Pain 72(1–2):261–267
20. Mojaverian P, Feddler IL, Vlasses PH, Rotmensch HH, Rocci ML, Swanson BN et al (1982) Cimetidine does not alter morphine disposition in man. Br J Clin Pharmacol 14(6):809–813
21. Eckhardt K, Ammon S, Hofmann U, Riebe A, Gugeler N, Mikus G (2000) Gabapentin enhances the analgesic effect of morphine in healthy volunteers. Anesth Analg 91(1):185–191
22. Drewe J, Ball HA, Beglinger C, Peng B, Kemmler A, Schachinger H et al (2000) Effect of P-glycoprotein modulation on the clinical pharmacokinetics and adverse effects of morphine. Br J Clin Pharmacol 50(3):237–246
23. Bhasker CR, McKinnon W, Stone A, Lo AC, Kubota T, Ishizaki T et al (2000) Genetic polymorphism of UDP-glucuronosyltransferase 2B7 (UGT2B7) at amino acid 268: ethnic diversity of alleles and potential clinical significance. Pharmacogenetics 10(8):679–685
24. Court MH, Krishnaswamy S, Hao Q, Duan SX, Patten CJ, von Moltke LL et al (2003) Evaluation of 3'-azido-3'-deoxythymidine, morphine, and codeine as probe substrates for UDP-glucuronosyltransferase 2B7 (UGT2B7) in human liver microsomes: specificity and influence of the UGT2B7*2 polymorphism. Drug Metab Dispos 31(9):1125–1133
25. Holthe M, Rakvag TN, Klepstad P, Idle JR, Kaasa S, Krokan HE et al (2003) Sequence variations in the UDP-glucuronosyltransferase 2B7 (UGT2B7) gene: identification of 10 novel single nucleotide polymorphisms (SNPs) and analysis of their relevance to morphine glucuronidation in cancer patients. Pharmacogenomics J 3(1):17–26
26. Holthe M, Klepstad P, Zahlsen K, Borchgrevink PC, Hagen L, Dale O et al (2002) Morphine glucuronide-to-morphine plasma ratios are unaffected by the UGT2B7 H268Y and UGT1A1*28 polymorphisms in cancer patients on chronic morphine therapy. Eur J Clin Pharmacol 58(5):353–536
27. Darbari DS, Van Schaik RH, Capparelli EV, Rana S, McCarter R, van den Anker J (2008) UGT2B7 promoter variant -840G>A contributes to the variability in hepatic clearance of morphine in patients with sickle cell disease. Am J Hematol 83(3):200–202
28. Sawyer MB, Innocenti F, Das S, Cheng C, Ramirez J, Pantle-Fisher FH et al (2003) A pharmacogenetic study of uridine diphosphate-glucuronosyltransferase 2B7 in patients receiving morphine. Clin Pharmacol Ther 73(6):566–574
29. Matic M, Norman E, Rane A, Beck O, Andersson M, Elens L et al (2014) Effect of UGT2B7 -900G>A (−842G>A; rs7438135) on morphine glucuronidation in preterm newborns: results from a pilot cohort. Pharmacogenomics 15(12):1589–1597
30. Dayer P, Desmeules J, Leemann T, Striberni R (1988) Bioactivation of the narcotic drug codeine in human liver is mediated by the polymorphic monooxygenase catalyzing debrisoquine 4-hydroxylation (cytochrome P-450 dbl/bufI). Biochem Biophys Res Commun 152(1):411–416

31. Caraco Y, Tateishi T, Guengerich FP, Wood AJ (1996) Microsomal codeine N-demethylation: cosegregation with cytochrome P4503A4 activity. Drug Metab Dispos 24(7):761–764
32. Gasche Y, Daali Y, Fathi M, Chiappe A, Cottini S, Dayer P et al (2004) Codeine intoxication associated with ultrarapid CYP2D6 metabolism. N Engl J Med 351(27):2827–2831
33. Eissing T, Lippert J, Willmann S (2012) Pharmacogenomics of codeine, morphine, and morphine-6-glucuronide: model-based analysis of the influence of CYP2D6 activity, UGT2B7 activity, renal impairment, and CYP3A4 inhibition. Mol Diagn Ther 16(1):43–53
34. Ammon S, Marx C, Behrens C, Hofmann U, Murdter T, Griese EU et al (2002) Diclofenac does not interact with codeine metabolism *in vivo*: a study in healthy volunteers. BMC Clin Pharmacol 27(2):2
35. Ammon S, von Richter O, Hofmann U, Thon KP, Eichelbaum M, Mikus G (2000) *In vitro* interaction of codeine and diclofenac. Drug Metab Dispos 28(10):1149–1152
36. Sindrup SH, Arendt-Nielsen L, Brosen K, Bierring P, Angelo HR, Eriksson B et al (1992) The effect of quinidine on the analgesic effect of codeine. Eur J Clin Pharmacol 42(6):587–591
37. Kathiramalainathan K, Kaplan HL, Romach MK, Busto UE, Li NY, Sawe J et al (2000) Inhibition of cytochrome P450 2D6 modifies codeine abuse liability. J Clin Psychopharmacol 20(4):435–444
38. Sindrup SH, Hofmann U, Asmussen J, Mikus G, Brosen K, Nielsen F et al (1996) Impact of quinidine on plasma and cerebrospinal fluid concentrations of codeine and morphine after codeine intake. Eur J Clin Pharmacol 49(6):503–509
39. Caraco Y, Sheller J, Wood AJ (1999) Impact of ethnic origin and quinidine coadministration on codeine's disposition and pharmacodynamic effects. J Pharmacol Exp Ther 290(1):413–422
40. Fernandes LC, Kilicarslan T, Kaplan HL, Tyndale RF, Sellers EM, Romach MK (2002) Treatment of codeine dependence with inhibitors of cytochrome P450 2D6. J Clin Psychopharmacol 22(3):326–329
41. Caraco Y, Sheller J, Wood AJ (1997) Pharmacogenetic determinants of codeine induction by rifampin: the impact on codeine's respiratory, psychomotor and miotic effects. J Pharmacol Exp Ther 281(1):330–336
42. Madadi P, Ross CJ, Hayden MR, Carleton BC, Gaedigk A, Leeder JS et al (2009) Pharmacogenetics of neonatal opioid toxicity following maternal use of codeine during breastfeeding: a case–control study. Clin Pharmacol Ther 85(1):31–35
43. Voronov P, Przbylo HJ, Jagannathan N (2007) Apnea in a child after oral codeine: a genetic variant - an ultra-rapid metabolizer. Paediatr Anaesth 17(7):684–687
44. Kelly LE, Rieder M, van den Anker J, Malkin B, Ross C, Neely MN et al (2012) More codeine fatalities after tonsillectomy in North American children. Pediatrics 129(5):e1343–e1347
45. Ciszkowski C, Madadi P, Phillips MS, Lauwers AE, Koren G (2009) Codeine, ultrarapid-metabolism genotype, and postoperative death. N Engl J Med 361(8):827–828
46. Dalen P, Frengell C, Dahl ML, Sjogvist F (1997) Quick onset of severe abdominal pain after codeine in an ultrarapid metabolizer of debrisoquine. Ther Drug Monit 19(5):543–544
47. Koren G, Cairns J, Chitayat D, Gaedigk A, Leeder SJ (2006) Pharmacogenetics of morphine poisoning in a breastfed neonate of a codeine-prescribed mother. Lancet 368(9536):704
48. Crews KR, Gaedigk A, Dunnenberger HM, Leeder JS, Klein TE, Caudle KE et al (2014) Clinical Pharmacogenetics Implementation Consortium guidelines for cytochrome P450 2D6 genotype and codeine therapy: 2014 update. Clin Pharmacol Ther 95(4):376–382
49. Sindrup SH, Brosen K, Bjerring P, Arendt-Nielsen L, Larsen U, Angelo HR et al (1990) Codeine increases pain thresholds to copper vapor laser stimuli in extensive but not poor metabolizers of sparteine. Clin Pharmacol Ther 48(6):686–693
50. Poulsen L, Brosen K, Arendt-Nielsen L, Gram LF, Elbaek K, Sindrup SH (1996) Codeine and morphine in extensive and poor metabolizers of sparteine: pharmacokinetics, analgesic effect and side effects. Eur J Clin Pharmacol 51(3–4):289–295

51. Poulsen L, Riishede L, Brosen K, Clemensen S, Sindrup SH (1998) Codeine in post-operative pain. Study of the influence of sparteine phenotype and serum concentrations of morphine and morphine-6-glucuronide. Eur J Clin Pharmacol 54(6):451–454
52. Yue QY, Hasselstron J, Svensson JO, Sawe J (1991) Pharmacokinetics of codeine and its metabolites in Caucasian healthy volunteers: comparisons between extensive and poor hydroxylators of debrisoquine. Br J Clin Pharmacol 31(6):635–642
53. Chen ZR, Somogyi AA, Reynolds G, Bochner F (1991) Disposition and metabolism of codeine after single and chronic doses in one poor and seven extensive metabolisers. Br J Clin Pharmacol 31(4):381–390
54. Mikus G, Trausch B, Rodewald C, Hofmann U, Richter K, Gramatte T et al (1997) Effect of codeine on gastrointestinal motility in relation to CYP2D6 phenotype. Clin Pharmacol Ther 61(4):459–466
55. Eckhardt K, Li S, Ammon S, Schanzle G, Mikus G, Eichelbaum M (1998) Same incidence of adverse drug events after codeine administration irrespective of the genetically determined differences in morphine formation. Pain 76(1–2):27–33
56. Kirchheiner J, Schmidt H, Tzvetkov M, Keulen JT, Lotsch J, Roots I et al (2007) Pharmacokinetics of codeine and its metabolite morphine in ultra-rapid metabolizers due to CYP2D6 duplication. Pharmacogenomics J 7(4):257–265
57. Lalovic B, Phillips B, Risler LL, Howald W, Shen DD (2004) Quantitative contribution of CYP2D6 and CYP3A to oxycodone metabolism in human liver and intestinal microsomes. Drug Metab Dispos 32(4):447–454
58. Liukas A, Hagelberg NM, Kuusniemi K, Neuvonen PJ, Olkkola KT (2011) Inhibition of cytochrome P450 3A by clarithromycin uniformly affects the pharmacokinetics and pharmacodynamics of oxycodone in young and elderly volunteers. J Clin Psychopharmacol 31(3):302–308
59. Nieminen TH, Hagelberg NM, Saari TI, Neuvonen M, Neuvonen PJ, Laine K et al (2010) Grapefruit juice enhances the exposure to oral oxycodone. Basic Clin Pharmacol Toxicol 107(4):782–788
60. Kummer O, Hammann F, Moser C, Schaller O, Drewe J, Krahenbuhl S (2011) Effect of the inhibition of CYP3A4 or CYP2D6 on the pharmacokinetics and pharmacodynamics of oxycodone. Eur J Clin Pharmacol 67(1):63–71
61. Saari TI, Gronlund J, Hagelberg NM, Neuvonen M, Laine K, Neuvonen PJ et al (2010) Effects of itraconazole on the pharmacokinetics and pharmacodynamics of intravenously and orally administered oxycodone. Eur J Clin Pharmacol 66(4):387–397
62. Nieminen TH, Hagelberg NM, Saari TI, Neuvonen M, Neuvonen PJ, Laine K et al (2010) Oxycodone concentrations are greatly increased by the concomitant use of ritonavir or lopinavir/ritonavir. Eur J Clin Pharmacol 66(10):977–985
63. Hagelberg NM, Nieminen TH, Saari TI, Neuvonen M, Neuvonen PJ, Laine K et al (2009) Voriconazole drastically increases exposure to oral oxycodone. Eur J Clin Pharmacol 65(3):263–271
64. Samer CF, Daali Y, Wagner M, Hopfgartner G, Eap CB, Rebsamen MC et al (2010) The effects of CYP2D6 and CYP3A activities on the pharmacokinetics of immediate release oxycodone. Br J Pharmacol 160(4):907–918
65. Heiskanen T, Olkkola KT, Kalso E (1998) Effects of blocking CYP2D6 on the pharmacokinetics and pharmacodynamics of oxycodone. Clin Pharmacol Ther 64:603–611
66. Gronlund J, Saari TI, Hagelberg NM, Neuvonen PJ, Olkkola KT, Laine K (2010) Exposure to oral oxycodone is increased by concomitant inhibition of CYP2D6 and 3A4 pathways, but not by inhibition of CYP2D6 alone. Br J Clin Pharmacol 70(1):78–87
67. Gronlund J, Saari TI, Hagelberg NM, Neuvonen PJ, Laine K, Olkkola KT (2011) Effect of inhibition of cytochrome P450 enzymes 2D6 and 3A4 on the pharmacokinetics of intravenous oxycodone: a randomized, three-phase, crossover, placebo-controlled study. Clin Drug Investig 31(3):143–153
68. Gronlund J, Saari TI, Hagelberg NM, Neuvonen PJ, Olkkola KT, Laine K (2011) Miconazole oral gel increases exposure to oral oxycodone by inhibition of CYP2D6 and CYP3A4. Antimicrob Agents Chemother 55(3):1063–1067

69. Gronlund J, Saari TI, Hagelberg NM, Martikainen IK, Neuvonen PJ, Olkkola KT et al (2010) Effect of telithromycin on the pharmacokinetics and pharmacodynamics of oral oxycodone. J Clin Pharmacol 50(1):101–108
70. Nieminen TH, Hagelberg NM, Saari TI, Pertovaara A, Neuvonen M, Laine K et al (2009) Rifampin greatly reduces the plasma concentrations of intravenous and oral oxycodone. Anesthesiology 110(6):1371–1378
71. Nieminen TH, Hagelberg NM, Saari TI, Neuvonen M, Laine K, Neuvonen PJ et al (2010) St John's wort greatly reduces the concentrations of oral oxycodone. Eur J Pain 14(8):854–859
72. Stamer UM, Zhang L, Book M, Lehmann LE, Stuber F, Musshoff F (2013) CYP2D6 genotype dependent oxycodone metabolism in postoperative patients. PLoS One 8(3), e60239
73. Zwisler ST, Enggaard TP, Noehr-Jensen L, Pedersen RS, Mikkelsen S, Nielsen F et al (2009) The hypoalgesic effect of oxycodone in human experimental pain models in relation to the CYP2D6 oxidation polymorphism. Basic Clin Pharmacol Toxicol 104(4):335–344
74. Zwisler ST, Enggaard TP, Mikkelsen S, Brosen K, Sindrup SH (2010) Impact of the CYP2D6 genotype on post-operative intravenous oxycodone analgesia. Acta Anaesthesiol Scand 54(2):232–240
75. Green MD, King CD, Mojarrabi B, MacKenzie PI, Tephly TR (1998) Glucuronidation of amines and other xenobiotics catalyzed by expressed human UDP-glucuronosyltransferase 1A3. Drug Metab Dispos 26(6):507–512
76. Radominska-Pandya A, Czernik PJ, Little JM, Battaglia E, MacKenzie PI (1999) Structural and functional studies of UDP-glucuronosyltransferases. Drug Metab Rev 31(4):817–899
77. Hagen N, Thirlwell MP, Dhaliwal HS, Babul N, Harsanyi Z, Darke AC (1995) Steady-state pharmacokinetics of hydromorphone and hydromorphone-3-glucuronide in cancer patients after immediate and controlled-release hydromorphone. J Clin Pharmacol 35(1):37–44
78. Wright AW, Mather LE, Smith MT (2001) Hydromorphone-3-glucuronide: a more potent neuro-excitant than its structural analogue, morphine-3-glucuronide. Life Sci 69(4): 409–420
79. McCann S, Yaksh TL, von Gunten CF (2010) Correlation between myoclonus and the 3-glucuronide metabolites in patients treated with morphine or hydromorphone: a pilot study. J Opioid Manag 6(2):87–94
80. Miners JO, MacKenzie PI, Knights KM (2010) The prediction of drug-glucuronidation parameters in humans: UDP-glucuronosyltransferase enzyme-selective substrate and inhibitor probes for reaction phenotyping and *in vitro-in vivo* extrapolation of drug clearance and drug-drug interaction potential. Drug Metab Dispos 42(1):196–208
81. Vandenbossche J, Richards H, Francke S, Van Den Bergh A, Lu CC, Franc MA (2014) The effect of UGT2B7*2 polymorphism on the pharmacokinetics of OROS?hydromorphone in Taiwanese subjects. J Clin Pharmacol 54(10):1170–1179
82. Stanley TH (2014) The fentanyl story. J Pain 15(12):1215–1226
83. Labroo RB, Paine MF, Thummel KE, Kharasch ED (1997) Fentanyl metabolism by human hepatic and intestinal cytochrome P450 3A4: implications for interindividual variability in disposition, efficacy, and drug interactions. Drug Metab Dispos 25(9):1072–1080
84. Feierman DE, Lasker JM (1996) Metabolism of fentanyl, a synthetic opioid analgesic, by human liver microsomes. Role of CYP3A4. Drug Metab Dispos 24(9):932–939
85. Palkama VJ, Neuvonen PJ, Olkkola KT (1998) The CYP 3A4 inhibitor itraconazole has no effect on the pharmacokinetics of i.v. fentanyl. Br J Anaesth 81(4):598–600
86. Kharasch ED, Whittington D, Hoffer C (2004) Influence of hepatic and intestinal cytochrome P4503A activity on the acute disposition and effects of oral transmucosal fentanyl citrate. Anesthesiology 101(3):729–737
87. Ibrahim AE, Feldman J, Karim A, Kharasch ED (2003) Simultaneous assessment of drug interactions with low- and high-extraction opioids: application to parecoxib effects on the pharmacokinetics and pharmacodynamics of fentanyl and alfentanil. Anesthesiology 98(4):853–861
88. Olkkola KT, Palkama VJ, Neuvonen PJ (1999) Ritonavir's role in reducing fentanyl clearance and prolonging its half-life. Anesthesiology 91(3):681–685

89. Saari TI, Laine K, Neuvonen M, Neuvonen PJ, Olkkola KT (2008) Effect of voriconazole and fluconazole on the pharmacokinetics of intravenous fentanyl. Eur J Clin Pharmacol 64(1):25–30
90. Takane H, Nosaka A, Wakushima H, Hosokawa K, Ieiri I (2005) Rifampin reduces the analgesic effect of transdermal fentanyl. Ann Pharmacother 39(12):2139–2140
91. Guitton J, Buronfosse T, Desage M, Lepape A, Brazier JL, Beaune P (1997) Possible involvement of multiple cytochrome P450S in fentanyl and sufentanil metabolism as opposed to alfentanil. Biochem Pharmacol 53(11):1613–1619
92. Subrahmanyam V, Renwick AB, Walter DG, Young PJ, Price RJ, Tonelli AP et al (2001) Identification of cytochrome P-450 isoforms responsible for cis-tramadol metabolism in human liver microsomes. Drug Metab Dispos 29(8):1146–1155
93. Volpe DA, McMahon Tobin GA, Mellon RD, Katki AG, Parker RJ, Colatsky T et al (2011) Uniform assessment and ranking of opioid? Receptor binding constants for selected opioid drugs. Regul Toxicol Pharmacol 59(3):385–390
94. Noehr-Jensen L, Zwisler ST, Larsen F, Sindrup SH, Damkier P, Brosen K (2009) Escitalopram is a weak inhibitor of the CYP2D6-catalyzed O-demethylation of (+)-tramadol but does not reduce the hypoalgesic effect in experimental pain. Clin Pharmacol Ther 86(6):626–633
95. Coller J, Michalakas JR, James HM, Farguharson AL, Colvill J, White JM et al (2012) Inhibition of CYP2D6-mediated tramadol O-demethylation in methadone but not buprenorphine maintenance patients. Br J Clin Pharmacol 74(5):835–841
96. Laugesen S, Enggaard TP, Pedersen RS, Sindrup SH, Brosen K (2005) Paroxetine, a cytochrome P450 2D6 inhibitor, diminishes the stereoselective O-demethylation and reduces the hypoalgesic effect of tramadol. Clin Pharmacol Ther 77(4):312–323
97. Nielsen AG, Pedersen RS, Noehr-Jensen L, Damkier P, Brosen K (2010) Two separate dose-dependent effects of paroxetine: mydriasis and inhibition of tramadol's O-demethylation via CYP2D6. Eur J Clin Pharmacol 66(7):655–660
98. Saarikoski T, Saari TI, Hagelberg NM, Neuvonen M, Neuvonen PJ, Scheinin M et al (2013) Rifampicin markedly decreases the exposure to oral and intravenous tramadol. Eur J Clin Pharmacol 69(6):1293–1301
99. Hagelberg NM, Saarikoski S, Saari TI, Neuvonen M, Neuvonen PJ, Turpeinen M et al (2013) Ticlopidine inhibits both O-demethylation and renal clearance of tramadol, increasing the exposure to it, but itraconazole has no marked effect on the ticlopidine-tramadol interaction. Eur J Clin Pharmacol 69(4):867–875
100. Poulsen L, Arendt-Nielsen L, Brosen K, Sindrup SH (1996) The hypoalgesic effect of tramadol in relation to CYP2D6. Clin Pharmacol Ther 60(6):636–644
101. Pedersen RS, Damkier P, Brosen K (2006) Enantioselective pharmacokinetics of tramadol in CYP2D6 extensive and poor metabolizers. Eur J Clin Pharmacol 62(7):513–521
102. Enggaard TP, Poulsen L, Arendt-Nielsen L, Brosen K, Ossig J, Sindrup SH (2006) The analgesic effect of tramadol after intravenous injection in healthy volunteers in relation to CYP2D6. Anesth Analg 102(1):146–150
103. Garcia-Quetglas E, Azanza JR, Sadaba B, Munoz MJ, Campanero MA (2007) Pharmacokinetics of tramadol enantiomers and their respective phase I metabolites in relation to CYP2D6 phenotype. Pharmacol Res 55(2):112–130
104. Halling J, Weihe P, Brosen K (2008) CYP2D6 polymorphism in relation to tramadol metabolism: a study of faroese patients. Ther Drug Monit 30(3):271–275
105. Stamer UM, Musshoff F, Kobilay M, Madea B, Hoeft A, Stuber F (2007) Concentrations of tramadol and O-desmethyltramadol enantiomers in different CYP2D6 genotypes. Clin Pharmacol Ther 82(1):41–47
106. Gan SH, Ismail R, Wan Adnan WA, Zulmi W (2007) Impact of CYP2D6 genetic polymorphism on tramadol pharmacokinetics and pharmacodynamics. Mol Diagn Ther 11(3):171–181
107. Kirchheiner J, Keulen JT, Bauer S, Roots I, Brockmoller J (2008) Effects of the CYP2D6 gene duplication on the pharmacokinetics and pharmacodynamics of tramadol. J Clin Psychopharmacol 28(1):78–83

108. Scott CC, Robbins EB, Chen KK (1948) Pharmacologic comparison of the optical isomers of methadon. J Pharmacol Exp Ther 93(3):282–286
109. Ebert B, Thorkildsen C, Andersen S, Christrup LL, Hjeds H (1998) Opioid analgesics as non-competitive N-methyl-D-aspartate (NMDA) antagonists. Biochem Pharmacol 56(5):553–559
110. Slotkin TA, Seidler FJ, Whitmore WL (1978) Methadone inhibits serotonin and norephinephrine uptake into rat brain synaptosomes and synaptic vesicles *in vitro* but not *in vivo*. Eur J Pharmacol 49(4):357–362
111. Fredheim OM, Moksnes K, Borchgrevink PC, Kaasa S, Dale O (2008) Clinical pharmacology of methadone for pain. Acta Anaesthesiol Scand 52(7):879–889
112. Bell J (2014) Pharmacological maintenance treatments of opiate addiction. Br J Clin Pharmacol 77(2):253–263
113. Gerber JG, Rhodes RJ, Gal J (2004) Stereoselective metabolism of methadone N-demethylation by cytochrome P4502B6 and 2C19. Chirality 16(1):36–44
114. Kharasch ED, Hoffer C, Whittington D, Sheffels P (2004) Role of hepatic and intestinal cytochrome P450 3A and 2B6 in the metabolism, disposition, and miotic effects of methadone. Clin Pharmacol Ther 76(3):250–269
115. Totah RA, Sheffels P, Roberts T, Whittington D, Thummel K, Kharasch ED (2008) Role of CYP2B6 in stereoselective human methadone metabolism. Anesthesiology 108(3):363–374
116. Moody DE, Alburges ME, Parker RJ, Collins JM, Strong JM (1997) The involvement of cytochrome P450 3A4 in the N-demethylation of L-alpha-acetylmethadol (LAAM), nor-LAAM, and methadone. Drug Metab Dispos 25(12):1347–1353
117. Iribarne C, Berthou F, Baird S, Dreano Y, Picart D, Bail JP et al (1996) Involvement of cytochrome P450 3A4 enzyme in the N-demethylation of methadone in human liver microsomes. Chem Res Toxicol 9(2):365–373
118. Foster DJ, Somogyi AA, Bochner F (1999) Methadone N-demethylation in human liver microsomes: lack of stereoselectivity and involvement of CYP3A4. Br J Clin Pharmacol 47(4):403–412
119. Chang Y, Fang WB, Lin SN, Moody DE (2011) Stereo-selective metabolism of methadone by human liver microsomes and cDNA-expressed cytochrome P450s: a reconciliation. Basic Clin Pharmacol Toxicol 108(1):55–62
120. Wang JS, DeVane CL (2003) Involvement of CYP3A4, CYP2C8, and CYP2D6 in the metabolism of (R)- and (S)-methadone *in vitro*. Drug Metab Dispos 31(6):742–747
121. Cobb MN, Desai J, Brown LS, Zannikos PN, Rainey PM (1998) The effect of fluconazole on the clinical pharmacokinetics of methadone. Clin Pharmacol Ther 63(6):655–662
122. Liu P, Foster G, Labadie R, Somoza E, Sharma A (2007) Pharmacokinetic interaction between voriconazole and methadone at steady state in patients on methadone therapy. Antimicrob Agents Chemother 51(1):110–118
123. Begre S, von Bardeleben U, Ladewig D, Jaquet-Rochat S, Cosendai-Savary L, Golay KP et al (2002) Paroxetine increases steady-state concentrations of (R)-methadone in CYP2D6 extensive but not poor metabolizers. J Clin Psychopharmacol 22(2):211–215
124. Uehlinger C, Crettol S, Chassot P, Brocard M, Koeb L, Brawand-Amey M et al (2007) Increased (R)-methadone plasma concentrations by quetiapine in cytochrome P450s and ABCB1 genotyped patients. J Clin Psychopharmacol 27(3):273–278
125. Hamilton SP, Nunes EV, Janal M, Weber L (2000) The effect of sertraline on methadone plasma levels in methadone-maintenance patients. Am J Addict 9(1):63–69
126. Hendrix CW, Wakeford J, Wire MB, Lou Y, Bigelow GE, Martinez E et al (2004) Pharmacokinetics and pharmacodynamics of methadone enantiomers after coadministration with amprenavir in opioid dependent subjects. Pharmacotherapy 24(9):1110–1121
127. McCance-Katz EF, Rainey PM, Friedland G, Jatlow P (2003) The protease inhibitor lopinavir-ritonavir may produce opiate withdrawal in methadone-maintained patients. Clin Infect Dis 37(4):476–482
128. Clarke S, Mulcahy F, Bergin C, Reynolds H, Boyle N, Barry M et al (2002) Absence of opioid withdrawal symptoms in patients receiving methadone and the protease inhibitor lopinavir-ritonavir. Clin Infect Dis 34(8):1143–1145

129. Kharasch ED, Stubbert K (2013) Cytochrome P4503A does not mediate the interaction between methadone and ritonavir-lopinavir. Drug Metab Dispos 41(12):2166–2167
130. Kharasch ED, Walker A, Whittington D, Hoffer C, Bedynek PS (2009) Methadone metabolism and clearance are induced by nelfinavir despite inhibition of cytochrome P4503A (CYP3A) activity. Drug Alcohol Depend 101(3):158–168
131. McCance-Katz EF, Rainey PM, Smith P, Morse G, Friedland G, Gourevitch M et al (2004) Drug interactions between opioids and antiretroviral medications: interaction between methadone, LAAM, and nelfinavir. Am J Addict 13(2):163–180
132. Hsyu PH, Lillibridge J, Daniels E, Kerr BM (2006) Pharmacokinetic interaction of nelfinavir and methadone in intravenous drug users. Biopharm Drug Dispos 27(2):61–68
133. Jamois C, Smith P, Morrison R, Riek M, Patel A, Schmitt C et al (2009) Effect of saquinavir/ritonavir (1000/100 mg bid) on the pharmacokinetics of methadone in opiate-dependent HIV-negative patients on stable methadone maintenance therapy. Addict Biol 14(3):321–327
134. Gerber JG, Rosenkranz S, Aberg J, D'Amico R, Mildvan D, Gulick R et al (2001) Effect of ritonavir/saquinavir on stereoselective pharmacokinetics of methadone: results of AIDS Clinical Trials Group (ACTG) 401. J Acquir Immune Defic Syndr 27(2):153–160
135. Friedland G, Andrews L, Schreibman T, Agarwala S, Daley L, Child M et al (2005) Lack of an effect of atazanavir on steady-state pharmacokinetics of methadone in patients chronically treated for opiate addiction. AIDS 19(15):1635–1641
136. Kharasch ED, Bedynek PS, Hoffer C, Walker A, Whittington D (2012) Lack of indinavir effects on methadone disposition despite inhibition of hepatic and intestinal cytochrome P4503A (CYP3A). Anesthesiology 116(2):432–447
137. Shelton MJ, Cloen D, DiFrancesco R, Berenson CS, Esch A, de Caprariis PJ et al (2004) The effects of once-daily saquinavir/minidose ritonavir on the pharmacokinetics of methadone. J Clin Pharmacol 44(3):293–304
138. Smith PF, Kearney BP, Liaw S, Cloen D, Bullock JM, Haas CE et al (2004) Effect of tenofovir disoproxil fumarate on the pharmacokinetics and pharmacodynamics of total, R-, and S-methadone. Pharmacotherapy 24(8):970–977
139. Schwartz EL, Brechbuhl AB, Kahl P, Miller MA, Selwyn PA, Friedland GH (1992) Pharmacokinetic interactions of zidovudine and methadone in intravenous drug-using patients with HIV infection. J Acquir Immune Defic Syndr 5(6):619–626
140. Song I, Mark S, Chen S, Savina P, Wajima T, Peppercorn A et al (2013) Dolutegravir does not affect methadone pharmacokinetics in opioid-dependent, HIV-seronegative subjects. Drug Alcohol Depend 133(2):781–784
141. Anderson MS, Mabalot Luk JA, Hanley WD, Jin B, Riesenberg RA, Wenning LA et al (2010) Effect of raltegravir on the pharmacokinetics of methadone. J Clin Pharmacol 50(12):1461–1466
142. Stocker H, Kruse G, Kreckel P, Herzmann C, Arasteh K, Claus J et al (2004) Nevirapine significantly reduces the levels of racemic methadone and (R)-methadone in human immunodeficiency virus-infected patients. Antimicrob Agents Chemother 48(11):4148–4153
143. Arroyo E, Valenzuela B, Portilla J, Climent-Grana E, Perez-Ruixo JJ, Merino E (2007) Pharmacokinetics of methadone in human-immunodeficiency-virus-infected patients receiving nevirapine once daily. Eur J Clin Pharmacol 63(7):669–675
144. Clarke SM, Mulcahy FM, Tjia J, Reynolds HE, Gibbons SE, Barry MG et al (2001) Pharmacokinetic interactions of nevirapine and methadone and guidelines for use of nevirapine to treat injection drug users. Clin Infect Dis 33(9):1595–1597
145. McCance-Katz EF, Rainey PM, Smith P, Morse GD, Friedland G, Boyarsky B et al (2006) Drug interactions between opioids and antiretroviral medications: interaction between methadone, LAAM, and delavirdine. Am J Addict 15(1):23–34
146. Vourvahis M, Wang R, Gruener DM, Bruce RD, Haider S, Tawadrous M (2012) Effect of lersivirine co-administration on pharmacokinetics of methadone in healthy volunteers. Drug Alcohol Depend 126(1–2):183–188
147. Eap CB, Broly F, Mino A, Hammig R, Deglon JJ, Uehlinger C et al (2001) Cytochrome P450 2D6 genotype and methadone steady-state concentrations. J Clin Psychopharmacol 21(2):229–234

148. Crettol S, Deglon JJ, Besson J, Croquette-Krokar M, Hammig R, Gothuey I et al (2006) ABCB1 and cytochrome P450 genotypes and phenotypes: influence on methadone plasma levels and response to treatment. Clin Pharmacol Ther 80(6):668–681
149. Cao YJ, Smith PF, Wire MB, Lou Y, Lancaster CT, Causon RC et al (2008) Pharmacokinetics and pharmacodynamics of methadone enantiomers after coadministration with fosamprenavir-ritonavir in opioid-dependent subjects. Pharmacotherapy 28(7):863–874
150. Rainey PM, Friedland G, Snidow JW, McCance-Katz EF, Mitra AK, Andrews L et al (2002) The pharmacokinetics of methadone following co-administration with a lamivudine/zidovudine combination tablet in opiate-dependent subjects. Am J Addict 11(1):66–74
151. Harnack LJ, Rydell SA, Stang J (2001) Prevalence of use of herbal products by adults in the Minneapolis/St Paul, Minn, metropolitan area. Mayo Clin Proc 76:688–694
152. Kiang TK, Wilby KJ, Ensom MHH (2015) Clinical Pharmacokinetic and pharmacodynamic drug interactions associated with antimalarials. Springer International Publishing, Switzerland. ISBN 978-3-319-10526-0

Chapter 21
Clinically Significant Interactions with Stimulants and Other Non-stimulants for ADHD

Rania S. Kattura and M. Lynn Crismon

Abstract The pharmacologic treatment of attention deficit and hyperactivity disorder (ADHD) involves the use of stimulant and non-stimulant agents. These agents have been implicated in various pharmacokinetic and pharmacodynamic interactions that could result in clinical outcomes that are either favorable or unfavorable to the patient's treatment. This chapter provides a discussion of such interactions and their management. Genetic polymorphisms associated with certain drug transporter systems and cytochrome P450 alleles have been shown to potentially alter treatment response when stimulant and non-stimulant agents are used for the management of ADHD. Some of the pharmacokinetic and pharmacodynamic interactions may not be considered clinically significant. However, patient-specific factors will often determine whether a potential drug interaction is clinically significant, and it is important for the treating physician to evaluate each patient's regimen to discern the significance of a potential interaction in that patient. Similarly, the area of pharmacogenomics continues to evolve, and as more becomes known in this area, treatment outcomes could be affected. After evaluation of the drug regimen and associated drug interaction, the clinician must determine whether therapy should be continued without changes or altered. Nonetheless, clinicians should adhere to recommended medication monitoring parameters and dose adjustments based on patient-specific parameters, as outlined by product labeling and clinical guidelines.

Keywords Stimulants • Non-stimulants • Pharmacokinetic interactions • Pharmacodynamic interactions • CES 1 • Atomoxetine • Methylphenidate • Amphetamines • Drug interactions • P-glycoprotein

R.S. Kattura, PharmD (✉)
Department of Pharmacy, Austin State Hospital, Austin, TX, USA
e-mail: rkattura@utexas.edu

M.L. Crismon, PharmD
Division of Health Outcomes and Pharmacy Practice, College of Pharmacy, The University of Texas at Austin, Austin, TX, USA
e-mail: lynn.crismon@austin.utexas.edu

M. Jann et al. (eds.), *Applied Clinical Pharmacokinetics and Pharmacodynamics of Psychopharmacological Agents*,
DOI 10.1007/978-3-319-27883-4_21

21.1 Introduction

Stimulant and non-stimulant agents are used for the management of ADHD in children, adolescents, and adults. While the use of these agents is effective in improving ADHD symptoms, pharmacokinetic and pharmacodynamic interactions have been reported when they are used in combination with other medications, foods, alcohol, or tobacco. Additionally, genetic polymorphisms at certain transporter protein sites and cytochrome P450 enzyme alleles have been implicated in potentially altering treatment response and producing clinical drug interactions associated with these agents. These interactions call for close attention to the prescribed medication regimen, as a change in therapy may be needed to reduce the potential for adverse events or to improve efficacy. This chapter details pharmacokinetic and pharmacodynamic drug interactions that occur with stimulant and non-stimulant agents and discusses genetic polymorphisms associated with these agents. This chapter also provides information on dose adjustment based on known patient factors and reviews recommended monitoring parameters and patient safety information for these agents.

21.2 Pharmacokinetic Interactions

This section details phase I drug interactions associated with stimulant and non-stimulant agents, p-glycoprotein-based interactions and interactions involving food, drink, tobacco, and herbals. Some of the interactions discussed in this section are theoretical and may not be clinically significant; others have both theoretical and clinical significance. To date, methylphenidate-containing agents have not been shown to be influenced by the pharmacokinetics of other drugs. However, numerous reports suggest that it affects the disposition of other drugs. Amphetamine has been shown to be affected by CYP2D6 inhibitors based on early studies involving quinidine. Those studies demonstrated a delay in the excretion of the metabolite (p-hydroxyamphetamine) [1, 2].

21.2.1 Phase I Mechanistic Interactions

The use of tricyclic antidepressants (TCAs) with methylphenidate- and amphetamine-containing products has yielded mixed data with regard to the significance of the interaction. Wharton and colleagues [3] reported methylphenidate 20 mg/d inhibiting the metabolism of the tertiary amine TCA imipramine and to a lesser extent the secondary amine desipramine, yielding higher steady-state concentration of the TCA being evaluated. Studies evaluating the effects of amphetamine on serum TCA concentrations yield no clinically significant interaction [4].

21.2.2 Atomoxetine Drug Interactions

Atomoxetine, a norepinephrine reuptake inhibitor, is a substrate for CYP2D6 enzyme which is capable of forming the major metabolite of atomoxetine, 4-hydroxyatomoxetine glucuronide [5]. Accordingly, there are potential interactions between this agent and CYP 2D6 inhibitors. Paulzen et al. [6] describe a 38-year-old male with uncontrolled ADHD and receiving treatment with atomoxetine 90 mg/d. While the patient's symptoms improved, they were not in remission, and the patient continued to have trouble at work. Low-dose paroxetine (10 mg/d), a selective serotonin reuptake inhibitor antidepressant (SSRI) and a potent CYP 2D6 inhibitor, was added to the regimen, and the patient reported improved symptoms and better work productivity. Paulzen et al. compared atomoxetine serum concentrations with and without the presence of paroxetine and showed a two- and threefold increase in atomoxetine serum concentrations, respectively, 120 and 240 min following paroxetine administration.

Dextromethorphan, an antitussive found in nonprescription cough suppressants, is metabolized via the CYP 2D6 pathway. In vitro studies suggest that atomoxetine, but not methylphenidate, inhibits metabolism of dextromethorphan. However, no clinical reports are available to confirm this drug interaction [7].

The protease inhibitors, ritonavir and darunavir, used for the management of human immunodeficiency virus (HIV), are potent CYP 2D6 inhibitors. Accordingly, a downward dose adjustment of atomoxetine is recommended, and close monitoring of the patient is advised [8]. No published case reports are available to support this interaction. However, as with dextromethorphan, clinicians should be vigilant when combining ritonavir or darunavir with atomoxetine due to the possibility of side effects associated with elevated atomoxetine serum concentrations.

21.2.3 P-glycoprotein-Based Interactions

P-glycoprotein is found in the blood–brain barrier among other body tissues. Accordingly, p-glycoproteins inhibit substrate penetration into the central nervous system (CNS) and hence result in reduced efficacy of medications [9]. There are no in vivo studies evaluating stimulant interactions with p-glycoprotein transporter but in vitro studies exist. In vitro studies show that of the agents used for the management of ADHD, l-methylphenidate and atomoxetine are the most potent p-glycoprotein inhibitors and potential interaction with p-glycoprotein substrates cannot be excluded. Isomers of methylphenidate and amphetamine show p-glycoprotein inhibitory effects at concentrations above 50–100 μM but are unlikely to affect the pharmacokinetics of co-administered p-glycoprotein substrates in vivo [9]. While in vivo studies evaluating p-glycoprotein interactions with agents used to manage ADHD are lacking, clinicians should be comfortable when prescribing such agents given that to date the p-glycoprotein effects on drug disposition are unlikely.

Guanfacine, a selective α-2 agonist used for the management of ADHD in combination with another agent or as monotherapy, has been shown to result in variable inter-patient response when used in children with ADHD and pervasive developmental disorder. As a result, guanfacine has been evaluated for possible p-glycoprotein activity as a way to explain the interindividual variability in response shown in available studies [10, 11]. Mahar et al. first showed that guanfacine is a weak p-glycoprotein substrate, and later, this was confirmed by Gillis et al. [12]. Results from the Gillis et al. [12] study do not support McCraken's findings in which response to guanfacine was correlated with the single nucleotide protein (SNP) MDRI gene [13]. This study suggests the variation in guanfacine response is not related to the p-glycoprotein transporter as previously thought.

21.3 Smoking, Food, and Other Types of Interactions

21.3.1 Methylphenidate Formulations

The pharmacokinetics of certain long-acting stimulant formulations can be affected by food or substances which alter the gastric pH, intestinal motility, or intestinal transit time. The extent of absorption of methylphenidate in any of its oral formulations is not affected in fasting conditions. However, as shown in Table 21.1, food delays time to peak concentration (T_{max}) which is likely due to delayed gastric emptying [14].

Table 21.1 Effects of food on stimulants

Stimulant type	Formulation	General food effect [14, 15]	Effect of high-fat meal [14, 15]
Methylphenidate	Metadate CD	T_{max} delayed by 1 h	↑C_{max} by 30 %
			↑AUC by 17 %
	Concerta		T_{max} delayed by 1 h
			↑C_{max} by 10–30 %
	Ritalin and ritalin LA		T_{max} delayed by 1 h
	Ritalin SR	↑C_{max} by 17 %, ↑AUC by 14 %	
Amphetamine	Adderall XR	↑renal excretion with acidic foods	↓AUC over the first 8 h post exposure
Dexmethylphenidate			T_{max} delayed by 1 h
Lisdexamphetamine	Vyvanse	T_{max} delayed by 1 h, AUC and C_{max} unaffected	
Amphetamine containing stimulants		↑renal excretion with acidic foods	
		↓renal excretion with urinary alkalizers	

AUC area under the curve, C_{max} maximum serum concentration, T_{max} time to reach maximum serum concentration (C_{max})

Depending on the formulation, peak methylphenidate serum concentrations (C_{max}) have been shown to either increase or decrease after eating, suggesting that rate of drug absorption may be affected by dietary food intake [14]. This is not the case for the methylphenidate formulations that can be mixed or sprinkled (Ritalin LA-SODAS formulation) into applesauce as no changes in bioavailability of the medication were detected; however, T_{max} is delayed by one hour if given with a high-fat meal.

Transdermal formulations of methylphenidate are not affected by fed and unfed states of the patient but are associated with inter-patient variability secondary to non-gastrointestinal factors such as surface area of the patch and duration that the patch is worn [15]. In contrast, lisdexamphetamine formulations have less inter-patient variability with respect to systemic amphetamine exposure largely due to its dependence on enzymatic cleavage, through hydrolysis in the blood, of the precursor molecule [15].

21.3.1.1 Age Effects

Preschool children treated with immediate release methylphenidate showed smaller treatment effect size compared to school-aged children receiving the same medication. Additionally, discontinuation due to side effects was reported more often in preschoolers receiving immediate release methylphenidate compared with school-aged children (11 % vs. < 1 %) [15]. However, this information should be interpreted carefully as the authors were comparing discontinuation rates from two different studies.

Bupropion has been shown to have a shorter half-life in adolescents (12 h) compared with adults (21 h), suggesting faster metabolism in adolescents. Based on this, divided dosing for bupropion in adolescents is recommended for optimal symptom coverage throughout the day [16].

21.3.1.2 Gender Effects

Although males tend to receive lower mg/kg/day doses of methylphenidate products (Concerta, Ritalin LA, Metadate CD) (approximately 30 % lower in males in one study), the mean area under the curve (AUC) between the genders did not differ [14, 15]. When methylphenidate dosing is normalized for body weight, it has been shown that females have lower systemic exposure based on a milligram per kilogram dosing regimen [15]. Of note, there is no difference in the half-life of methylphenidate between genders; accordingly, it is possible that females have greater first-pass metabolism of methylphenidate compared to males. In children, girls demonstrate superior responses compared to boys after 1.5 to 3 h from receiving methylphenidate (Concerta, Metadate CD) with inferior responses seen later in the day, i.e., 7.5 to 12 h post dose [17, 18]. These differences where independent of the once-daily long-acting stimulant used, each having their own pharmacokinetic and delivery system [18]. Nonetheless, more studies are needed to further explain this phenomenon and whether it has any implications for drug interactions.

21.3.2 Methylphenidate and Alcohol

Methylphenidate metabolism primarily yields the inactive metabolite, ritalinic acid, a de-esterification product [18]. However, when administered with ethanol, the presence of the transesterification product ethylphenidate has been detected. Additionally, methylphenidate serum concentrations and AUC were shown to be increased in the presence of alcohol in normal metabolizers [18]. The concentration of ethylphenidate after administration of a single dose of methylphenidate (20 mg) and moderate alcohol consumption (1.6 mg/kg) was noted to correlate with methylphenidate and not with that of alcohol. Ethylphenidate produces a stimulatory effect, though less active than methylphenidate. Ethanol is expected to potentiate the effects of methylphenidate when co-administered, with magnified effects seen in individuals who do not clear methylphenidate at normal rates, are receiving higher doses of methylphenidate, or are abusing methylphenidate [19, 20]. Table 21.2 highlights interactions between alcohol and stimulants and non-stimulant agents. Other miscellaneous interactions are also listed in the table.

21.4 Pharmacodynamic Drug Interactions with Stimulants and Non-stimulant Agents Used for the Management of ADHD

Earlier in this chapter, potential pharmacokinetic interactions with stimulants and non-stimulant ADHD agents were highlighted. These interactions suggest a dose–concentration relationship; however, an overview of the response–concentration relationship is just as important. Table 21.3 illustrates pharmacodynamic interactions that may occur with stimulant and non-stimulant agents used in ADHD treatment.

The use of monoamine oxidase inhibitors (MAOIs) is contraindicated with stimulant agents, atomoxetine and bupropion due to the risk for hypertensive crisis. Should stimulant therapy, atomoxetine, or bupropion be needed in a patient receiving a MAOI, MAOI discontinuation and a 14-day washout period is recommended prior to initiating the ADHD medication [5, 23]. A similar approach is recommended when using the anti-infective linezolid. However, if a patient is already receiving bupropion, it should be held for the duration of linezolid treatment and, if needed, reinitiated 24 h after completion of linezolid treatment.

Similarly, atomoxetine is contraindicated with MAOIs or within 2 weeks of discontinuation of a MAOI, or other medications which change the concentration of monoamines in the brain [5]. Serious and sometimes fatal reactions have been reported when atomoxetine was taken with a MAOI. Such reactions include hyperthermia, rigidity, myoclonus, autonomic instability with possible rapid fluctuations of vital signs, and mental status changes, including extreme agitation progressing to delirium and coma. Aggarwal et al. discuss a 10-year-old stabilized on atomox-

Table 21.2 Stimulant/non-stimulant miscellaneous interactions

Interacting agent	Medication	Effect	Notes
Alcohol	Methylphenidate [15, 21, 22]	↑d-methylphenidate C_{max} 40 %	Effect may be more pronounced with Ritalin LA and Metadate CD
		↑d-methylphenidate AUC 25 %	
	Bupropion [23]	↑risk for seizures	
	Guanfacine/clonidine [24]	Potentiates hypotensive effects; CNS depression	
Caffeine [25, 26]	Stimulants	Additive CNS effects E.g., ↑irritability, nervousness, insomnia, cardiac side effects	Caffeine-containing natural products include: coffee, guarana, cola nut, green tea, Yerba mate
		↑blood pressure	
	Bupropion	↑risk for seizures	
	Guanfacine/clonidine	↓antihypertensive effects	
St. John's wort [24, 27]	Guanfacine/clonidine	↓serum guanfacine concentrations	Twofold increase in guanfacine dose is recommended
Ephedrine [28, 29]	Guanfacine/clonidine	↓antihypertensive effects	Ephedrine containing natural products include: Ma huang
Yohimbine [30]	Guanfacine/clonidine	↓antihypertensive effects	
	Stimulants	↑risk of hypertensive crisis	
Kava-kava	Atomoxetine	↑atomoxetine levels via CYP 2D6 inhibition	
Eucalyptus [31]	Amphetamines	↓amphetamine plasma levels	
Urinary alkalinizing agents (e.g., citric acid, sodium lactate, acetazolamide) [32]	Amphetamines	↓urinary excretion of amphetamine, increasing the half-life and therapeutic action of amphetamines	Avoid combination if possible. If combination used however, monitor the patient's blood pressure
Urinary acidifier (e.g. ammonium chloride)	Amphetamines, dexamphetamines	↑elimination of dexamphetamine in urine by 20 times [4]	Avoid combination if possible
		Amphetamine clearance is accelerated and duration of effect reduced [32]	

etine 40 mg/d who was initiated on linezolid 310 mg IV every 8 h for the management of an infection [33]. Based upon the mechanism of action of the antibiotic, the authors suspected a possible drug interaction. Atomoxetine was held during the

Table 21.3 Pharmacodynamic interactions with stimulant and non-stimulant agents

Agent	Offending agent	Effect of the combination	How to manage this interaction
Stimulants (methylphenidate and amphetamine-containing agents)	Antidepressants (e.g., nefazodone, SSRIs, and SNRIs)	Risk for serotonin syndrome	Use with caution and monitor patient. Antidepressants are frequently used with stimulants, and the clinical significance of this interaction is questionable
	Antidepressants: imipramine	Increased agitation, aggression and violence [35]	Closely monitor patients for mood changes and adjust dose based on tolerability and response. The clinical significance of this interaction remains questionable
	First-generation antipsychotics	Diminished clinical effect of either agent (decreased attention to task and/or worsening psychosis) due to opposing effects on dopamine [4]	Avoid combination. If combination necessary, patients' mood should be closely monitored for worsening psychosis. Similarly, efficacy of the stimulant should be evaluated in controlling ADHD symptoms.
	Methylene blue	Risk for serotonin syndrome [21]	Avoid combination if possible; otherwise, monitor patient for signs and symptoms of serotonin syndrome
	Antihypertensives (e.g., clonidine, guanfacine)	Negate hypotensive effects, attributed to decrease in norepinephrine tone in locus ceruleus [4]	Monitor blood pressure
	Monoamine oxidase inhibitors (MAOIs)	Hypertensive crisis and serotonin syndrome	Avoid combination.
	Linezolid		A 14-day washout period is required before a stimulant is initiated if patient is on MAOI treatment
	Atomoxetine	Increase risk for noradrenergic effect (tachycardia and/or hypertension) [5]	Caution if this combination is used, and monitor patient's blood pressure and heart rate
	Dopamine agonists	Increase dopaminergic effects	Monitor patient for nausea, weight loss, nervousness, tremors, insomnia

Atomoxetine [5]	Amitriptyline	Enhanced efficacy of atomoxetine reported, and lower doses of atomoxetine utilized [36]	Monitor patient for symptom improvement over time. If amitriptyline added later in therapy to atomoxetine, a lower dose of atomoxetine may be warranted
	MAOIs	Hypertensive crisis	Combination contraindicated
	Beta-agonists	Potentiate CV effects (increased heart rate and blood pressure), more likely to occur with systemic beta-agonists rather than inhaled beta-agonists	Monitor patients' blood pressure and heart rate
	Oral decongestants (i.e., sympathomimetics)	Risk for blood pressure and heart rate increase due to sympathomimetic activity	Monitor patient blood pressure and heart rate
Bupropion [23]	MAOIs	Hypertensive crisis	Combination contraindicated, a 14-day washout period needed prior to initiating bupropion in patients exposed to MAOI
	Linezolid	Hypertensive crisis	Combination should be avoided. If linezolid is the only anti-infective option, bupropion should be held until antibiotic course completed. Bupropion may be restarted after 24 h of last linezolid dose. Patient's blood pressure should be monitored during combination treatment
	Stimulants, ethanol, tramadol	Lowering of seizure threshold	Monitor patient for seizure; educate patient on risk
	Dopamine agonists (e.g., levodopa)	CNS toxicity: restlessness, agitation, tremor, ataxia, gait disturbance, vertigo, and dizziness	Monitor patient for CNS toxicity
			If taking levodopa concurrently, low initial dosing and slow titration of bupropion is recommended

(continued)

Table 21.3 (continued)

Agent	Offending agent	Effect of the combination	How to manage this interaction
Alpha-agonist (guanfacine and clonidine) [24, 37, 38]	MAOIs	Increased risk for hypotension after initial hypertension	Monitor blood pressure
	TCAs	Reduce hypotensive effects of guanfacine	Monitor blood pressure
	Beta-blockers	Bradycardia	Monitor heart rate
	CNS depressants	Increased sedation, reduced concentration, respiratory depression	Monitor patient and educate on effect
	Antipsychotics	Hypotensive effects and exacerbation of sedation	Monitor patient's blood pressure and alertness
	Sympathomimetic	Loss of antihypertensive effect	Monitor blood pressure

CNS central nervous system, *MAOIs* monoamine oxidase inhibitors, *SNRIs* serotonin norepinephrine reuptake inhibitor, *SSRIs* selective serotonin reuptake inhibitors, *TCAs* tricyclic antidepressants hospital stay, and the patient was instructed to restart it 14 days after discontinuation of the antibiotic. This case exemplifies the importance of anticipating potential drug interactions that may be serious and being proactive in managing patients who could be at risk for this or similar drug interactions.

Methylene blue has been reported to cause serotonin syndrome when combined with antidepressants [34]. While not reported clinically, stimulants have been proposed to cause the same when combined with methylene blue, but the interaction is theoretical [21].

21.5 Genetic Polymorphisms

21.5.1 Carboxylesterase 1 (CES 1) Gene

The Carboxylesterase 1 (CES 1) enzyme is responsible for the metabolism of methylphenidate as well as other medications and illicit substances such as cocaine and heroin by cleavage of the ester group [39]. This metabolic pathway results in both inactive and active metabolites. A single nucleotide protein (SNP) can significantly influence metabolism and disposition of medications metabolized via the CES 1 enzyme. With regard to methylphenidate, Zhu et al. reported an increase in hemodynamic measures [blood pressure and heart rate] after administration of racemic methylphenidate to a subject of European descent. Upon further investigation, mutations on the CES 1 gene were identified as contributors to the pharmacokinetic changes and alterations in drug response observed in this patient [18, 39]. The CES 1 gene variants result from an amino acid substitution on exon 4 and a deletion on exon 6. These mutations have been shown to yield high serum methylphenidate concentrations (up to a sevenfold increase). Pharmacodynamically, higher systolic blood pressure, diastolic blood pressure, heart rate, and mean arterial pressure were recorded in those with the CES 1 gene variants compared to those without the gene variant [39]. Although this suggests an increased risk of adverse events in individuals with any of the CES 1 gene variants, further studies are needed to confirm this finding.

The hepatic enzyme CES 1 is considered the major source for the metabolism of methylphenidate and likely the reason for drug–drug interactions occurring independent of the CYP P450 metabolic pathways. Zhu et al. demonstrated this in an in vitro study in which an overexpressing CES 1 enzyme cell line was used in the presence of medications known to inhibit the CES 1 metabolic pathway and by extension methylphenidate metabolism [40]. The study identified aripiprazole, perphenazine, thioridazine, and fluoxetine as most potent CES 1 inhibitors. These CES 1 inhibitors identified by Zhu et al. may be used with methylphenidate in patients being treated for ADHD comorbid with other psychiatric disorders. The investigators combined aripiprazole with methylphenidate in vivo and found an increased plasma concentration of total methylphenidate, suggesting an alteration of methylphenidate pharmacokinetics [40]. This is considered a novel explanation for drug–

drug interactions involving methylphenidate which is primarily metabolized via CES 1 enzyme pathway. Based upon this described interaction pathway, increased adverse effects could occur [41, 42]. For example, psychosis occurred in an adolescent who was switched from risperidone to aripiprazole while also taking methylphenidate. The etiology for the psychosis in this patient was proposed to be related to the increase in methylphenidate concentration [41]. While Ekinci proposed the psychosis to be related to increase methylphenidate concentration, it is difficult to conclude that this is a pharmacokinetic interaction as serum drug concentrations were not collected.

Another potent inhibitor of the CES 1 enzyme identified is nelfinavir, a protease inhibitor used in the management of patients with HIV. When combined with methylphenidate, nelfinavir inhibited hydrolysis of methylphenidate in a concentration-dependent manner which could result in clinically significant drug–drug interactions; however, in vivo studies are needed to confirm this [43].

21.6 Monitoring Recommendations and Safety Parameters for Stimulants

In pediatric patients, stimulants have been implicated in causing weight loss and increase in blood pressure (mean 2–4 mmHg) and heart rate (mean 3–6 bpm). Accordingly, baseline weight, height, blood pressure, and heart rate should be obtained, and weight, height, blood pressure, and pulse should be checked at every follow-up visit [21, 22, 32, 44]. An electrocardiogram (ECG) is recommended if the patient or their family history suggests an increased risk for cardiovascular disorders. Co-occurring mental disorders are common in individuals with ADHD. A thorough mental status assessment should be performed before beginning stimulants. If a co-occurring mental disorder exists, then the clinician needs to consider whether additional pharmacological or psychosocial treatment needs to be targeted toward the co-occurring disorder. Mild depression and anxiety is often secondary to ADHD and may likely improve with improvement in ADHD symptoms [45]. Although concern exists regarding stimulants exacerbating the course of bipolar disorder, available research does not substantiate this as long as the patient is receiving an appropriate regimen for the bipolar disorder [46]. Although parents are often concerned about the potential of abuse in adolescents prescribed stimulants, available research indicates that the risk of substance abuse in individuals with ADHD is lower if they are taking stimulants [47]. However, adolescents and young adults prescribed stimulants may divert stimulants by selling or giving them to others [48]. Educating the patient and their family is one way to help deter abuse and diversion with stimulants, and prescribers are encouraged to keep careful prescription records for prescribed stimulants. No established correlation has been found between serum concentrations and clinical response; accordingly, therapeutic drug monitoring for stimulants is not recommended [15].

Severe cases of liver injury have been reported with atomoxetine; therefore, liver function tests should be obtained at baseline and the patient and caregiver taught to monitor for signs of jaundice during treatment. If jaundice develops, atomoxetine should be discontinued [5]. Weight and height as well as blood pressure and heart rate should be monitored at baseline and throughout treatment according to the manufacturer package insert [5]. Reports of sudden cardiac death with atomoxetine are available; therefore, a thorough history of the patient's cardiovascular health and family history of cardiovascular disease should be completed prior to initiating treatment. Atomoxetine carries a boxed warning regarding increased risk for suicidal ideation; however, no completed suicides have been reported in clinical trials. Nonetheless, patients started on atomoxetine should be monitored for potential mood changes and suicidality [5].

Bupropion, like atomoxetine, carries a boxed warning for suicidal ideation, and patients should be screened and monitored for potential suicidal thoughts and behaviors and mood changes throughout treatment [23]. Patients should be screened for potential risk or history of seizure disorders or eating disorders prior to initiating bupropion therapy. No specific laboratory measures are needed during bupropion treatment; however, measuring blood pressure during treatment is recommended by the manufacturer [23].

Clonidine and guanfacine do not have any required laboratory testing prior to their initiation. As both of these medications were originally developed as antihypertensives, the package insert recommends baseline measurement of vital signs, at dose increase and periodically as necessary for the patient. Patients who are receiving concomitant sympathomimetics should have their blood pressures measured frequently [24, 44].

References

1. Tomkins DE, Otten SV, Joharchi N et al (1997) Effect of CYP 2D1 inhibition on the behavioral effects of D-amphetamine. Behav Pharmacol 8:223–235
2. Moody DE, Ruangyuttikarn W, Law MY (1990) Quinidine inhibits in vivo metabolism of amphetamine in rats: impact upon correlation between GC/MS and immunoassay findings in rat urine. J Anal Toxicol 14:311–317
3. Wharton RN, Perel JM, Dayton PG et al (1971) A potential clinical use of methylphenidate with tricyclic antidepressants. Am J Psychiatry 127:57–62
4. Markowitz JS, Patrick KS (2001) Pharmacokinetic and pharmacodynamic drug interactions in the treatment of attention deficit hyperactivity disorder. Clin Pharmacokinet 40(10):753–772
5. Strattera® [package insert] (2014) Indianapolis, IN: Eli Lilly and Company
6. Paulzen M, Clement HW, Gründer G (2008) Enhancement of atomoxetne serum levels by co-administration of paroxetine. Int J Neuropsychopharmacol 11(2):289–291
7. Ciccone PR, Ramabadran K, Jessen LM (2006) Potential interactions of methylphenidate and atomoxetine with dextromethorphan. J Am Pharm Assoc 46(4):472–478
8. Piscitelli SC, Gallicano KD (2001) Interactions among drugs for HIV and opportunistic infections. N Engl J Med 344:984–996
9. Zhu HJ, Wang JS, Donovan JL et al (2008) Interactions of attention deficit/hyperactivity disorder therapeutic agents with the efflux transporter P-glycoprotein. Eur J Pharmacol 578:148–158

10. Scahill L, Aman MG, McDougle CJ et al (2006) A prospective open label trial of guanfacine in children with pervasive developmental disorders. J Child Adolesc Psychopharmacol 16(5):589–598
11. Mahar Doan KM, Humphreys JE, Webster LO et al (2002) Passive permeability and P-glycoprotein-mediated efflux differentiate central nervous system (CNS) and non-CNS marked drugs. J Pharmacol Exp Ther 303(3):1029–1037
12. Gillis NK, Zhu HJ, Markowitz J (2011) An in vitro evaluation of guanfacine as a substrate for P-glycoprotein. Neuropsychiatr Dis Treat 7:501–505
13. McCracken JT, Aman MG, McDougle CJ et al (2010) Possible influence of variant of the P-glycoprotein gene (MDRI/ABCB1) on clinical response to guanfacine in children with pervasive developmental disorder and hyperactivity. J Child Adolesc Psychopharmacol 20(1):1–5
14. Patrick KS, Gonzalez MA, Straughn AB, Markowitz JS (2005) New methylphenidate formulations for the treatment of attention deficit/hyperactivity disorder. Expert Opin Drug Deliv 2(1):121–143
15. Ermer J, Adeyi B, Pucci M (2010) Pharmacokinetic variability of long-acting stimulants in the treatment of children and adults with attention-deficit hyperactivity disorder. CNS Drugs 24(12):1009–1025
16. Dopheide JA, Pliszka SR (2009) Attention-deficit-hyperactivity disorder: an update. Pharmacotherapy 29(6):656–679
17. Sonuga-Barke EIS, Coghill D, Markowitz JS et al (2007) Sex differences in the response of children with ADHD to once daily formulations of methyiphenidate. J Am Acad Child Adolesc Psychiatry 46(6):701–710
18. Patrick KS, Straughn AB, Minhinnett RR et al (2007) Influence of ethanol and gender on methylphenidate pharmacokinetics and pharmacodynamics. Clin Pharmacol Ther 81(3):346–353
19. Williard RL, Robin L, Middaugh LD et al (2007) Methylphenidate and its ethanol transesterification metabolite ethylphenidate: brain disposition, monoamine transporters and motor activity. Behav Pharmacol 18(1):39–51
20. Markowitz JS, Devane L, Boulton DW et al (2000) Ethylphenidate formation in human subjects after the administration of a single dose of methylphenidate and ethanol. Drug Metab Dispos 28(6):620–624
21. Ritalin LA (2013) Prescribing information. Novartis AG, East Hanover
22. Metadate CD (2013) Prescribing information. UCB, Inc., Smyrna
23. Wellbutrin (2013) Prescribing information. GlaxoSmithKline, Research Triangle Park
24. Intuniv (guanfacine) (2013) Prescribing information. Shire Inc., Wayne
25. Caffeine (2014) In: Natural medicines comprehensive database. Therapeutic Research Faculty, Stockton. http://naturaldatabase.therapeuticresearch.com.ezproxy.lib.utexas.edu/nd/Search.aspx?cs=UTEX~CPCE&s=ND&pt=100&id=979&ds=. Last Updated 17 Oct 2014, Accessed 16 Dec 2014
26. Institute of Medicine (2001) Caffeine for the sustainment of mental task performance: formulations for military operations. National Academy Press, Washington, DC, Available at: http://www.nap.edu/openbook.php?record_id=10219&page=R1
27. St. John's Wort (2014) In: Natural medicines comprehensive database. Therapeutic Research Faculty, Stockton. http://naturaldatabase.therapeuticresearch.com.ezproxy.lib.utexas.edu/nd/Search.aspx?cs=utex~cpce&s=ND&pt=100&id=329&fs=ND&searchid=49589760. Last Updated 14 Oct 2014, Accessed 16 Dec 2014
28. Ephedra. In: Natural medicines comprehensive database. Therapeutic Research Faculty, Stockton. http://naturaldatabase.therapeuticresearch.com/nd/Search.aspx?cs=UTEX~CPCE&s=ND&pt=100&id=847&ds=&name=EPHEDRA&searchid=49588695. Last Updated 5 Nov 2014, Accessed 16 Dec 2014
29. Haller CA, Benowitz NL (2000) Adverse cardiovascular and central nervous system events associated with dietary supplements containing ephedra alkaloids. N Engl J Med 343:1833–1838

30. Yohimbine. In: Natural medicines comprehensive database. Therapeutic Research Faculty, Stockton. http://naturaldatabase.therapeuticresearch.com.ezproxy.lib.utexas.edu/nd/Search.aspx?cs=UTEX~CPCE&s=ND&pt=100&id=759&ds=&name=Yohimbine+%28YOHIMBE%29&searchid=49589760. Last Updated 27 Oct 2014, Accessed 16 Dec 2014
31. Jori A, Bianchetti A, Prestini PE, Gerattini S (1970) Effect of eucalyptol (1,8-cineole) on the metabolism of other drugs in rats and in man. Eur J Pharmacol 9(3):362–366
32. Adderall XR (2014) (Amphetamine; dextroamphetamine) package insert. Shire US Inc., Wayne
33. Aggarwal A, Kulkarni G, Jahan S (2012) Potential serious adverse interactions between linezolid and atomoxetine. J Child Adolesc Psychopharmacol 22(5):406
34. Food and Drug Administration (US FDA) Drug Safety Communication (2015) Updated information about the drug interaction between methylene blue (methylthioninium chloride) and serotonergic psychiatric medications. Retrieved 15 Jan 2015. Available on the World Wide Web at http://www.fda.gov/Drugs/DrugSafety/ucm276119.htm
35. Grob C, Coyle JT (1986) Suspected adverse methylphenidate-imipramine interactions in children. J Dev Behav Pediatr 7:265–267
36. Niederhoder H (2008) Tricyclic antidepressants (TCA) may improve atomoxetine's efficacy. Int J Neuropsychopharmacol 11(6):877
37. Cocco G, Ague C (1977) Interactions between cardioactive drugs and antidepressants. Eur J Clin Pharmacol 11:389–393
38. Chua SS, Benrimoj SI (1988) Non-prescription sympathomimetic agents and hypertension. Med Toxicol Adverse Drug Exp 3:387–417
39. Zhu HJ, Patrick KS, Yuan HJ et al (2008) Two CES 1 Gene mutations lead to dysfunctional carboxylesterase Q activity in man: clinical significance and molecular basis. Am J Hum Genet 82:1241–1248
40. Zhu HJ, Appel DI, Peterson YK, Wang Z, Markowitz JS (2010) Identification of selected therapeutic agents as inhibitors of caboxylesterase 1: potential source of metabolic drug interactions. Toxicology 270:59–65
41. Ekinci O, Sabuncuoglu O (2011) Psychosis associated with switching from risperidone to aripirazole in an adolescent on methylphenidate treatment. Prog Neuropsychopharmacol Biol Psychiatry 35(2):648–649
42. McLaren JL, Cauble S, Barnett RJ (2010) Aripirazole induced acute dystonia after discontinuation of a stimulant medication. J Clin Psychopharmacol 30(1):77–78
43. Rhoades JA, Peterson YK, Zhu HJ, Appel DI, Peloquin CA, Markowitz JS (2012) Prediction and *In Vitro* evaluation of selected protease inhibitor antiviral drugs as inhibitors of Caroboxylesterase I: a potential source of drug-drug interactions. Pharm Res 29(4):972–982
44. Vyvanse (2015) (lisdexamfetamine dimesylate) [package insert]. Shire US Inc., Wayne
45. Pliszka SR, Crismon ML, Hughes CW, Conners CK, Emslie GJ, Jensen PT, McCracken JT, Swanson JM, Lopez M, Texas Consensus Conference Panel on Pharmacotherapy of Childhood Attention Deficit/Hyperactivity Disorder (2006) The Texas Children's Medication Algorithm Project: a revision of the algorithm for the pharmacotherapy of childhood attention deficit/hyperactivity disorder. J Am Acad Child Adolesc Psychiatry 45:642–657
46. Bond DJ, Hadjipavlou G, Lam RW et al (2012) The Canadian Network for Mood and Anxiety Treatments (CANMAT) taskforce recommendations for the management of patients with mood disorders and comorbid attention-deficit/hyperactivity disorder. Ann Clin Psychiatry 24:23–37
47. Groenman AP, Oosterlaan J, Rommelse NN et al (2013) Stimulant treatment of attention-deficit hyperactivity disorder and risk of developing substance abuse disorder. Br J Psychiatry 203:112–119
48. McCabe SE, West BT, Teter CJ, Boyd CK (2003) Trends in medical use, diversion, and nonmedical use of prescription medications among college students from to 2013: connecting the dots. Addict Behav 2014(39):1176–1182

Chapter 22
Clinically Significant Interactions with Cholinesterase Inhibitors and Other Antidementia Agents

Chad M. VanDenBerg

Abstract Cholinesterase inhibitors (ChEIs) and the NMDA receptor antagonist memantine are the currently approved treatment options for patients diagnosed with Alzheimer's disease (AD). Due largely to the lack of alternatives, these same medications are consequently used off-label to treat the many other forms of dementia, too. Future treatments for AD may include disease-modifying agents targeting amyloid beta production or aggregation including several immunotherapies. Potential drug interactions with these medications are limited since neither the ChEIs nor memantine is known for strong inhibition or induction of the cytochrome P450 (CYP) enzymes. Inhibitors of CYP3A4 or CYP2D6 may increase the concentrations of donepezil or galantamine leading to increased or reappearance of adverse events, typically GI related. Clinically significant interactions due to protein binding, glucuronidation, and p-glycoprotein are unlikely. Pharmacodynamic interactions may occur with ChEIs when other drugs affecting the cholinergic system are administered concomitantly. Similar pharmacodynamic interactions with memantine are unlikely. The clinical consequences of drug interactions with any of the ChEIs or memantine would most likely present as increased adverse events typical for these medications. Clinicians should monitor for increased cholinergic effects and potentially adjust dosage of ChEIs when drugs with potential pharmacokinetic or pharmacodynamic interactions are added to patient therapy for dementia.

Keywords Alzheimer's disease • Dementia • Cognitive disorders • Antidementia • Cholinesterase inhibitors • NMDA antagonists • Memantine • Donepezil • Galantamine • Rivastigmine

---

C.M. VanDenBerg, PharmD
Institute for Healthcare Innovation, Midwestern University,
Glendale, AZ, USA
e-mail: cvande@midwestern.edu

M. Jann et al. (eds.), *Applied Clinical Pharmacokinetics and Pharmacodynamics of Psychopharmacological Agents*,
DOI 10.1007/978-3-319-27883-4_22

Alzheimer's disease (AD), the most common form of dementia, is characterized by a gradual decline in cognition, activities of daily living, and behavior and produces characteristic symptoms such as memory loss, confusion, agitation, and difficulties performing the activities of daily living. The prevalence of AD is strongly correlated with increasing age and is a consequence of progressive neurodegeneration of the brain occurring over a period of several years or even decades. As the neurodegeneration progresses, the symptoms become more severe over time, creating a decline in independence and an increasing reliance on caregiver support. By the end stages of AD, patients are frequently bedridden due to substantial impairments or complete loss of motor abilities, continence, swallowing, eating, and speech.

Loss of cholinergic neurons in areas of the brain associated with learning, executive functioning, and memory is central to the symptomatology of Alzheimer's disease. The exact mechanism for the loss of these neurons remains unclear; however, amyloid plaques and neurofibrillary tangles in the brain of AD patients are two key pathological features of the disease. Amyloid plaques consist mainly of insoluble amyloid beta peptide; however, it has been proposed that the soluble oligomers of amyloid beta, rather than the insoluble deposits, are primarily responsible for cholinergic neurodegeneration and the impairment of synaptic function [1, 2]. Neurofibrillary tangles consisting of hyperphosphorylated tau proteins which are deposited in neuronal cell bodies and dystrophic neurites also correlate with the loss of cholinergic function. These observations form the basis of the cholinergic hypothesis of AD [3]. In addition to the neurotoxic proteins, dysfunction in the glutamatergic system leading to overstimulation of NMDA receptors may lead to the direct impairment of cognition and further long-term neuronal loss [4, 5].

Based on these pathological observations, the two drug classes that are current standard therapy for patients diagnosed with AD are cholinesterase inhibitors (donepezil, rivastigmine, and galantamine), which increase levels of acetylcholine in the brain, and the NMDA receptor antagonist, memantine. None of these agents modify the course of the disease, but rather have been approved based on symptomatic improvement. All agents are approved specifically for the treatment of AD at various stages, but their use in other forms of dementia (vascular, Lewy body dementia), neurological diseases (cerebral ischemia, traumatic brain injury, Parkinson's disease), and psychiatric disorders (cognitive impairment in schizophrenia, attention deficit disorders) is common. With regard to AD, the ChEIs produce modest improvements over time in cognition versus placebo with adverse effects mainly due to excessive cholinergic stimulation causing gastrointestinal, neurological, or cardiovascular abnormalities. A majority of the drug interactions with these medications arise from the exacerbation of the known adverse effects through either pharmacodynamic or pharmacokinetic properties. Other consequences of drug interactions including loss of efficacy due to decreases in concentration of ChEIs or memantine are less problematic mainly due to the already small clinical effect on cognition and the difficulty in demonstrating differences in clinical effect of individual patients over time.

Although none have been approved, there are several mechanistically different strategies that may provide treatment targets for AD in the future. Since there is evidence to indicate that aberrant amyloid beta production or clearance is an early component in the pathogenesis of AD, treatments targeting the amyloid cascade may be effective as disease-modifying agents and include passive and active immunotherapies, antiaggregation approaches, and γ- and β-secretase inhibitors. Several trials of immunotherapies designed to increase the clearance of amyloid beta by means of prolonged treatment with monoclonal antibodies directed against this peptide to reducing brain amyloid have proven ineffective. Since amyloid accumulation probably starts many years before the onset of symptoms, initiation of anti-amyloid treatments only after dementia develops, as was the case for the failed studies, may be too late to affect the clinical course of the disease. Other strategies based on the pathophysiology of AD include neurotransmitter-based therapies, metabolic or neurotrophic drugs, regenerative approaches, glial cell modulators, and tau protein modulator approaches. Drug interactions with these novel agents will be based on each treatment's proposed mechanism of action and or specific physical properties or effects. In the case of immunotherapies, drug interactions are unlikely due to the specificity of the antibodies for specific proteins of interest.

For the purpose of this chapter, the known, clinically significant drug interactions with the ChEIs and memantine will be addressed. Section 22.1.1 will address each medication individually. Sections 22.1.2, 22.1.3, 22.1.4, and 22.1.5 will address existing evidence on other specific pharmacokinetic drug interactions, while Sect. 22.2 will address the clinically relevant drug interactions based on drug class.

22.1 Pharmacokinetic Drug Interactions

Pharmacokinetic drug interactions involving the ChEIs and memantine are reviewed below. The potential phase I interactions for each individual agent are evaluated from both the potential of other agents to cause changes in the CYP metabolism of the antidementia drugs and the potential for the antidementia drugs to cause changes in the CYP metabolism of other drugs. Information on phase II drug interactions, protein binding interactions, and other mechanistic interactions is also evaluated where evidence exists.

22.1.1 Phase I Mechanistic Interactions (CYP)

Interactions with ChEIs through the CYP system are mainly due to the inhibition of enzymes by other drugs added to therapy causing decreased metabolism of the ChEI resulting in excessive cholinergic stimulation and related toxicities. Interactions caused by ChEIs due to their effect on the CYP system are less common but will be addressed where applicable.

Table 22.1 Potential pharmacokinetic interactions with ChEIs and memantine

Mechanism	Drug/drug class	Interaction
CYP3A4 inhibition	Amiodarone, cimetidine, clarithromycin, erythromycin, azole antifungals (e.g., ketoconazole, etc.), fluoxetine, fluvoxamine, sertraline, conivaptan, nefazodone, cobicistat, delavirdine, protease inhibitors (e.g., indinavir, etc.), suboxone, telithromycin, aprepitant, grapefruit juice, verapamil, diltiazem, chloramphenicol, ciprofloxacin, delavirdine, diethyldithiocarbamate, gestodene, imatinib, mibefradil, mifepristone, norfloxacin	↑ Donepezil concentrations ↑ Galantamine concentrations
CYP2D6 inhibition	Bupropion, cinacalcet, fluoxetine, paroxetine, quinidine, duloxetine, sertraline, terbinafine, amiodarone, cimetidine, celecoxib, chlorpheniramine, chlorpromazine, citalopram, clemastine, clomipramine, diphenhydramine, doxepin, doxorubicin, escitalopram, haloperidol, hydroxyzine, methadone, metoclopramide, midodrine, moclobemide, perphenazine, ranitidine, ritonavir, ticlopidine, tripelennamine	↑ Donepezil concentrations ↑ Galantamine concentrations
P-glycoprotein inhibition	Clarithromycin, erythromycin, ritonavir, and verapamil	↑ Galantamine concentrations
P-glycoprotein induction	Rifampicin and St. John's wort	↓ Galantamine concentrations
Urinary alkalization	Carbonic anhydrous inhibitors (e.g., acetazolamide) and sodium bicarbonate	↑ Memantine concentrations
Competitive renal secretion	Hydrochlorothiazide, triamterene, metformin, cimetidine, ranitidine, quinidine, nicotine	↑ Memantine concentrations

22.1.1.1 Donepezil

Donepezil is metabolized primarily through the CYP3A4 subsystem and to a lesser extent through the CYP2D6 subsystem; therefore, drugs that either inhibit or induce those CYP subsystems (Table 22.1) have the potential to affect the plasma concentrations of donepezil [6, 7]. In a study of healthy volunteers, ketoconazole 200 mg, a potent inhibitor of CYP3A4, administered concomitantly with donepezil 5 mg, significantly increased donepezil concentrations (AUC and Cmax) after both single and multiple doses with an estimated increase of 23–30 % at steady state [8]. Clinically significant pharmacokinetic effects were not demonstrated in a study with sertraline, a CYP2D6 subsystem inhibitor [9]; however, case reports for the potent CYP2D6 inhibitors paroxetine [10] and fluoxetine [11, 12] suggest that an interaction is possible. Two patients previously receiving paroxetine exhibited increased gastrointestinal adverse effects when concomitantly administered with donepezil 5 mg/day. Symptoms in both patients persisted until donepezil was discontinued [10]. A patient with a 3-year history of donepezil 10 mg treatment was initiated on fluoxetine and developed signs of cholinergic excess including excessive salivation, lacrimation, and fecal incontinence. Upon discontinuation of both drugs, symptoms resolved [12].

Although no clinical studies have been completed to identify an effect of donepezil on other drugs metabolized through the CYP3A4 or CYP2D6 subsystems, in vitro studies demonstrate a low rate of binding to these enzymes suggesting that drug interactions of this type are unlikely [6].

No significant pharmacokinetic interactions or clinical adverse events have been reported when donepezil was coadministered with memantine, risperidone, or anti-Parkinson's disease medications [13–15].

22.1.1.2 Galantamine

Similar to donepezil, galantamine is metabolized through the CYP3A4 and CYP2D6 subsystems. In addition to the CYP metabolic routes of elimination, galantamine is also glucuronidated and excreted unchanged, with no single pathway appearing to be predominant. To determine the effects of the inhibition of CYP on the bioavailability of galantamine, studies were conducted in healthy volunteers who were coadministered with the potent CYP2D6 inhibitor paroxetine 20 mg/day or the CYP3A4 inhibitor ketoconazole 200 mg BID or erythromycin 500 mg QID. Plasma levels of galantamine were increased by 40 %, 30 %, and 10 % by paroxetine, ketoconazole, and erythromycin, respectively [16]. A population pharmacokinetic study of patients coadministered with galantamine with amitriptyline, fluoxetine, fluvoxamine, or quinidine demonstrated decreases in galantamine clearance between 25 and 33 % [16].

Although no clinical studies have been completed to identify an effect of galantamine on other drugs metabolized through the CYP subsystems, in vitro studies demonstrate a low rate of binding to CYP1A2, CYP2A6, CYP3A4, CYP4A, CYP2C, CYP2D6, or CYP2E1 enzymes indicating that the inhibitory potential of galantamine toward the major forms of cytochrome P450 is very low, and drug interactions of this type are unlikely.

22.1.1.3 Rivastigmine

Rivastigmine is primarily metabolized through hydrolysis by esterases and not significantly metabolized through the CYP system; therefore, clinically significant, phase I drug interactions are not expected [17]. In vitro studies with different CYP subsystems including CYP1A2, CYP2D6, CYP3A4/5, CYP2E1, CYP2C9, CYP2C8, CYP2C19, or CYP2B6 support this expectation [17]. Studies conducted with healthy volunteers coadministered with rivastigmine with diazepam or fluoxetine also demonstrated no significant interactions [17]. Population pharmacokinetic analysis showed that the pharmacokinetics of oral rivastigmine were not influenced by commonly prescribed medications such as antacids, antihypertensives, ß-blockers, calcium channel blockers, antidiabetics, nonsteroidal anti-inflammatory drugs, estrogens, salicylate analgesics, antianginals, and antihistamines [17]. Retrospective analysis of clinical trials revealed no increase in adverse effects compared with placebo (16 % versus 14 %) in patients who were taking ß-blockers, antianginal agents, antacids, antihypertensive agents, antiemetics, calcium channel blockers, estrogens, antihistamines, benzodiazepines, and nonsteroidal anti-inflammatory agents [18]. Finally, a pharmacodynamic analysis of rivastigmine did not reveal any significant increases in adverse events that would indicate a drug interaction when administered concomitantly with medications from 22 different therapeutic classes [19].

22.1.1.4 Memantine

Memantine is predominantly eliminated unchanged in the urine, and therefore clinically significant, phase I interactions with the CYP system affecting memantine are not expected [20].

Memantine has been shown to significantly inhibit the activity of CYP2B6 at physiologic relevant concentrations in vitro [21]. Although no clinically significant interactions have been reported between memantine and drugs metabolized by CYP2B6, this enzyme plays an important role in the metabolism of cyclophosphamide, tamoxifen, S-mephenytoin, and diazepam and therefore has the potential to increase the concentrations of these drugs if used concomitantly. Other interactions are unlikely since memantine only minimally inhibits CYP1A2, CYP2A6, CYP2C9, CYP2D6, CYP2E1, or CYP3A4 and does not induce the activity of CYP1A2, CYP2C9, CYP2E1, or CYP3A4/5 [21].

A clinical study investigating the additive antidepressant effects of memantine to citalopram, a weak inhibitor of CYP1A2, CYP2D6, and CYP2C19, did not reveal any significant difference in adverse events between the addition of memantine and placebo [22]. A clinical pharmacokinetic/pharmacodynamic study of the concomitant use of memantine and the combination product dextromethorphan/quinidine demonstrated that quinidine, a CYP2D6 inhibitor, did not affect the plasma concentrations of memantine [23].

22.1.2 *Phase II Mechanistic Interactions (Glucuronidation)*

Of the four currently prescribed antidementia agents, both galantamine and memantine undergo glucuronidation. In addition to glucuronidation, galantamine also undergoes metabolism by the CYP3A4 and CYP2D6 subsystems and is excreted unchanged. Memantine is largely excreted unchanged in the urine, but a smaller portion is converted via glucuronidation. Since glucuronidation of galantamine and memantine is not considered a predominant route of elimination, clinically significant interactions are unlikely.

22.1.3 P-Glycoprotein-Based Interactions

Galantamine is a substrate of the P-glycoprotein [24]. Although no studies have been completed to define the effect of P-glycoprotein inhibitors or inducers on the pharmacokinetics of galantamine, clinicians should be aware of the potential for altered pharmacokinetics of galantamine when used concomitantly with drugs that inhibit or induce P-glycoprotein (Table 22.1). An in vitro study showed that donepezil was not a substrate of P-glycoprotein [25].

22.1.4 Protein Binding Interactions

Protein binding with galantamine (18 %), rivastigmine (40 %), or memantine (45 %) is relatively low; therefore, interactions with drugs that are highly protein bound are unlikely [16–18, 20]. Indeed, clinical interaction studies have demonstrated that neither the protein binding of warfarin nor the pharmacodynamics of warfarin as assessed by prothrombin INR was affected by daily administration of galantamine 24 mg [26] or rivastigmine [18, 27].

Donepezil is the only ChEI that has an appreciable amount of protein binding. Although donepezil is highly protein bound (96 %), the portion bound to albumin is only 75 %, while 21 % is bound to α_1-acid glycoprotein; therefore, protein displacement interactions with donepezil are unlikely [28]. Clinical interaction studies confirm that concurrent administration of donepezil 10 mg/day did not alter the pharmacokinetics or pharmacodynamics of a single dose of warfarin 25 mg in healthy male volunteers [29]. Donepezil also did not have any significant effects on the pharmacokinetics of theophylline (titrated to therapeutic range) or digoxin 0.375 mg once daily which are also highly protein bound [30, 31]. Similarly, the binding of donepezil to human albumin was not affected by furosemide, digoxin, and warfarin [6].

22.1.5 Smoking, Food, and Other Types of Interactions

Memantine is eliminated renally and the clearance is dependent upon urinary pH. Alkaline urine with pH 8 reduces memantine clearance by 80 % which may lead to accumulation of the drug and an increase in adverse events [20]. Drugs that have an alkalizing effect on the urinary pH such as carbonic anhydrous inhibitors and sodium bicarbonate may cause increased adverse effects due to memantine accumulation (Table 22.1). Concomitant use of drugs that are eliminated by the same renal cationic system as memantine (Table 22.1) has the potential to interfere with the clearance of memantine; however, no interaction was noted when memantine was used concomitantly with the combination products hydrochlorothiazide/triamterene or glyburide/metformin HCl [20].

22.2 Pharmacodynamic Drug Interactions

The following section will review the potential pharmacodynamic drug interactions that may occur with either the ChEIs or memantine. Since each of the ChEIs has a very high specificity to the cholinesterase enzyme and relatively little influence over other enzymes or receptor systems, the potential pharmacodynamic interactions may be considered inclusive of the class. Memantine is considered separately and has distinct potential pharmacodynamic interactions.

22.2.1 ChEIs

Based on the mechanism of action of the ChEIs, interactions with drugs that have an effect on the cholinergic system may be expected. Anticholinergic drugs are of particular interest due to the many drug classes that possess these properties (Table 22.1). Anticholinergic drugs may already have a negative effect on elderly patients producing clinically significant mental status changes ranging from mild cognitive impairment to delirium. Patients with AD and other dementias are especially sensitive to these effects. Therefore, drugs with anticholinergic activity should be avoided in patients taking ChEIs. For patients already receiving an anticholinergic agent, ChEIs may also interfere with the activity of anticholinergic medications, although due to the potential negative consequences of anticholinergic agents, regardless of whether the patient is receiving a ChEI, substitution or discontinuation of the anticholinergic is recommended.

Increased cholinergic effects may be expected when ChEIs are administered with other cholinomimetic drugs (Table 22.2). A synergistic effect may be expected when cholinesterase inhibitors are given concurrently with succinylcholine, similar neuromuscular blocking agents, or cholinergic agonists such as bethanechol.

Seizure activity can be induced or exacerbated by cholinomimetic drugs [32], and there have been occasional but not systematic reports of seizure activity due to donepezil [33], rivastigmine [34], and memantine [35]. Concomitant use of ChEIs or memantine with other drugs that are known to lower the seizure threshold may result in seizure activity (Table 22.2). It should be noted that seizure activity may also be a manifestation of AD [36], and these conclusions are based on uncontrolled, retrospective case reports in patients who may have other risk factors for seizures as well.

ChEIs can cause bradycardia and heart block due to vagotonic effects on the sinoatrial and atrioventricular nodes, and additive effects may occur with other

Table 22.2 Potential pharmacodynamic interactions with ChEIs and memantine

Mechanism	Example drugs/drug classes	Interaction
Anticholinergic	Sedating antihistamines, antispasmodics, neuroleptics, phenothiazines, skeletal muscle relaxants, tricyclic antidepressants, class IA antiarrhythmics, carbamazepine, cimetidine, ranitidine	↓ Response to ChEIs
Cholinergic	Succinylcholine or other similar neuromuscular blocking agents, cholinergic agonists (e.g., bethanechol, carbachol)	↑ Adverse effects of ChEIs
Ionotropic	Beta-blockers, calcium channel blockers, digoxin, protease inhibitors (i.e., atazanavir, lopinavir-ritonavir, saquinavir), amiodarone, dronedarone, moricizine, lacosamide, and mefloquine	↑ Bradycardia effect of ChEIs
Epilogenic	Selective serotonin reuptake inhibitors, monoamine oxidase inhibitors, neuroleptic agents, central nervous system stimulants, opioids, tricyclic antidepressants, other tricyclic compounds (e.g., cyclobenzaprine, phenothiazines), carbapenems, cholinergic agents, fluoroquinolones, interferons, chloroquine, mefloquine, lindane, theophylline, iodinated contrast media	↓ Seizure threshold

agents that also possess bradycardic effects (Table 22.2). A retrospective analysis of spontaneous adverse drug reaction reports to the French Pharmacovigilance Database associated with use of donepezil, galantamine, and rivastigmine revealed 205 cases of potential drug interactions with bradycardic drugs of which 73 were associated with serious ADRs including five deaths due to syncope, bradycardia, arrhythmia, or cardiac arrest [37]. Confirmation of a definitive drug interaction in these cases was not possible since details on the individual cases such as patient characteristics or concomitant risk factors were not provided. In contrast, a phase III trial of donepezil consisting of 1,035 patients reported no significant increase in risk ratios for bradycardia during concomitant use of beta-blockers, nondihydropyridine calcium channel blockers, or digoxin [38].

22.2.2 Memantine

Dextromethorphan, the active agent of the combination product dextromethorphan/quinidine, is a low-affinity, uncompetitive N-methyl-D-aspartate (NMDA) receptor antagonist approved for the treatment of pseudobulbar affect (PBA), a condition affecting as much as 39 % of AD patients. In addition dextromethorphan is a common active ingredient in many formulations of cough suppressants. Since both memantine and dextromethorphan are NMDA receptor antagonists, concomitant use could theoretically lead to an additive effect and increased rates or severity of adverse events [23]. In addition to the pharmacokinetic interaction (see Sect. 22.1.1), the pharmacodynamic interaction between memantine and the combination product dextromethorphan/quinidine was investigated. Concomitant use of memantine and dextromethorphan did not affect the incidence of adverse events or measured pharmacodynamic variables when compared to the use of either product alone [23].

22.3 Clinical Significance of PK and PD Interactions

The major consequence of pharmacokinetic drug interactions with the ChEIs (specifically donepezil or galantamine) is the potential for cholinergic toxicity resulting from concomitant use of a drug that inhibits the CYP2D6 or CYP3A4 (see Sect. 22.1.1) or agents that produce a synergistic effect. The signs and symptoms of these types of interactions are likely to be increases or reappearance of the known adverse events of the ChEIs (Table 22.3). The clinical significance of the interactions seems to be rather small since the symptoms are non-life threatening, easily identified, and readily controlled with either a decrease in dosage or elimination of the interacting agent. Since rivastigmine does not undergo CYP metabolism, pharmacokinetic interactions are not thought to occur.

Agents that possess anticholinergic activity may negate the pharmacologic effects of ChEIs and diminish the already small clinical benefits of ChEIs in the treatment of dementia. Regardless of whether the patient is receiving a ChEI, clinically significant mental status changes may be associated with anticholinergic agents and should generally be avoided in patients with AD or other cognitive impairment.

The clinical effectiveness of ChEIs and memantine in delaying or improving cognition is likely very small and difficult to measure; therefore, the clinical significance of decreases in the concentration of the ChEIs or memantine due to inducers of CYP system is likely negligible. It may be possible to retitrate the dosage of these medications to tolerability if a CYP2D6 or CYP3A4 enzyme inducer is required for long-term concomitant therapy.

Table 22.3 Signs and symptoms of toxicities resulting from drug interactions with ChEIs or memantine

Mechanism	Result	Sign/symptoms
↑ ChEI concentrations Synergistic PD effect with ChEIs	Cholinergic excess	GI upset/cramping, nausea, vomiting, sweating, weakness, salivation, lacrimation, dizziness, syncope, or slowed respirations
Concomitant use of anticholinergic agent	↓ Clinical effect of ChEIs	↑ Confusion, ↑ memory loss, ↑ agitation
↑ Urinary pH ↓ Renal tubular secretion	↑ Memantine concentrations	Dizziness, headache, confusion, constipation

22.3.1 *Dosage Adjustments*

When adding a ChEI or memantine to an existing treatment which may have either a pharmacokinetic (Table 22.1) or pharmacodynamic interaction (Table 22.2), dosage adjustment is not necessary as the dose of each of these drugs is individually titrated to tolerability up to the maximum recommended dose. However, there may be a need to decrease or retitrate the dosage of donepezil or galantamine when a potent CYP2D6 or CYP3A4 inhibitor (Table 22.1) is added to therapy if intolerable adverse events emerge.

22.3.2 *Monitoring Recommendations and Patient Safety*

Clinicians and patients should be aware of the potential for increased adverse cholinergic effects (Table 22.3) when a potent inhibitor of CYP2D6 or CYP3A4 is added to either donepezil or galantamine therapy or a medication with additive cholinergic effects is used concomitantly.

Cholinergic agents, including ChEIs, may be individually epileptogenic, and there may be a theoretical risk of increased seizure potential when used with any substance that can reduce the seizure threshold (Table 22.2).

Caution is advised if acetylcholinesterase inhibitors are used concomitantly with bradycardic drugs (Table 22.2). Patients should be advised to notify their physician if they experience dizziness, light-headedness, fainting, or irregular heartbeat.

22.4 Conclusions

Although they are typically used in an elderly population that may be at higher risk of drug interactions, both the ChEIs and memantine are relatively well tolerated. Consequences of drug interactions with the ChEIs are relatively minor and generally well explained either by the pharmacokinetic interaction with the CYP system or pharmacodynamically through synergistic cholinergic effects. Typical symptoms of both the pharmacokinetic and pharmacodynamic interactions consist of increased gastrointestinal complaints such as nausea and vomiting due to the increase in cholinergic activity. These symptoms can be easily managed with a slower titration or decrease in dosage. Additional care is merited when ChEIs are used concomitantly with ionotropic agents as there is an increased potential for bradycardia. Increases in memantine concentration may occur when agents that alter the urinary pH are used concomitantly, but resulting adverse events are relatively minor and can be easily managed with a dose reduction or discontinuation of the interacting agent. It is unlikely that the ChEIs or memantine will cause interactions with other medications when added to therapy since they have little inhibitory or induction potential of the CYP system and low protein binding potential.

References

1. De Felice FG, Velasco PT, Lambert MP et al (2007) Abeta oligomers induce neuronal oxidative stress through an N-methyl-D-aspartate receptor-dependent mechanism that is blocked by the Alzheimer drug memantine. J Biol Chem 282(15):11590–11601
2. Lacor PN, Buniel MC, Furlow PW et al (2007) Abeta oligomer-induced aberrations in synapse composition, shape, and density provide a molecular basis for loss of connectivity in Alzheimer's disease. J Neurosci (Off J Soc Neurosci) 27(4):796–807
3. Perry EK, Tomlinson BE, Blessed G, Bergmann K, Gibson PH, Perry RH (1978) Correlation of cholinergic abnormalities with senile plaques and mental test scores in senile dementia. Br Med J 2(6150):1457–1459
4. Cacabelos R, Takeda M, Winblad B (1999) The glutamatergic system and neurodegeneration in dementia: preventive strategies in Alzheimer's disease. Int J Geriatr Psychiatry 14(1):3–47
5. Danysz W, Parsons CG (2003) The NMDA receptor antagonist memantine as a symptomatological and neuroprotective treatment for Alzheimer's disease: preclinical evidence. Int J Geriatr Psychiatry 18(S1):S23–S32
6. Eisai (2015) ARICEPT® (donepezil hydrochloride) tablets: prescribing information. Eisai Inc. Woodcliff Lake, NJ.
7. Wilkinson DG (1999) The pharmacology of donepezil: a new treatment for Alzheimer's disease. Expert Opin Pharmacother 1(1):121–135
8. Tiseo PJ, Perdomo CA, Friedhoff LT (1998) Concurrent administration of donepezil HCl and ketoconazole: assessment of pharmacokinetic changes following single and multiple doses. Br J Clin Pharmacol 46(Suppl 1):30–34
9. Nagy CF, Kumar D, Perdomo CA, Wason S, Cullen EI, Pratt RD (2004) Concurrent administration of donepezil HCl and sertraline HCl in healthy volunteers: assessment of pharmacokinetic changes and safety following single and multiple oral doses. Br J Clin Pharmacol 58:25–33
10. Carrier L (1999) Donepezil and paroxetine: possible drug interaction. J Am Geriatr Soc 47(8):1037
11. Chew AP, Lim WS, Tan KT (2014) Donepezil-induced hepatotoxicity in an elderly adult taking fluoxetine. J Am Geriatr Soc 62(10):2009–2011
12. Marshall K, Fritz K, Thom W, Xiong G (2012) Toxic interaction between fluoxetine and donepezil: a case of cholinergic toxidrome. J Neuropsychiatry Clin Neurosci 24(2):E50
13. Zhao Q, Xie C, Pesco-Koplowitz L, Jia X, Parier J-L (2003) Pharmacokinetic and safety assessments of concurrent administration of risperidone and donepezil. J Clin Pharmacol 43(2):180–186
14. Molino I, Colucci L, Fasanaro AM, Traini E, Amenta F (2013) Efficacy of memantine, donepezil, or their association in moderate-severe Alzheimer's disease: a review of clinical trials. Scientific World Journal 2013:925702
15. Dubois B, Tolosa E, Katzenschlager R et al (2012) Donepezil in Parkinson's disease dementia: a randomized, double-blind efficacy and safety study. Mov Disord 27(10):1230–1238
16. Janssen (2013) RAZADYNE® ER (galantamine hydrobromide) full prescribing information. Janssen Pharmaceuticals, Inc. Titusville, NJ.
17. Novartis (2015) Exelon® Patch (rivastigmine transdermal system), Full Prescribing Information. Novartis Pharmaceuticals Corporation, East Hanover, NJ.
18. Polinsky RJ (1998) Clinical pharmacology of rivastigmine: a new-generation acetylcholinesterase inhibitor for the treatment of Alzheimer's disease. Clin Ther 20(4):634–647
19. Grossberg GT, Stahelin HB, Messina JC, Anand R, Veach J (2000) Lack of adverse pharmacodynamic drug interactions with rivastigmine and twenty-two classes of medications. Int J Geriatr Psychiatry 15(3):242–247
20. Forest (2014) Namenda (memantine HCl) Full prescribing information. Forest Pharmaceuticals, Inc. St. Louis, MO.

21. Micuda S, Mundlova L, Anzenbacherova E et al (2004) Inhibitory effects of memantine on human cytochrome P450 activities: prediction of in vivo drug interactions. Eur J Clin Pharmacol 60(8):583–589
22. Omranifard V, Shirzadi E, Samandari S, Afshar H, Maracy MR (2014) Memantine add on to citalopram in elderly patients with depression: a double-blind placebo-controlled study. J Res Med Sci (The Official Journal of Isfahan University of Medical Sciences) 19(6):525–530
23. Pope LE, Schoedel KA, Bartlett C, Sellers EM (2012) A study of potential pharmacokinetic and pharmacodynamic interactions between dextromethorphan/quinidine and memantine in healthy volunteers. Clin Drug Investig 32(8):e1–e15
24. Noetzli M, Guidi M, Ebbing K et al (2013) Relationship of CYP2D6, CYP3A, POR, and ABCB1 genotypes with galantamine plasma concentrations. Ther Drug Monit 35(2):270–275
25. McEneny-King A, Edginton AN, Rao PP (2015) Investigating the binding interactions of the anti-Alzheimer's drug donepezil with CYP3A4 and P-glycoprotein. Bioorg Med Chem Lett 25(2):297–301
26. Scott L, Goa K (2000) Galantamine. Drugs 60(5):1095–1122
27. Spencer CM, Noble S (1998) Rivastigmine. A review of its use in Alzheimer's disease. Drugs Aging 13(5):391–411
28. Defilippi JL, Crismon ML (2003) Drug interactions with cholinesterase inhibitors. Drugs Aging 20(6):437–444
29. Tiseo PJ, Foley K, Friedhoff LT (1998) The effect of multiple doses of donepezil HCl on the pharmacokinetic and pharmacodynamic profile of warfarin. Br J Clin Pharmacol 46(Suppl 1):45–50
30. Tiseo PJ, Foley K, Friedhoff LT (1998) Concurrent administration of donepezil HCl and theophylline: assessment of pharmacokinetic changes following multiple-dose administration in healthy volunteers. Br J Clin Pharmacol 46(Suppl 1):35–39
31. Tiseo PJ, Perdomo CA, Friedhoff LT (1998) Concurrent administration of donepezil HCl and digoxin: assessment of pharmacokinetic changes. Br J Clin Pharmacol 46(Suppl 1):40–44
32. Friedman A, Behrens CJ, Heinemann U (2007) Cholinergic dysfunction in temporal lobe epilepsy. Epilepsia 48(Suppl 5):126–130
33. Babic T, Zurak N (1999) Convulsions induced by donepezil. J Neurol Neurosurg Psychiatry 66(3):410
34. Kumlien E, Lundberg PO (2010) Seizure risk associated with neuroactive drugs: data from the WHO adverse drug reactions database. Seizure 19(2):69–73
35. Peltz G, Pacific DM, Noviasky JA, Shatla A, Mehalic T (2005) Seizures associated with memantine use. Am J Health Syst Pharm 62(4):420–421
36. Bird TD (1998) Alzheimer disease overview. In: Pagon RA, Adam MP, Ardinger HH et al (eds) GeneReviews(R). University of Washington, Seattle
37. Tavassoli N, Sommet A, Lapeyre-Mestre M, Bagheri H, Montrastruc JL (2007) Drug interactions with cholinesterase inhibitors: an analysis of the French pharmacovigilance database and a comparison of two national drug formularies (Vidal, British National Formulary). Drug Saf 30(11):1063–1071
38. Relkin NR, Reichman WE, Orazem J, McRae T (2003) A large, community-based, open-label trial of donepezil in the treatment of Alzheimer's disease. Dement Geriatr Cogn Disord 16(1):15–24

Chapter 23
Clinically Significant Interactions with Anti-addiction Agents

Janet K. Coller, Daniel T. Barratt, and Andrew A. Somogyi

Abstract Anti-addiction agents are important psychopharmacological agents used to treat addiction to opioids (illicit and licit), alcohol and nicotine. The goal of treatment is to eliminate further use of the addicted drug by either preventing addicted drug reward or managing withdrawal symptoms experienced when the addicted drug is no longer used. Treatment success relies on adequate plasma and brain concentrations to produce the required pharmacodynamic response without toxic adverse effects. In this chapter, we describe clinically significant drug-drug interactions caused by changes in pharmacokinetics (induction or inhibition of metabolism) and pharmacodynamics (inhibited, additive or synergistic activity at the drug target) of the anti-addiction agents that alter treatment success, cause harmful effects and/or have led to recommendations from regulatory bodies regarding dosage adjustments or additional monitoring for patient safety. Clinicians need to be aware of the potential for these drug-drug interactions and prescribe and monitor patients for safety and efficacy as needed.

Keywords Opioid • Alcohol • Nicotine • Pharmacodynamic • Pharmacokinetic

23.1 Pharmacokinetic Drug Interactions

The pharmacokinetics (PK) of anti-addiction agents, like all medicines, can influence patient response, treatment success and adverse effects. There is a wide body of literature that discusses changes in pharmacokinetics due to drug-drug interactions involving phase I and II metabolism, efflux transport by P-glycoprotein and as a result of other patient environmental characteristics including smoking of tobacco

J.K. Coller, BSc (Hon), PhD, GCert. Ed (✉) • D.T. Barratt, PhD • A.A. Somogyi, PhD
Discipline of Pharmacology, School of Medicine, The University of Adelaide,
Adelaide 5005, Australia
e-mail: janet.coller@adelaide.edu.au

M. Jann et al. (eds.), *Applied Clinical Pharmacokinetics and Pharmacodynamics of Psychopharmacological Agents*,
DOI 10.1007/978-3-319-27883-4_23

Table 23.1 Summary of important drug interactions that alter PK of anti-opioid, anti-alcohol and anti-nicotine addiction agents

Anti-addiction agent	Impact of PK interaction on anti-addiction agent	PK consequence
Methadone and buprenorphine	Induction of metabolism	Reduced plasma concentrations
	Inhibition of metabolism	Increased plasma concentrations
Acamprosate	Increased rate and extent of absorption	Increased plasma concentrations
Bupropion	Induction of metabolism	Reduced plasma concentrations
	Inhibition of metabolism	Increased plasma concentrations

and cannabis (refer to Tables 23.1 and 23.3). This section will summarise the current knowledge on how the PK of anti-addiction agents are altered and how anti-addiction agents themselves alter the PK of concomitant medications.

23.1.1 Anti-opioid Addiction Agents

23.1.1.1 Methadone

Methadone (Dolophine®, Methadose®, Biodone Forte®, Physeptone®) is highly bound (90 %) by alpha-acid glycoprotein [1] and extensively metabolised by phase I reactions mediated predominantly by CYP3A4 and CYP2B6. It also has significant inhibitory activity of phase I and II metabolism via CYP2D6 and UGT2B7, respectively, and is a substrate and inhibitor of P-glycoprotein (P-gp). Methadone's inhibition of CYP2D6 and UGT2B7 alters the PK of co-medications that are substrates for these enzymes; for example, the metabolism of codeine via CYP2D6 and UGT2B7 is significantly reduced with co-administration of methadone [2]. Similarly, co-administration of many other drugs (including herbal medicines such as St. John's wort) that induce or inhibit metabolism by these enzymes can decrease or increase, respectively, plasma methadone concentrations [3–5]. These interactions can result in significant clinical effects of CNS and cardiac toxicities if methadone concentrations are too high and opioid withdrawal and treatment failure if concentrations are too low. Consequently the FDA has comprehensive recommendations regarding co-administration of these medications with methadone (summarised in Table 23.3).

23.1.1.2 Buprenorphine

Buprenorphine (Buprenex®, Suboxone®, Subutex®) is highly (95 %) plasma protein bound [6] and undergoes phase I and II metabolism by CYP3A4 and 2C8, and UGT1A1, 1A3 and 2B7, respectively. Whilst it is not a substrate for P-gp, its main metabolite, norbuprenorphine, is a substrate. Buprenorphine is a weak inhibitor of CYP2D6 and CYP3A4, but this is not likely to be clinically significant due to the relative low inhibitory potential [4]. However, co-administration of several drugs has revealed potential PK interactions that increase or decrease buprenorphine concentrations, in particular inhibitors and inducers of CYP3A4 [3–5]. For example, ketoconazole, erythromycin and HIV-protease inhibitors (ritonavir, atazanavir) can inhibit the CYP3A4 metabolism to increase concentrations, whilst rifampin and St. John's wort can induce the CYP3A4 metabolism to reduce concentrations. Similarly, buprenorphine can decrease concentrations of atazanavir, but only when given alone, and not when in combination with ritonavir.

23.1.2 Anti-alcohol Addiction Agents

23.1.2.1 Acamprosate

Acamprosate (Campral®) does not undergo phase I or II metabolism, is not an inducer or inhibitor of CYP450 enzymes and is not plasma protein bound (for review see [7]). As acamprosate is used for alcohol addiction, potential acamprosate PK changes when combined with alcohol, disulfiram and diazepam (drugs commonly co-administered) have been investigated, with no significant interactions observed. However, co-administration of acamprosate with naltrexone significantly increased acamprosate AUC and C_{max} by 25 and 33 %, respectively [8]. The mechanism by which this occurs is likely due to the interaction altering acamprosate absorption parameters from the gastrointestinal tract, although this is yet to be confirmed. With regard to its impact on PK of co-medications, acamprosate did not alter the PK of alcohol, diazepam and its metabolite nordiazepam, imipramine and its metabolite desipramine, or naltrexone and its metabolite 6-beta naltrexol [7].

23.1.2.2 Disulfiram

Disulfiram (Antabuse, Antabus) is rapidly reduced to its metabolite diethyldithiocarbamate (DDC) which is further metabolised via glucuronidation, methylation, oxidation and non-enzymatic degradation [9]. It is highly (96 %) bound to albumin [10]. It inhibits CYP2E1 and CYP2C9 enzyme activity, therefore altering the PK of drugs that are metabolised by these enzymes (e.g. phenytoin, warfarin) [11, 12].

23.1.2.3 Naltrexone

Naltrexone (Revia®, Vivitrol®) undergoes reduction to form 6-beta naltrexol mediated by dihydrodiol dehydrogenase [4, 13], and both the parent and metabolite are glucuronidated. Its very low plasma protein binding, at <20 % [14], will not cause PK interactions clinically. In comparison to other anti-alcohol addiction agents, there are relatively few reports regarding naltrexone altering PK drug interactions, being limited to the following: naltrexone increased diazepam C_{max} [15]; and naltrexone increased the rate and extent of acamprosate absorption (as discussed above) [8].

23.1.3 *Anti-nicotine Addiction Agents*

23.1.3.1 Bupropion

Bupropion (Zyban®) undergoes phase I reduction to hydroxybupropion mediated by CYP2B6. It is not a substrate for P-gp, but is highly plasma protein bound (75–85 %) [16, 17]. A number of drugs have been reported to alter the PK of bupropion and genetic polymorphism of the *CYP2B6* enzyme can also alter its metabolism. For example, drugs that inhibit or induce CYP2B6 enzyme function increase or decrease, respectively, bupropion concentrations. Similarly, bupropion and its metabolites are inhibitors of CYP2D6 that results in significant potential to alter PK of co-medications that are substrates of CYP2D6 (including a number of drugs from the following drug classes: antidepressants, antipsychotics, beta-blockers, antiarrhythmics, immunosuppressants).

23.1.3.2 Nicotine Replacement Therapy

Nicotine in nicotine replacement therapy (NRT, Nicorette®, Nicabate®, Nicotinell®, QuitX®) undergoes phase I and II metabolism by CYP2A6, CYP2B6 and FMO, and UGT1A4, 1A9 and 2B10, respectively. It is not protein bound (<20 %) [18] and is not a substrate/inhibitor of P-gp. Studies have shown that nicotine can induce brain expression of CYP2D [19] that can result in enhanced central metabolism of substrates for this enzyme (e.g. tramadol a human CYP2D6 substrate that is metabolised by CYP2D in an animal model) [20]. However, the implications of this induction in humans are yet to be investigated.

23.1.3.3 Varenicline

Varenicline (Chantix®, Champix®) is not extensively metabolised by phase I and II reactions, with only minor glucuronidation (<10 %) to varenicline *N*-carbamoylglucorinide by UGT2B7 [21]. There are no reports of exposure causing enzyme induction or inhibition; it is not a substrate or inhibitor of P-gp and is poorly bound to plasma proteins (<20 %) thus unlikely to result in clinically significant interactions (for review see [22]). A few studies have investigated potential impact of varenicline on co-medication PK with no significant interaction reported for warfarin [23], digoxin [24], cimetidine, metformin, bupropion and nicotine (transdermal patch).

23.2 Pharmacodynamic Drug Interactions

Patient variability in pharmacodynamics (PD) of anti-addiction agents can have a substantial impact on response, toxicity and treatment success (refer to Tables 23.2 and 23.3). There are three main consequences of drug interactions at a PD level: inhibited, additive or synergistic responses. This section will summarise the current knowledge on how the PD of anti-addiction agents are altered and how anti-addiction agents themselves alter the PD of concomitant medications.

23.2.1 Anti-opioid Addiction Agents

23.2.1.1 Methadone

Methadone is an agonist at mu opioid and antagonist at NMDA receptors. Co-administration of mu opioid receptor partial agonists and antagonists (e.g. buprenorphine and naltrexone, respectively) will cause loss of methadone PD and clinical response. At high doses (and plasma concentrations), methadone (principally the mu receptor inactive S enantiomer) causes prolongation of the QT_c interval that can result in a PD additive effect when combined with other drugs that prolong this interval (e.g. SSRIs, psychotropics and drugs that alter electrolyte balance) [4].

Table 23.2 Summary of important drug interactions that alter PD of anti-opioid, anti-alcohol and anti-nicotine addiction agents

Anti-addiction agent	Impact of PD interaction on anti-addiction agent	PD consequence
Methadone	Additive PD response with benzodiazepines and alcohol	Overdose symptoms (sedation, coma)
	Additive PD response with SSRIs, psychotropics and drugs that alter electrolyte balance	QTc interval prolongation (*Torsades des pointes*)
Buprenorphine	Additive PD response with benzodiazepines	Overdose symptoms (sedation, coma)
Disulfiram	Additive PD response with metronidazole or other alcohol-containing drug formulations	Increased toxicity due to accumulation of acetaldehyde
Naltrexone	Blocks PD response of opioids; additive PD response with THC	Prevent analgesia/precipitate withdrawal with opioids; increase THC PD-positive effects
Bupropion	Additive PD effect with seizure threshold lowering drugs, dopaminergic drugs, MAOIs	Increased toxicity of drugs, including lowering of seizure threshold, hypertensive events
NRT	Additive PD effect with alcohol, cannabis, antipsychotics	Decreased locomotor performance, increased anxiolytic effect
Varenicline	Additive PD effect with NRT	Increased adverse effects

Table 23.3 FDA recommendations regarding the co-administration of anti-addiction agents with drugs that are likely to cause a PK/PD drug interaction

Anti-addiction agent	Co-medication	PK/PD cause	Dosage adjustment recommendation	Webpage reference
Methadone	Fluvoxamine, voriconazole, acyclovir, amitriptyline, erythromycin, ketoconazole	PK inhibition by co-medications	May require dosage reduction, monitor for toxicity	[45]
	Carbamazepine, efavirenz, HCV protease inhibitors, ritonavir, nevirapine, phenobarbital, phenytoin, rifampin, St. John's wort	PK induction by co-medications	May require dosage increase, monitor for withdrawal, avoid co-administration	
	Codeine, tramadol	PK inhibition by methadone	Choose alternative analgesic	
	Zidovudine (AZT)	PK inhibition by methadone	Monitor for toxicity	
	Antiarrhythmics, psychotropics, calcium channel blockers, medicines that cause electrolyte imbalance (e.g. diuretics, laxatives)	PD additive effect on QT_c interval	Use caution when co-administering	
	Benzodiazepines	PD additive effect on CNS depressant effects	Warn patient of potential effects	
Buprenorphine	Atazanavir, delavirdine	PK inhibition by co-medications	May require dosage reduction, monitor for toxicity	[46]
	Phenobarbital, carbamazepine, phenytoin rifampin, St. John's wort	PK induction by co-medications	May require dosage increase, monitor for withdrawal, avoid co-administration	
	Benzodiazepines	PD additive effect on CNS depressant effects	Warn patient of potential effects	
Disulfiram	Alcohol	ALDH inhibition by disulfiram	Contraindicated use	[47]
	Metronidazole, isoniazid, alcohol-containing drug formulations	ALDH inhibition by disulfiram	Contraindicated use	
	Phenytoin	CYP2C9 inhibition by disulfiram	May require dosage adjustment	
	Warfarin	CYP2C9 inhibition by disulfiram	May require dosage adjustment	
	Theophylline	PK inhibition by disulfiram	May require dosage adjustment	

Naltrexone	Opioids	PD inhibition by naltrexone	Use alternative analgesic; contraindicated with methadone and buprenorphine	[48]
	Thioridazine	PD additive effect	No recommendation	
Bupropion	Ritonavir, lopinavir, efavirenz, rifampicin, carbamazepine, phenobarbital, phenytoin	CYP2B6 induction by co-medication	Increase bupropion, but not > maximum recommended dose	[49]
	Ticlopidine, clopidogrel, prasugrel	CYP2B6 inhibition by co-medication	Decrease bupropion	
	Antidepressants (imipramine/desipramine, fluoxetine, nortriptyline, paroxetine, sertraline, venlafaxine), antipsychotics (haloperidol, risperidone, thioridazine), beta-blockers (metoprolol), antiarrhythmics (propafenone, flecainide), immunosuppressants (cyclosporine)	CYP2D6 inhibition by bupropion and its metabolites	Decrease dose of co-medications	
	Tamoxifen	CYP2D6 inhibition by bupropion and its metabolites to limit conversion to active PD metabolite	Increase dose of co-medication or use alternative medication if available	
	Antipsychotics, antidepressants, theophylline, systemic corticosteroids	PD additive effect to lower seizure threshold	Low initial dose of bupropion, gradual dose increase	
	Laevcdopa, amantadine	PD additive effect on dopaminergic system to cause adverse effects	Use caution when co-administering	
	Alcohol	PD additive adverse effect, reduction in alcohol tolerance	Minimal/avoid use of alcohol	
	Moncamine oxidase inhibitors (MAOIs)	PD hypertensive effects	Contraindicated use, stop bupropion >14 days before MAOI use	

Further, at high doses it results in sedation and respiratory depressant PD effects such that administration with alcohol and benzodiazepines can result in a PD additive effect that in some cases precipitates overdose symptoms. Methadone is also a competitive antagonist of human $\alpha4\beta2$ and $\alpha3$ nicotinic acetylcholine receptors (nAChRs) and an agonist at $\alpha7$ nAChRs [25] and consequently has the ability to alter nicotine response in cigarette smokers (majority of patients being treated with methadone are smokers) and patients using NRT. Anecdotally, the majority of patients being treated with methadone are smokers [26], and the PD interaction may explain why methadone patients crave nicotine more and experience enhanced nicotine withdrawal symptoms [27]. Currently, there are no recommendations regarding changes in methadone dosages due to the methadone-nicotine interaction or transfer to buprenorphine therapy.

Aside from drug interactions, genetic polymorphisms of *CYP2B6*, *ABCB1* and *OPRM1* that encode for CYP2B6, P-gp and the mu opioid receptor, respectively, have been reported to result in altered dose requirements to prevent opioid withdrawal [28–30].

23.2.1.2 Buprenorphine

Buprenorphine is a partial agonist at the mu and kappa opioid receptors, whilst norbuprenorphine is also an agonist at the mu opioid receptors (for review see [5]). As it is a partial agonist, with a high affinity, it has the ability to block the PD actions of co-administered opioids and precipitate withdrawal in opioid addicted patients receiving methadone [3]. In addition, it can cause CNS depressant additive PD effects, including coma and overdose, when administered with benzodiazepines.

23.2.2 Anti-alcohol Addiction Agents

23.2.2.1 Acamprosate

Acamprosate (Campral®) enhances the uptake of the inhibitory neurotransmitter GABA and also displays some activity at NMDA receptors [7]. It does not alter the CNS effects of alcohol nor precipitate withdrawal symptoms of addicted patients.

23.2.2.2 Disulfiram

Disulfiram non-competitively inhibits aldehyde dehydrogenase [12] to prevent enzymatic breakdown of the acetaldehyde metabolite following alcohol consumption, resulting in toxicity from accumulation of acetaldehyde (symptoms including facial flushing, sweating, nausea, vomiting and seizures in some cases). It is this inhibition that prevents co-administration of metronidazole or other alcohol-containing drug formulations (e.g. cough syrups) with disulfiram due to additive PD effects.

23.2.2.3 Naltrexone

Naltrexone is a mu opioid receptor antagonist to reduce the craving and pleasurable PD effects of alcohol in addiction (potentially via blocking endogenous opioid binding). Due to its antagonist action, co-administration with any opioid will result in loss of opioid PD response and, in the case of opioids used to treat addiction, will precipitate withdrawal. In addition, a toxic PD response of lethargy has been reported when naltrexone was co-administered with thioridazine, although the exact mechanism underlying this interaction is unknown [31], and it has also been reported to have a PD additive effect on tetrahydrocannabinol (THC)-positive effects (increased subjective responses of "good drug effect", "high" and "stimulated") [32]. Aside from drug interactions, PD response and treatment success with naltrexone have been linked with genetic variability in *OPRM1*, the gene encoding for the mu opioid receptor. However, results have been contradictory [33–36], and hence, the impact of genetic variability requires further investigation in prospective trials.

23.2.3 *Anti-nicotine Addiction Agents*

23.2.3.1 Bupropion

Bupropion acts to inhibit the neuronal uptake of dopamine, noradrenaline and serotonin. Interaction with neurotransmission has the ability to lower seizure threshold (co-administration with other drugs that have similar PD response causes an additive PD effect) and cause dopamine additive adverse effects (co-administration with other dopaminergic drugs) and other adverse effects (alcohol, rare adverse effects and a reduction in alcohol tolerance; St. John's wort, rare adverse effect of orofacial dystonia) [37]. Finally, co-administration of monoamine oxidase inhibitors (MAOIs) and bupropion is contraindicated due to the occurrence of hypertensive adverse effects.

23.2.3.2 Nicotine Replacement Therapy

Nicotine is an agonist of nicotinic acetylcholine receptors (nAChRs). Nicotine and alcohol have a combined PD effect to exacerbate reward pathways but have opposing actions on other PD effects such as locomotor performance [38], whilst nicotine and cannabis also have an additive anxiolytic PD effect. Other PD interactions have been reported with antipsychotics (e.g. clozapine) [39].

Aside from drug interactions, genetic polymorphisms in *CYP2A6* and *CHRNA5* (encodes for the α5 subunit of the nicotinic receptor) have been linked to successful outcome of NRT [40–42].

23.2.3.3 Varenicline

Varenicline is a partial agonist of central nicotinic acetylcholine receptors ($\alpha_4\beta_2$ nAChR). Given its mode of action, it is not surprising that when administered with nicotine replacement therapy (transdermal patch), an increase in adverse effects was reported. However, there was no increase in cardiovascular parameters. These outcomes are reported in varenicline's label [43].

23.3 Clinical Significance of Pharmacokinetic and Pharmacodynamic Interactions

Not all PK and PD drug interactions are deemed to be of clinical significance. That is, not all interactions will result in recommendations for dosage adjustments or additional monitoring for patient safety from regulatory bodies such as the Food and Drug Administration USA (FDA). This section will highlight dosing precautions recommended by the FDA as a result of post-marketing surveillance of anti-addiction agents. In addition, dosage reduction recommendations are particularly important for drugs with a narrow therapeutic index to limit toxicity.

For methadone, buprenorphine, disulfiram, naltrexone and bupropion, there are significant PK/PD interactions that impact not only on these agents but also on co-medications. Therefore, the FDA have recommended dosage reductions, use of alternative drugs and increased patient monitoring that are summarised on the drug labels (from FDA or Pharmaceutical Company) and are presented in Table 23.3.

23.3.1 Acamprosate

Despite the reported increase in C_{max} and AUC of acamprosate when co-administered with naltrexone, no dosing adjustments have been recommended by the FDA [44].

23.3.2 Nicotine Replacement Therapy

Although there is the potential for PK and PD interactions with nicotine, no dosage adjustments are recommended as a result of co-administration.

23.3.3 Varenicline

Varenicline does not have significant PK or PD interactions with the exception of increased adverse effects when co-administered with nicotine replacement therapy. No dosage adjustments are recommended in this case [43].

23.4 Conclusions

For a number of the anti-addiction agents discussed in this chapter, i.e. methadone, buprenorphine, disulfiram, naltrexone and bupropion, there are clinically significant drug-drug interactions that occur due to altered PK or PD. With regard to PK, the mechanisms are largely a result of inhibition or induction of metabolism; whilst for PD, the mechanisms are a result of inhibited, additive or synergistic activity at the drug target. The clinical consequences of these interactions are sufficient in many cases for the FDA to have made recommendations regarding contraindications, dosage adjustments and additional monitoring to ensure patient safety. Clinicians need to be aware of the potential for these drug-drug interactions and prescribe and monitor patients for safety as needed.

References

1. Romach MK, Piafsky KM, Abel JG, Khouw V, Sellers EM (1981) Methadone binding to orosomucoid (alpha 1-acid glycoprotein): determinant of free fraction in plasma. Clin Pharmacol Ther 29:211–217
2. Gelston EA et al (2012) Methadone inhibits CYP2D6 and UGT2B7/2B4 in vivo: a study using codeine in methadone- and buprenorphine-maintained subjects. Br J Clin Pharmacol 73:786–794
3. McCance-Katz EF, Sullivan LE, Nallani S (2010) Drug interactions of clinical importance among the opioids, methadone and buprenorphine, and other frequently prescribed medications: a review. Am J Addict 19:4–16
4. Saber-Tehrani AS, Bruce RD, Altice FL (2011) Pharmacokinetic drug interactions and adverse consequences between psychotropic medications and pharmacotherapy for the treatment of opioid dependence. Am J Drug Alcohol Abuse 37:1–11
5. Moody DE (2013) Metabolic and toxicological considerations of the opioid replacement therapy drugs: methadone and buprenorphine. Expert Opin Drug Metab Toxicol 9:675–697
6. Garrett ER, Chandran VR (1985) Pharmacokinetics of morphine and its surrogates VI: bioanalysis, solvolysis kinetics, solubility, pK'a values, and protein binding of buprenorphine. J Pharm Sci 74:515–524
7. Saivin S et al (1998) Clinical pharmacokinetics of acamprosate. Clin Pharmacokinet 35:331–345
8. Mason BJ et al (2002) A pharmacokinetic and pharmacodynamic drug interaction study of acamprosate and naltrexone. Neuropsychopharmacology 27:596–606
9. Eneanya DI, Bianchine JR, Duran DO, Andresen BD (1981) The actions and metabolic fate of disulfiram. Annu Rev Pharmacol Toxicol 21:575–596

10. Johansson B (1990) Plasma protein binding of disulfiram and its metabolite diethylthiocarbamic acid methyl ester. J Pharm Pharmacol 42:806–807
11. Chick J (1999) Safety issues concerning the use of disulfiram in treating alcohol dependence. Drug Saf 20:427–435
12. Barth KS, Malcolm RJ (2010) Disulfiram: an old therapeutic with new applications. CNS Neurol Disord Drug Targets 9:5–12
13. Porter SJ, Somogyi AA, White JM (2000) Kinetics and inhibition of the formation of 6beta-natrexol from naltrexone in human liver cytosol. Br J Clin Pharmacol 50:465–471
14. Gonzalez JP, Brogden RN (1988) Naltrexone: a review of its pharmacodynamic and pharmacokinetic properties and therapeutic efficacy in the management of opioid dependence. Drugs 35:192–213
15. Swift R, Davidson D, Rosen S, Fitz E, Camara P (1998) Naltrexone effects on diazepam intoxication and pharmacokinetics in humans. Psychopharmacology (Berl) 135:256–262
16. Schroeder DH (1983) Metabolism and kinetics of bupropion. J Clin Psychiatry 44:79–81
17. Findlay JW et al (1981) Pharmacokinetics of bupropion, a novel antidepressant agent, following oral administration to healthy subjects. Eur J Clin Pharmacol 21:127–135
18. Svensson CK (1997) Clinical pharmacokinetics of nicotine. Clin Pharmacokinet 12:30–40
19. Yue J, Miksys S, Hoffmann E, Tyndale RF (2008) Chronic nicotine treatment induces rat CYP2D in the brain but not in the liver: an investigation of induction and time course. J Psychiatry Neurosci 33:54–63
20. Wang Q et al (2015) Regulation of cerebral CYP2D6 alters tramadol metabolism in the brain: interactions of tramadol with propranolol and nicotine. Xenobiotica 45:335–344
21. Obach RS et al (2006) Metabolism and disposition of varenicline, a selective alpha4beta2 acetylcholine receptor partial agonist, in vivo and in vitro. Drug Metab Dispos 34:121–130
22. Faessel HM et al (2010) A review of the clinical pharmacokinetics and pharmacodynamics of varenicline for smoking cessation. Clin Pharmacokinet 49:799–816
23. Burstein AH et al (2007) Lack of pharmacokinetic and pharmacodynamic interactions between a smoking cessation therapy, varenicline, and warfarin: an in vivo and in vitro study. J Clin Pharmacol 47:1421–1429
24. Faessel HM et al (2008) Lack of pharmacokinetic interaction between a new smoking cessation therapy, varenicline, and digoxin in adult smokers. Eur J Clin Pharmacol 64:1101–1109
25. Talka R, Salminen O, Tuominen RK (2015) Methadone is a non-competitive antagonist at the α4b2 and α3* nicotinic acetylcholine receptors and an agonist at the α7 nicotinic acetylcholine receptor. Basic Clin Pharmacol Toxicol 116:321–328
26. Clemmey P, Brooner R, Chutuape MA, Kidorf M, Stitzer M (1997) Smoking habits and attitudes in a methadone maintenance treatment population. Drug Alcohol Depend 44:123–132
27. Story J, Stark MJ (1991) Treating cigarette smoking in methadone maintenance clients. J Psychoactive Drugs 23:203–215
28. Coller JK, Barratt DT, Dahlen K, Loennechen MH, Somogyi AA (2006) ABCB1 genetic variability and methadone dosage requirements in opioid-dependent individuals. Clin Pharmacol Ther 80:682–690
29. Barratt DT et al (2012) *ABCB1* haplotype and *OPRM1* 118A>G genotype interaction in methadone maintenance treatment pharmacogenetics. Pharmgenomics Pers Med 5:53–62
30. Levran O et al (2013) CYP2B6 SNPs are associated with methadone dose required for effective treatment of opioid addiction. Addict Biol 18:709–716
31. Maany I, O'Brien CP, Woody G (1987) Interaction between thioridazine and naltrexone. Am J Psychiatry 144:966
32. Haney M, Bisaga A, Foltin RW (2003) Interaction between naltrexone and oral THC in heavy marijuana smokers. Psychopharmacology (Berl) 166:77–85
33. Coller JK et al (2011) OPRM1 A118G genotype fails to predict the effectiveness of naltrexone treatment for alcohol dependence. Pharmacogenet Genomics 21:902–905
34. Chamorro AJ et al (2012) Association of μ-opioid receptor (OPRM1) gene polymorphism with response to naltrexone in alcohol dependence: a systemative review and meta-analysis. Addict Biol 17:505–512

35. Garbutt JC et al (2014) Clinical and biological moderators of response to naltrexone in alcohol dependence: a systematic review of the evidence. Addiction 109:1274–1284
36. Jonas DE et al (2014) Genetic polymorphisms and response to medications for alcohol use disorders: a systematic review and meta-analysis. Pharmacogenomics 15:1687–1700
37. Milton JC, Abdulla A (2007) Prolonged oro-facial dystonia in a 58 year old female following therapy with bupropion and St John's Wort. Br J Clin Pharmacol 64:717–718
38. Lajtha A, Sershen H (2010) Nicotine: alcohol reward interactions. Neurochem Res 35:1248–1258
39. Levin ED, Rezvani AH (2007) Nicotinic interactions with antipsychotics drugs, models of schizophrenia and impacts on cognitive function. Biochem Pharmacol 74:1182–1191
40. Ray R, Tyndale RF, Lerman C (2009) Nicotine dependence pharmacogenetics: role of genetic variation in nicotine-metabolizing enzymes. J Neurogenet 23:252–261
41. Chen LS et al (2014) Pharmacotherapy effects on smoking cessation vary with nicotine metabolism gene (CYP2A6). Addiction 109:128–137
42. Chen LS et al (2014) CHRNA5 variant predicts smoking cessation in patients with acute myocardial infarction. Nicotine Tob Res 16:1224–1231
43. FDA USA (2014) Highlights of prescribing information CHANTIX® (varenicline). http://www.accessdata.fda.gov/drugsatfda_docs/label/2014/021928s033s034s037lbl.pdf
44. FDA USA (2014) Campral (acamprosate calcium) tablets label. http://www.accessdata.fda.gov/drugsatfda_docs/label/2010/021431s013lbl.pdf
45. FDA USA (2014) Highlights of prescribing information for Dolophine®. http://www.accessdata.fda.gov/drugsatfda_docs/label/2014/006134s035lbl.pdf
46. FDA USA (2014) SUBUTEX (buprenorphine HCl sublingual tablets). http://www.fda.gov/downloads/Drugs/DrugSafety/PostmarketDrugSafetyInformationforPatientsandProviders/UCM191529.pdf
47. Teva Women's Health Inc. (2014) ANTABUSE – disulfiram tablet. http://dailymed.nlm.nih.gov/dailymed/drugInfo.cfm?setid=f0ca0e1f-9641-48d5-9367-e5d1069e8680
48. FDA USA (2014) Highlights of prescribing information VIVTROL®. http://www.accessdata.fda.gov/drugsatfda_docs/label/2010/021897s015lbl.pdf
49. FDA USA (2014) ZYBAN® (bupropion hydrochloride) sustained-release tablets. http://www.accessdata.fda.gov/drugsatfda_docs/label/2014/020711s043lbl.pdf

Chapter 24
Clinically Significant Interactions with Anesthetic Agents

Michael W. Jann

Abstract Induction and maintenance of anesthesia require multiple medications where drug-drug interactions form the basis of clinical practice. Drug-drug interactions with anesthetic agents can take place by pharmacokinetic mechanisms leading to enhanced or reduced pharmacodynamic effects or by only pharmacodynamic mechanism that promotes anesthetic outcomes such as pain and sedative actions. Ketamine, midazolam, and alfentanil are metabolized by the CYP3A4 enzyme system and various drug-drug interactions with agents that are well-known CYP3A4 inhibitors have been reported to alter their pharmacokinetic disposition. Antibiotics erythromycin and clarithromycin were found to significantly reduce ketamine and midazolam disposition. Grapefruit juice was reported to significantly increase ketamine and midazolam bioavailability. Antifungal drugs such as ketoconazole and fluconazole were shown to significantly reduce alfentanil clearance and prolong its pharmacodynamic actions. Drug interactions with opioid anesthetics fentanyl and sufentanil may be less prone to due to their high extraction ratio. The opioid-propofol interactions have been described in various articles. Propofol interactions were also presented with midazolam and interestingly counteracted the effects of droperidol-induced prolonged QTc effects. Thiopental protein-binding displacement was shown to occur with a variety of agents, thereby increasing free drug concentrations. An enhanced pharmacodynamic effect with thiopental was found when combined with midazolam and other central nervous system depressants.

Keywords CYP3A4 inhibitors • Grapefruit juice • Etomidate • Ketamine • Midazolam • Opioids • Alfentanil • Propofol • Thiopental

M.W. Jann, PharmD
Department of Pharmacotherapy, University of North Texas System College of Pharmacy (UNTSCP) and University of North Texas Health Science Center (UNTHSC), Fort Worth, TX, USA
e-mail: Michael.jann@unthsc.edu

M. Jann et al. (eds.), *Applied Clinical Pharmacokinetics and Pharmacodynamics of Psychopharmacological Agents*,
DOI 10.1007/978-3-319-27883-4_24

24.1 Introduction

Drug-drug interactions form the basis of anesthetic clinical practice. The current anesthetic agents typically require a minimum of two different classes of drugs to achieve adequate anesthesia [1]. Concomitant use of anesthetic agents that act pharmacodynamically in a synergistic manner creates the anesthetic state. General anesthesia can be defined as the prevention of autonomic signs (e.g., tearing, lacrimation) and purposeful movement (e.g., sedation) achieved with appropriate hemodynamic control during the surgical procedure [2]. Clear physical features include monitoring somatic muscle tone, respiratory patterns, and ocular signs. Various pharmacodynamic (PD) biomarkers like the minimum alveolar concentrations (MAC) and hemodynamic measures (e.g., blood pressure, heart rate) are easily quantified and carefully monitored during anesthesia, in addition to the body's physiological parameters that can be assessed. The central nervous system (CNS) activity via the EEG can be another biomarker approach to monitor patients. Quantifying drug-drug interactions using the pharmaco-EEG method has been accomplished with various CNS-acting agents [3]. Therefore, clinical research with anesthetics offers the investigator a variety of pharmacodynamic measures to determine accurate drug dosing and optimizing patient care during the surgery.

Utilization of the pharmacodynamic principles with the anesthetics in clinical practice predated the discovery of their pharmacokinetic (PK) drug interaction mechanisms. Mathematical models using PD biomarkers have been developed to evaluate anesthetic drug-drug interactions [4]. However, with the advent of the cytochrome P450 (CYP) enzyme system, the understanding of drug-drug PK interactions has increased and can be applied to the anesthetic drugs. Ultimately, use of the drug interactions with anesthetics is designed to enhance the anesthesia while minimizing unwanted medication adverse effects. The mean PK and PD effects of the anesthetic agents are presented in Table 24.1. A wide interpatient variability in the PK parameters was reported for the anesthetic agents that range between 70 and 80 %, while even a considerably larger interpatient variability of 300–400 % in the PD parameters has been described [2, 5].

This chapter will not cover the inhalation volatile agents unless a significant drug interaction study was conducted with an agent presented in this chapter and focused only on the intravenous or oral anesthetics discussed in Chap. 15. Few anesthetics are administered orally, and where appropriate, these agents will be included in this chapter as an oral agent that may be given with another anesthetic drug administered intravenously. It is beyond this chapter's scope to cover every anesthetic drug-drug interaction reported. However, select key articles were identified and will be presented to provide fundamental information on various anesthetic drug-drug interactions. Unlike the other drug-drug interaction chapters, this chapter will combine the PK and the PD sections together as the anesthetic agents are clinically used in various drug combinations to achieve optimal anesthesia.

Table 24.1 Summary of the pharmacokinetic parameters of selected anesthetic agents

Drug	Vd (L/kg)	CL (mL/kg/min)	Protein binding (%)	Metabolism	$T_{1/2\beta}$ (h)	Action duration (min)
Alfentanil[a]	0.3–1.0	3–7.6	92	CYP3A4[b]	0.6–1.5	5–10
Etomidate	2.5–4.5	18–25	77	Hydrolysis[c]	2.9–5.3	3–5
Ketamine	3.1	12–17	12	CYP3A4[d]	2–4	5–10
Midazolam	1.1–1.7	6.4–11	94	CYP3A4[e]	1.7–2.6	15–20
Propofol	2–10	20–30	97	CYP2B6[f]	4–23	3–5
Thiopental	2.5	3.4	83	N.R.	11	5–10

Adapted from Eilers and Niemann [2]
[a]Davis and Cook [121]
[b]Kharasch et al. [67]
[c]Geise and Staney [6]
[d]Santamaria et al. [16]
[e]Kronbach et al. [27]
[f]Turpeinen and Zanger [77]
Vd volume of distribution at steady state, *CL* clearance, $T_{1/2}$ elimination half-life, *N.R.* not reported

24.2 Etomidate

Etomidate (ETD) is a very short-acting anesthetic agent (see Table 24.1) that is rapidly hydrolyzed in the plasma and its metabolic clearance almost equal to hepatic blood flow. ETD binds to human plasma protein albumin 76 % [6]. The two factors of rapid hydrolysis and protein binding <90 % indicate the likelihood of significant pharmacokinetic drug-drug interactions to have a low or modest effect. Very few studies have examined potential drug-drug interactions with ETD. A small study with twelve patients undergoing spinal surgery was given premedications and an initial ETD infusion of 100 μg/kg/min for 10 min with the dose lowered to 10 μg/kg/min [7]. After a neuromuscular blocker was given, patients were administered either 67 % nitrous oxide (NO) in oxygen or enriched oxygen (O_2). Blood samples for ETD were obtained during infusion for PK analysis. The PD effects assessed were the time to open the eyes upon command (t_1) and time of giving the correct date of birth (t_2). Both t_1 and t_2 times were significantly longer (by almost fourfold) in the NO group compared to the O_2 group (e.g., t_1 NO 37.9 min versus O_2 9.0 min, $p<0.01$). The PK analysis revealed that the mean (±SEM) area under the concentration time curve (AUC) was significantly greater in the NO group (85.3 μg/mL/min ± 7.9 versus 64.7 μg/mL/min ± 4.4, $p<0.05$). Although mean ETD clearance was lower in the NO group compared to the O_2 group, it was found not to be significant (20.9 mL/kg/min ± 2.6 versus 27.3 mL/kg/min ± 4.2, p = n.s). Post-infusion blood samples were not obtained. As the ETD AUC for the NO group was greater than the O_2 group without a significant difference in clearance, the suggestion was that NO may influence ETD volume of distribution and or elimination half-life. Another small ETD study with patients ($N=19$) examined the effects of alfentanil (Alf) on ETD infusion

[8]. PD effects were not assessed. ETD blood samples were obtained in only five subjects and the few data could not be analyzed due to large variability. The mean (±S.D) ETD elimination half-life was 29.4 min ± 6.2 with a range of 23.9–38.5 min. Since the ETD elimination half-life for these five subjects was considerably shorter than the reported population norm (see Table 24.1), the suggestion was that Alf reduced ETD elimination half-life but a mechanism was not proposed due to the small number of subjects with further investigation that was suggested.

24.3 Ketamine (KTM)

Ketamine (KTM) is an N-methyl-D-aspartate (NMDA) antagonist that blocks the glutamatergic receptor and is widely used in veterinary medicine for the past several decades. It has gained acceptance for oral, IM, and IV administration for sedation and anesthesia in humans [9]. KTM is often given with other anesthetic agents to induce and maintain sedation and analgesia. KTM IV was used in the 1970s with nondepolarizing agents (e.g., d-tubocurarine, pancuronium, and succinylcholine) to potentiate their neuromuscular blocking actions [10]. The PD effect was assessed by the force of thumb adduction in response to the stimulation of the ulnar nerve. As KTM blood concentrations remained the same for the three neuromuscular blockers, the ED_{50} for only the d-tubocurarine was significantly reduced from 4.9 to 2.8 mf/m^2 ($p<0.01$) while the ED_{50} other agents were not altered. KTM is commonly given with a diazepam or lorazepam [11, 12]. KTM is also given with morphine (MOR) to induce anesthesia and analgesic effects in various surgical procedures [13]. Physostigmine was reported in animal models to antagonize the anesthetic actions of KTM but not the analgesia effects, which can suggest that this agent can be possibly used as pharmacologic antidote [14, 15].

24.4 KTM and CYP3A4 and CYP2B6 Inducers and Inhibitors

KTM is metabolized by N-demethylation to nor-KTM via CYP3A4, CYP2A6, and CYP2B6 [16, 17]. KTM is a chiral agent which comprises of R and S isomers where the S isomer has greater analgesic potency than the R isomer [18]. Rifampicin was shown to significantly reduced the AUC of IV and oral S-KTM in 11 healthy volunteers by 14 % ($p<0.005$) and 86 % ($p<0.001$), respectively [19]. Rifampicin also significantly decreased the AUC ratio of nor-KTM/KTM by 66 % ($p<0.001$). The C_{max} of oral KTM was significantly reduced by 81 % ($p<0.001$) but not IV KTM. The mechanism of the rifampicin-KTM was suggested to occur via CYP induction during the first-pass metabolic phase. St. John's wort (SJW) is a CYP3A4 inducer and was reported to significantly decrease the oral S-KTM AUC by 58 % ($p<0.001$) in twelve healthy volunteers [20]. The mean S-KTM elimination half-life decreased from 6.5 to 4.2 h ($p=0.001$). The nor-KTM metabolite pharmacokinetic parameters also were significantly affected with a decrease in mean AUC by 2.23-fold ($p<0.001$) and mean elimination half-life from 7.0 to 5.2 h ($p=0.017$). Significant PD effects were not found measured by using a 100 mm visual analogue scale (VAS).

GFJ was shown to significantly increase the mean AUC of oral S-KTM by 3.0-fold ($p<0.001$) in twelve healthy volunteers [21]. Other S-KTM PK parameters significantly increased were C_{max} by 2.1-fold ($p<0.001$) and elimination half-life by 24 % ($p<0.05$). The nor-KTM/KTM AUC ratio was significantly decreased by 57 % ($p<0.001$). The PD effects of self-relaxation and digit symbol-substitution test (DSST) were significantly decreased ($p<0.05$) but other behavioral or analgesic actions were not affected. Clarithromycin was shown to significantly inhibit oral S-KTM in ten healthy volunteers [22]. The S-KTM mean C_{max} and AUC significantly increased by 3.6-fold ($p<0.001$) and 2.6-fold ($p<0.001$), respectively. The nor-KTM/KTM AUC ratio was significantly decreased by 54 % ($p=0.004$). Significant changes in the PD effects were not found in analgesia (cold pressor test) or the psychomotor VAS test. Itraconazole (a potent CYP3A4 inhibitor) was found not to significantly affect oral S-KTM but ticlopidine (a potent CYP2B6 inhibitor) was reported to significantly increased the AUC by 2.4-fold ($p<0.001$) in 11 healthy volunteers [23]. The nor-KTM/KTM AUC ratio was significantly reduced by 47 % ($p<0.001$) and the mean nor-KTM C_{max} from 56.9 ng/mL ± 22.3 to 46.2 ng/mL ± 11.9 ($p<0.05$). The PD effects using the VAS and drowsiness were significantly increased by both itraconazole and ticlopidine ($p<0.05$). The lack of interaction by itraconazole raises interesting questions and theories where the authors suggested that itraconazole may modulate another drug transport system (e.g., P-glycoprotein) that masks the CYP3A4-mediated inhibition although no evidence is offered. This study demonstrated that CYP2B6 inhibition can play significant role drug interactions with oral S-KTM besides CYP3A4.

24.5 KTM and Other Potential Drug Interactions

In vitro studies with perfused rat liver preparations indicated that KTM inhibited the conversion of MOR to its glucuronidated metabolite MOR-3-glucuronide (M3G) with the mean fractional conversion of MOR to M3G that was significantly decreased from 0.46 ± 0.17 to 0.28 ± 0.14 ($p<0.05$) [24]. Phase II glucuronidation is a major route of MOR metabolism and is catalyzed by the UDP-glucuronosyltransferase (UGT) system [24]. The conversion from MOR to M3G occurs via UGT2B7, UGT1A1, and UGT1A8 but the major influence occurs with the UGT2B7 system. KTM using Michaelis-Menten kinetics inhibited M3G formation via glucuronidation. Using human hepatic microsomes, the effect of KTM on MOR and codeine (COD) was examined [25]. COD conversion to codeine-6-glucuronide (C6G) also occurs by UGT2B7 [25]. KTM was shown to inhibit recombinant human UGT enzymes in a dose-dependent manner with <100 μM to inhibit UGT2B7 activity. KTM administration to human hepatic microsome preparations inhibited the MOR conversion to M3G and COD to C6G with Ki values derived from the enzyme kinetics using the Dixon plots [24, 25]. These in vitro studies indicate that possible interactions with KTM could occur with other drugs that are significantly metabolized the UGT2B7 and possibly by these other UGT2B4 and UGT2B15 enzymes systems.

24.5.1 *Midazolam (MDZ)*

Diazepam, lorazepam, and other older benzodiazepines have given way to midazolam as the most commonly used benzodiazepine agents used in anesthesia. MDZ can be used to induce anesthesia in surgery and dental procedures that can be administered orally or by IV [26]. MDZ shown in Table 24.1 is a short-acting benzodiazepine metabolized by the intestinal and hepatic CYP3A4 enzymes to 4-hydroxy MDZ and α –OH MDZ [27]. The pharmacodynamics actions of severe respiratory depression can be successfully treated with benzodiazepine antagonist flumazenil [28]. MDZ was reported to have an intermediate extraction ratio of 0.38 [29], which indicates the likelihood of significant drug-drug interactions involving the CYP enzyme system. In vitro models with Caco-2 cells reported that MDZ was a P-gp inhibitor but not a P-gp substrate [30]. Grapefruit juice (GFJ) is a CYP3A4 inhibitor and was given to healthy male subjects ($N=8$) with MDZ oral 15 mg or IV 5 mg [31]. GFJ was shown to increase mean MDZ bioavailability from 24 % ± 3 % to 35 % ± 3 % ($p<0.01$). GFJ did not significantly affect IV MDZ disposition but significantly increased mean oral MDZ AUC from 143 μg • h/L ± 26 to 217 μg • h/L ± 31 ($p<0.01$). The PD effects of sedation assessed by the subject and the investigator, which noted an increase in sedation with the oral MDZ + GFJ compared to the MDZ + water (placebo). GFJ was reported to increase the oral MDZ bioavailability by 35 % in a pediatric population undergoing dental procedures but this effect was not found in the adult population [32, 33]. Clinicians should exercise caution when MDZ is used and it should be included in the patient history if GFJ is a regular part in the patient's diet.

24.6 MDZ: Antibiotic and Antifungal Interactions

Macrolide antibiotics are well-known CYP3A4 inhibitors, and with human hepatic microsomes, in vitro models examined the effects of preincubation with erythromycin, clarithromycin, and azithromycin on MDZ metabolic hydroxylation [34]. The kinetic parameter for enzyme inactivation was most potent with erythromycin (ERY) and clarithromycin (CLY) noted to occur at 12.6 mM and 41.6 nM, respectively. The least potent was azithromycin at 623 nM. Therefore, the in vitro model predicts significant drug interactions with ERY and CLY but not azithromycin. Erythromycin is commonly used in a preoperative agent prior to anesthesia to prevent increased gastric pH and decrease residual gastric volume as well as an antibiotic effective against gram (+) and gram (−) bacteria [35].

A case report in an 8-year-old patient given with oral erythromycin and oral MDZ noted lost consciousness and awoke 45 min later where the MDZ samples obtained at the same time noted a concentration of 134 ng/mL [36]. The authors then entered six children into a pharmacokinetic study given with oral MDZ alone and noted the mean MDZ C_{max} was 73 ng/mL (range of 31–114 ng/mL) at 2.5 h and concluded that a significant drug interaction likely occurred between ERY and MDZ agents. An in-depth study with healthy volunteers ($N = 12$) was conducted, which were given with 500 mg ERY TID or placebo for 1 week or placebo [37]. Six subjects were then given with oral MDZ 15 mg and a ERY 500 mg dose followed by 4 months, the study was repeated with the other six subjects administered IV MDZ 0.05 mg/kg 2 h after a 500 mg dose of ERY. Both oral and IV MDZ pharmacokinetics were significantly increased when ERY was given (mean oral MDZ AUC 12 μg • h/min ± 1 versus 53 μg • h/min, $p < 0.003$; mean IV MDZ CL 7.8 mL/min/kg ± 0.6 versus 3.6 mL/min/kg ± 0.3, $p < 0.028$). Six different PD effects were assessed (e.g., sedation) and each parameter was significantly increased ($p < 0.05$) during coadministration of ERY and MDZ. The recommendation was that either MDZ dose be reduced by 50–75 % or prescriptions of MDZ and ERY be avoided for patient safety.

A similar finding was found when CLY and MDZ were given in the elderly (aged 65–75 years, $N = 16$) patients with an increase of 3.2-fold and 8.0-fold in MDZ AUC given orally and IV, respectively [38]. Significantly lower mean [95 % C.I.] MDZ CL occurred with both oral and IV MDZ with CLY (121 L/h [88,154] versus 17.4 L/h [12.3, 22.5]; 33.2 L/h [28.7, 37.8] versus 11.5 L/h [8.7, 14.4], $p < 0.0001$), respectively. Azithromycin was found not to significantly affect human performance (e.g., digit symbol-substitution test) when given with MDZ in 64 healthy volunteers [39]. A modest PK and PD interaction between roxithromycin and MDZ was reported in ten healthy volunteers [40]. Although a significant MDZ AUC was found (8.3–12.2 μg • mL/min, $p < 0.05$), only a minor increase psychomotor impairment occurred (p = n.s.). Unlike the interaction with ERY, roxithromycin appears less likely to be clinically significant.

Itraconazole 100 mg given for 4 days was reported to significantly increase by sixfold the MDZ AUC ($p < 0.001$) when given with oral MDZ 7.5 mg in 12 healthy volunteers [40]. Other PK parameters significantly have increased elimination half-life by twofold ($p < 0.001$) and C_{max} 2.5-fold ($p < 0.001$). A similar finding was found with itraconazole 200 mg that was given with MDZ [41]. This study also included an additional interaction with rifampicin 600 mg for 5 days and MDZ AUC was dramatically reduced to only 2.3 % of the original MDZ AUC when given alone. Itraconazole 200 mg for 6 days and fluconazole 200 mg for 5 days were evaluated in healthy volunteers given with oral MDZ 7.5 mg and IN DZ 0.05 mg/kg [42]. Both itraconazole and fluconazole significantly reduced MDZ by CL 69 % and 51 % ($p < 0.01$), respectively. A lower fluconazole single dose of 150 mg did not substantially affect oral MDZ 10 mg effects on both PK and PD parameters (p = n.s.) [43]. Itraconazole at 100 and 200 mg produced a significant change in MDZ PK and PD effects.

24.7 MDZ and Other Anesthetic Drug Interactions

MDZ has been combined synergistically to promote PD effects with other anesthetic agents such as Ppf (see Propofol section) to lower dosage requirements of the other agents while enhancing patient recovery time. MDZ is commonly used with Ppf in adults and children for various surgical procedures [44, 45]. The combined actions of MDZ and Alf were examined in female patients ($N=90$) scheduled for various gynecologic procedures [46]. Patients were randomized into three different groups ($N=30$ per group) – Alf alone, MDZ alone, and MDZ-Alf. The ED_{50} dose for Alf alone (0.13 mg/kg) and MDZ alone (0.22 mg/kg) was designated as the baseline effect of 1.00 to induce anesthesia. The MDZ-Alf combination had a lower ED_{50} fraction of 0.33 and 0.21, respectively, compared to each agent alone. The MDZ-Alf doses used to induce anesthesia were 0.028 mg/kg and 0.07 mg/kg, respectively, indicating a supradditive effect ($p<0.0001$). Since both MDZ and Alf are metabolized by CYP3A4, the possibility of a PK interaction of these two agents was examined in the rat model [47]. The combined MDZ-Alf yielded no significant increase in either agent in plasma or brain concentrations. However, the PD effects of analgesia and tail compression test for pain were significantly increased ($p<0.01$) indicating the enhanced PD effects without a PK interaction.

Subhypnotic MDZ doses of 0.02 mg/kg were reported to significantly potentiate the anesthetic effects of thiopental in fifty patients requiring eye surgery [48]. The combined effects of MDZ-thiopental in female patients ($N=90$) undergoing minor gynecologic procedures were studied [49]. Patients were randomized into three different groups ($N=30$ per group) – MDZ alone, thiopental alone, and MDZ-thiopental. The ED_{50} for MDZ alone (0.19 mg/kg) and thiopental alone (2.9 mg/kg) was designated as the baseline effect of 1.00 to induce anesthesia. The combined MDZ-thiopental had an ED_{50} of 0.26 and 0.24, respectively, compared to each agent alone. The MDZ-thiopental doses used to induce anesthesia were 0.05 mg/kg and 0.70 mg/kg, respectively, indicating a supradditive effect ($p<0.0001$). Thiopental is a barbiturate, which can have additive PD effects at the BZ-GABA-CL receptor complex with MDZ. Anesthetic drug interaction studies rarely assess greater than two drugs coadministered due to the complexity of the drug-drug interactions and when the multiple PD factors are included in either healthy volunteers or patients undergoing surgery. Effects of MDZ, Alf, and Ppf alone, the two-drug combination, and finally the three-drug combination were evaluated in 130 undergoing different surgeries [50]. The baseline ED_{50} doses of each agent alone were used to compare the various effects of the different drug combinations. The two-drug combinations were shown to act synergistically significantly lowering the doses of each agent to induce anesthesia. The three-drug MDZ-Alf-Ppf combination ED_{50} did not significantly from any of the two-drug combinations (e.g., MDZ-Alf or MDZ-Ppf) suggesting that greater than two drugs that included MDZ with another agent is adequate to induce anesthesia.

24.8 MDZ and Other Drug Interactions

Saquinavir is a protease inhibitor and a potent CYP3A4 inhibitor [51]. The PK and PD effects of saquinavir on oral and IV MDZ were examined in 12 healthy volunteers [52]. Saquinavir significantly increased the oral MDZ bioavailability from 41 to 90 % ($p<0.001$), MDZ AUC by fivefold ($p<0.001$), and C_{max} greater than two-fold ($p<0.001$). Five of six PD psychomotor tests reported impaired skills and increased sedative effects ($p<0.05$). Saquinavir significantly decreased IV MDZ CL by 56 % ($p<0.001$) and increased elimination half-life from 4.1 to 9.5 h ($p<0.01$). The recommendation was that the oral MDZ dose be reduced by 50 %. When parecoxib 40 mg IV was given to the subjects, it was reported not to significantly alter PK and PD parameters [53].

24.8.1 Muscle Relaxant Anesthetic Drug Interactions

As muscle relaxants are commonly used during anesthesia, specific drug-drug interaction studies are lacking due to their different pharmacologic actions and PD effects that focus on the skeletal muscles [54]. In two small studies with Ppf, a significant PD interaction with vecuronium and rocuronium was not found [55, 56]. Smoking (>10 cigarettes/day) was not found to significantly effect rocuronium PD effects compared to nonsmokers ($N=10$ per group) as nicotine has stimulant effects on the cardiovascular system [57]. Patients ($N=60$) undergoing laryngoscopy were randomly assigned to receive either TPL or etomidate for a rapid anesthetic induction given with rocuronium [58]. All patients were given with Alf for induction and then followed by two agents. The etomidate-rocuronium groups had a more pronounced effect on muscle relaxation than rocuronium-alone group and the TPL-rocuronium group ($p<0.05$).

24.8.2 Opioid Anesthetic Drug-Drug Interactions

The most commonly used opioid agents used in anesthesia are Alf, fentanyl, and sufentanil due to their quick onset of action and short elimination half-life [59]. Factors that may affect opioid disposition include age, protein binding, cardiopulmonary bypass, and renal and hepatic dysfunction. The drug interaction between opioids and Ppf has been previously described (see the Propofol: Opioid section). The majority of opioids including Alf are metabolized by the hepatic CYP3A4 and CYP2D6 (see Chap. 11) [60]. Alf and fentanyl are metabolized by CYP3A4 [61] and Alf has been used as a validated probe for CYP3A4 activity [62]. Although sufentanil is metabolized by CYP3A4, its PK profile was not significantly changed when oral ERY, a well-known CYP3A4 metabolic inhibitor, was given to six healthy volunteers [63]. Itraconazole, an antifungal agent and also a well-known CYP3A4 inhibitor, was shown not to influence IV fentanyl pharmacokinetics (mean CL fentanyl alone 23.9 mL/kg/min ± 9.9 versus itraconazole + fentanyl 22.0 mL/kg/min ± 12.7) in ten healthy volunteers [64]. The difference between Alf and these two other opioid anesthetic agents can be explained by drug's extraction ratio. Alf has a low extraction ratio (0.14), and in contrast, both fentanyl and sufentanil have a high extraction ratio >0.8 [29]. As Alf disposition is dependent on hepatic blood flow, changes in CYP3A4 activity can exert significant effects upon its pharmacokinetic profile, whereas fentanyl and sufentanil are unaffected by intrinsic hepatic CL [29]. Alf, fentanyl, and sufentanil were reported not to be substrates for P-glycoprotein (P-gp) [65]. Drug interactions with the P-gp system remain to be identified with these agents.

24.9 Opioid: Antibiotic/Antifungal Drug Interactions

Oral ERY was administered to six healthy volunteers and it was reported to significantly inhibit Alf metabolism [66]. Alf mean elimination half-life significantly increased by about 25 % from 105.9 min ± 41.5 to 131.4 min ± 43.5 ($p < 0.01$) and mean CL significantly decreased from 3.9 mL/kg/min ± 0.8 to 2.9 mL/kg/min ± 1.2 ($p < 0.01$). Volume of distribution did not significantly change. From these results, a recommendation was that either ERY not be used or the Alf dose be significantly reduced. The effects of CYP3A4 activity was reported in healthy volunteers ($N = 9$) when given with intravenous Alf 20 mcg/kg and also given with rifampin (inducer) and troleandomycin (inhibitor) [67]. Alf mean CL given alone (control) was significantly increased with rifampin (5.8 mL/kg/min, $p < 0.05$) and significantly decreased with troleandomycin (1.1 mL/kg/min, $p < 0.05$). A later study compared the effects of parecoxib and troleandomycin on Alf and fentanyl in 12 healthy volunteers [29]. Parecoxib is a prodrug that is metabolized to valdecoxib, which is a compound that is a CYP3A4 substrate and then may interact with Alf or fentanyl. However, Parecoxib was shown not to significantly alter Alf and fentanyl disposition. Troleandomycin was reported not to significantly affect fentanyl pharmacokinetics but significantly decreased the mean Alf CL from 5.53 mL/kg/min ± 2.16 to 0.64 mL/kg/min ± 0.25 ($p < 0.05$). Other Alf pharmacokinetic parameters were significantly changed (AUC, C_{max}, K_{el}, and elimination half-life, $p < 0.05$). However, Alf T_{max} and volume of distribution were found not to be unchanged.

The antifungal agent ketoconazole (potent CYP3A4 inhibitor) was reported to significantly decrease Alf CL by 82 % ($p < 0.05$) [68]. Fluconazole is another antifungal agent and a less potent in vitro CYP3A4 inhibitor than ketoconazole or itraconazole [69]. Nine healthy volunteers were given with oral fluconazole 400 mg or placebo and then followed by either intravenous fluconazole 60 mg or saline. Alf 20 mcg/kg was given after fluconazole or placebo [70]. Fluconazole led to a significant decrease in

Alf CL from 3.1 mL/min/kg ± 1.1 to 1.4 mL/min/kg ($p < 0.001$) with a subsequent increase in Alf AUC from 117.8 ng/mL/h ± 41.1 to 231.5 ng/mL/h ± 62.2 ($p < 0.001$) and mean elimination half-life from 1.5 h ± 0.5 to 2.5 h ± 0.7 ($p < 0.001$). Alf volume of distribution remained unchanged. Voriconazole is a recently new antifungal agent that inhibits CYP3A4, CYP2C9, and CYP2C19 enzyme activity [71]. Like with fluconazole, voriconazole was given orally and intravenously, which significantly decreased mean the Alf CL from 4.4 mL/min/kg ± 2.4 to 0.67 mL/min/kg ± 0.27 ($p < 0.001$) in 12 healthy volunteers [72]. Alf mean elimination half-life was dramatically increased from 1.5 h ± 0.49 to 6.6 h ± 1.8 ($p < 0.001$). Alf + voriconazole led to nausea in five persons and vomiting in four subjects which was not reported with Alf given alone. Terbinafine (CYP2D6 inhibitor) was also tested with Alf ($N = 12$) and did not lead to any significant changes in Alf pharmacokinetics. These results indicate that CYP3A4 inhibition and not CYP2D6 inhibition produced significant drug-drug interactions with Alf.

24.10 Opioid and Other Drug Interactions

Patients ($N = 30$) undergoing coronary bypass surgery were randomly assigned either diltiazem or placebo with Alf anesthesia induction [73]. Diltiazem inhibits CYP3A4 and its actions on Alf disposition were examined. Besides the Alf pharmacokinetics, the time for the drug plasma level to decrease by 50 % after cessation of the infusion (t_{50}) was also reported. Diltiazem significantly increased the mean Alf AUC by 40 % ($p < 0.05$), mean elimination half-life by 50 % ($p < 0.05$), and mean t_{50} by 40 % ($p < 0.05$). Patients that received diltiazem had tracheal extubation performed on the average 2.5 h later ($p = 0.054$) compared to those that received the placebo. Atorvastatin is a CYP3A4 substrate and inhibitor prescribed for hypercholesterolemia. Concurrent use with Alf was reported not to affect Alf pharmacokinetics in sixteen patients undergoing elective surgery [74]. The effects of fentanyl and Alf on minimum alveolar concentration (MAC) when isoflurane inhalation was administered in patients ($N = 79$) that had various surgical procedures [75]. Isoflurane alone reported a MAC of 1.25 % and when combined with fentanyl (0.5 ng/mL, 95 % C.I. 0–4.6 ng/mL) and Alf (28.8 ng/mL, 95 % C.I. 0–79 ng/mL) resulted in a 50 % isoflurane MAC reduction ($p < 0.05$). Due to the combined PD actions, a decreased amount of isoflurane administration was recommended when Alf or fentanyl is given.

Ritonavir is a protease inhibitor that is a potent CYP3A4 and CYP2D6 inhibitor but a less potent CYP2C9/10 inhibitor [76]. Healthy volunteers ($N = 12$) were given with ritonavir up to 900 mg after 2 days and then 300 mg or placebo in the morning of the third day. On the second day, fentanyl 5 μg/kg was given intravenously (IV) and naloxone 0.1 mg IV administered to prevent respiratory depression. Ritonavir significantly reduced the mean fentanyl CL from 15.6 mL/kg/min ± 8.2 to 5.2 mL/kg/min ± 2.0 ($p < 0.01$) and increased the mean fentanyl AUC from 4.8 ng/mL/h ± 2.7 to 8.8 ng/mL/h ± 2.3 ($p < 0.01$). Caution was recommended when ritonavir is added to persons taking fentanyl for anesthesia induction or pain management.

24.10.1 Propofol-Opioid Interactions

Propofol (Ppf) can be given by target-controlled infusion (TCI) to maintain anesthesia as some patients may lose consciousness at a concentration of 1.0 μg/mL as other patients may need higher concentrations of 4–5.0 μg/mL when used as the sole agent [5]. Ppf given with other anesthetics acts synergistically with the opioids that lead to lower Ppf concentrations to induce anesthesia. Ppf is metabolized by the hepatic CYP1A1, CYP1A2, and CYP2B6 [77, 78]. CYP2B6 enzymes are also expressed in the brain which can be an additional source of possible PD variability [79]. Ppf possesses a high hepatic extraction ratio of 0.76 in the large intestine and a smaller extraction ratio of 0.24 in the small intestine [80]. Opioids combined with Ppf include fentanyl, sufentanil, alfentanil, and remifentanil [81]. When Ppf is combined with remifentanil, a Ppf plasma concentration of 2.5–3.0 μg/mL is needed to achieve an anesthetic therapeutic effect. When Ppf is used with the other three opioids, the optimal plasma Ppf concentration is about 3.5 μg/mL [80, 82]. All of these opioids are primarily metabolized by CYP3A4. Based upon these results, Ppf may then also be metabolized by CYP3A4.81 Using data from clinical trials and employing computer simulations, it was reported that anesthesia induction occurred <5 min with the three opioids, whereas the peak induction effect of 8.5 min was longer with sufentanil [83]. Computer simulation analysis of Ppf-opioid drug interactions has been used in various surgeries and examination procedures such as upper endoscopy [84].

The drug interaction between Ppf and opioids has been mostly evaluated with alfentanil (Alf). The pharmacokinetic drug interaction between Ppf and Alf (and also fentanyl) was described in 1993 where the opioids increased the Ppf volume of distribution (Vd) in the central compartment and clearance (CL) [85]. Ppf was reported to increase the mean Alf plasma concentrations by about 15 % by decreasing Alf CL to 15 %. When Ppf and Alf were used together, the mean arterial pressure and system vascular resistance was significantly lower ($p<0.05$) suggesting that the PD changes resulted from the PK interaction [86]. A subsequent study showed that Alf significantly reduced Ppf CL (2.1–1.9 L/min, $p<0.05$) and the peripheral Vd from 179 to 141 L ($p<0.05$) [86]. The PD effects reported heart rate as a significant covariable where bradycardia occurred with an increased Ppf plasma concentration, while tachycardia took place with reduced Ppf plasma concentrations. These results indicate that Ppf and Alf effects each other's distribution and elimination by changes in hepatic perfusion and not by the hepatic CYP enzyme system.

The Prf-Alf PK and PD interaction for anesthesia induction was extensively studied in patients ($N=20$) undergoing general surgery [83]. The study reported a significant PD effects when using the eyelash reflex and state of consciousness: (1) Increasing Alf plasma concentrations from 0 to 500 ng/ml, the EC_{50} of Ppf decreased from 2.07 to 0.83 μg/mL for the loss of eyelash reflex and from 3.62 to 1.55 μg/mL for the loss of consciousness; (2) the Ppf EC_{50} for a 10 % decrease from baseline in systolic blood pressure and heart rate dropped from 1.68 μg/mL to 0.17 μg/mL and from 2.36 μg/mL to 0.04 μg/mL, respectively. These PD interactions were nonlinear as when the Ppf concentration increased, the decrease in Alf dose was not proportional to the change in Ppf concentrations due to their synergistic actions. This was evident when plasma Ppf concentrations were plotted against the plasma Alf concentrations and the combined PD effects reduced the mean heart rate by 10 %, 20 %, and 30 %. The steepness of the nonlinear curve progressively increased from 10 % to 30 % with a dramatic decrease in heart rate. This study and subsequent studies have recommended the optimal Ppf-Alf combination to target concentrations of 3.5 μg/mL for Ppf and 85 ng/mL for Alf. After a 5-h TCI with these agents at these target concentrations, 50 % of the patients should regain consciousness after about 16 min [87].

Remifentanil (Rfl) is another short-acting opioid used for general anesthesia. Like Alf, Rfl can be coadministered with Ppf and act in a PD synergistic manner [88]. Female patients ($N=38$) undergoing elective gynecologic surgery were randomly assigned Rlf doses of 0, 0.5 μg/kg, or 1.0 μg/kg with Ppf given via TCI of 4 μg/mL [89]. The PD effects monitored included hemodynamic (e.g., HR) and the EEG bispectral index (BIS). Rlf at a concentration of 1.0 μg/mL was reported to significantly increase Ppf concentrations ($p<0.001$) due to the decreased in cardiac output and heart rate induced by Rlf. Lower Rlf concentrations did not produce this effect on Ppf concentrations. A significant change in BIS activity was not found with the Rlf addition and the suggested reasons were the relatively low and burst EEG suppression and that the increase in Ppf concentrations may not have been sufficient to effect BIS changes while the subjects were under deep anesthesia. Like Alf, Rlf produced similar effects on the PK and PD parameters when combined with Ppf.

24.11 Propofol: Sedative/Hypnotics

Ppf interacts in a synergistic mode with the sedative-hypnotics midazolam (MDZ) or thiopentone by suppressing neuronal actions on the neurotransmitter γ-aminobutyric acid (GABA) activity and enhancing various PD effects required for anesthesia [81]. MDZ coadministration significantly reduces the Ppf dosage requirements but may prolong postoperative recovery [90]. The drug interaction between Ppf and MDZ occurs by various mechanisms. Both Ppf and MDZ are highly protein bound to albumin >90 % (see Table 24.1). An in vitro study reported that when MDZ was added to Ppf, Ppf significantly raised the amount of free MDZ concentrations by 4–5 % ($p<0.05$) [91]. A clinical study in patients ($n=19$) undergoing cardiopulmonary bypass surgery where MDZ was used for anesthesia induction [92]. Ppf was continuously infused at a rate of 4 mg/kg/h and blood samples taken at predetermined intervals. The total Ppf plasma concentrations remained unchanged during surgery, but the plasma free Ppf concentrations increased by twofold 15 min after coadministration. Erythrocytes' Ppf concentrations also increased by 1.6-fold. Both plasma and erythrocyte Ppf concentrations returned to the baseline amounts upon surgery completion.

MDZ is extensively metabolized by CYP3A4 and suggestion of Ppf reducing MDZ CL by competitive hepatic CYP inhibition was proposed [27, 29]. The effects of Ppf on MDZ CL were evaluated in eight healthy volunteers [93]. Subjects received MDZ starting dose of – and then an infusion of – 0.035–0.05 mg/kg/h for 59 min. Ppf was added under TCI conditions at 0.6 or 1.0 μg/mL 15 min before the MDZ start and then for the next 6 h. Both PK and PD variables were analyzed using population PK (NONMEM version VI 1.2) method. Ppf was shown to significantly reduce MDZ volume of distribution from 5.37 to 2.98 L ($p<0.05$) and CL from 0.39 to 0.31 L/min ($p<0.05$). Inclusion of the heart rate the covariate improved the model, whereas other cardiovascular hemodynamics (e.g., cardiac output) had no significant effects. However, all cardiovascular effects were significantly effected ($p<0.05$) when both drugs were coadministered. In another study with healthy volunteers ($N=8$) that received MDZ with an initial dose 0.035–0.050 mg/kg/h and then an infusion 0.035–0.050 mg/kg/h 59 min [94]. Ppf was given at a target concentration at 0.6 or 1.0 mg/mL MDZ was administered under TCI (target concentration of 125 ng/mL) at 15 min before Ppf was given and until 6 h after Ppf termination. MDZ presence resulted in a mean increased Ppf blood concentration by 25.1 % ± 13.3 % and reduced Ppf elimination CL 1.94–1.64 L/min ($p<0.05$). Heart rate, mean arterial pressure (MAP), and stroke volume as PD effects were shown to be significantly effected ($p<0.05$), but only the mean arterial pressure (MAP) was reported to improve the population model.

24.12 Propofol: Other Drug Interactions

The EC_{50} of Ppf when given with nitrous oxide 60 % was found to be significantly reduced from 14.3 to 3.85 μg/mL for suppression of movements to skin incision [95]. Similar findings were reported with Ppf and nitrous oxide 67 % that suppressed a 50 % response to skin incision with a Ppf EC_{50} reduction from 6.0 to 4.5 μg/mL [96]. A case report described profound hypotension when two doses of rifampin 600 mg were given prior to surgery and when Ppf was used for anesthesia induction. This led to a retrospective case-control study that examined the effects of rifampin on Ppf ($n=25$) and thiopential ($N=25$) versus Ppf alone ($N=25$) as this antibiotic can be given for prophylaxis of infection prior to surgery [97]. Patients given with rifampin + Ppf combination had a significant effect in changing the MAP with a longer duration of hypotension (odds ratio 11.0 and 95 % C.I. 3–39, $p<0.005$) compared to other two groups. A mechanism for a Ppf-rifampin interaction was not explored but suggested to occur by enhancement of venous smooth muscle through increased production and release of endothelial nitric oxide. This is an interesting hypothesis that needs clarification, and until further information is available, the use of rifampin prior to Ppf anesthesia induction is cautioned and other antibiotics are recommended to be used.

Patients ($N=72$) that underwent upper limb surgery reported prolonged QTc intervals when Ppf and droperidol 1.25 and 2.5 mg were coadministered [98]. Droperidol prevents postoperative nausea and vomiting (PONV) and doses of 0.625 and 1.25 mg are recommended. For severe PONV cases, a maximum droperidol dose of 2.5 mg is recommended. However, droperidol 2.5 mg can lead to significant QTc prolongation and it was found that Ppf counteracted the droperidol-induced prolonged QTc actions. The mechanism for this counteracting effect was suggested to occur as droperidol inhibits the cardiac K+ current rectifier (I_{Kr}) and Ppf shortens the QTc interval by suppression of L-type calcium currents (I_{Ca}). Ppf would be useful for anesthesia induction in patients needing droperidol for PONV. Parecoxib is a prodrug converted to valdecoxib, which inhibits CYP2C9 and possibly interacts with Ppf. A balanced crossover study with 12 healthy volunteers received Ppf 2 mg/kg bolus 1 h after an intravenous parecoxib 40 mg dose or placebo [99]. The single-bolus parecoxib dose was shown not to significantly affect Ppf pharmacokinetic parameters (C_{max}, CL, elimination half-life, and volume of distribution) or pharmacodynamics parameters (VAS, Ppf EC_{50}, and BIS scores).

24.12.1 Thiopental (TPL)

Thiopental is a barbiturate anesthetic agent used for many years to induce sedation and commonly combined with other agents to maintain anesthesia in patients undergoing surgery. As a barbiturate, TPL pharmacologic actions occur allosterically on the BZ-GABA-CL ion receptor complex producing its sedative actions [100]. TPL metabolism remains relatively unknown due to its early use in anesthesia and PK interactions have not been well studied. However, an in vitro study reported that protein-binding displacement of TPL from albumin may occur with diazepam, desmethyldiazepam, fentanyl, and other agents increasing free TPL concentrations [101].

PD interactions are likely to occur when used with other anesthetics due to their differing pharmacologic mechanism of action and the increased free TPL concentrations promote sedation while, maintaining analgesia, and optimal cardiovascular effects.

24.13 TPL: Other CNS Depressant Agents

TPL combined with Ppf in unpremedicated patients ($N=120$) was assessed where the PD endpoint was anesthesia induction and a patient's inability to open their eyes to command after 60 s [102]. Patients were randomly assigned to one of three groups – TPL and Ppf alone and combined TPL-Ppf. The ED50 for the TPL-Ppf group was significantly lower than the TPL and Ppf alone groups ($p<0.05$) suggesting a synergistic action between the two agents. The TPL and Ppf doses when used alone were 1.9 and 1.17 mg/kg, respectively, to induce anesthesia. To achieve similar effects, the combined TPL-Ppf doses were significantly lower and reported to synergistically induce anesthesia using multiple endpoints that included EEG measurements, analgesia maintenance, and reflex assessments [102]. TPL was given and patients ($N=22$) were assigned either no MDZ or MDZ with the ED_{50}'s calculated for the multiple endpoints. For each endpoint, the combined TPL-MDZ ED_{50} was significantly lower than the TPL-alone group ($p<0.05$). Even a subtherapeutic MDZ dose of 0.02 mg/kg was shown to potentiate TPL anesthesia when evaluated in 50 patients scheduled for eye surgery [103].

Fentanyl was combined with TPL, and in the animal model, an enhanced lethal effect was found that was greater than the hypnotic effects (loss of righting reflex) [104]. However, when evaluated in patients ($N=46$), it was reported that no significant changes in TPL plasma concentrations were found when fentanyl was added. Further, the hypnotic and analgesic effects did not differ between TPL-fentanyl and TPL alone. Although earlier in vitro study indicated increased free TPL concentrations from protein-binding displacement from albumin when fentanyl was added, this effect may not be clinically significant under in vivo conditions (see Table 24.1). Melatonin is a sedative-hypnotic agent and was evaluated in combination with TPL [105]. Melatonin premedication significantly decreased the TPL ED_{50} value for the PD effect of loss of response to verbal command (3.4 mg/kg versus 2.7 mg/kg, $p<0.05$) and eyelash reflex (3.7 mg/kg versus 2.6 mg/kg, $p<0.05$). Alcohol was shown to enhance TPL effects 4 h after TPL administration under ambulatory surgery conditions [106]. Psychomotor effects and body sway were significantly altered ($p<0.05$) and caution is suggested for patient who may consume alcohol shortly after an outpatient surgery when TPL is used as anesthetic agent.

24.14 TPL: Other Drug Interactions

Clonidine is an α-adrenergic receptor agonist acting in the CNS to decrease sympathetic outflow and when orally administered was reported to decrease the fentanyl anesthetic dose requirements [107]. Patients ($N=60$) undergoing elective surgery were randomly assigned to TPL (50 mg every 15 s) alone, TPL-clonidine 2.5 μg/kg, and TPL-clonidine 5.0 μg/kg groups [108]. It was reported that the TPL-clonidine groups produced more sedation than TPL alone. Clonidine 2.5 and 5.0 μg/kg resulted in a significantly lower ($p<0.05$) TPL dose by 25 % and 37 %, respectively. A significantly lower blood pressure was found with the clonidine 2.5 μg/kg versus the 5.0 μg/kg dose ($p<0.05$) but not with heart rate. Clonidine can be safely given with TPL but the higher 5.0 μg/kg offered no advantages over the lower 2.5 μg/kg dose. Dexmedetomidine (DXD) is another α-adrenergic receptor agonist with a shorter elimination half-life than clonidine (1.6 h versus 7.5 h) and a more selective α-adrenergic agent [109]. Patients ($N=14$) with elective surgery were randomized to receive infusions of either TPL alone (100 mg/min) or TPL-DXD (100 mg/min+6 ng/kg/min) [110]. EEG burst suppression was used as the main PD effect. DXD use reduced the TPL dose by 30 % needed to achieve the EEG burst suppression. Using a three compartment PK model, a significant decreased in volume of distribution and intercompartmental volume of distribution of TPL was noted. Interestingly, TPL clearance and elimination half-life were not different between the two groups. The volume of distribution change for TPL likely accounts for the need of lower TPL doses when used with DXD.

TPL and KTM interactions were found to differ depending upon the KTM dose. The anesthetic effects of TPL-KTM combination were additive (not synergistic) at the endpoints for anesthesia (e.g., open-eye command) in patients ($N=150$) undergoing various surgeries [111]. However, KTM at a subhypnotic dose of 0.4 mg/kg had reported antagonistic effects to TPL anesthesia in female patients ($N=30$) with elective surgery [112]. The different dose KTM effects may be related to its NMDA actions compared the TPL BZ-GABA-CL receptor complex. KTM used with TPL requires further assessment prior to routine therapeutic application in anesthesia. A case report of a patient with an acute amphetamine abuse noted that the usual anesthetic dosages of TPL 350 mg and succinylcholine 80 mg were insufficient, and in less than 30 s, the patient was wide awake. Diazepam 7.5 mg IV was given to calm the agitated patient and discharged to the recovery room [113]. Prior stimulant use may increase the anesthetic dosage requirements in some patients with psychiatric conditions.

Ondansetron, a selective 5HT3 antagonist, is an effective agent for prophylaxis as an antiemetic treatment postsurgery [114]. TPL dose requirements were found not to be influenced by ondansetron in adult female patients ($N=168$) completing surgery and based upon the PD effects of ability to open eyes on command [115]. Esomeprazole (ESP), a proton pump inhibitor, was used to treatment stress-induced esophageal ulcers in critically ill patients ($N=52$) placed under TPL-induced coma to reduce intracranial pressure (ICP) [116]. A population PK model using the nonlinear mixed effects model (NONMEM, version 7.2) was employed to estimate the PK TPL parameters. ESP was shown to significantly increase ($p<0.05$) TPL volume of distribution (3.46 L/kg) and decrease clearance (1.19 mL/min/kg) compared to the population norms (see Table 24.1) and TPL dosage adjustments may be necessary. Metoclopramide (MET) is a dopamine receptor subtype two antagonist used for postsurgery antiemetic effects [117]. MET reduced the TPL ED50 for anesthesia by 44 % ($p<0.001$) in female patients ($N=48$) and significantly lowered the mean TPL dose requirement for hypnotic activity from 5.3 mg/kg ± 0.3 to 3.2 mg/kg ± 0.2 ($p<0.001$). Droperidol, like MET, also significantly lowered TPL dose requirement by the same magnitude in another group of female patients ($N=48$).

24.15 Conclusions

Anesthetic agents are commonly used in various combinations to induce hypnosis and analgesia. Taken into account that patients are likely prescribed medications for various chronic medical conditions (e.g., hypertension, diabetes), the chances of drug-drug interactions between anesthetics and other drugs can easily occur. Although this chapter did not focus on the inhalation anesthetic drugs, these volatile gases can produce a variety of drug interactions [118]. Different PK interactions can occur with anesthetic agents when given either by inhalation, oral, intramuscular, or intravenous routes of administration. Certain premedication drugs such as morphine and anticholinergics can delay gastric emptying time that can affect drug absorption. Anesthetics may alter protein binding of other drugs and displacement reactions can occur, which can alter a drug's volume of distribution. Hepatic CYP drug interactions (induction or inhibition) and alterations in hepatic blood flow can significantly change anesthetic drug clearance and elimination half-life, which may prolong patient recovery or modify other PD endpoints [119]. The main PD effects of the general anesthetics are to promote immobility (analgesia, pain reflex) and hypnosis (sleep induction and maintenance). Of the different anesthetics covered in this chapter, the majority of the drug interactions occur in a synergistic manner with or without a PK interaction. The PD synergistic actions are explained by their different pharmacologic mechanisms of action that each agent produces to induce anesthesia. Only KTM differed as when combined with another anesthetic drug, it can lead to a dose-dependent additive or antagonistic manner. Inhaled anesthetics characteristically display a synergetic action with the IV anesthetics nitrous oxide and isoflurane and produce additive PD effects [120]. The PD effects can be quantified by a variety of methods that assess the analgesic, hypnotic, and cardiovascular factors providing clinicians with substantial amounts of data to measure anesthetic drug accomplishments. Sophisticated mathematical models have been developed to unite the complex PK and PD interactions that occur with anesthetic drugs to improve their clinical efficacy, patient recovery, and minimize adverse effects.

References

1. Stanski DR, Shafer SL (1995) Quantifying anesthetic drug interaction. Anesthesiology 83:1–5
2. Eilers H, Niemann CU (2003) Clinically important drug interactions with intravenous anesthetics in older patients. Drugs Aging 20:969–980
3. Barbanoj MJ, Antonijoan RM, Riba J, Valle M, Romero S, Jane F (2006) Quantifying drug-drug interactions in pharmaco-EEG. Clin EEG Neurosci 37:108–120
4. Minto CF, Schnider TW, Short TG et al (2000) Response surface model for anesthetic drug interactions. Anesthesiology 92:1603–1616
5. Valle M, Barbanoj MJ, Jane F (2002) Pharmaco-EEG and pharmacokinetic/pharmacodynamics modeling in basic research: focus on human pharmacology. Methods Find Exp Clin Pharmacol 24(Suppl D):129–137
6. Giese JL, Stanley TH (1983) Etomidate: a new intravenous anesthetic induction agent. Pharmacotherapy 3:251–258
7. Sear JW, Walters FJ, Wilkins DG, Willatss SM (1984) Etomidate by infusion for neuroanesthesia kinetic and dynamic interactions with nitrous oxide. Anaesthesia 39:12–18
8. Richter O, Klatte A, Abel J et al (1985) Pharmacokinetic data analysis of Alfentanil after multiple injections and Etomidate-infusion in patients undergoing orthopedic surgery. Int J Clin Pharmacol Ther Toxic 23:11–15
9. Tawfic QA (2013) A review of the use of ketamine in pain management. J Opioid Manag 9:379–388
10. Johnston RR, Miller RD, Way WL (1974) The interaction of ketamine with d-tubocurarine, pancuronium, and succinylcholine in man. Anesth Analg 53:496–501

11. Wathen JE, Roback MG, Mackenzie T, Bothner JP (2000) Does midazolam alter the clinical effects of intravenous ketamine sedation in children? A double-blind, randomized, controlled, emergency department trial. Ann Emerg Med 36:579–588
12. Pechter EA (2005) Safety of ketamine and diazepam in anesthesia. Plast Reconstr Surg 115:1781–1782
13. Bossard AE, Guirmand F, Fletcher D et al (2002) Interaction of a combination of morphine and ketamine on the nociceptive flexion reflex in human volunteers. Pain 98:47–57
14. Lawrence D, Livingston A (1979) The effect of physostigmine and neostigmine on ketamine anesthesia and analgesia. Br J Pharmacol 67:426P
15. Mimura M, Namiki A, Kishi R, Ikeda T, Miyake H (1990) Antagonistic effect of physostigmine on ketamine-induced anesthesia. Psychopharmacology 102:399–403
16. Santamaria R, Pailleux F, Beaudry F (2013) In vitro ketamine CYP3A4 mediated metabolism study using mammalian liver S9 fractions, cDNA expressed enzymes and liquid chromatography tandem mass spectrometry. Biomed Chromatogr, 1002/bmc3199
17. Hijazi Y, Boulieu R (2002) Contribution of CYP3A4, CYP2B6, CYP2C19 isoforms to N-demethylation of ketamine in human liver microsomes. Drug Metab Dispos 30:853–858
18. Desta Z, Moaddel R, Ogburn ET et al (2012) Stereoselective and regiospecific hydroxylation of ketamine and norketamine. Xenobiotica 42:1076–1087
19. Peltoniemi Saari TI, Hagelberg NM et al (2012) Rifampicin has a profound effect on the pharmacokinetics of oral S-ketamine and less on intravenous S-ketamine. Basic Clin Pharmacol Toxic 111:325–332
20. Peltoniemi MA, Saari TI, Hagelberg NM et al (2012) St. John's Wort greatly decreases the plasma concentrations of oral S-ketamine. Fundam Clin Pharmacol 26:743–750
21. Peltoniemi MA, Saari TI, Hagelberg NM et al (2012) S-ketamine concentrations are greatly increased by grapefruit juice. Eur J Clin Pharmacol 68:979–986
22. Hagelberg NM, Peltoniemi MA, Saari TI et al (2010) Clarithromycin, a potent inhibitor of CYP3A, greatly increases exposure to oral S-ketamine. Eur J Pain 14:625–629
23. Peltoniemi MA, Saari TI, Hagelberg NM et al (2011) Exposure to oral S-ketamine is unaffected by itraconazole but greatly increased by ticlopidine. Clin Pharmacol Ther 90:296–302
24. Qi X, Evans AM, Miners JO, Upton RN, Miline RW (2010) Inhibition of morphine metabolism by ketamine. Drug Metab Dispos 38:728–731
25. Uchaipichat V, Raungrut P, Chau N et al (2011) Effects of ketamine on human UDP-glucuronosyltransferases in vitro predict potential drug-drug interactions arising from ketamine inhibition of codeine and morphine glucuronidation. Drug Metab Dispos 39:1324–1328
26. Broderick D, Clarke M, Stassen L (2014) Midazolam and drug-drug interactions in dental conscious sedation. J Ir Dent Assoc 60:38–43
27. Kronbach T, Mathys D, Umeno M, Gonzalez FJ, Meyer UA (1989) Oxidation of midazolam and triazolam by human liver microsomes cytochrome IIIA4. Mol Pharmacol 36:89–96
28. Merry AF, Clapham GJ, Walker JS (1988) The reversal of midazolam sedation with the benzodiazepine antagonist flumazenil. NZ Med J 101:571–572
29. Ibrahim AE, Feldman J, Karim A, Kharasch ED (2003) Simultaneous assessment of drug interactions with low – high extraction opioids. Anesthesiology 98:853–861
30. Takano M, Hasegawa R, Fukuda T et al (1998) Interaction with P-glycoprotein and transport of erythromycin, midazolam and ketoconazole in Caco-2 cells. Eur J Pharmacol 358:289–294
31. Kupferschmidt HH, Ha HR, Ziegler WH, Meier PJ, Krahenbuhl S (1995) Interaction between grapefruit juice and midazolam in humans. Clin Pharmacol Ther 58:20–28
32. Vanakoski J, Mattila MJ, Seppala T (1996) Grapefruit juice does not enhance the effects of midazolam and triazolam in man. Eur J Clin Pharmacol 50:501–508
33. Goho C (2001) Oral midazolam-grapefruit juice drug interaction. Pediatr Dent 23:365–366

34. Ito K, Ogihara K, Kanamitsu S, Itoh T (2003) Prediction of in vivo interaction between midazolam and macrolides based upon in vitro studies using human liver microsomes. Drug Metab Dispos 31:945–954
35. Narchi P, Benhamou D, Elhaddoury M, Locatelli C, Fernandez H (1993) Interactions of preoperative erythromycin administration with general anesthesia. Can J Anesth 40:444–447
36. Hiller A, Olkkola KT, Isohanni L, Saarnivaara A (1990) Unconsciousness associated with midazolam and erythromycin. Br J Anesth 65:826–828
37. Olkkola KT, Aranko K, Luurila H et al (1993) A potentially hazardous interaction between erythromycin and midazolam. Clin Pharmacol Ther 53:298–305
38. Quinney SK, Haehner BD, Rhoades M et al (2007) Interaction between midazolam and clarithromycin in the elderly. Br J Clin Pharmacol 65:98–109
39. Mattila MJ, Vanakoski J, Idanpaan-Heikkila JJ (1994) Azithromycin does not alter the effects of oral midazolam on human performance. Eur J Clin Pharmacol 47:49–52
40. Ahonen J, Olkkola KT, Neuvonen PJ (1995) Effect of itraconazole and terfinafine on the pharmacokinetics and pharmacodynamics of midazolam in healthy volunteers. Br J Clin Pharmacol 40:270–272
41. Backman JT, Kivisto KT, Olkkola KT, Neuvonen PJ (1998) The area under the plasma concentration-time curve for oral midazolam is 400-fold larger during treatment with itraconazole than with rifampicin. Eur J Clin Pharmacol 54:53–58
42. Olkkola KT, Ahonen J, Neuvonen PJ (1996) The effect of the systemic antimycotics, itraconazole, and fluconazole, on the pharmacokinetics and pharmacodynamics of intravenous and oral midazolam. Anesth Analg 82:511–516
43. Vanakoski J, Mattila MJ, Vanio P, Idaanpaan-Heikkila JJ, Tornwall M (1995) 150 mg fluconazole does not substantially increase the effects of 10 mg midazolam or plasma midazolam concentrations in healthy subjects. Int J Clin Phrmacol Ther 33:518–523
44. Reinhart DJ, Grum DR, Berry J et al (1997) Outpatient general anesthesia: a comparison of a combination of midazolam plus propofol and propofol alone. J Clin Anesth 9:130–137
45. Paspatis GA, Charoniti I, Manolaraki M et al (2006) Synergistic sedation with oral midazolam as a premedication and intravenous propofol versus intravenous propofol alone in upper gastrointestinal endoscopies in children: a prospective randomized study. J Pediatr Gastroenterol Nutr 43:195–199
46. Vinil HR, Bradley EL, Kissin I (1989) Midazolam-alfentanil synergism for anesthetic induction in patients. Anesth Analg 69:213–217
47. Kissin I, Lee SS, Arthur GR et al (1997) Effect of midazolam on development of acute tolerance to alfentanil: the role of pharmacokinetic interactions. Anesth Analg 85:182–187
48. Kissin I, Vinik HR, Bradley EL (1991) Midazolam potentiates thiopental sodium anesthetic induction in patients. J Clin Anesth 3:367–370
49. Tverskoy M, Fleyshman G, Bradley EL, Kissin I (1988) Midazolam-thiopental anesthetic induction in patients. Anesth Analg 67:342–345
50. Vinik HR, Bradley EL, Kissin I (1994) Triple anesthetic combination: propofol-midazolam-alfentanil. Anesth Analg 78:354–358
51. Li F, Lu J, Ma X (2014) CYP3A4 mediated α-hydroxyaldehyde formation in saquinavir metabolism. Drug Metab Dispos 42:213–220
52. Palkama VJ, Ahonen J, Neuvonen PJ, Olkkola KT (1999) Effect of saquinavir on the pharmacokinetics and pharmacodynamics of oral and intravenous midazolam. Clin Pharmacol Ther 66:33–39
53. Ibrahim A, Karim A, Feldman J, Kharasch E (2002) The influence of parecoxib, a parenteral cyclooxygenase-2 specific inhibitor on the pharmacokinetics and clinical effects of midazolam. Anesth Analg 95:667–673
54. Drague A, Varin F, Plaud B, Donati F (2002) Rocuronium pharmacokinetic and pharmacodynamics relationship under stable propofol or isoflurane anesthesia. Can J Anesth 49:353–360

55. Miller RD, Way WL, Dolan WM et al (1971) Comparative neuromuscular effects of pancuronium, gallamine, and succinylcholine during Forane and halothane anesthesia in man. Anesthesiology 35:509–514
56. McCarthy GJ, Mirakhur RK, Pandit SK (1992) Lack of interaction between propofol and vecuronium. Anesth Analg 75:536–538
57. Latorre F, de Almeida MC, Stanek A, Kleemann PP (1997) The interaction between rocuronium and smoking. The effect of smoking on neuromuscular transmission after rocuronium. Anaesthesist 46:493–495
58. Fuchs-Buder T, Sparr HJ, Ziegenfub T (1998) Thiopental or etomidate for rapid sequence induction with rocuronium. Br J Anesth 80(4):504–506
59. Scholz J, Steinfath M, Schulz M (1996) Clinical pharmacokinetics of alfentanil, fentanyl, and sufentanil. An update. Clin Pharmacokinet 31:275–292
60. Overholsen BR, Foster DR (2011) Opioid pharmacokinetic drug-drug interactions. Am J Manag Care 17(Suppl 11):S276–S287
61. Labroo RB, Paine MF, Thummel KE, Kharasch ED (1997) Fentanyl metabolism by human hepatic and intestinal cytochrome P450 3A4: implications for interindividual variability in disposition, efficacy, and drug interactions. Drug Metab Dispos 25:1072–1080
62. Kharasch ED, Francis A, London A et al (2011) Sensitivity of intravenous and oral alfentanil and pupillary miosis as minimal and noninvasive probes for hepatic and first-pass CYP3A induction. Clin Pharmacol Ther 90:100–108
63. Bartkowski RR, Goldberg ME, Huffnagle S, Epstein RH (1993) Sufentanil disposition. Is it affected by erythromycin administration? Anesthesiology 78:260–265
64. Palkama VJ, Neuvonen PJ, Olkkola KT (1998) The CYP3A4 inhibitor itraconazole has no effect on the pharmacokinetics of iv fentanyl. Br J Anaesth 81:598–600
65. Wandel C, Kim R, Wood M, Wood A (2002) Interaction of morphine, fentanyl, sufentanil, alfentanil, and loperamide with the efflux drug transporter P-glycoprotein. Anesthesiology 96:913–920
66. Bartkowski RR, Goldberg ME, Larijani GE, Boerner T (1989) Inhibition of alfentanil metabolism by erythromycin. Clin Pharmacol Ther 46:99–102
67. Kharasch ED, Russell M, Mautz D et al (1997) The role of cytochrome P450 3A4 in alfentanil clearance. Implications for interindividual variability in disposition and perioperative drug interactions. Anesthesiology 87:36–50
68. Clotz MA, Nahata MC (1991) Clinical uses of fentanyl, sufentanil, and alfentanil. Clin Pharm 10:581–593
69. Bruggemann RJ, Alffenaar JW, Blijilevens NM et al (2009) Clinical relevance of the pharmacokinetic interactions of azole antifungal drugs with other coadministered agents. Clin Infect Dis 48:1441–1458
70. Palkama VJ, Isohanni MH, Neuvonen PJ, Olkkola KT (1998) The effect of intravenous and oral fluconazole on the pharmacokinetics and pharmacodynamics of intravenous alfentanil. Anesth Analg 87:190–194
71. Geist MJ, Eqerer G, Burhenne J et al (2013) Steady-state pharmacokinetics and metabolism of voriconazole in patients. J Antimicrob Chemother 68:2592–2599
72. Saari TI, Laine K, Leino K et al (2006) Voriconazole, but not terbinafine, markedly reduces alfentanil clearance and prolongs its half-life. Clin Pharmacol Ther 80:502–508
73. Ahonen J, Olkkola KT, Salmenpera M, Hynyen M, Neuvonen PJ (1996) Effect of diltiazem on midazolam and alfentanil disposition in patients undergoing coronary artery bypass grafting. Anesthesiology 85:1246–1252
74. McDonnell CG, Malan D, Van Pelt FD, Shorten GD (2003) Elimination of alfentanil delivered by infusion is not altered by the chronic administration of atorvastatin. Eur J Anaesthesiol 20:662–667
75. Westmoreland CL, Sbel PS, Gropper A (1994) Fentanyl or alfentanil decreases the minimum alveolar anesthetic concentration of isoflurane in surgical patients. Anesth Analg 78:23–28

76. Olkkola KT, Palkama VJ, Neuvonen PJ (1999) Ritonavir's role in reducing fentanyl clearance and prolonging its half-life. Anesthesiology 91:681–685
77. Turpeinen M, Zanger M (2012) Cytochrome P4502B6: function, genetics, and clinical relevance. Drug Metabol Drug Interact 27:185–197
78. Vanlersberghne C, Camu F (2008) Prpofol. Handb Exp Pharmacol 182:227–252
79. Khokhar JY, Tyndale RF (2011) Drug metabolism within the bran changes drug response: selective manipulation of brain CYP2B alters propofol effects. Neuropsychopharmacology 36:692–700
80. Vuyk J (1998) TCI: supplementation and drug interactions. Anesthesia 53(Suppl 1):35–41
81. Vuyk J (2001) Clinical interpretation of pharmacokinetic and pharmacodynamics propofol-opioid interactions. Acta Anaesthesiol Belg 52:445–451
82. LaPierre CD, Johnson KB, Randall BR, Egan TD (2012) A simulation study of common propofol and propofol-opioid dosing regimens for upper endoscopy. Anesthesiology 117:252–262
83. Vuyk J, Engbers FH, Burn AG et al (1996) Pharmacodynamic interaction between propofol and alfentanil when given for induction of anesthesia. Anesthesiology 81:288–299
84. Schutter J, Ihmsen H (2000) Population pharmacokinetics of propofol: a multicenter study. Anesthesiology 92:727–738
85. Fenkel C, Schutter J, Ihmsen H, Heye H, Rommelsheim K (1995) Pharmacokinetics and pharmacodynamics of propofol/alfentanil infusions for sedation in ICU patients. Intensive Care Med 21:981–988
86. Mertens MJ, Olofsen E, Burn AG, Bovill JG, Vuyk J (2004) Mixed-effects modeling of the influence of alfentanil on propofol pharmacokinetics. Anesthesiology 100:795–805
87. Pavlin DJ, Coda B, Shen DD et al (1996) Effects of combining propofol and alfentanil on ventilation, analgesia, sedation, and emesis in human volunteers. Anesthesiology 84:23–37
88. Kern SE, Xie G, Whiye D, Egan TD (2004) A response surface analysis of propofol-alfentanil pharmacodynamics interaction. Anesthesiology 100:1377–1381
89. Yufune S, Takamatsu I, Masui K, Kazama T (2011) Effect of remifentanil on plasma propofol concentration and bispectral during propofol anesthesia. Br J Anesth 106:208–214
90. McClune S, McKay AC, Wright PM et al (1992) Synergistic interaction between midazolam and propofol. Br J Aneasth 69:240–245
91. Ohmori J, Maeda S, Higuchi H et al (2011) Propofol increases the rate of albumin-unbound free midazolam in serum albumin solution. J Anesth 25:618–620
92. Hiraoka H, Yamamoto K, Okano N et al (2004) Changes in drug plasma concentrations of an extensively bound and highly extracted drug, propofol, in response to altered plasma binding. Clin Pharmacol Ther 75:324–330
93. Vuyk J, Lichtenbelt BJ, Olofsen E, van Kleef JW, Dahan A (2009) Mixed-effects modeling of the influence of midazolam on propofol pharmacokinetics. Anesth Analg 108:1522–1530
94. Lichtenbelt BJ, Olofsen E, Dahan A et al (2010) Propofol reduces the distribution and clearance of midazolam. Anesth Analg 110:1597–1606
95. Johnson JW, Flaishon R, Sebel PS (1997) Esmolol reduces anesthetic requirement for skin incision during propofol/nitrous oxide/morphine anesthesia. Anesthesiology 86:364–371
96. Davison JA, MacLeod AD, Howie JC, White M, Kenny GN (1993) Effective concentration 50 for propofol with and without 67% nitrous oxide. Acta Anesthesiol Scand 37:458–464
97. Mirzakhani H, Nozari A, Ehremfeld JM et al (2013) Profound hypotension after anesthetic induction with propofol in patients treated with rifampin. Anesth Analg 117:61–64
98. Toyoda T, Terao Y, Oji M et al (2013) The interaction of antiemetic dose of droperidol with propofol on QT interval during anesthetic induction. J Anesth 27:885–889
99. Ibrahim A, Park S, Feldman J, Karin A, Kharasch ED (2002) Effects of parecoxib, a parenteral COX-2 specific inhibitor, on the pharmacokinetics and pharmacodynamics of propofol. Anesthesiology 96:88–95
100. Skolnick P, Moncada V, Barker JL, Paul SM (1981) Pentobarbital: dual actions in increase benzodiazepine receptor affinity. Science 211:1448–1450

101. Russo H, Audran M, Bressolle F, Bres J, Mailols H (1993) Displacement of thiopental from human serum albumin by associated drugs. J Pharm Sci 82:493–497
102. Naguib M, Sari-Kouzel AS (1991) Thiopental-propofol hypnotic synergism in patients. Br J Anesth 67:4–6
103. Wilder-Smith OH, Rvussin PA, Decosterd LA et al (1999) Midazolam premedication and thiopental induction of anesthesia: interactions at multiple end-points. Br J Anesth 83:590–595
104. Telford R, Glass PSA, Goodman D, Jacobs JR (1992) Fentanyl does not alter the "sleep" plasma concentration of thiopental. Anesth Analg 75:523–529
105. Naguib M, Samarkandi AH, Moniem MA et al (2006) The effects of melatonin premedication on propofol and thiopental induction dose-response curves: a prospective, randomized, double-blind study. Anesth Analg 103:1448–1452
106. Lichtor JL, Zacny JP, Coalson DW et al (1993) The interaction between alcohol and the residual effects of thiopental anesthesia. Anesthesiology 79:28–35
107. Ghigone M, Quintin L, Duke PC et al (1986) Effects of clonidine on narcotic requirements and hemodynamic response during induction of fentanyl anesthesia and endotracheal intubation. Anesthesiology 64:36–42
108. Leslie K, Mooney PH, Silbert BS (1992) Effect of intravenous clonidine on the dose of thiopental required to induce anesthesia. Anesth Analg 75:530–535
109. Schein H, Karhuvaara S, Olkkola KT et al (1992) Pharmacodynamics and pharmacokinetics of intramuscular dexmedetomidine. Clin Pharmacol Ther 52:537–546
110. Buhrer M, Mappes A, Lauber R, Stanski DR, Mailtre PO (1994) Dexmedetomidine decreases thiopental dose requirements and alter distribution pharmacokinetics. Anesthesiology 80:1216–1227
111. Roytbalt L, Katz J, Rozentsveig V (1992) Anesthetic interaction between thiopentone and ketamine. Eur J Anesth 9:307–312
112. Manani G, Valenti S, Vincenti E et al (1992) Interaction between thiopentone and subhypnotic doses of ketamine. Eur J Anesth 9:43–47
113. Stibolt O, Wachowiak-Andersen G (2002) Altered response to intravenous thiopental and succinylcholine in acute amphetamine abuse. Acta Anesthesiol Scand 46:609–610
114. Christofaki M, Papaionnou A (2014) Ondansetron: a review of pharmacokinetic and clinical experience in postoperative nausea and vomiting. Exp Opin Drug Metab Toxic 10:437–444
115. Kostopanagiotou G, Pouriezis T, Theodoraki K et al (1998) Influence of ondansetron on thiopental hypnotic requirements. J Clin Pharmacol 38:825–829
116. Marsot A, Goirand F, Milesi N et al (2013) Interaction of thiopental with esomeprazole in critically ill patients. Eur J Clin Pharmacol 69:1667–1672
117. Mehta D, Bradley EL, Kissin I (1993) Metoclopramide decreases thiopental hypnotic requirements. Anesth Analg 77:784–787
118. Christensen LQ, Bonde J, Kampmann JP (1993) Drug interactions with inhalational anaesthetics. Acta Anaesthesiol Scand 37:231–244
119. Wood M (1991) Pharmacokinetic drug interactions in anaesthetic practice. Clin Pharmacokinet 21:285–307
120. Hendricks JF, Eger EI, Sonner JM, Shafer SL (2008) Is synergy the rule? A review of anesthetic interactions producing hypnosis and immobility. Anesth Analg 107:494–506
121. Davis PJ, Cook DR (1986) Clinical pharmacokinetics of the newer intravenous anaesthetic agents. Clin Pharmacokinet 11:18–35

The manufacturer's authorised representative in the EU is Springer Nature Customer Service Centre GmbH, Europaplatz 3, 69115 Heidelberg, Germany. If you have any concerns regarding our products, please contact ProductSafety@springernature.com

Printed and bound by CPI Group (UK) Ltd, Croydon, CR0 4YY
25/09/2026
02222880-0003